Pediatric Nursing

CONTENT REVIEW **PLUS** PRACTICE QUESTIONS

MARGOT R. DE SEVO, PHD, LCCE, IBCLC, RNC
Associate Professor
Adelphia University
Garden City, NY

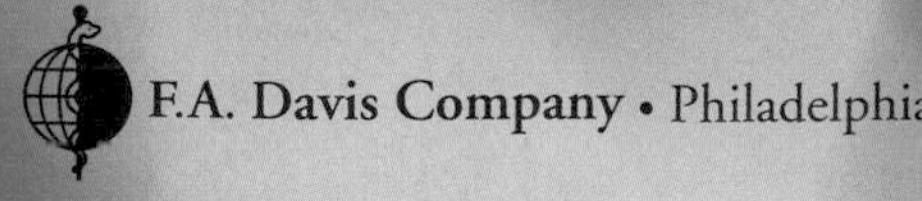

F.A. Davis Company
1915 Arch Street
Philadelphia, PA 19103
www.fadavis.com

Printed in the United States of America

Last digit indicates print number: 10 9 8 7 6 5 4 3 2 1

Publisher, Nursing: Robert G. Martone
Director of Content Development: Darlene D. Pedersen
Content Project Manager: Elizabeth Hart
Electronic Product Manager: Tyler R. Baber
Design & Illustration Manager: Carolyn O'Brien

As new scientific information becomes available through basic and clinical research, recommended treatments and drug therapies undergo changes. The author(s) and publisher have done everything possible to make this book accurate, up to date, and in accord with accepted standards at the time of publication. The author(s), editors, and publisher are not responsible for errors or omissions or for consequences from application of the book, and make no warranty, expressed or implied, in regard to the contents of the book. Any practice described in this book should be applied by the reader in accordance with professional standards of care used in regard to the unique circumstances that may apply in each situation. The reader is advised always to check product information (package inserts) for changes and new information regarding dose and contraindications before administering any drug. Caution is especially urged when using new or infrequently ordered drugs.

Library of Congress Cataloging-in-Publication Data

De Sevo, Margot, author.
Pediatric nursing: content review plus practice questions / Margot De Sevo.
p.; cm.
Includes bibliographical references and index.
ISBN 978-0-8036-3042-0 – ISBN 0-8036-3042-5
I. Title.
[DNLM: 1. Nursing Care–methods–Examination Questions. 2. Adolescent. 3. Child. 4. Infant. 5. Pediatric Nursing–methods–Examination Questions. WY 18.2]
RJ245
618.92′00231–dc23

2014015702

In respect and admiration for the circle of life, I dedicate this book to the memory of my beloved parents, Eleanor and J. Warren Rauscher, and to the bright and vital lives of my cherished grandchildren, Cameron, Abigail, and Aaron.

Why This Book Is Necessary

Most beginning nursing students have information overload. They must possess knowledge about a variety of subjects, including anatomy and physiology, psychology, sociology, medical terminology, diagnostic and laboratory tests, and growth and development, to mention a few. In addition, with the expanding roles and responsibilities of the nursing profession, the nursing information that beginning nursing students must learn is growing in depth and breadth exponentially. The quantity of information is more than any nursing student can possibly absorb, remember, and apply. Pediatric Nursing: Content Review PLUS Practice Questions provides nursing students with additional educational support!

Who Should Use This Book

Pediatric Nursing: Content Review PLUS Practice Questions provides beginning nursing students with need-to-know information as well as questions to practice their ability to apply the information in a simulated clinical situation. This textbook is designed to:

- Be required or recommended by a nursing program to be used in conjunction with a traditional pediatric nursing textbook.
- Be used by nursing students who want to focus on the essential information contained in a pediatric nursing course.
- Be used by nursing students to learn how to be more successful when answering National Council Licensure Examination (NCLEX)–type multiple-choice and alternate-item format nursing questions early in their nursing education.
- Be used by nursing students preparing for the NCLEX-RN examination to review pediatric nursing theory and practice.

What Information Is Presented in This Textbook

This textbook begins with an introduction, which includes information to help students maximize their ability to study effectively and achieve success when studying pediatric content and when taking nursing examinations. General study strategies, specific study strategies, test-taking tips for answering multiple-choice questions and alternate-format questions, and the test plan categories for the NCLEX examinations are discussed.

The pediatric content is divided into 25 chapters. In addition, a comprehensive final exam is included in Chapter 26.

- The first group of chapters—Chapters 1 to 9—focus on foundational information needed by the pediatric nurse.
  - The first chapter discusses the child in the context of a family because families differ in relation to such aspects as composition, cultural norms, and religion. Brief descriptions of these differences are discussed.
  - Chapters 2 through 6 focus on the five stages of child growth and development. Unless the nurse is familiar with the norms of each stage, he or she may miss important assessments or intervene in inappropriate ways.
  - Chapters 7 to 9 include essential skills required of the nurse in relation to child physical assessment, care of the sick child, and medication administration.
- Chapters 10 through 25 focus on specific content areas related to care of the child. They begin with an examination of children who are in imminent danger and, therefore, in need of emergent care, and progress through the many systems of the body, concluding with care of the child with sensory deficits.
- Each chapter ends with a "Putting It All Together" case study, encouraging students to put the content into practice. Students are quizzed on the relevant objective and subjective information presented in a scenario and asked to identify a primary nursing diagnosis and interventions and to provide patient evaluation at discharge.
- Chapter 26 is a comprehensive final exam containing a 75-item pediatric nursing examination that integrates questions spanning content from throughout the textbook. Each question contains rationales for correct and incorrect answers and the NCLEX-RN test plan categories.

Each chapter presents need-to-know information in an outline format, eliminating nice-to-know, extraneous information. Just essential information is included, limiting the challenge of wading through excessive material. This approach assists students to focus on what is most important. The chapters include definitions of key words and practice questions specific to their content. Multiple-choice questions as well as all the alternate-type questions included on NCLEX examinations are incorporated. Of the approximately 450 questions in the textbook, almost one-fifth of them are alternate-format questions. Each question is coded according to the NCLEX-RN test plan categories: Integrated Processes, including the Nursing Process, Client Need, and Cognitive Domain. In addition, every question has the rationale for correct and incorrect answers. Studying rationales for the right and wrong answers to practice questions helps students learn new information or solidify previously learned information.

To provide even more opportunities to practice NCLEX-type questions, the book includes an additional 152-question comprehensive test, which is posted online at www.DavisPlus.com. Like the practice questions in the book, each question includes the rationale for correct and incorrect answers and coding for the NCLEX test plan categories.

Students should use every resource available to facilitate the learning process. I believe that this textbook will meet the needs of beginning nursing students who experience information overload!

Reviewers

Dawn Babbage, RN, MS, CNE
Associate Professor of Nursing
Jamestown Community College
Jamestown, New York

Vicky H. Becherer, PhD, RN
Assistant Teaching Professor
University of Missouri-St. Louis
Education Consultant
Cardinal Glennon Children's Medical Center
St. Louis, Missouri

Kate K. Chappell, MSN, APRN, CPNP
Clinical Assistant Professor
University of South Carolina College of Nursing
Columbia, South Carolina

Julie C. Chew, RN, MS, PhD
Resident Faculty
Mohave Community College
Lake Havasu, Arizona

Georgina Colalillo, MS, RN, CNE
Associate Professor, Nursing Department
Queensborough Community College/CUNY
Bayside, New York

Leslie Collins, MS, RN
Assistant Chair/Instructor
Division of Nursing
Northwestern Oklahoma State University
Alva, Oklahoma

Fleurdeliza Cuyco, BS
Instructor/Compliance Director
Preferred College of Nursing, Los Angeles
Los Angeles, California

Nancy Danou, RN, MSN, CPN
Professor Emeritus and Adjunct Associate Professor, Child Health Nursing
Viterbo University
La Crosse, Wisconsin

Peggy Dermer, RNC, MSN, WHCNS
Faculty/Nursing Instructor
Tri-County Technical College
Pendleton, South Carolina

Debbie Diamond, MSN, ARNP, FNP-BC
Assistant Professor
Nova Southeastern University
Miami, Florida

Judith Drumm, DNS, RN, CPN
Associate Professor
Palm Beach Atlantic University
West Palm Beach, Florida

Patricia Durham-Taylor, RN, PhD
Faculty
Truckee Meadows Community College
Reno, Nevada

Joyce Estes, RN, BSN, MSN
Nursing Faculty
Catawba Valley Community College
Hickory, North Carolina

Catherine Folker-Maglaya, MSN, APN/CNM, IBCLC
Assistant Professor, Nursing
Truman College/City Colleges of Chicago
Chicago, Illinois

Norene Gachignard, RN, MSN, CNE
Professor
North Shore Community College
Danvers, Massachusetts

Debora L. Geis, MS, RN, CNE
Professor
Rhodes State College
Lima, Ohio

Sharlene Georgesen, RN, MSN
Assistant Professor, Nursing
Morningside College
Sioux City, Iowa

Wanda Golden, RN, CCRN, PhD(C)
Associate Professor of Nursing
Abraham Baldwin Agricultural College
Tifton, Georgia

Mindy L. Herrin, PhDc, RN
Director of Assessment and Associate Professor
Lakeview College of Nursing
Danville, Illinois

Jill Holmstrom, Ed.D., RN, CNE
Associate Professor
Concordia College
Moorhead, Minnesota

Susan L. Hutton, MSN, RNC
Assistant Professor of Nursing
State College of Florida Manatee–Sarasota
Venice, Florida

Lenetra Jefferson, PhD, RN, CNE, LMT
Assistant Professor of Nursing
Dillard University
New Orleans, Louisiana

Kathryn M.L. Konrad, MS, RNC-OB, LCCE, FACCE
Instructor
The University of Oklahoma College of Nursing
Oklahoma City, Oklahoma

Jerrie Kirksey, RN; MSN Woman-Child Health
Associate Professor of Nursing
Gulf Coast State College
Panama City, Florida

Susan G. Lawless, MSN, RN, CNE
Nursing Faculty
Calhoun Community College
Decatur, Alabama

Cynthia Mailloux, PhD, RN, CNE
Professor and Chairperson Department of Nursing
Misericordia University
Dallas, Pennsylvania

Maria Angela Medina, RN, MSN
Nursing Instructor
Trinidad State Junior College
Alamosa, Colorado

Kathleen J. Murray, MSN, RNC, CFN, CHS III
Nursing Faculty and ACEN Evaluator
Henry Ford Community College
Dearborn, Michigan

Valerie Myers, MSN, RN
Nursing Faculty/Instructor
Pennsylvania College of Technology
Williamsport, Pennsylvania

Margery Orr, RN, DNS
Nursing Education Specialist
Becker College
Worcester, Massachusetts

Helen Papas-Kavalis, RN, C; MA
Professor of Nursing
Bronx Community College
Bronx, New York

Gloanna Peek, CPNP, MSN, RN
Clinical Associate Professor
University of Arizona College of Nursing
Tucson, Arizona

Cindy D. Phillips, MSN, RN (DrPh Candidate)
Assistant Professor, Nursing
Northeast State Community College
Kingsport, Tennessee

Malinda Poduska, MSN, RN
Assistant Professor of Nursing
Mount Mercy University
Cedar Rapids, Iowa

Sami Rahman, Med, MSN, RN
Director of Simulation and Clinical Labs
Blinn College
Bryan, Texas

Chassity Speight-Washburn, MSN, RN, CNE
Director of Nursing
Stanly Community College
Locust, North Carolina

Diane Taylor, MSN, RNC-MNN
Assistant Professor/Nursing
State College of Florida Manatee–Sarasota
Venice, Florida

Theresa Turick-Gibson, MA, PNP-BC
Professor
Hartwick College
Oneonta, New York

Blair Whitley, RN, MSN
Second Level Course Coordinator, ADN Program
Stanly Community College
Locust, North Carolina

Erica R. Williams-Woodley, RN, PNP, MSN
Professor
Bronx Community College
Bronx, New York

Mary Wunnenberg, MSN, RN, CNE
Assistant Professor of Nursing
Atlantic Cape Community College
Mays Landing, New Jersey

Acknowledgments

I would like to thank a number of individuals without whom this book would never have been published:

The assistance of Mary T. Hickey, EdD, WHNP-BC, Clinical Associate Professor at NYU College of Nursing, was invaluable when writing the chapter entitled, "Pediatric Medication Administration." Her expertise markedly strengthened the chapter content. The support of faculty with whom I teach at Adelphi University College of Nursing and Public Health was vital for the book's success.

F.A. Davis Publisher Robert Martone's faith in me has now extended to the publication of a second text. I thank him for his confidence in me and for this opportunity. Elizabeth (Liz) Hart, F.A. Davis Content Product Manager II, and, while Liz was on maternity leave, Catherine Carroll, F.A. Davis Manager of Project and eProject Management, were wonderfully supportive and helpful while overseeing the entire project. I could not have completed the book without the expertise and guidance of John Tomedi, Developmental Editor at Spring Hollow Press. His many suggestions made the book clearer and more complete. His assistance and patience throughout the process were invaluable. Marsha Hall and the copyediting staff at Progressive Publishing Alternatives edited the prose and made the book more readable for future students. Daniel Domzalski, F.A. Davis Illustration Coordinator, and the staff at Graphic World Illustration Services created beautiful images that bring many of my words to life.

Finally, these words of acknowledgment would not be complete without a thank you to the members of my family, who are always there when I need them.

Table of Contents

This book is one piece in a series published by F.A. Davis designed to assist student nurses successfully to graduate from nursing school and, ultimately, successfully to pass the NCLEX-RN examination. In particular, the book focuses on pediatric nursing care (i.e., the nursing care of children). Children are different from adults. In fact, children have different physiological characteristics, behave differently, think differently, and, in a number of cases, experience different illnesses than do adults. Not only is the large group of children different from the large group of adults, each subgroup of children—infant, toddler, preschooler, school-age child, and adolescent—exhibits differences from each other subgroup. In addition, children are members of a family, and families exist within cultural, ethnic, and religious contexts. To disclose those differences, this book presents chapters on the nursing care of each of those age groups as well as chapters on important considerations that nurses must take into account when caring for and administering medications to children. To provide comprehensive information, the book includes a chapter on each system of the body and the nursing care required of children suffering from diseases of each system.

In each chapter, the reader finds brief descriptions of the chapter's focus as well as a summary, in outline form, of the important content related to that focus. Each chapter is followed by two critical thinking sections. First is a case study, entitled "Putting It All Together," that relates directly to the content in that chapter. At the end of the case is a series of critical thinking questions, requiring the student nurse to determine how he or she would act in that situation. Answers to those questions follow the case. After the case study are a number of NCLEX-RN-style questions, with correct responses, rationales, and test-taking tips, related to the chapter content. Although the majority of the questions are multiple choice, the reader will also find multiple-response, fill-in-the-blank, drag-and-drop, and ordered-response items in the text.

It is important for the reader to realize that this book is not meant to be a primary nursing text on pediatrics. Rather, it has been written to supplement comprehensive pediatric texts. For the book to be of best use to the student nurse, therefore, he or she must have a foundational understanding of pediatric nursing. To gain that understanding, the student nurse must read and study an inclusive, pediatric nursing textbook.

Use This Book as One Educational Strategy

The first step to take when studying pediatric content is to study and learn the relevant material. Learning does not mean simply reading textbooks and/or attending class. Learning is an active process that requires a number of complex skills, including reading, discussing, and organizing information.

Read Assignments

Students must first read their assignments. By far the best time to read the assigned material is before the class in which the information will be discussed. Then, if students have any questions about what was read, they can ask the instructor during class and clarify anything that is confusing. In addition, students will find discussions much more meaningful when they have a basic understanding of the material.

Discuss the Information

During class time, material should be discussed with students rather than fed to them. Teachers have an obligation to provide stimulating and thought-provoking classes, but students also have an obligation to be prepared to engage in discussions on entering the classroom.

Although facts must be learned, nursing is not a fact-based profession. Nursing is an applied science. Nurses must use information. When a nurse enters a client's room, the client rarely asks the nurse to define a term or to recite a fact. Rather, the client presents the nurse with a set of data that the nurse must interpret and act on. In other words, the nurse must think critically. Students, therefore, must discuss client-based information by asking "why" questions rather than simply learning facts by asking "what" questions.

Organize the Information

While reading and discussing information, nursing students must begin to organize their knowledge. Nursing knowledge cannot be memorized. There is too much information, and, more important, memorization negatively affects the ability to use information. Nurses must be able to analyze data critically to determine priorities and actions. To think critically, nurses develop connections between and among elements of information.

There are several steps for organizing basic information, including understanding the pathophysiology of a problem; determining its significance for a particular client; identifying signs and symptoms; and using the steps of the nursing process.

Use the Nursing Process

The nursing process is foundational to nursing practice. To provide comprehensive care to their clients, nurses must understand and use each part of the nursing process—assessment, formulation of a nursing diagnosis, development of a plan of care, implementation of that plan, and evaluation of the outcomes.

Assess

Nurses gather a variety of information during the assessment phase of the nursing process. Some of the information is objective, or fact-based. For example, a client's hematocrit level and other blood values in the chart are facts that the nurse can use to determine a client's needs. Nurses also must identify subjective data, or information as perceived through the eyes of the client. A client's rating of pain is an excellent example of subjective information. Nurses must be aware of which data must be assessed because each client situation is unique. In other words, nurses must be able to use the information taught in class and individualize it for each client interaction to determine which objective data must be accessed and which questions should be asked of the client. Once the information is obtained, the nurse analyzes it.

Formulate Nursing Diagnoses

After the nurse has analyzed the data, a diagnosis is made. Nurses are licensed to treat actual or potential health problems. Nursing diagnoses are statements of the health problems that the nurse, in collaboration with the client and the primary health-care provider, has concluded are critical to the client's well-being.

Develop a Plan of Care

The nurse develops a plan of care, including goals of care, expected client outcomes, and interventions necessary to achieve the goals and outcomes. The nurse determines what he or she wishes to achieve in relation to each of the diagnoses and how to go about meeting those goals.

One very important part of this process is the development of the priorities of care. The nurse must determine which diagnoses are the most important and, consequently, which actions are the most important. For example, a client's physical well-being must take precedence over emotional well-being. It is essential that the nurse consider the client's priorities and the goals and orders of the client's primary health-care provider.

Implement the Care

Once the plan is established, the nurse implements it. The plan may include direct client care by the nurse and/or care that is coordinated by the nurse but performed by other practitioners. If assessment data change during implementation, the nurse must reanalyze the data, change diagnoses, and reprioritize care.

One very important aspect of nursing care is that it be evidence based. Nurses are independent practitioners. They are mandated to provide safe, therapeutic care that has a scientific basis. Nurses, therefore, must engage in lifelong learning. It is essential that nurses realize that much of the information in textbooks is outdated before the text was even published. To provide evidence-based care, nurses must keep their knowledge current by accessing information from reliable sources on the Internet, in professional journals, and at professional conferences.

Evaluate the Care

The evaluation phase is usually identified as the last phase of the nursing process, but it also could be classified as another assessment phase. When nurses evaluate, they are reassessing clients to determine whether the actions taken during the implementation phase met the needs of the client. In other words, "Were the goals of the nursing care met?" If the goals were not met, the nurse is obligated to develop new actions to meet the goals. If some of the goals were met, priorities may need to be changed, and so on. As can be seen from this phase, the nursing process is ongoing and ever changing.

Types of Questions

There are four integrative processes upon which questions in the NCLEX-RN examination are based: "Nursing Process," "Caring," "Communication and Documentation," and "Teaching/Learning" (*2013 NCLEX-RN Detailed Test Plan, Candidate Version*, 2013, p 5). The test taker must determine which process(es) is (are) being evaluated in each question. The test taker must realize that because nursing is an action profession, the NCLEX-RN questions simulate, in a written format, clinical situations. Therefore, critical reading is essential.

Most of the questions on the NCLEX-RN exam are multiple choice. Other types of questions, known as alternate-type questions, include fill-in-the-blank questions, multiple-response questions, drag-and-drop questions, and hot-spot items. In addition, any one of the types of questions may include an item to interpret, including lab data, images, and/or audio or video files (*2013 NCLEX-RN Detailed Test Plan*, 2013, p 46). The types of questions and examples of each are discussed below.

Multiple-Choice Questions

In these questions, a stem is provided (i.e., a situation is presented, and a question is asked). The test taker must then choose the best answer to the question among four possible responses. Sometimes, the test taker is asked to choose the best response, sometimes to choose the first action that should be taken, and so on. There are numerous ways that multiple-choice questions may be asked. Following is one example:

The nurse is assessing the growth and development of a 12-month-old child. Which of the following behaviors would the nurse expect the child to exhibit?

1. *Sits with assistance*
2. *Walks independently*
3. *Feeds self bite-sized foods using a neat pincer grasp*
4. *Holds a cup with one hand without spilling the contents*

Answer: 3

The test taker must know, for example, that although many children walk independently at 12 months of age, the majority of children are expected to walk independently by 15 months of age.

Fill-in-the-Blank Questions

These are calculation questions. The test taker may be asked to calculate a medication dosage, an intravenous (IV) drip rate, a minimum urinary output, or other factor. Included in the question are the units that the test taker should have in the answer.

The nurse is caring for a 2-year-old child who saturated her blanket with vomitus. To determine the volume of emesis, the nurse weighed a clean blanket (2,223 g) and the soiled blanket (2,338 g). How many milliliters of emesis has the client vomited?

______________ *mL*

Answer: 115 mL

The test taker must subtract 2,223 g from 2,338 g to determine that the client has vomited 115 g of emesis. Then, knowing that 1 g of fluid is equal to 1 mL of fluid, the test taker knows that the client has lost 115 mL of emesis.

Drag-and-Drop Questions

In drag-and-drop questions, the test taker is asked to place four or five possible responses in chronological or rank order. The responses may be related to such things as actions to be taken during a nursing procedure or steps in growth and development. The items are called drag-and-drop questions because the test taker will move the items with his or her computer mouse. Needless to say, in this book, the test taker will simply be asked to write the responses in the correct sequence.

A nurse is studying the psychosocial development of children. Place the following stages, as defined by Erik Erikson, into the correct chronological order:

1. *Trust versus mistrust*
2. *Initiative versus guilt*
3. *Industry versus inferiority*
4. *Identity versus role confusion*
5. *Autonomy versus shame and doubt*

Answer: 1, 5, 2, 3, 4

The correct order, as developed by Erikson, is trust versus mistrust in the infancy period, autonomy versus shame and doubt in the toddler period, initiative versus guilt in the preschool period, industry versus inferiority in the school age period, and identity versus role confusion in the adolescent period.

Multiple-Response Questions

The phrase "Select all that apply" following a question means that the examiner has included more than one correct response to the question. Usually, there will be five responses given, and the test taker must determine which of the five responses are correct. There may be two, three, four, or even five correct responses.

A nurse is caring for a 3-year-old child who has had 6 loose, green stools in the past 12 hr. Which of the following assessments should the nurse perform at this time? ***Select all that apply.***

1. *Height*
2. *Weight*
3. *Skin turgor*
4. *Patellar reflex*
5. *Fontanel tension*

Answer: 2 and 3

Because this child is at high risk for dehydration, the nurse should assess for weight loss and poor skin turgor. Neither the child's height nor patellar reflexes are directly related to the diagnosis of dehydration. In addition, both fontanels are closed by the time a child reaches 3 years of age.

Hot-Spot Items

These items require the test taker to identify the correct response to a question about a picture, graph, or other image. For example, a test taker may be asked to place an "X" on a picture of an infant.

A nurse is assessing an infant's rooting reflex. Place an "X" on the following image of the infant at the site where the nurse would assess the infant's rooting reflex.

Answer: The test taker should place an "X" on one of the infant's cheeks. When an infant exhibits a rooting reflex, he or she moves his or her head toward the cheek that is stroked. (See image.)

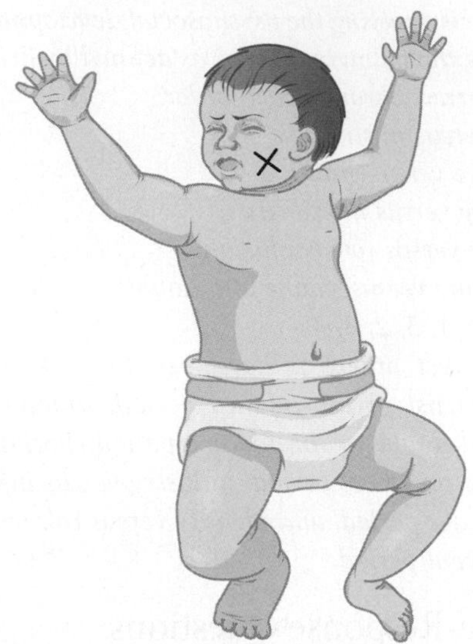

Items for Interpretation

Some questions may include an item to interpret. For example, the test taker is asked to interpret the sound on an audio file as tachycardia, recognize that a client is becoming progressively more anemic by interpreting laboratory results, or perform a calculation based on information given on an intake and output sheet.

A nurse assesses a laboratory report on a 16-year-old patient on the adolescent clinical unit each day during the patient's hospitalization. The nurse should report to the primary health-care provider that the patient's lab data are abnormal on which of the following days? ***Select all that apply****.*

	Day 1	Day 2	Day 3	Day 4	Day 5
K (mEq/L)	3.7	3.7	3.5	3.2	3.6
Na (mEq/L)	130	133	139	140	141
Hct (%)	35	38	40	38	37
Hgb (g/dL)	12.9	13.1	13.2	13.1	13.0

1. *Day 1*
2. *Day 2*
3. *Day 3*
4. *Day 4*
5. *Day 5*

Answer: 1, 2, and 4

Not only is this question a multiple-response item but also an item that requires the test taker to interpret a laboratory report. The nurse must be able to interpret the results of four different laboratory tests.

Know-How to Approach Exam Questions

There are several techniques that a test taker should use when approaching examination questions.

- **Pretend that the examination is a clinical experience:** First and foremost, test takers must approach critical-thinking questions as if they were in a clinical setting and the situation were developing on the spot. If the test taker pretends he or she is in a clinical situation, the importance of the response becomes evident. In addition, the test taker is likely to prepare for the examination with more commitment. That is not to say that students are rarely committed to doing well on examinations, but rather that they often approach examinations differently than they approach clinical situations. It is a rare nurse who goes to clinical not having had sufficient sleep to care for his or her clients, and yet students often enter an examination room after only 2 or 3 hours of sleep. The student taking an exam and a nurse working on a clinical unit both need the same critical-thinking ability that sleep provides. It is essential that test takers be well rested before all exams.
- **Read the stem carefully before reading the responses:** As discussed earlier, there are a number of different types of questions on the NCLEX-RN examination, and most faculty are including alternate-format questions in their classroom examinations as well. Before answering any question, the test taker must be sure, therefore, what the questioner is asking. This is one enormous drawback to classroom examinations. A test taker standing in a client's room is much less likely to misinterpret the situation when he or she is facing a client than when reading a question on an examination.
- **Consider possible responses:** After clearly understanding the stem of the question, *but before reading the possible responses*, the test taker should consider possible correct answers to the question. It is important for the test taker to realize that test writers include only plausible answer options. A test writer's goal is to determine whether the test taker knows and understands the material. The test taker, therefore, must have an idea of what the correct answer might be before beginning to read the possible responses.
- **Read the responses:** Only after clearly understanding what is being asked and after developing an idea of what the correct answer might be should the test taker read the responses. The one response that is closest in content to the test taker's guess should be the answer that is chosen, and the test taker should not second-guess himself or herself. One's first

impression is usually the correct response. Only if the test taker knows that he or she misread the question should the answer be changed.

- **Read the rationales for each question:** In this book, rationales are given for each answer option. The student should take full advantage of this feature. Read why the correct answer is correct. The rationale may be based on content, on interpretation of information, or on a number of other bases. Understanding why the answer to one question is correct is likely to transfer over to other questions with similar rationales. Next, read why the wrong answers are wrong. Again, the rationales may be based on a number of different factors. Understanding why answers are wrong also may transfer over to other questions.
- **Read all test-taking tips:** Some of the tips relate directly to test-taking skills, whereas others include invaluable information for the test taker.

If the test taker uses this text as recommended above, he or she should be well prepared to be successful when taking an examination in any or all of the content areas represented. As a result, the test taker should be fully prepared to care for children as a beginning registered professional nurse.

The Child as a Member of the Family

KEY TERMS

Bar mitzvah—In the Jewish faith, a coming-of-age ceremony for a 13 year old boy, after which he is responsible, morally and ethically, for his actions.

Bat mitzvah—In the Jewish faith, a coming-of-age ceremony for a 12-year-old girl, after which she is responsible for her actions, morally and ethically.

Blended family—A type of nontraditional family in which one or both parents is single, divorced, or widowed, and children from former relationship(s) may live together.

Bris—The ritual circumcision of the penis, practiced by members of the Jewish faith.

Communal family—A type of nontraditional family in which several family units live together.

Curandero—Among Hispanics and Latinos, a faith healer.

Haj—A journey to the holy city Mecca, which a member of the Muslim faith is expected to make once in his or her lifetime.

Halal—The types of foods members of the Muslim faith are permitted to eat; non-Halal foods include pork and alcohol, among others.

I. The Child as a Member of a Family

A. Description.

Children do not live independently. Rather, they live and are cared for in the context of a family structure. Families are responsible for meeting children's physical and emotional needs to enable them to grow and become healthy, mature, and ethical adults. To achieve those goals, adult family members are expected to provide children with such things as clothing, food, medical and dental needs, moral guidance, and love. However, the way those needs are provided is not universal. Indeed, families are diverse. They exist in cultural, racial, ethnic, and religious contexts, and nurses must have an understanding of those differences in order to provide holistic, empathic care when assessing children during well-child visits, when educating or providing care to children in a school system, when children are hospitalized, and in any other setting. Below is a review of many of the diverse family units that nurses may encounter. If, however, the nurse should care for a family that he or she is not familiar with, it is expected that the nurse will ask the parents and/or child regarding any specific needs that they may have.

II. Family Structures

Children's family experiences are as diverse as the types of families that exist. Nurses must be understanding and accepting of each type of family to minimize the need for explanations by either the parents or child and to minimize each family's stressors. The major types of family structures are:

A. Traditional family.

1. Mother, father, and one or more children.

B. Nontraditional family.

1. Single parent: either mother or father with one or more children.

2. Adoptive family.
   a. Traditional or single parent family.
   b. One or more children is adopted.
   c. Adopted children may or may not be of the same ethnicity or race as the parent(s) or siblings.
3. **Blended family.**
   a. One or both parents are single, divorced, or widowed.
   b. Children from former relationships live together.
4. Multigenerational family.
   a. Traditional or single parent family with one or more children.
   b. Grandparents of one or both parents live in the same household.
5. Same-sex family.
   a. Both parents are of the same sex.
   b. Remainder of family structure may be comprised of an adoptive, blended, or multigenerational structure.
6. Grandparent-led family.
   a. Because of death, incarceration, or other reason, the parents are not able to care for the children.
   b. Grandparents assume the responsibility of parenthood.
7. **Communal family.**
   a. Many family units living together.

III. Culture

A family's culture is defined by the values, principles, and convictions espoused by the family members. The culture of the family guides many decisions and practices as well as dietary preferences, financial priorities, and other choices made within the family. When two or more adults in a family come from different cultures, conflicts may arise. In addition, families whose members were raised in a country other than the United States often have unique cultural beliefs. One of the most important factors that influences cultural beliefs is religion. Some of the more important issues guided by culture that impact pediatric nursing care are birth practices; developmental rites of passage, such as baptism, ritual circumcision, and first communion; dietary preferences; and death rituals.

A. Major religions practiced in the United States.
1. Christianity: there are a number of different Christian sects, each with its unique perspective. Although differences exist, the major tenets of Christianity are universal.
   a. Fundamental principles.
      i. Jesus was the Son of God and the Messiah.
      ii. Jesus' works while on Earth, as well as his death and resurrection, guarantee believers posthumous heavenly salvation.
   b. Basics.
      i. Christian clergy's titles are dependent on the specific faith, for example:
         (1) Priest: Roman Catholic and Episcopalian.
         (2) Minister: Methodist and Lutheran.
         (3) Preacher: Baptist.
      ii. A Christian house of worship is called a church or a cathedral.
   c. Practices common to Christians.
      i. Scripture study of the Old and New Testaments of the Bible.
      ii. Baptism.
      iii. Prayer.
      iv. Communion.
      v. Performing good deeds.
      vi. Funerals.
2. Judaism: the three main branches of the Jewish faith, in which followers are often called the People of the Book, from most traditional in beliefs to the most liberal, are Orthodox, Conservative, and Reform.
   a. Fundamental principles.
      i. Monotheism: one God to whom the people pray directly.
      ii. Messiah has yet to arrive on Earth.
      iii. Information written in the Hebrew language in the Old Testament, Torah, and Talmudic scriptures guide choices and actions of daily life.
   b. Basics.
      i. Jewish clergy are called rabbis or rebbes.
      ii. Jewish houses of worship are called temples or synagogues.
   c. Practices common to Jews.
      i. Ritual circumcision, or **bris**.
      ii. **Bar mitzvah:** coming of age ceremony for 13-year-old boys.
      iii. **Bat mitzvah:** coming of age ceremony for 12-year-old girls.
      iv. Dietary restrictions (i.e., kosher eating practices) prohibit, for example, the ingestion of pork and shellfish.
      v. Giving of charity to others less fortunate.
      vi. Death rituals and burial within 24 hours of death.
3. Islam: Islam is practiced by a number of peoples, called Muslims, throughout the world, most predominantly among those from Arabic countries in the Middle East.
   a. Fundamental principles.
      i. Monotheism: one God, Allah, to whom the people pray directly.

ii. Based on the teachings of the prophet, Mohammed.
   (1) Mohammed received God's word.
   (2) Teachings are written in the Book of Quran.

b. Basics.
   i. Although there is no ordained clergy in Islam, those who lead Muslim communities are often referred to as imams.
   ii. Muslim houses of worship are called mosques.

c. Practices common to Muslims, of which the majority are guided by the five pillars of the faith:
   i. Male is the head of household and the decision maker.
   ii. Recitation of the principles of Islam.
   iii. Five mandatory times for prayer during each day.
   iv. Providing charity to those in need.
   v. Fasting during the sacred month of Ramadan.
   vi. Performing **Haj** or making the pilgrimage to Holy City of Islam—Mecca in the current country of Saudi Arabia—at least once during one's lifetime.
   vii. Dietary restrictions (i.e., **Halal**) prohibit, for example, the consumption of pork and alcoholic beverages.

4. Hinduism is the primary religion of the majority of individuals living in or from India and Nepal. Hindu practices are quite diverse (e.g., some Hindus are polytheistic, while others believe in one Supreme Being).

a. Fundamental principles.
   i. Most believe in *Dharma* (there is no direct translation into English), a Hindu word loosely translated as guiding principle or duty.
   ii. The four Vedas are the scriptures of Hinduism: Rig Veda, Sama Veda, Yajur Veda, and Atharva Veda. The Vedas help to guide the daily lives of Hindus.

b. Basics.
   i. There is no one clergyperson who leads Hindu worship but rather a number of priests and teachers.
   ii. A Hindu house of worship is called a temple.

c. Practices common to Hindus.
   i. Personal sacrifice and purification.
   ii. Pregnancy and birthing rituals, including a naming ceremony.
   iii. Rituals at many developmental periods of a child's life.
   iv. Marriage rituals.
   v. Death rituals, including cremation with transition to the next life.
   vi. Vegetarianism commonly is practiced.

B. Ethnic and racial groups: customs based on a family member's country of origin and/or racial background often markedly influence his or her cultural practices. In addition, the child's or parent's primary language, if other than English, can affect care. If communication is hampered, children's and family members' comfort levels can be negatively affected as well as the children's ultimate recovery. Based on the 2010 U.S. census, it is determined that as of 2012, in addition to the predominant non-Hispanic or Latino white population, i.e., the "original peoples of Europe, the Middle East, or North Africa," who comprise 63% of the U.S. population (U.S. Census, 2012), the following groups reside in the United States:

1. Asian and Pacific Islanders.
   a. 5.3% of the U.S. population.
   b. Individuals whose origins have their roots in the "Far East, Southeast Asia, or the Indian subcontinent including, for example, Cambodia, China, India, Japan, Korea, Malaysia, Pakistan, the Philippine Islands, Thailand, and Vietnam" (U.S. Census, 2012). Those from the Islands of the Pacific (e.g., Hawaii, Guam, Samoa) also often identify with the Asian culture.
   c. Common beliefs among many Asian and Pacific Islanders.
      i. Importance of and respect for the family, especially the wisdom of the elderly.
      ii. Importance of self-control and personal honor.
      iii. Diet primarily comprised of vegetables, rice, and fish.

2. Blacks.
   a. 13.1% of the U.S. population.
   b. Individuals whose "origins [are] in any of the Black racial groups of Africa" (U.S. Census, 2012).
   c. Common beliefs among many Blacks.
      i. Precepts of Christianity and the guidance of the preacher are followed while some Blacks follow the Muslim faith.
      ii. Illnesses are often viewed as having been sent by God.

3. Native Americans.
   a. 1.2% of the U.S. population.
   b. People who adhere to the rituals and beliefs of the "original peoples of North and South

America (including Central America)" and who identify with their native tribe (U.S. Census, 2012).

c. Common beliefs among many Native Americans.
   i. Supremacy of the family and especially the elders of the community.
   ii. Often wish to consult with the Native American healer who may employ rituals and the consumption of herbs as healing practices.

4. Hispanics and Latinos.
   a. 16.9% of the U.S. population.
   b. Those whose origins are from "Spain, the Spanish-speaking countries of Central or South America, or the Dominican Republic" (U.S. Census, 2012).
   c. Hispanic people may be of any racial background.
   d. Common beliefs among many Hispanics.
      i. Extended families are common and provide great comfort during periods of stress.
      ii. The male, who is usually the head of household, should be consulted when decisions are made.
      iii. Hispanics are usually Christian, with Catholicism being the primary faith practiced.
      iv. Faith healers, or **curanderos**, may be consulted when a child is ill, and traditional remedies are often used.

IV. Parent-Child Relationships

The relationships between parents and children, as well as parents' disciplinary practices, are grounded in the cultural practices of the family. Parenting is not learned in a classroom, rather one learns to parent from watching the behaviors of one's parents.

A. Discipline (see also "Growth and Development," Chapters 2–6).

V. Nursing Considerations

A. Nursing diagnoses: based on a nurse's assessment, a number of nursing diagnoses may be important for the nurse to identify.

DID YOU KNOW?

The development of nursing diagnoses is one of the key components of the nursing process—assessment, diagnosis, planning, implementation, evaluation. The diagnoses are determined by the nurse after he or she identifies the subjective and objective assessments in collaboration with his or her client. Throughout this text, nursing diagnoses are identified. The diagnoses in this text are based on those developed by the North American Nursing Diagnosis Association (NANDA). Other diagnostic terms (e.g., those of Nursing Interventions Classifications [NIC] or simple problem statements) may also be used.

1. Parental role conflict, characterized by, for example:
   a. A parent whose child is ill feels incapable of caring for the child.
   b. A parent who feels that a child's illness is adversely affecting him or herself or other members of the family.
2. Interrupted Family Processes characterized by, for example:
   a. Siblings who are assuming parental roles because their parents must care for a sick brother or sister.
   b. Siblings who resent the time spent by parents caring for a sick brother or sister.
   c. Changes in the distribution of resources because of the expense of a child's health care.
3. Caregiver Role Strain characterized by, for example:
   a. Physical and/or emotional fatigue experienced by the parents of a hospitalized child or a child at home who needs extensive care.
   b. Physical and/or emotional fatigue experienced by parents of the sandwich generation—those who must care for their children as well as their elderly parents.
   c. Abuse of substances in response to the stress of the severe illness or death of a child.
4. Deficient Knowledge related to inability to speak or understand English, characterized by, for example:
   a. Parents and/or child falsely communicating—by the nod of the head, for example—that the health-care regimen is understood.
   b. Anger and/or frustration with the inability to communicate or understand what is being said.

B. Interventions: specific interventions are dependent on individual circumstances, but many include any or all of the following:

1. Educating the parents and family members regarding the child's illness and health-care needs.
2. Providing emotional support to parents and family members during periods of stress.
3. Assisting parents and family members to identify coping mechanisms for times of stress, including prayer or other religious practices, meditation, and exercise.

4. Providing grief counseling to parents and family members when appropriate.
5. Identifying support systems for parents and family members for times of stress, including extended family members, community leaders, members of religious organizations, and siblings' educators.
6. Assisting parents to access available community resources by referring parents to social services and government agencies (e.g., Women, Infants, and Children nutrition services and neighborhood clinics).
7. Providing the parents and/or child with a language interpreter.

CASE STUDY: Putting It All Together

An 8-year-old boy is seen in the emergency department accompanied by his parents, maternal grandparents, two younger siblings aged 2 and 5, and his mother's sister

Subjective Data

- Multiple people are speaking at once, some in English and others in Spanish.
- The father, in a Spanish accent, tells the nurse, "My son, he fell down. *Es en mucho dolor.*"
- A certified medical interpreter is at the child's bedside.
- In Spanish, the child communicates that he fell when riding his bicycle and has injured his right leg. He rates his pain at 5 out of 10 on a numeric pain scale.
- When queried about his immunization history, neither the child nor any of the adults know when or if the child has received his immunizations.

Objective Data

- Abrasion and bruise, 2 in. by 2 in. in size, noted on outer aspect of right leg distal to the knee
- Abrasion is dirt covered
- X-rays performed—no fracture seen

Vital Signs	
Temperature:	98.6°F
Heart rate:	90 bpm
Respiratory rate:	24 rpm
Blood pressure:	100/60 mm Hg

Health-Care Provider's Orders

- Administer ibuprofen 200 mg PO every 6 hr for pain
- Cleanse wound with soap and water
- Apply triple antibiotic (bacitracin/neomycin/polymyxin B) ointment after cleansing
- Administer Tdap (Tetanus, Diphtheria, Pertussis) vaccine IM STAT
- Educate child and parents regarding need for helmet protection when riding bicycle
- Refer to pediatric clinic for follow-up

Case Study Questions

A. What *subjective* assessments indicate that the client is experiencing a health alteration?

1. ______
2. ______
3. ______
4. ______

B. What *objective* assessments indicate that the client is experiencing a health alteration?

1. ______
2. ______
3. ______
4. ______

Continued

CASE STUDY: Putting It All Together *cont'd*

Case Study Questions

C. After analyzing the data that has been collected, what **primary** nursing diagnosis should the nurse assign to this client?

1. ______________________________

D. What interventions should the nurse plan and/or implement to meet this child's and his family's needs?

1. ______________________________
2. ______________________________
3. ______________________________
4. ______________________________
5. ______________________________
6. ______________________________
7. ______________________________
8. ______________________________
9. ______________________________
10. ______________________________

E. What client outcomes should the nurse evaluate regarding the effectiveness of the nursing interventions?

1. ______________________________
2. ______________________________
3. ______________________________
4. ______________________________

F. What physiological characteristics should the child exhibit after treatment?

1. ______________________________

G. What psychological characteristics should the child and family exhibit before being discharged home?

1. ______________________________

REVIEW QUESTIONS

1. A 3-year-old Native American child is admitted to the pediatric unit for emergency surgery. Which of the following questions should the nurse include when taking the admission history from the child's parents?
   1. "Does your Indian tribe believe in immunizing children?"
   2. "Do you attend Native American powwows with the family?"
   3. "Have you consulted with your tribal healer about your child's illness?"
   4. "What herbal remedies have you given your child today?"

2. The parents of an infant have just been informed by the infant's primary health-care provider that their child has an aggressive form of cancer. The parents have previously communicated that they are Jewish. Which of the following statements would be appropriate for the nurse to make? "It is often comforting for parents of very sick children to:
   1. speak with their rabbis."
   2. read the sacred scriptures of Jesus."
   3. go to their church to pray."
   4. consult with members of the mosque."

3. The nurse notes in a toddler's medical record that the child was adopted internationally at 1 week of age. The child has been diagnosed with a terminal autosomal dominant genetic disease. Which of the following statements would be appropriate for the nurse to make?
   1. "I will provide you with a referral for a meeting with a genetic counselor regarding your pregnancy risks."
   2. "It is very important that the mother be notified of the baby's genetic condition."
   3. "What a shame that you adopted a sick child rather than a healthy child."
   4. "If you would like to learn more about your child's disease, I can refer you to a genetic counselor."

4. A second grader enters the school nurse's office crying and states, "I feel sick. My belly hurts." The nurse replies, "I'll call your mommy or daddy to pick you up." The child replies, "I don't have a mommy, I have 2 daddies." Which of the following comments by the nurse is appropriate?
   1. "That's right. I forgot that your parents are gay."
   2. "Of course you have a mommy. You just don't live with your mommy."
   3. "I'll call one of your daddies to pick you up."
   4. "It must be interesting to live with two men and no women in the house."

5. A 10-year-old Hindu child who has just been diagnosed with diabetes is admitted to the pediatric clinical unit. The nurse is counseling the parents and child regarding the child's dietary needs. Which of the following statements by the nurse would be appropriate?
   1. "It is very important for you to eat protein at each meal. Meat is an excellent source of protein."
   2. "I understand that you do not usually eat fruit, but because you are diabetic, it will be essential for you to eat fruit."
   3. "To be able to provide you with the best information about dietary needs, I need to ask whether you follow a vegan diet."
   4. "Diabetes is a very serious illness. It may be necessary for you to consume foods that you are unaccustomed to eating."

REVIEW ANSWERS

1. ANSWER: 3
Rationale:
1. This is an inappropriate question. It should not be asked.
2. This is an inappropriate question. It should not be asked.
3. This question should be included when the nurse is taking the admission history.
4. This is an inappropriate question. It should not be asked.
TEST-TAKING TIP: Because Native American families often seek counseling from a tribal healer, it is important to include that question. Questions that could be construed as insulting or that make assumptions about care should not be asked.
Content Area: *Pediatrics*
Integrated Processes: *Nursing Process: Assessment*
Client Need: *Psychosocial Integrity: Cultural Diversity*
Cognitive Level: *Application*

2. ANSWER: 1
Rationale:
1. This statement is appropriate. The Jewish spiritual leader is called a rabbi.
2. This statement is not appropriate. Jews do not read the scriptures that discuss Jesus.
3. This statement is not appropriate. The Jewish house of worship is called either a temple or a synagogue.
4. This statement is not appropriate. The Muslim holy sanctuary is called a mosque.
TEST-TAKING TIP: It is appropriate to suggest to clients that they seek counsel with their religious advisor or clergyperson. The nurse must, however, be aware that there are differences in clients' belief systems. For example, the nurse should never make parents feel uncomfortable if they should decide not to seek counsel from a clergyperson. In addition, if the nurse is not familiar with the clients' beliefs, it is best to use generic terms or to consult someone who is knowledgeable.
Content Area: *Pediatrics*
Integrated Processes: *Nursing Process: Implementation*
Client Need: *Psychosocial Integrity: Cultural Diversity*
Cognitive Level: *Application*

3. ANSWER: 4
Rationale:
1. This statement is inappropriate. This child has been adopted. The child's adoptive mother is not the child's biological mother.
2. This statement is inappropriate. The adoption was performed in another country. It is probable that the adoptive parents are unaware of the identity of the biological mother.
3. This statement is inappropriate. The nurse must always communicate an understanding that an adopted child is cherished as much as a biological child.
4. This statement is appropriate. Because the disease is genetic, the professionals who are most knowledgeable about the disease are genetic counselors.
TEST-TAKING TIP: It must be assumed that adopted children are cherished as much as biological children. The nurse should refer to the child as the parent's child, not as the parent's adopted child.
Content Area: *Pediatrics*
Integrated Processes: *Nursing Process: Implementation*
Client Need: *Psychosocial Integrity: Cultural Diversity*
Cognitive Level: *Application*

4. ANSWER: 3
Rationale:
1. This statement is inappropriate.
2. Although this statement is accurate, it is inappropriate.
3. The nurse should respond with this statement.
4. This statement is inappropriate.
TEST-TAKING TIP: Nurses must be prepared to care for children with same-sex parents. The children should never be made to feel that the family structure is abnormal.
Content Area: *Pediatrics*
Integrated Processes: *Nursing Process: Implementation*
Client Need: *Psychosocial Integrity: Cultural Diversity*
Cognitive Level: *Application*

5. ANSWER: 3
Rationale:
1. This statement is not appropriate. Although not universal, many Hindus are vegetarians.
2. This statement is inaccurate. Hindus do eat fruit.
3. This statement is correct. Although some vegetarians eat eggs and drink milk, others follow a more restrictive, vegan diet.
4. This statement is not appropriate. Vegetarian diets are compatible with diabetic diets.
TEST-TAKING TIP: Many Hindus are vegetarians. The nurse should assume, unless advised by a licensed nutritionist, that the vegetarian diet is compatible with the diets required of medical illnesses, including diabetes.
Content Area: *Pediatrics*
Integrated Processes: *Nursing Process: Implementation*
Client Need: *Psychosocial Integrity: Cultural Diversity*
Cognitive Level: *Application*

Preface to Growth and Development in Pediatric Nursing

It is the goal of health-care providers to promote health and to prevent illness in their clients. When caring for children, that goal is translated into four main actions:

- To monitor children's biological growth and maturational development on a regular basis in order to identify alterations from the norm.
- To intervene when needed to return children to normal growth and development.
- To provide interventions that increase children's likelihood of maintaining health.
- To educate caregivers regarding ways to provide children with healthy and safe lifestyles.

The next five chapters discuss the five major age periods in a child's development: infancy, toddlerhood, preschool age, school age, and adolescence. While outlining the milestones of each period of development, these chapters provide information that enables nurses to achieve the stated goals. To that end, these chapters are divided into four sections: "Biological Development," "Language and Social Development," "Nursing Considerations: Health Promotion/Parent Education," and "Nursing Considerations: Disease Prevention/Parent Education."

The section "Biological Development," which concerns growth in size, shape, and function of the body, covers a number of important concepts, including the height, weight, and normal vital signs for children at the designated ages, as well as the motor development that is expected of children at each age level. Although these chapters provide benchmarks, it is important to note that for complete and objective assessments of a child's development, standardized tools should always be used. The growth charts published by the Centers for Disease Control and Prevention (CDC) (www.cdc.gov/growthcharts/clinical_charts.htm) as well as the Denver Developmental Screening Test II (DDST-II) (www.denverii.com/), the Ages and Stages Questionnaires (http://agesandstages.com/), and the Parents' Evaluation of Developmental Status (PEDS) (www.pedstest.com/default.aspx) are but a few of those tools.

The section "Language and Social Development" covers a number of concepts, of which three are based on the research conducted by well-known theorists:

- Language development, or the maturation in growth and function of a child's ability to communicate.
- Psychosocial development, or the changes in children's emotional and social growth, based on the work of Erik Erikson.
- Cognitive development, or the maturation in relation to a child's intellectual abilities, based on the work of Jean Piaget.
- Moral development, or the maturation of a child's understanding of his and others' ethical behaviors, as discussed by Lawrence Kohlberg.

In addition, the chapters on growth and development include important information related to health-promotion strategies (e.g., healthy eating and exercise) that help children to stay well and disease prevention protocols (e.g., immunization administration and dental hygiene) that help to keep children from becoming sick. Nursing considerations and parent education related to both health promotion and disease prevention are included.

Chapter 2

Normal Growth and Development: Infancy

KEY TERMS

Biological development—Growth in size, shape, and function of the body.

Cognitive development—Maturation in intellectual abilities of the child; this text references the work of cognitive theorist Jean Piaget.

Deciduous teeth—A baby's first teeth, also called primary teeth or baby teeth, usually appearing between 6 and 9 months of age.

Dental caries—Cavities.

Disease prevention—Actions, such as immunizations and dental hygiene, that help to keep children from becoming sick.

Fine motor development—Maturation in size and function of the small muscles of the body, such as development in the dexterity of the hands and fingers.

Fontanels—The soft spots on a baby's head.

Gross motor development—Maturation in size and function of the large muscles of the body, that is, development of the muscles that enable the child to sit, crawl, and walk.

Head circumference—Measurement of the size of a child's head. The measurement is taken at the point just above the ears and at the level of the child's eyebrows.

Health promotion—Actions, such as eating healthy and exercise, that help children to stay well.

Infancy period—The period of a child's life between his or her birth and 1 year of age.

Language development—Maturation in growth and function of a child's ability to communicate.

Moral development—Ethical development, or the maturation of a child's understanding of his and others' behaviors that are right versus wrong. This text references the work of moral theorist Lawrence Kohlberg.

Neonatal period—A child's age period from the time of his or her birth to 28 days of life.

Object permanence—A baby's ability to realize that objects, including his or her parents, exist even when they cannot be seen.

Plagiocephaly—Also called flat head syndrome, a flattening of the back of the baby's head due to sleeping on his or her back.

Pseudostrabismus—The false appearance of crossed or wandering eyes, commonly seen in babies until 6 months of age.

Psychosocial development—Changes in an individual's emotional and social growth; this text references the work of psychosocial theorist Erik Erikson.

Shaken baby syndrome (SBS)—A condition that can result when an infant is violently shaken, causing permanent damage, including mental retardation and physical disability, or death from bleeding in the brain.

I. Description

The **infancy period** is defined as the age period between a child's birth and first birthday. The first 28 days of life, however, are called the **neonatal period.** This age period is considered separate because the characteristics and behaviors of the newborn are impacted by the newborn's fetal environment and transition to extrauterine life. The neonatal period is discussed in depth in maternity texts. This chapter focuses on the remainder of the infancy period, from 28 days to 1 year of life.

DID YOU KNOW?

Children change dramatically during their infancy. They begin the period as persons who are unable to perform any independent actions. They must rely on their caregivers for food, warmth, transport, and safety. By the time they reach their first birthday, however, infants are able to walk, albeit often with some assistance; feed themselves; and speak in a rudimentary language. The transition is quite astounding.

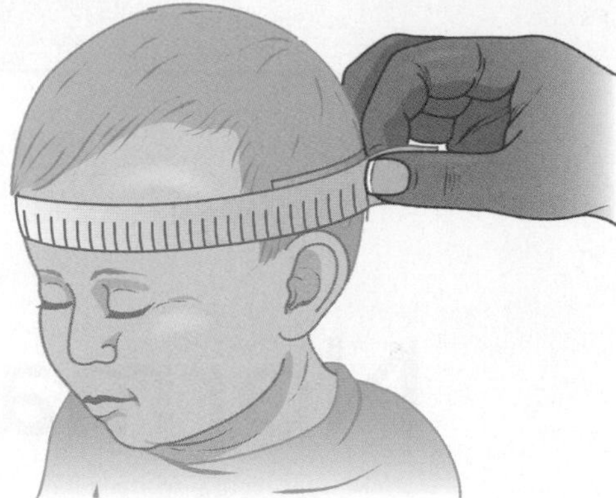

Fig 2.1 Measurement of head circumference.

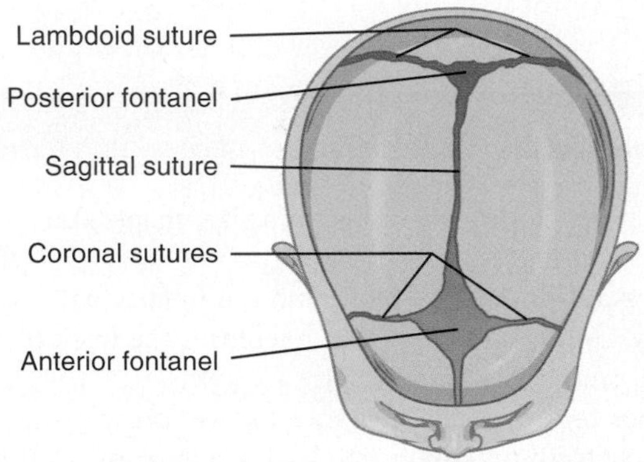

Fig 2.2 Anterior and posterior fontanels.

II. Biological Development

A. Growth: rapid in the first 6 months and slows during the second 6 months.
1. Weight.
   a. During the first 6 months of life, babies gain approximately 1.5 lb (680 g) per month and often double their birth weight by 6 months.
   b. Babies usually triple their birth weight by 1 year.
2. Height.
   a. During the first 6 months of life, babies grow on average 1 in. (2.5 cm)/month.
   b. During the second 6 months, growth slows to 0.5 in. (1.25 cm)/month.
3. **Head circumference** is a measurement of the size of a child's head, which is an indicator of brain growth. The measurement is taken at the point just above the ears and at the level of the child's eyebrows (see Fig. 2.1).
   a. During the first 6 months of life, babies' head circumference grows on average 0.6 in. (1.5 cm)/month.
   b. During the second 6 months, growth slows to 0.2 in. (0.5 cm)/month.
4. **Fontanels** are the soft spots on a baby's head (see Fig. 2.2).
   a. Posterior fontanel.
      i. Triangular in shape.
      ii. Closes between 1 and 3 months of age.
   b. Anterior fontanel.
      i. Diamond shaped.
      ii. Closes between 12 and 18 months of age.

MAKING THE CONNECTION

Because the pattern of a child's growth is as important as his or her exact measurements, each time a child is examined, weight and height are measured, and the values are charted on a standardized growth chart. The health-care provider monitors the child's growth pattern to see whether the child is following the anticipated growth path. For example, if a child's height and weight pattern consistently is on the 25th percentile path, the child is proportional and is growing consistently. If, however, a child's height and weight move from the 60th percentile to the 50th to the 25th, the health-care practitioner would be obligated to assess the reason for the growth alteration (see growth charts from the Centers for Disease Control and Prevention [CDC] in the Appendices).

B. Vital signs: should be taken and compared with normal ranges at each contact with an infant.
1. Temperature.
   a. Normal range is 97.7° to 99.0°F (36.5° to 37.3°C).

b. Rectal method.
   i. Method that provides the most accurate temperature.
   ii. To prevent trauma to the rectum, the tip of the thermometer should be well lubricated and inserted into the anus no farther than 0.5 in.
c. Axillary, or armpit, method.
   i. Used most frequently because the rectal method can cause injury to the anus.

DID YOU KNOW?

When taking an axillary temperature, the bulb of the thermometer must be placed directly into the axilla, or armpit, of the baby. The arm of the child should then be held firmly against the side of his or her body so that the thermometer remains in place. If the thermometer moves out of the axilla, an inaccurate temperature will be recorded.

2. Heart rate.
   a. Normal range is 80 to 150 bpm.
   b. Apical method should always be used and, to obtain an accurate rate, it should be taken for one full minute.
3. Respiratory rate.
   a. Normal range is 25 to 55 rpm.
   b. Respirations should also be counted for a full minute.
4. Blood pressure.
   a. Normal range is 65 to 100/45 to 65 mm Hg.
   b. Rarely taken until children reach 3 years of age.
   c. If taken, an electronic method should be used.

C. Dentition: the growth and eruption of infants' **deciduous teeth**, also called primary or baby teeth, usually occurs in a predictable pattern.
1. Drooling starts at about 4 months of age.
2. First teeth usually appear between 6 and 9 months of age, and by 12 months of age, children usually have six to eight teeth. Teeth erupt in the following order:
   a. First: lower central incisors.
   b. Next: upper central incisors.
   c. Last: upper and lower lateral incisors.
3. Parent education.
   a. Teeth should be cleaned daily either with a washcloth or a soft child's toothbrush.
   b. No toothpaste should be used until the child, usually in late toddlerhood, is able to spit on command.
   c. Infants should never be put to sleep with a bottle filled with formula, breast milk, or juice because of the potential for the development of **dental caries** (i.e., cavities).

D. Senses.
1. Hearing.
   a. All babies should be assessed for hearing deficit in the newborn period.
      i. By 4 months of age, babies should turn their heads toward a sound.
      ii. By 10 months of age, babies should respond to their names.
   b. To prevent speech delay, if a hearing deficit exists, intervention should begin as early as possible and no later than 6 months of age.
2. Vision.
   a. Vision acuity progresses rapidly from 20/100 at birth.
      i. Babies prefer black and white and primary colors early in infancy.
      ii. Babies are able to see pastels by 6 months of age.
   b. **Pseudostrabismus**, what appears to be crossed or wandering eyes, commonly is seen in babies until 6 months of age when binocular vision is established.

E. Motor development.
1. **Gross motor development:** expected milestones in gross motor development are included in Table 2.1.
2. **Fine motor development:** expected milestones in fine motor development are included in Table 2.2.

III. Language and Social Development

A. Language development comprises two aspects: the ability to understand others, and the ability to express oneself. *Receptive language development* refers to a child's ability to understand words. *Expressive language development* refers to the child's ability to communicate via speech or, eventually, via the written word. Expected milestones in language development are included in Table 2.3.

MAKING THE CONNECTION

Parents must be advised that children are unable to learn and grow if they are not given the opportunity to practice important skills. To enable children to crawl and walk, they must be placed on the floor where those actions can be practiced. To enable children to develop fine motor skills, they must be provided with rattles, blocks, and small finger foods so that they can practice those skills. Some parents are reluctant to put their children on the floor or to allow them to feed themselves because they might get dirty. Good suggestions that the nurse might give the parents are to put a blanket on the floor for play and to schedule the baby's bath right after a messy meal.

Table 2.1 Gross Motor Development

Age	Expected Milestones in Development
1–2 months	Rudimentary reflexes still present (see Chapter 7, "Physical Assessment of Children" for images of rudimentary reflexes), for example: *Grasp reflex: when an item (e.g., the parent's finger) is placed in the palm, the baby's fingers encircle it. The reflex is very endearing to parents who often interpret the reflex as a loving gesture.* *Tonic neck reflex: when the baby's head is turned toward one side, the baby's arm that is on that same side will straighten, and the baby's other arm will bend. The reflex is often called the fencing reflex because the baby appears to be in a fencing pose.* *Rooting reflex: when a baby's cheek is stroked, the baby will turn toward that side. This reflex is especially important for breastfeeding babies to entice them to turn toward their mothers' breast.* *Moro reflex: when a baby is startled or dropped suddenly, the baby's arms and legs extend and then retract. The reflex, also called the startle reflex, usually ends with the baby crying as if in fear. Because the baby's entire body is involved, a Moro response informs the health-care practitioner that the baby's central nervous system is intact.* *Babinski reflex: when the sole of the baby's foot is stroked from heel to toe, the baby's great toe dorsiflexes, and the remaining toes flare out. This sign is also an important indicator of central nervous system integrity.* *Head lag: backward slumping of the head when a baby is picked up by the arms from the supine position.* 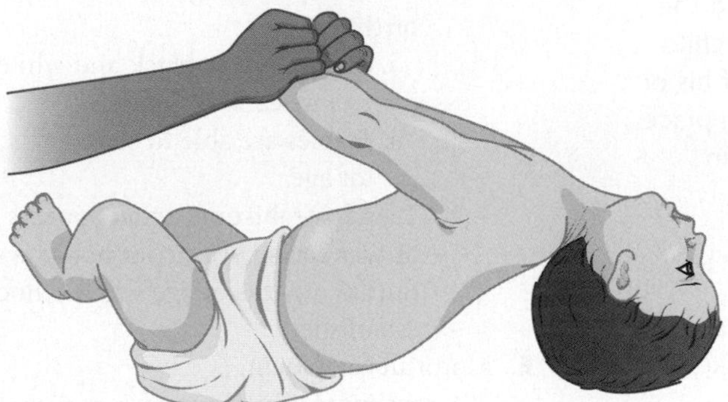
3 months	*Lifts head from bed when prone* *Head lag diminishing* *Moves hand to mouth*
4–5 months	*Majority of rudimentary reflexes have disappeared* *Plays with feet* *Puts weight on feet when held* *May turn from tummy to back*
6–7 months	*Sits in tripod positioning, with hands supporting body while leaning forward* 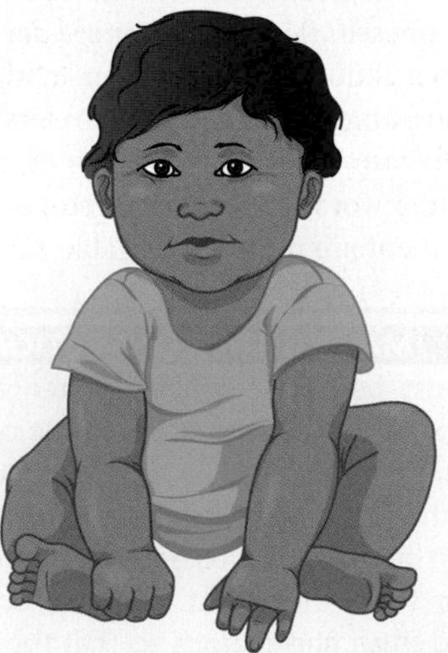 *Head lag has disappeared* *May turn from back to tummy*
8–9 months	*Sits well* *Crawls and pulls self to standing position*
10–12 months	*Babinski reflex disappears* *Stands independently* *Walks while holding on with one hand*

Table 2.2 Fine Motor Development

Age	Expected Milestones in Development
1–2 months	*Follows objects with eyes to midline* *Grasp reflex still present* *Drops rattle*
3 months	*Grasp reflex diminishing or absent* *Holds object if placed in hands*
4–5 months	*Begins to reach and grasp voluntarily*
6–7 months	*Independently can transfer objects from one hand to the other* *Uses palmar grasp well—holding an object with the palm of the hand rather than in the fingers*
8–9 months	*Develops a crude pincer grasp—grasping an object between the thumb and the other fingers of the hand* *Is able purposefully to drop objects*
10–12 months	*Feeds self finger foods, moving from putting fistfuls of food in the mouth at about 10 months to using fine pincer feeding by 12 months—neatly picking up food between the thumb and the index finger* *Begins to use a spoon*

Table 2.3 Language Development

Age	Expected Milestones in Development
1–2 months	*Cries but soon quiets when needs are met* *Social smile between 6 and 8 weeks (i.e., smiles when he sees Mommy's or Daddy's face)*
3 months	*Makes cooing and babbling sounds* *Watches others*
4–5 months	*Cries are different, depending on needs and wants* *Begins to make sounds—hard consonant and some vowels sounds—that are understandable*
6–7 months	*Repeats sounds (e.g., "da da da da") with no specific meaning* *Laughs out loud* *Babbles purposefully (e.g., "talks" to toys, siblings, or an image in a mirror)*
8–9 months	*Starts to "speak" words (e.g., "bye-bye," "ma ma") with no specific meaning* *Begins to respond to simple commands (e.g., waves when told "bye-bye")* *Understands the word "no"*
10–12 months	*Two or more words now have definite meaning (e.g., "ba ba" means bottle but may also mean "blanket" and "bye-bye")* *Responds to his or her own name*

MAKING THE CONNECTION

Just as children must be provided with the opportunity to develop their muscles for gross and fine motor development, they need caregivers to speak with them and respond to their sounds in order for them to learn to speak and to become social beings. Children will not learn language unless they hear language. They will not become socially interactive if no one interacts with them.

B. Psychosocial development.
1. Babies in the infancy period are experiencing Erik Erikson's first stage of **psychosocial development,** trust versus mistrust.
   a. Baby learns whether or not to trust his or her caregivers.
      i. Successful completion of this stage is foundational for future healthy psychosocial interactions.
2. Parent education.
   a. Infants should not be allowed to cry for extended periods, especially during the first few months of life.
   b. Young babies will not become "spoiled" if they are held and their needs are met.
   c. Babies thrive when they are consoled and comforted in times of stress.

C. Cognitive development.
1. Babies in the infancy age period are going through the early sensorimotor stage, as defined by Jean Piaget.
   a. Children learn through their senses and their ability to move and explore.
      i. In early infancy, babies' reflexes predominate.
      ii. At 4 to 5 months, babies recognize their parents and have a memory that lasts 4 to 5 minutes.
         (1) By this age, they learn to wait for a few minutes for their needs to be met.
      iii. At 6 to 7 months.
         (1) Babies begin to develop the concept of **object permanence** (i.e., they begin to realize that objects, including their parents, exist even when they cannot be seen).
         (2) They also progressively develop stranger anxiety. The bond with their parents has become so strong that they do not trust strangers to hold or care for them.
      iv. At 10 to 12 months.
         (1) Will actively hunt for a hidden toy.

2. Parent education.
   a. Parents should be encouraged to play hide and seek games with their child. For example, playing peek-a-boo and encouraging the child to find a toy hidden under a blanket or pillow help children to develop object permanence.
   b. Parents should be advised that stranger anxiety can be very stressful for babies. Having a stranger give the child a favorite toy or read a favorite book may help to reduce the child's response.

D. Moral development.

1. In infancy, babies are too young for **moral development**. This developmental process, as defined by Lawrence Kohlberg, does not begin until children reach toddlerhood.
2. Parent education.
   a. Parents should be reminded that although babies begin to understand the word "no," they do not yet understand the difference between being good and being bad.
      i. It is too early, therefore, to discipline a child.

IV. Nursing Considerations: Health Promotion/Parent Education

A. Nutrition: for babies to grow into healthy toddlers, they must be fed foods that meet their caloric and nutritional needs.

1. Breast milk is the ideal food.
   a. Human product comprised of human carbohydrates, fats, and proteins for human babies.
   b. Contains substances (e.g., antibodies and white blood cells) that protect babies from infection and disease.
   c. If the mother is having difficulty with breastfeeding, she should be encouraged to consult a certified lactation consultant.

DID YOU KNOW?

A policy statement from the American Academy of Pediatrics (AAP) recommends that all healthy babies be exclusively breastfed for the first 6 months of life. During the second half of the first year, the AAP recommends that solid foods be added but that the baby continue to consume breast milk.

2. If parents choose not to breastfeed, the baby should be fed a commercially produced formula.
   a. Feeding guidelines.
      i. By 1 month of age, babies consume, on average, 4 oz. every 3 to 4 hr.
      ii. By 6 months, they drink approximately 8 oz. at each feeding.
   b. Parent education.
      i. To prevent choking, parents should be advised never to prop bottles and never to add cereal to the formula in bottles.
      ii. To prevent obesity, parents should be advised never to overfeed babies.

(!) Because water is devoid of electrolytes, it should not be served to babies under 6 months of age. If young babies are thirsty, they should be served breast milk or formula. Sodas and other concentrated sweet drinks should never be served to infants. They are high in sugar and calories, with little to no nutritional value.

      iii. Parents may be educated that sterilization of bottles is not necessary, but that bottles should be thoroughly scrubbed and washed. Formula should be thrown out when it has been unrefrigerated for over 1 hr.
      iv. To prevent injury, parents should be warned to warm bottles in a pan of water and never in the microwave.
      v. Advise parents to prepare formula exactly as stated in the instructions on the can or jar.

(!) Parents, especially breastfeeding mothers, must be taught the indicators of sufficient nutritional intake for young babies. The most accurate and objective method of evaluating nutritional intake is weight gain. At each well visit, babies are weighed, and their weight is plotted on a growth chart. In addition, especially for young babies, the number of soiled and wet diapers should be counted. Young infants should have a minimum of six very wet diapers and a minimum of four stools in a 24-hr period.

3. Solid foods should be added to the diet at approximately 6 months of age, when babies' weight curves begin to flatten and/or when babies' hematocrits and hemoglobins drop.
   a. By 6 months of age, babies' iron stores become depleted. Parents should begin by feeding babies iron-rich cereals.
      i. Rice cereal usually is an infant's first food.
   b. To reduce the potential for choking, babies should be fed while sitting in an infant seat or high chair.
   c. During meals, water and breast milk or formula should be offered to babies from a cup.
4. New foods should be added to the diet slowly.
   a. For example, rice cereal should be served for 2 to 3 days, then barley cereal for 2 to 3 days.
   b. If the baby should develop an allergic response (rash, vomiting, or other symptoms), the parents will then know to which food the baby is sensitive.

5. Finger foods should be added at about 9 months of age, and the baby should be watched carefully for signs of choking.
    a. All foods should be soft and cut into small bites.

Foods such as popcorn, carrot chunks, hot dog chunks, and whole grapes should NEVER be given to babies under the age of 2. Babies are unable to chew the items effectively and, therefore, are at high risk for choking. If parents wish to serve these foods, the items should be cut up into very small pieces, and the baby should be watched carefully for signs of choking.

6. Nutritional supplements that should be administered to infants.
    a. Because babies should be kept out of direct sunlight, they need vitamin D supplementation. Four hundred international units of vitamin D per day should be administered to breastfed infants and to formula-fed babies who consume less than 16 oz. of formula each day.
    b. Fluoride supplementation should be administered beginning at 6 months of age to any child who is not drinking fluoridated water.

B. Play and toys: play is a child's "work." It is essential for growth and development.

1. Toys must be safe and should be consistent with the child's growth and development.
    a. Parents should be encouraged to use the toilet paper roll test (see the following box) to determine whether an object is too small for the child to play with.

DID YOU KNOW?

Toilet paper roll test: a cheap and easy way to determine whether an object poses a choking threat to a child under 3 years of age is the toilet paper roll test. Advise parents to place small objects into a toilet paper roll. If the objects fit inside the roll, they are too small to be safe. Only if the objects lie completely outside of the roll can the objects be considered safe.

2. Toys and play activities should be appropriate for the child at his or her developmental stage. Toys should be safe and should promote cognitive development. They should not, however, be so challenging that they frustrate the child. Table 2.4 lists appropriate toys by age range.
3. Babies should engage in supervised "tummy time" a few times each day. Because babies are always put to sleep on their backs, they can develop **plagiocephaly** (i.e., flat head syndrome) when the back of the head flattens, and the face takes on a lopsided appearance. Tummy time—only when under constant supervision—helps to prevent plagiocephaly.

Table 2.4 Recommended Toys and Activities by Age

Age	Recommended Toys and Play Activities
1–2 months	*Items for visual and auditory stimulation (e.g., mobiles, music)* *Sing and talk to baby*
3–4 months	*Continue earlier play* *Rattles* *Supervised floor play*
5–6 months	*Continue earlier play* *Play peek-a-boo and pat-a-cake* *Mirrors* *Large balls* *Soft toys* *Small blocks* *Shape sorters (e.g., nesting blocks, stacking rings)* *Supervised water play*
9 months	*Continue earlier play* *Play hide and go seek with toys* *Pots and pans*
12 months	*Play dates because children begin parallel play* *Push and pull toys* *Picture books* *Activity centers* *Supervised sand play*

C. Sleep.

1. To prevent sudden infant death syndrome (SIDS)—90% of deaths occur before 6 months of age—parents should be advised that babies should:
    a. Be breastfed, if possible.
    b. Be put to sleep:
        i. In a crib or other infant sleep location and never on a sofa, lounge chair, futon, or an adult bed (Fig. 2.3).
        ii. On a firm surface.
        iii. In the same room as the caregivers but not in the same bed as other children or adults.
        iv. Either clothed in a sleep sack with no blanket or have the blanket placed well below the face with the bottom of the blanket tucked under the mattress.
        v. With nothing soft placed in the crib (e.g., no bumpers, soft toys, or pillows).
        vi. In an environment that is not overheated.
    c. Be kept away from cigarette smoke.
    d. Be offered a pacifier at the beginning of nap and bedtime (it need not be reintroduced into the mouth once the baby has dropped it).

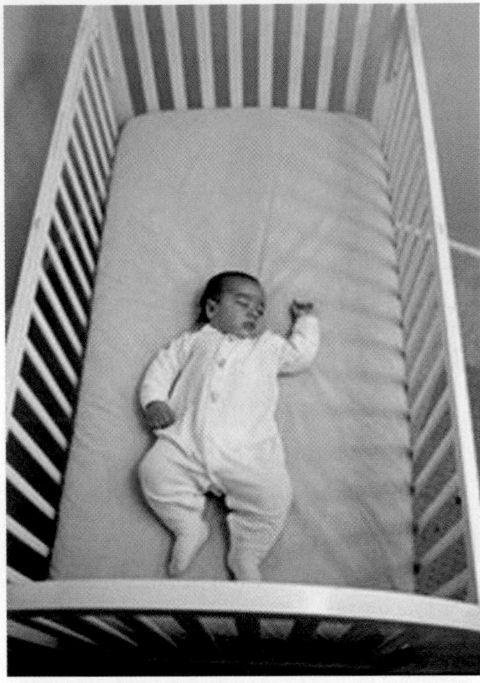

Fig 2.3 Always educate parents to put babies to sleep on their backs to help prevent SIDS.

2. To prevent strangulation, parents should be advised that:
   a. Slats of a crib should be no wider than 2⅜ in. apart.
   b. Cribs should have rigid sides (i.e., the sides of the crib should not move up and down).
   c. Sleep areas should be placed away from blinds and curtain strings that can be wrapped around the neck.

V. Nursing Considerations: Disease Prevention/Parent Education

A. It is important for nurses to educate parents about baby-care skills, including diapering, feeding, and bathing.
1. Diapers should be changed frequently to prevent diaper rash.
2. When bathing an infant:
   a. The baby should never be left alone in or near water to prevent drowning.
   b. All needed supplies should be collected before immersing baby in the water.
   c. The bath water should be approximately 105°F to prevent chilling and burns.

B. Safety issues should be emphasized.
1. Childproofing the home should be started by 4 months of age.
   a. Parents should be encouraged to crawl on their hands and knees and look for unsafe conditions.
   b. Possible poisoning threats that parents should be reminded of:
      i. Plants: should be kept out of baby's reach.
      ii. Medicines: should be kept out of reach in a locked cabinet.
      iii. Cleaning supplies: should be kept in locked cabinets.
      iv. Lead: the importance of keeping their home clean should be emphasized in order to prevent the ingestion of potentially harmful objects, such as lead from dust and paint chips.
   c. Drowning threats.
      i. Buckets of water should be emptied.
      ii. Bathtubs should only be filled for bathing, and children should be supervised in their bath at all times.
      iii. Toilets should be locked.

(!) When educating parents about activities that will enable their children to grow and develop, it is essential that the nurse stress the importance of safety. When the baby is placed on the floor, the area must be free of small objects, electrical cords, and other hazards that could injure the infant. In the same way, objects given to the child for small motor development must not pose a choking threat.

   d. Burn threats.
      i. Safety plugs should be inserted into all electrical sockets.
      ii. Electrical cords should be kept out of reach. Infants can pull on the cords and dislodge appliances that then can land on their heads (e.g., an iron can be pulled off from an ironing board or a lamp off from a side table).
   e. Possible falls.
      i. Babies require constant supervision when lying on elevated surfaces and when in such apparatuses as strollers and high chairs.
      ii. Gates should be placed at tops and bottoms of all stairs and should be attached to all windows.
      iii. Infant walkers should never be used.
   f. Choking hazards (see the previous section, "Nursing Considerations: Health Promotion/Parent Education"):
      i. Toys of older siblings are potential dangers.
   g. Possible strangling.
      i. Pacifiers should never be tied to a string that could encircle the neck.

ii. Never place cribs next to blinds or curtain cords.
iii. Children should never be put to sleep with a bib in place.

Parents should be encouraged to learn emergency action skills for choking, infant and child CPR, and first aid. Parents will become guilt ridden if they are unable to help their children during a life-threatening emergency.

2. Travel safety.
   a. In cars.
      i. Parents should only use car seats that have been designed for infant use. Many bucket seats are safely used only until a baby reaches 20 lb.
      ii. Children's car seats should be placed rear facing in the back seat of the car—for 2 full years—or until the child has reached the weight limit for the seat.
      iii. Child safety door latches should be in place at all times.

Children should NEVER be left unattended in a car, even for a few minutes. They may be abducted or may be locked in the car by mistake. Children left in a car may die from overheating or freezing.

   b. In airplanes, it is not required to restrain a child who is under 2 years of age, but both the Federal Aviation Administration (FAA) and the AAP recommend that children be in a child restraint system until they are 4 years of age.
3. Burn safety and sun exposure.
   a. Children should be kept out of direct sunlight, especially between 10 a.m. and 4 p.m.
      i. For the first 6 months of life, infants should have no sun exposure unless it is unavoidable.
   b. Methods should be used to protect children from sun exposure (e.g., they should wear clothing covering the skin, UVA and UVB protectants, and sunglasses).
      i. Sun protectants:
         (1) Should be applied at least every 2 hours and always reapplied if child gets wet.
   c. Fire and smoke alarms should be located throughout the home.
   d. Yearly fire drills should be conducted with all members of the family.
   e. Dangerous items (e.g., matches, electrical cords, and electrical sockets) should be kept out of reach of children.
   f. Hot water heaters should be set at 120°F or lower.
   g. Pot handles should be turned away from the front of the stove.
   h. The knobs on stoves and ovens should be covered with child covers.
   i. Adults should stay away from children when eating or drinking hot substances or when smoking cigarettes.
   j. Children should be kept away from such things as grills, fireplaces, stoves, and radiators.
4. Lead poisoning prevention (see Chapter 10, "Pediatric Emergencies").
   a. At 9 months of age, blood lead screening should be performed, with hematocrit and hemoglobin assessments and with blood lead levels.
   b. Parent education.
      i. Parents should be advised to wash their children's hands and face frequently, especially before eating, to prevent ingestion of lead.
      ii. Parents should be advised to clean their homes regularly to remove potential sources of lead.
5. Personal safety: infants are much too young to protect themselves. They need constant supervision at all time, including when in the presence of strangers.
6. Other.
   a. In addition to smoke and fire detectors, houses should also be equipped with carbon monoxide detectors.
   b. Poison control hotline and other emergency numbers should be placed by every telephone (see Box 2.1 for a list of indications regarding when parents should call their child's health-care provider).

C. Immunizations: the latest immunization schedule published by the Advisory Committee on Immunization Practices (ACIP) of the CDC should always be checked (www.cdc.gov/vaccines/

Box 2.1 When to Have an Infant Seen by a Health-Care Professional

When the child:

1. *Has a temperature of 100°F or higher.*
2. *Has a rash.*
3. *Refuses to eat.*
4. *Is not able to be roused from sleep.*
5. *Has fewer than the recommended numbers of wet or soiled diapers.*
6. *Has diarrhea or is vomiting.*
7. *Has yellow-tinged (jaundice) skin or sclerae.*

schedules/hcp/child-adolescent.html). The current recommended immunizations for infants are shown in Table 2.5.

D. Child abuse issues (see also Chapter 23, "Nursing Care of the Child With Psychosocial Disorders").

1. **Shaken baby syndrome (SBS).**
   a. A serious syndrome that can result when an infant is violently shaken.
   b. It can result in permanent damage, including mental retardation and physical disability, or death from bleeding in the brain.
   c. Parents should be educated regarding actions that can lead to SBS.
2. Normal growth and development.
   a. One of the most significant causes of child abuse is parental misunderstanding of normal child behavior.
   b. Nurses must educate parents regarding normal growth and development, including psychosocial and cognitive norms.
   c. If child abuse is suspected, the nurse must report the abuse to the appropriate child protective agency.

Table 2.5 Recommended Immunizations for the First Year of Life

Age	Recommended Immunization
1 month	*Hep B (hepatitis B): first of series (if not received in newborn nursery) or second of the series (if first received in nursery)*
2 months	*DTaP (diphtheria/tetanus/acellular pertussis)* *IPV (inactivated polio vaccine)* *Hep B: second of the series (if not received at 1 month of age)* *Hib (*Hemophilus influenza *type b)* *PCV (pneumococcal vaccine)* *RV (rotavirus)*
4 months	*DTaP, IPV, Hib, PCV, and RV (second in the series for all)*
6 months	*Hep B (last of the series by 7 months)* *DTaP, Hib, PCV, and RV (third in the series for all)* *Influenza (should be administered yearly beginning at 6 months of age)*
12 months	*DTaP, Hib, PCV, and IPV (all may be given at 12 months or later)* *MMR (measles, mumps, and rubella), varicella, hepatitis A (all may be given at 12 months or later)*

CASE STUDY: Putting It All Together

10-month-old, African American male, mother accompanying the child for his well-baby checkup

Subjective Data

- Child dressed in clean outfit that is appropriate to the weather.
- Child begins to cry as soon as the nurse enters the room. In response, mother states, "The only people he doesn't cry at are me, his dad, and his day-care teacher."
- When queried about diet, mother states,
  - "He's still taking his formula. He does love that bottle! He won't go to sleep without it."
  - "He eats just about everything, except for peas. I make sure to cut everything up really small, but when I feed him, he is always getting his hands into the food. Then he puts his hands in his hair and on his clothes. I can't keep this child clean!"
- When asked about other issues, mother states,
  - "He's such a bad boy. He is forever getting into things. I have to scold him all the time."
  - "He has to ride on my lap when my girlfriend drives me places. She doesn't have a car seat in her car."

Objective Data

Nursing Assessments

- Birth statistics
  - 39 weeks' gestation, no complications during pregnancy, vaginal delivery, Apgar 9/10
  - Weight: 3.2 kg
  - Length: 49 cm
  - Head circumference: 34 cm
- Current statistics
  - Weight: 9 kg
  - Length: 73 cm
  - Head circumference: 45.35 cm
- Other current data
  - Dentition: two lower incisors
  - Responded to his name twice
  - No strabismus noted, red reflex present

Vital Signs

Axillary temperature:	36.9°C
Apical heart rate:	144 bpm
Respiratory rate:	50 rpm

CASE STUDY: Putting It All Together *cont'd*

- Physical assessment: all within normal limits
- Immunizations: up to date
- DDST-II results
  - Gross motor
    - Gets himself to a sitting position without assistance
    - Falls when placed in a standing position by mother
  - Fine motor
    - Exhibits a crude pincer grasp
    - Bangs two blocks together
  - Language
    - Jabbers constantly while crying (e.g., "da da da ba da ba")
  - Personal-social
    - Refuses to wave "bye-bye," but mother states, "He waves to me all the time. What's wrong with that boy?"

Health-Care Provider's Orders

- Continue infant care
- Provide needed education

Case Study Questions

A. Which *subjective* assessments are important in this scenario?

1. ______
2. ______
3. ______
4. ______
5. ______

B. Which *objective* assessments are important in this scenario?

1. ______
2. ______
3. ______

C. After analyzing the data that has been collected, what **primary** nursing diagnosis should the nurse assign to this client?

1. ______

D. What interventions should the nurse plan and/or implement to meet this child's and his family's needs?

1. ______
2. ______
3. ______
4. ______
5. ______
6. ______
7. ______
8. ______

E. What client outcomes should the nurse evaluate regarding the effectiveness of the nursing interventions?

1. ______
2. ______

F. What physiological characteristics should the child exhibit before being discharged home?

1. ______
2. ______

REVIEW QUESTIONS

1. The mother of a 1-month-old states that she is curious as to whether her infant is developing normally. Which of the following developmental milestones would the nurse inform the mother that the infant is expected to perform at this age?
   1. Rolling from back to front
   2. Smiling and laughing out loud
   3. Turning head from side to side
   4. Holding a rattle for ten seconds

2. An 8-month-old is seen in the well-child clinic. Which of the following behaviors would the nurse expect to see? **Select all that apply.**
   1. Plays peek-a-boo
   2. Walks independently
   3. Feeds self with a spoon
   4. Stacks two blocks into a tower
   5. Transfers objects from hand to hand

3. A nurse is educating a parent regarding the immunizations that a child is to receive during the first year of life. Which of the following immunizations did the nurse discuss?
   1. Measles
   2. Mumps
   3. Rubella
   4. Polio

4. A nurse is educating a parent regarding the psychosocial stage of development of the infancy period. Which of the following information did the nurse include in the discussion?
   1. Infants should have their needs met in a timely fashion.
   2. Mothers should let their babies cry themselves to sleep each night.
   3. Infants should be scolded for bad behavior whenever they break objects.
   4. Mothers should sneak out of the room when they must leave their babies.

5. The parent of a 10-month-old is being interviewed by the nurse preceding an examination by the pediatric nurse practitioner and states, "My baby loves all kinds of food, and he always drinks his milk from a sippy cup, except in the evening when he wants a bottle." Which of the following follow-up questions is most important for the nurse to ask?
   1. "Have you decided when you will wean your child from the bottle entirely?"
   2. "Is your child drinking cow's milk from the sippy cup and bottle?"
   3. "Which fruits and vegetables have you fed your child so far?"
   4. "Have you fed your child any foods that he can feed himself, like cereal or peas?"

6. The mother of a 2-month-old who is being seen in the pediatrician's office states, "I am really worried because my child's head is not shaped right." The nurse should ask a question to obtain which of the following information?
   1. Is the child yet able to roll over by himself?
   2. Do the parents put the child on his stomach during supervised play?
   3. Is the child turning his head to follow an object?
   4. Do the parents elicit a smile from the child when they speak to him?

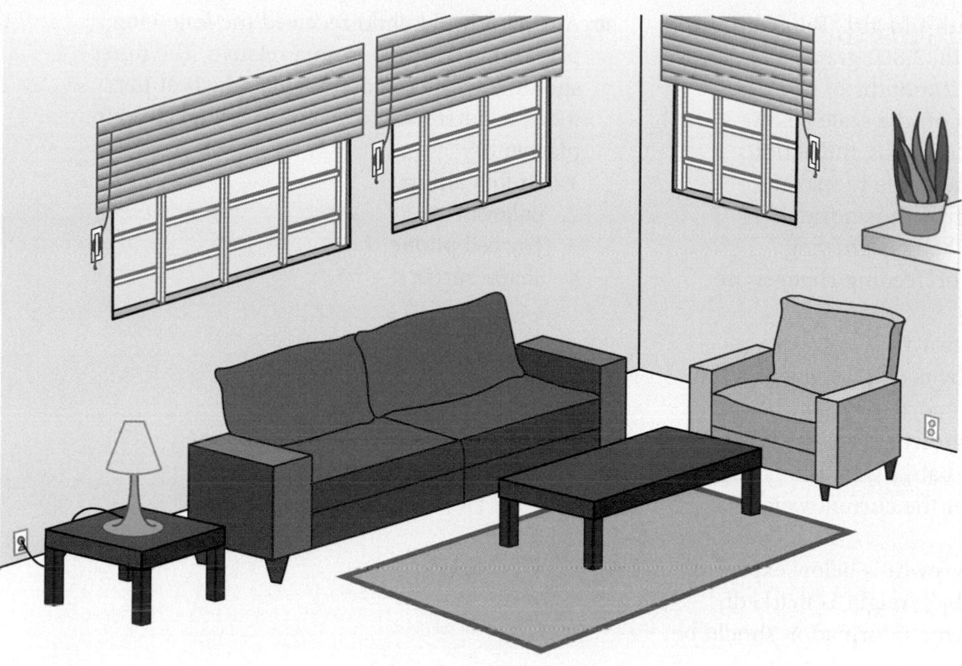

7. The nurse is visiting the home pictured above. A 6-month-old child lives in the home. Please select the image in the picture that the nurse should inform the parents presents a potential danger to the child.

8. A mother visits her child's primary health-care provider for the child's 12-month visit. The child weighed 2,800 grams at birth. Which of the following weights is most consistent with the expected weight for this child?
   1. 7,500 grams
   2. 8,000 grams
   3. 8,500 grams
   4. 9,000 grams

9. The nurse assesses a 2-month-old girl. The baby weighed 3,400 grams at birth, 3,800 grams at 1 month, and 4,000 grams at 2 months of age. The nurse plots the information on the scale below. Which of the following conclusions and actions would be appropriate for the nurse to make?

1. Conclusion: the child's growth is normal. Action—no change: the baby is growing appropriately, therefore no feeding changes are needed.
2. Conclusion: the child's growth is excessive. Action—change: the baby is overweight, and the information should be reported.
3. Conclusion: the child's growth is inconsistent. Action—no change: the baby's weight was larger than normal at birth, but the current weight is appropriate.
4. Conclusion: the child's growth is below expected. Action—change: the baby's weight is markedly lower than normal, and the information should be reported.

10. A 6-month-old child received the following play things as a gift from a relative. The nurse should advise the parents that which of the items is potentially dangerous for the child to play with?

1. Stuffed animal
2. Balloon
3. Toy cell phone
4. Shape sorter

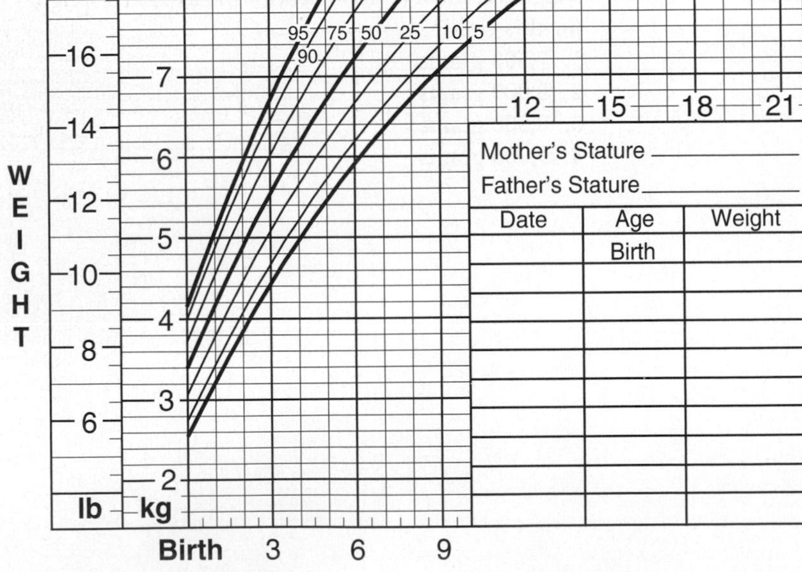

11. A mother of an 8-month-old boy states that the family is vacationing in a beach house for the next 2 weeks. Which of the following information should the nurse educate the mother about in relation to sun exposure? **Select all that apply.**
1. Reapply sun lotions to all exposed skin every 4 to 6 hours.
2. Use sun lotions that protect against both UVA and UVB rays.
3. Have the baby wear child-sized sunglasses whenever he is in the sun.
4. Avoid exposing the child to the sun between the hours of 12 and 2 p.m.
5. Dress the child in lightweight clothing that covers the majority of his skin.

12. The mother of an 11-month-old states, "My child has 8 teeth. I brush them every morning with bubble gum-flavored toothpaste. My child loves it." Which of the following responses by the nurse is appropriate?
1. "That is great. Even though they are baby teeth, it is very important to brush them with toothpaste."
2. "I am so glad to hear that your child loves the toothpaste. So many babies get cavities because they refuse to use toothpaste."
3. "I am very happy to know that you are cleaning your baby's teeth, but I am afraid that the bubble gum flavor will spoil him."
4. "It is wonderful that you are brushing your child's teeth, but it is recommended for you not to use toothpaste."

13. A mother questions the nurse regarding car seat safety for her infant. Which of the following information should the nurse include in the discussion?
1. Place the infant car seat rear facing in the back seat of the car.
2. Move the car seat to the forward-facing position when the child reaches 1 year of age.
3. Keep the child in a bucket seat until the child is at least 12 months of age.
4. Tighten the straps of the seat so that only an adult fist fits under the straps.

REVIEW ANSWERS

1. ANSWER: 3
Rationale:
1. Infants roll from back to front at about 6 to 7 months of age.
2. Infants smile when they are 1½ to 2 months of age and laugh out loud when they reach 6 to 7 months of age.
3. At one month of age, children still perform basic skills like moving their heads from side to side.
4. Infants begin to hold rattles, if placed in their hands, at about 3 months of age.
TEST-TAKING TIP: Development is progressive. Although babies develop a social smile at 6 to 8 weeks of age, they usually do not laugh out loud until they are much older.
Content Area: *Pediatrics—Infant*
Integrated Processes: *Nursing Process: Implementation; Teaching/Learning*
Client Need: *Health Promotion and Maintenance: Developmental Stages and Transitions*
Cognitive Level: *Application*

2. ANSWER: 1 and 5
Rationale:
1. 8-month-old children do play peek-a-boo with their parents.
2. Children are not expected to walk independently until they reach 15 months of age.
3. It is too early for a child to be expected to feed him/herself with a spoon.
4. Children are able to stack blocks into a 2-block tower at about 18 months of age.
5. Babies can transfer objects from hand to hand at 7 months of age.
TEST-TAKING TIP: The key to answering multiple response items correctly is to view each response independently. In other words, read the first response after carefully reading the stem of the question. If it is accurate, it should be chosen. Then read the second response, and compare it to the stem. If it is accurate, then it should be chosen. Continue to compare each response independently until all responses have been reviewed.
Content Area: *Pediatrics—Infant*
Integrated Processes: *Nursing Process: Assessment*
Client Need: *Health Promotion and Maintenance: Developmental Stages and Transitions*
Cognitive Level: *Application*

3. ANSWER: 4
Rationale:
1. Because the antibodies cross the placenta and may inhibit the active immune response in infants, measles, mumps, rubella, and varicella vaccines are all administered in the second year of life.
2. Because the antibodies cross the placenta and may inhibit the active immune response in infants, measles, mumps, rubella, and varicella vaccines are all administered in the second year of life.
3. Because the antibodies cross the placenta and may inhibit the active immune response in infants, measles, mumps, rubella, and varicella vaccines are all administered in the second year of life.
4. The polio vaccine is administered in infancy.
TEST-TAKING TIP: It is important to note that because of potential serious side effects, the Sabin oral polio vaccine is no longer being administered in the United States. Rather, the injectable vaccine is being administered at 2, 4, and 6 months of age during the first year of life.
Content Area: *Pediatrics—Infant*
Integrated Processes: *Nursing Process: Implementation; Teaching/Learning*
Client Need: *Health Promotion and Maintenance: Health Promotion/Disease Prevention*
Cognitive Level: *Application*

4. ANSWER: 1
Rationale:
1. This response is correct. Infants should have their needs met in a timely manner.
2. It is not recommended that infants cry themselves to sleep each night.
3. It is not recommended that infants be disciplined for breaking items.
4. Mothers who sneak out when they are leaving their children are not promoting a sense of trust in their children.
TEST-TAKING TIP: The Eriksonian psychosocial stage of the infancy period is trust versus mistrust. Infants develop trust when they become assured that their parents will meet their needs (e.g., feed them when they are hungry, change their diapers when they are wet or soiled). Parents who meet their children's needs in a timely fashion are promoting a sense of trust in their children.
Content Area: *Pediatrics—Infant*
Integrated Processes: *Nursing Process: Implementation; Teaching/Learning*
Client Need: *Health Promotion and Maintenance: Developmental Stages and Transitions*
Cognitive Level: *Application*

5. ANSWER: 2
Rationale:
1. This is an appropriate question to ask, but it is not the priority.
2. This is the priority question. Babies should consume either breast milk or a commercially prepared formula until 1 year of age.
3. This is an appropriate question to ask, but it is not the priority.
4. This is an appropriate question to ask, but it is not the priority.
TEST-TAKING TIP: Pure cow's milk contains fats, proteins, and carbohydrates that are in much different proportions than those found in breast milk and formula. Children are unable to digest the nutrients in cow's milk effectively until they have reached 1 year of age.

Content Area: *Pediatrics—Infant*
Integrated Processes: *Nursing Process: Implementation; Teaching/Learning*
Client Need: *Health Promotion and Maintenance: Health Promotion/Disease Prevention*
Cognitive Level: *Application*

6. **ANSWER: 2**
Rationale:
1. Two months of age is too early to expect a child to roll over independently.
2. This is an appropriate question to ask.
3. This question, although related to the child's development, will not elicit information needed to respond to the mother's concerns.
4. This question, although related to the child's development, will not elicit information needed to respond to the mother's concerns.
TEST-TAKING TIP: Babies often develop plagiocephaly when they are placed on their backs all day every day. To prevent this disfigurement, parents are strongly encouraged to place their babies on their tummies each day. Tummy time should only occur, however, when a caregiver is directly supervising the child.
Content Area: *Pediatrics—Infant*
Integrated Processes: *Nursing Process: Implementation; Teaching/Learning*
Client Need: *Health Promotion and Maintenance: Health Promotion/Disease Prevention*
Cognitive Level: *Application*

7. **ANSWER: The test taker should select the image of the electrical cord hanging from the table.**
Rationale:
TEST-TAKING TIP: Once babies develop the ability to grasp objects, they explore their environment by grasping and playing with items within their reach. If the child were placed near the table, he or she could grasp the cord and attempt to chew it or to pull down on the cord and topple the lamp. Babies do not understand the potential dangers that cords present.
Content Area: *Pediatrics—Infant*
Integrated Processes: *Nursing Process: Assessment*
Client Need: *Health Promotion and Maintenance: Health Promotion/Disease Prevention*
Cognitive Level: *Application*

8. **ANSWER: 3**
Rationale:
1. The nurse would expect the baby to weigh about 8,500 g.
2. The nurse would expect the baby to weigh about 8,500 g.
3. The nurse would expect the baby to weigh about 8,500 g.
4. The nurse would expect the baby to weigh about 8,500 g.
TEST-TAKING TIP: Infants usually triple their birth weights by 12 months of age. 2,800 × 3 = 8,400 g. A weight of 8,500 g is most consistent with the expected weight for this child.
Content Area: *Pediatrics—Infant*
Integrated Processes: *Nursing Process: Analysis*
Client Need: *Health Promotion and Maintenance: Health Screening*
Cognitive Level: *Analysis*

9. **ANSWER: 4**
Rationale:
1. The infant's weight is not increasing at the appropriate rate. A complete assessment is needed.
2. The infant's weight is not increasing at the appropriate rate. A complete assessment is needed.
3. The infant's weight is not increasing at the appropriate rate. A complete assessment is needed.
4. The infant's weight is not increasing at the appropriate rate. A complete assessment is needed.

Girls — birth to 21 months of age

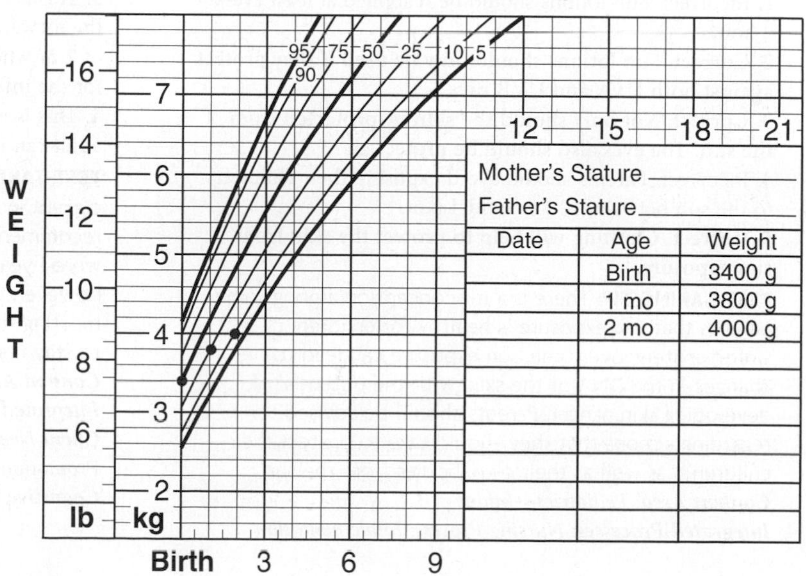

TEST-TAKING TIP: After plotting the weights on the girl's weight chart, the test-taker would see that the percentiles dropped from the 50th at birth to about the 25th percentile at 1 month to about the 10th percentile at 2 months. This baby needs to have a thorough physical assessment, and the parents need to be thoroughly queried regarding the child's feeding, urinary, and stooling patterns.
Content Area: *Pediatrics—Infant*
Integrated Processes: *Nursing Process: Analysis*
Client Need: *Health Promotion and Maintenance: Health Screening*
Cognitive Level: *Analysis*

10. ANSWER: 2
Rationale:
1. Stuffed animals are safe toys for infants to play with as long as they are not placed in the crib when the child is put to sleep.
2. Balloons are potentially dangerous items for young children.
3. Toy cell phones are safe and appropriate toys for infants to play with.
4. Shape sorters are safe and appropriate toys for infants to play with.
TEST-TAKING TIP: It is very important to be aware of toys that are safe and appropriate to the growth and development of the child. Although older children can safely play with balloons, infants and toddlers should not play with them. A young child could easily inhale either an uninflated or a broken balloon and suffocate when putting the item in his/her mouth during play.
Content Area: *Pediatrics—Infant*
Integrated Processes: *Nursing Process: Implementation*
Client Need: *Health Promotion and Maintenance: Health Promotion/Disease Prevention*
Cognitive Level: *Application*

11. ANSWER: 2, 3, and 5
Rationale:
1. Incorrect. Sun lotions should be reapplied at least every 2 hours.
2. Correct. Sun lotions should only be used if they protect against both UVA and UVB rays.
3. Correct. Not only should the skin be protected from the sun. The eyes also should be protected.
4. Incorrect. Parents should avoid exposing their children to the sun between 10 a.m. and 4 p.m.
5. Correct. Clothing will help to protect the skin from sun exposure.
TEST-TAKING TIP: There is a misconception among some parents that sun exposure is healthy for children. Unfortunately, over time, sun exposure can lead to changes in the DNA of the skin, with the potential of developing skin cancer. Parents should be advised regarding actions that they should take to protect their children's, as well as their own, bodies from the sun.
Content Area: *Pediatrics—Infant*
Integrated Processes: *Nursing Process: Implementation*
Client Need: *Health Promotion and Maintenance: Health Promotion/Disease Prevention*
Cognitive Level: *Application*

12. ANSWER: 4
Rationale:
1. This response is not appropriate. Until children can spit out the toothpaste on command, they should not have their teeth brushed with toothpaste.
2. This response is not appropriate. Until children can spit out the toothpaste on command, they should not have their teeth brushed with toothpaste.
3. This response is not appropriate. Although the bubble gum-flavored toothpaste may result in the child only allowing the sweet toothpaste to be used, until children can spit out the toothpaste on command, they should not have their teeth brushed with toothpaste.
4. This response is correct. Until children can spit out the toothpaste on command, they should not have their teeth brushed with toothpaste.
TEST-TAKING TIP: The vast majority of toothpaste on the market contains fluoride. When exposed to toothpaste, no matter which flavor, infants will swallow it simply because they have yet to learn how to spit out on command. To prevent a fluoride overdose, it is recommended that toothpaste not be used until the child is able to spit out on command.
Content Area: *Pediatrics—Infant*
Integrated Processes: *Nursing Process: Implementation*
Client Need: *Health Promotion and Maintenance: Health Promotion/Disease Prevention*
Cognitive Level: *Application*

13. ANSWER: 1
Rationale:
1. This is the correct response.
2. This is incorrect. An infant's car seat should be moved to the forward-facing position when the child reaches the age of 2 or when the child reaches the weight limit for the infant seat.
3. This is incorrect. An infant's car seat should be moved to the forward-facing position when the child reaches the age of 2 or when the child reaches the height or weight limit for the infant seat.
4. This is incorrect. The straps should be tightened until an adult can just insert the fingers under the straps.
TEST-TAKING TIP: It is important for test takers to be current in their practice. Prior to 2012, it was recommended that infants remain rear facing until they were 1 year of age. As a result of further research, however, the recommendation was changed for those still meeting the height and weight requirements of the seats to stay rear facing until 2 years of age.
Content Area: *Pediatrics—Infant*
Integrated Processes: *Nursing Process: Implementation*
Client Need: *Health Promotion and Maintenance: Health Promotion/Disease Prevention*
Cognitive Level: *Application*

Chapter 3

Normal Growth and Development: Toddlerhood

KEY TERMS

Parallel play—A form of play exhibited by toddlers in which children play side by side but independently.

Physiological anorexia—Reduced appetite seen in toddlers due to slower growth in this age period.

Telegraphic speech—Shortened, simple speech consisting of two or more words (e.g., "Me do it").

Toddlerhood—The age period between a child's first birthday and third birthday.

Transition object—A large number of toddlers have one or two objects to which they are especially attached (e.g., blanket, doll, pacifier). During times of stress, toddlers hold the transition objects close in order to feel more secure.

I. Description

The period of **toddlerhood** spans the ages of 1 to 3 years. Toddlers normally appear short and squat because they have relatively short legs with naturally pendulous bellies. In addition, because they are just learning to walk, to provide as secure a stance as possible, they walk with a wide gait and also with their arms raised above their waist (see Fig. 3.1).

Toddlerhood is characterized by an intense inquisitiveness that often gets the children into trouble. As a result, mothers and fathers are constantly saying "No" to their toddlers, with the toddlers responding with stamping of the feet and violent outbursts. These tantrums are the reason why this age period is often called "the terrible twos." Just as characteristic of the age period, however, is a child who is a fascinating mini-scientist, thoroughly exploring his or her environment in order to learn exactly how everything works. The successful culmination of the toddler period is often cited as a fully toilet-trained child. Many children, however, especially boys, do not toilet train until 3½ to 4 years of age.

II. Biological Development

A. Growth: the toddler period is characterized by less rapid growth as compared with infancy. As a result, children tend to eat less food during this period, which can confuse and concern many parents. As during the infancy period, all measurements should be plotted on growth charts (see Appendix A).

1. Weight.
   a. During the toddler period, children gain approximately 2.25 kg/year (5 lb/year).
   b. Toddlers' birth weight usually quadruples during the third year of life.

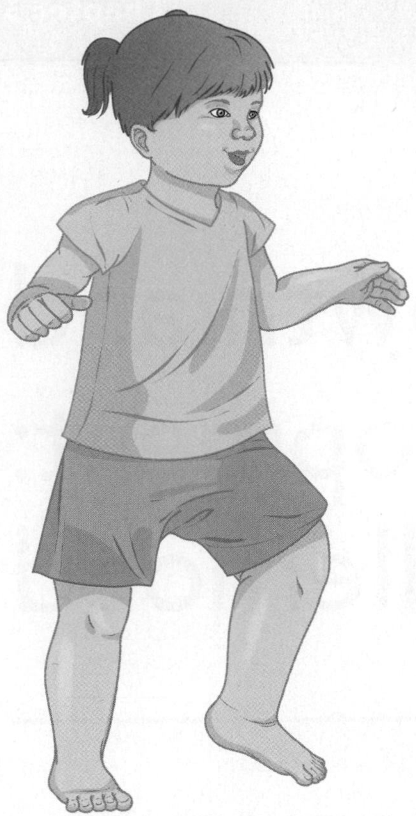

Fig 3.1 A toddler walking.

2. Height.
   a. Toddlers grow on average 7.5 cm/year (3 in./year).
3. Body mass index (BMI).
   a. BMI should be calculated for all children 2 years of age and older.
   b. The following criteria should be used to interpret BMIs:
      i. BMI less than the 5th percentile: child is defined as underweight.
      ii. BMI between the 5th and the 85th percentiles: healthy weight for the child's height.
      iii. BMI greater than the 85th percentile: child is defined as overweight.
      iv. BMI greater than the 95th percentile: child is defined as obese.

MAKING THE CONNECTION

To calculate the BMI, the following formula should be used:

Child's weight in kilograms divided by the child's height in meters squared, that is, BMI = kg/m^2

4. Head circumference.
   a. Anterior fontanel: closes between 12 and 18 months of age (posterior fontanel is already closed).
   b. By age 2, the toddler's head is approximately 90% of the size of the adult head.

B. Vital signs (average).

1. Temperature.
   a. 98.6°F (36°C).
   b. Except oral, any method of measuring temperature is acceptable (e.g., axillary, aural, temporal artery) unless absolutely accurate reading is required. Then rectal is considered to be the most accurate.
   c. Safe insertion with a rectal probe is critical to prevent injury.
2. Apical heart rate.
   a. 70 to 110 bpm.
   b. Radial artery may be used to assess pulse rates in children over 2 years of age.
3. Respiratory rate.
   a. 20 to 30 rpm.
4. Blood pressure.
   a. At 3 years of age: 100/59 mm Hg for boys; 100/61 mm Hg for girls.
   b. Pressures above these values should be considered hypertension.
   c. Blood pressures are rarely taken until children reach 3 years of age. If taken, an electronic method, including the correct size cuff, should be used.

C. Dentition.

1. After 1 year of age, teeth erupt slowly over time.
2. By 2½ years, toddlers should have a full set of 20 teeth.
3. Parent education.
   a. By 2½ years of age, children should have their first dental exam and should be seen every 6 months thereafter.
   b. Teeth should be cleaned at least twice daily by the parent with a soft child's toothbrush—no toothpaste should be used until child can spit out on command.
      i. It is recommended that children's teeth also be flossed daily.
      ii. After the parent cleans the teeth, the child can practice doing so.
   c. Prevent dental caries.
      i. Dental caries can endanger the development of the secondary teeth.
      ii. Children should never be put to sleep with a bottle filled with anything other than water.
   d. Fluoride supplementation.
      i. If water is not supplemented, children should receive 0.25 mg/day.

D. Senses.
1. Hearing, smell, and touch are fully developed.
2. Vision.
   a. Toddlers have full binocular vision at 20/40 acuity.
3. Taste:
   a. Is well developed, and toddlers become very discriminating in relation to their food choices. They clearly declare which foods they like and which they do not.

E. Motor development.
1. Gross motor development.
   a. By 15 months of age, toddlers:
      i. Walk well independently.
      ii. Enjoy crawling up stairs.
   b. By 18 months of age, toddlers:
      i. Climb stairs while holding hands.
      ii. Jump in place.
   c. By 2 years of age, toddlers:
      i. Run and kick a ball.
      ii. Walk well backward.
      iii. Climb stairs, one foot at a time, while holding onto a railing.
2. Fine motor development.
   a. By 15 months of age, toddlers:
      i. Drink from a cup using both hands.
      ii. Scribble.
      iii. Put a block in a cup.
   b. By 18 months of age, toddlers:
      i. Throw a ball overhand.
      ii. Build a tower of two blocks.
      iii. Take off their own clothes.
      iv. Try to use a spoon when eating, but often tip it upside down.
   c. By 2 years of age, toddlers:
      i. Feed themselves fairly well with a spoon.
      ii. Build a tower of six blocks.

III. Language and Social Development

A. Language development.
1. By 15 months of age, toddlers:
   a. Say two to three words together.
   b. Understand the meaning of approximately 15 words.
2. By 2 years of age, toddlers:
   a. Possess a vocabulary of approximately 300 words.
   b. Use **telegraphic speech** consisting of short, simple sentences.
      i. Telegraphic speech is understandable, although children do not use all parts of speech (e.g., "get milk," "want baby," "mine bottle," "me do it").

B. Psychosocial development.
1. Toddlers are in Erik Erikson's second stage of psychosocial development, autonomy versus shame and doubt.
   a. Toddlers develop a form of egocentrism and independence, characterized by:
      i. Statements like: "Me do it" and "No."
      ii. Expressing a desire to choose—from a small selection—things such as which outfit to wear, what to eat, and where to sit.
      iii. Ability to leave parents without expressing stranger anxiety.
      iv. For many, becoming toilet trained.
   b. Potential problem: toddlers can develop a sense of shame when they are punished for toileting accidents or other types of accidents, especially when they are not physically or emotionally ready for the behavior.
2. Parent education: striving for independence is exhilarating for the toddler but also a bit scary. To minimize the potential for negative outcomes, the parents should be encouraged to employ:
   a. Actions to reduce stress in toddlers.
      i. Play hide and go seek in a small area so that the child is able to find the parent quickly. The game helps the child to feel secure and helps to solidify the development of object permanence.
      ii. Provide the child with his/her **transition objects** (e.g., favorite toy or blanket), especially during periods of high stress for the child.
      iii. Establish rituals (see the next section) for activities such as sleeping, bathing, and eating.
         (1) Rituals are comforting to toddlers. They enable toddlers to try out autonomous behavior without increasing their stress level.
   b. Actions to help the child to develop independence.
      i. Parents should be encouraged to give their children choices—of two or three items because more than that is too confusing to a toddler—when appropriate, for example:
         (1) "Would you like a grilled cheese sandwich or a tuna sandwich for lunch?" rather than "What kind of sandwich would you like for lunch?"
         (2) "Would you like to go to the park or the beach today?" rather than "What would you like to do today?"
      ii. When giving choices, parents must be reminded to make sure the choices are realistic, for example:

(1) "Would you like to take your nap now or in 10 minutes?" rather than "Would you like to take a nap?" If the child were to say "No" to taking a nap, the parent must either ignore the child's response or forgo the nap.

c. If a new baby is born into a toddler family, the parents must be forewarned that the toddler may act out in a number of ways, for example, temper tantrums, regressing, refusing to go to bed.

C. Cognitive development.

1. Toddlerhood is defined by Piaget as the stage of preoperational thought.
   a. Toddlers view and experience the world directly—they are unable to conceptualize things or events.
   b. Language development speeds up during this period but is very "me" oriented.
      i. Language as self-entertainment: toddlers often talk simply because they find it is enjoyable to hear themselves.
      ii. Language as interpersonal communication.
         (1) Toddlers do talk with others, but their language is still egocentric.
         (2) To toddlers, "I" and "me" are the most important words in the vocabulary.
   c. Ritualism: toddlers begin to learn that certain actions occur at the same time or same sequence each day (e.g., stories and bath precede bedtime every night).
   d. Animism: toddlers believe things such as toys and dolls possess human abilities. For example, a toddler will scold a toy or a chair for getting in his or her way.
   e. Toddlers begin to see differences between many things.
      i. They learn that some children are boys and some are girls and often imitate the behavior of the same-sex parent.
      ii. They begin to notice the differences between such things as colors, shapes, and clothes.
2. Parent education.
   a. Parents should be encouraged to incorporate learning into play, daily conversation, and everyday activities, for example:
      i. "You are wearing a red shirt today."
      ii. "What color is dolly's dress?"
      iii. "Look, you are eating sandwich triangles!"
      iv. "Look, your waffle is a circle!"
   b. Parents should establish rituals and inform their children of patterns. In addition, parents as well as health-care providers should connect the information to an understandable event or concept such as:
      i. "You eat your breakfast at the same time that Sesame Street is on the TV."
      ii. "We eat dinner every night right after Mommy and Daddy get home from work."
      iii. "You brush your teeth every morning right before we go to day care."
   c. When providing toddlers with explanations, parents as well as health-care providers should use understandable language, for example:
      i. "The doctor is going to take a picture of your insides," rather than "You are going to have an x-ray."
         (1) The word x-ray is too abstract for the child to understand.
      ii. "The hairdresser is putting paint on Mommy's hair," rather than "Mommy's hair is going to be dyed."
         (2) The child will hear the word "died" rather than "dyed."

D. Moral development.

1. Stage 1, or premorality, is described by Kohlberg.
   a. Toddlers believe that actions are only wrong if they are punished. Similarly, they believe that actions are good if they are not punished or if they are rewarded.
2. Parent education.
   a. It is important for parents to begin to use appropriate means of limit setting and discipline (see the section "Toddler Behavior and Discipline") in preparation for later, more sophisticated stages of moral development.

IV. Nursing Consideration: Health Promotion/Parent Education

A. Nutrition.

1. The toddler period is characterized by what is called **physiological anorexia,** marked by slower growth and decreased appetite.
   a. Growth slows and interest in the environment grows.
   b. Toddlers often stop eating regular meals, becoming finicky eaters who snack and graze.
2. Parent education.
   a. Parents should be forewarned that toddlers often refuse to sit to eat.
      i. They stand at the table to eat or walk while eating.
      ii. If they are allowed to walk and eat, safety concerns must be considered (see below).

b. Food fads are very common in this population (e.g., a child might eat only blueberries and crackers on Monday and eat only cheese and peas on Tuesday).
   i. Parents should be advised that they should not worry.
   ii. After a few days, the vast majority of children somehow consume a balanced diet.

c. The important principle to teach parents is that they should always serve their children nutritious foods.
   i. Foods that are high in calories, fat, and/or sodium and low in nutritional value should be served as infrequently as possible.

d. Parents should be advised to give their toddlers child-size portions.
   i. If too much food is put on a young toddler's plate, he or she will often not even try to eat. The quantity is simply too overwhelming.

e. Parents should be advised to continue to be concerned about choking hazards.
   i. Popcorn, carrot chunks, and hot dog chunks should not be served to toddlers.
   ii. All foods should be soft and cut into small bites, especially if the child is allowed to eat on the run.

f. Information should be conveyed to parents regarding milk intake.
   i. Once children reach 1 year of age, they have developed the ability to digest unaltered cow's milk, although if the mother is still breastfeeding, that certainly is still appropriate.
   ii. To take in the fats needed for optimal brain growth, parents should be advised to feed their children whole milk until at least the age of 2.
   iii. After age 2, depending on the child's growth pattern, children may continue to consume whole milk or may be switched to low fat, skim, or soy.
   iv. During the toddler period, children should ingest most of their calories from food rather than from milk. Those who drink large quantities of milk often become anemic because iron is not found in milk.

DID YOU KNOW?

As long as they are safe to eat, toddlers should be eating most of the same foods as the rest of the family—just in bite-size portions. Although milk should be consumed as a calcium and protein source, it should no longer be the child's primary source of nutrition.

   v. If the child is still using a bottle at night, only water, never milk, should be put into the bottle to prevent dental caries.

g. Parents should be advised that vitamin and mineral supplements, other than fluoride, as discussed earlier, are not required but, if given safely, are not harmful either. However:
   i. Parents must be reminded never to leave vitamin pills where their child can access them.
      (1) A child may consume an entire bottle of vitamins because he or she thinks, "If the one vitamin that Mommy gives me is good, more is probably better."
   ii. Parents must be advised never to call vitamin pills "candy."
      (1) Simply because vitamins are sweet to taste and often look like cartoon characters is enough incentive for toddlers to want to consume more than one.

B. Sleep.

1. The risk of SIDS is no longer an issue. Toddlers may have such things as pillows, soft toys, and quilts in their beds.
2. Toddlers need up to 14 hours of sleep per day and usually take at least one nap per day.
3. Parent education.
   a. To prevent tantrums (see the section "Toddler Behavior and Discipline"), forewarning a child that bed or nap time is coming is often helpful (e.g., 30 minutes before, state, "Bedtime in 30 minutes," then 15 minutes before, state, "Bedtime in 15 minutes").
   b. To prevent injury, parents should be advised to move their children from a crib to a bed once they can climb out.
   c. If parents establish a bedtime routine and stick to it, they rarely have bedtime difficulties.
      i. Toddlers find rituals comforting, enabling them to assert their autonomy without becoming too anxious.
         (1) A sample routine that should remain consistent every night is: bath (fun and relaxing), read two books, brush teeth, have one sip of water, hugs and kisses, get tucked in with special blanket, and sleep.

C. Toilet training.

1. Parents must be advised that child readiness is essential.

a. Both physical and emotional readiness are needed.
b. If child is not ready, frustration and possible abuse, verbal or/and physical, may result.

2. Girls often train before boys.
3. Bowel training usually precedes bladder training.
4. Day training usually precedes night training—night training may not occur until many years later.
5. Toileting accidents are very common, especially when toddlers are engaged in active play.
6. Parent education.
   a. Parents should obtain a potty chair or toilet potty seat.
      ii. Sitting on an adult toilet can be scary for toddlers. They fear that they may fall in.
   b. Parents should be advised to be attentive to cues from the child that he or she is ready.
      i. Some children want their diaper changed immediately after wetting or soiling.
      ii. Some children communicate, verbally or behaviorally, when they are wetting or soiling their diapers.
      iii. Some children want to be like an older sibling, a parent, or a friend at preschool.
   c. Parents should be encouraged to place their child onto the potty seat shortly after eating or when their child usually has a bowel movement.
   d. Parents should be encouraged to praise their child for success but not to punish the child if he or she is not successful or if he or she has an accident.
   e. If accidents are frequent, it is advisable to recommend to parents to abandon the training until the child is more ready.
   f. Problem: children who are repeatedly punished for accidents may develop feelings of shame toward themselves and/or fear of their parents.

D. Play and toys.

1. Toddlers engage in **parallel play**, in which two or more toddlers will play independently but side by side.
   a. They love to play with other toddlers, but they rarely interact with each other during the play.
   b. They often grab toys from one another, exhibiting their egocentrism.
2. Parent education.
   a. If a toddler needs to be taught that taking a toy or hitting is unacceptable, the child should be reprimanded using very simple language, for example:
      i. "No, you must not grab the toy from Johnny," or "You must not hit."
      ii. Toddlers do not understand long explanations.
   b. Toys should always be safe and consistent with the child's development.
      i. Parents should be encouraged to check the Consumer Product Safety Commission's Web site regarding the safety of children's toys (www.cpsc.gov).
      ii. The toilet paper roll test should still be used to assess the safe size of toys (see Chapter 2).
   c. Appropriate toys that parents should be encouraged to provide for their toddlers include:
      i. Push-pull toys, large blocks, balls, and trucks that help to promote and reinforce gross motor development.
      ii. Paint, sand and water play (all supervised), large crayons, and large puzzles that help to promote and reinforce small motor development.
      iii. Musical toys and books that help to promote and reinforce language development.

E. Toddler behavior and discipline.

1. Tantrums.
   a. They are relatively common but need not persist.
   b. Tantrums usually occur when:
      i. Toddlers are abruptly told that they must leave an activity.
      ii. Limit setting is inconsistent.
      iii. The child simply cannot get his feelings across verbally because his or her language skills are so immature.
   c. Parent education.
      i. Suggestions that should be provided to parents as means of preventing a tantrum. Parents should be encouraged to:
         (1) Forewarn their child that an activity will end soon (e.g., "In 10 minutes, we will be leaving the park," then 5 minutes later, "In 5 minutes, we will be leaving the park"). The change in activity is no longer a surprise.
         (2) Consistently limit the child's behavior (e.g., bedtime is always at 8 p.m. preceded by a bath and book reading).
         (3) Be patient when the child is trying to communicate something.
      ii. Suggestions for limiting the length of a tantrum.
         (1) The parent should ignore the behavior. The parent should NOT abandon the child but simply turn his or her

attention somewhere else (i.e., say, "I will speak with you when you stop screaming"), then turn around and say nothing more.

(2) Once the child is acting appropriately, the parent should then quickly provide a hug and verbal praise for the appropriate behavior.

If an activity is unsafe, a child must not be allowed to engage in that activity, even though a tantrum may be triggered.

iii. Parents must be advised that limit setting and discipline (see the section "Discipline") are very important, but the form of discipline must be appropriate to the child's age and understanding.

2. Sexual exploration: toddlers often engage in masturbation and body exploration.
   a. Very natural.
   b. Parent education.
      i. Parents should be advised to try not to discipline their child for sexual exploration because the negative remarks may lead to feelings of guilt or shame.
      ii. Rather, parents should be encouraged to:
         (1) Advise the child that masturbation should be performed in private.
         (2) Redirect the child to another activity.
3. Discipline.
   a. Limit setting: parents must be encouraged to set realistic limits on their children's behavior beginning in the toddler period.
      i. There are certain items that children may not play with or touch.
         (1) Parents should be encouraged to move the items, if possible.
         (2) Parents should consistently advise their child to refrain from playing or touching those items.
      ii. There are certain behaviors that are not acceptable (e.g., biting, hitting, throwing sand in someone's face, running into the street).
      iii. Parents' responses to unacceptable behaviors should be consistent.
   b. Time out is an excellent form of discipline for toddlers.
      i. Moving and exploring are important to children of this age.
      ii. The time out should only last for a few minutes (usually the same number of minutes as the age of the child).
   c. Parents should be encouraged to redirect the child to an acceptable activity (e.g., if the child grabs a toy from another child, provide the child with an alternative).
   d. Once the child is exhibiting appropriate behavior, or once time out is complete, the child should be praised (hugging is a wonderful action) for correct/appropriate behavior.
   e. Spanking is not recommended because toddlers may interpret the spanking as, "If Mommy and Daddy can hit, then it must be acceptable for me to hit."

F. Day care and nursery school.
1. Often very positive experiences for children.
   a. Provides opportunity for interacting with children and adults.
   b. Provides opportunity for learning.
2. Parent education.
   a. Before sending the child, the parents should be advised to inspect the facility carefully and interview the staff.
   b. Before sending the child, parents must be advised fully to prepare the child.
      i. The child should be given a simple, clear rationale for the experience.
      ii. The parents should tell the child that day care is not a punishment.
      iii. The parents should let the child take his or her transition object for security.

V. Nursing Considerations: Disease Prevention and Parent Education

A. Safety.
1. Toddlers as "mini-scientists."
   a. Toddlers are highly inquisitive. It is exhausting, challenging, potentially dangerous, and fun to watch young children.
   b. Parent education.
      i. Parents must be advised that toddlers must be watched at all times because they may endanger themselves and/or others during their explorations. Examples of potential dangers include the following:
         (1) Toddlers often play with light switches—in every room—to make sure that the same thing happens in each location. However, one of those switches may be for a portable heater or a portable fan—either of which could seriously injure the child.
         (2) Toddlers often remove everything from places such as closets and drawers to check out what treasures they contain. However, dry cleaner

bags that are fun to play with are potential suffocation hazards.

ii. An appropriate response to parents who become frustrated by toddler behaviors might be, "Toddlers do not get in trouble because they are defying their parents. They get in trouble because they simply cannot help it."

iii. If parents are well educated about toddler behavior, they likely will refrain from punishing the child for actions that are related to growth and development.

2. Childproofing the home.
   a. Toddlers are at high risk for accidental injury.
   b. There are a number of possible poisoning threats in a toddler's environment.
      i. Plants should be kept out of reach.
      ii. Medicines should be kept out of reach in a locked cabinet.
      iii. Cleaning supplies should be kept in locked cabinets.
      iv. Other: homes should be kept clean to prevent ingestion of such harmful materials as lead from dust and paint chips.
   c. Drowning threats.
      i. Buckets of water should be emptied.
      ii. Bathtubs should only be filled for bathing, and children should be supervised in the bath at all times.
      iii. Bathrooms should be locked.
   d. Burn threats.
      i. Electrical sockets: safety plugs should be inserted into all sockets.
      ii. Electrical cords: should be kept out of reach because a toddler could pull on a cord, and the appliance could land on the child's head (e.g., an iron could fall from an ironing board).
   e. Possible falls.
      i. Constant supervision is needed when young children are lying on elevated surfaces and when they are in such items as strollers and high chairs.
      ii. Gates should be placed at the tops and bottoms of all stairs.
      iii. Gates should be attached to all windows.
   f. Choking hazards (see the section "Nutrition"):
      i. Small toys and toys of older siblings are potential dangers.
   g. Possible strangling.
      i. Cribs should never be placed next to blinds and curtain cords.
      ii. Children should never be put to sleep wearing a bib.
      iii. Toy phones and pull toys with long strings should never be given to toddlers, unless the children are supervised.
   h. If they have not already done so, parents should be encouraged to learn or be recertified in emergency action skills for choking, infant and child CPR, and first aid.
3. Travel safety.
   a. In cars.
      i. Infant seats: toddlers should remain rear facing in the back seat of the car in an infant seat for 2 full years, unless the child has reached the weight limit on the seat before age 2.
      ii. Forward-facing car seats: 2-year-old and older children should be in forward-facing car seats until they reach the weight limit on that seat.
         (1) Forward-facing seats should always be placed in the back seat of the car.
         (2) It is recommended that seat placement be checked at a designated police facility.
      iii. Child safety car door latches should be in place at all times.

Children should NEVER be left unattended in a car, even for a few minutes. They may be abducted or may be locked in the car by mistake. Children left in a car may die from overheating or freezing.

   b. As pedestrians:
      i. Toddlers must be supervised at all times and, if anywhere near traffic, must always hold hands.
      ii. Young children can dart quickly behind and/or in front of a moving vehicle.
   c. In airplanes.
      i. The FAA (Federal Aviation Administration) does not require a child to be restrained in an airplane until the child is 2 years of age.
      ii. However, both the FAA and the American Academy of Pediatrics (AAP) recommend that children be in a child restraint system on airplanes until they are 4 years of age.
         (1) Not all car seats are compatible with airline seats.
4. Burn safety and sun exposure.
   a. Cigarette smoking should not be allowed within the vicinity of the child.
      i. Many toddlers have been burned when accidentally running into a lit cigarette that is held by an adult.

b. All homes should be equipped with fire, smoke, and carbon monoxide detectors.
   i. Families should have periodic fire drills for home safety.
      (1) The child must be taught where to meet his/her parents if an alarm is sounded.
      (2) Children must be instructed not to hide under the bed or in a closet during a fire.
c. Water heaters should be set to no higher than 120°F.
   i. Toddlers are often able to turn on the water. Higher temperatures can burn a toddler's skin.
   ii. Bath water should be approximately 105°F to prevent both chilling and burns.
d. Children should be kept out of direct sunlight, especially between 10 a.m. and 4 p.m.
e. Methods should be used to protect children from sun exposure (e.g., clothing covering the skin, UVA and UVB protectants, and sunglasses).
   i. Sun protectants should be applied at least every 2 hours and always reapplied if children get wet.
f. Dangerous items, such as matches, electrical cords, and electrical sockets, should be kept out of the reach of children.
   i. Children should be kept away from such things as grills, fireplaces, stoves, and radiators.
   ii. In the kitchen, pot handles should be turned away from the front of the stove.
      (1) Toddlers love to "help" Mommy and, therefore, may try to move pots and pans on the stove.
   iii. Stove and oven knobs should be covered to prevent toddlers from accidentally or purposefully turning on the oven or a burner.
g. Parents should be advised to stay away from their children when eating or drinking hot substances or when smoking cigarettes.

5. Poisonings (see Chapter 10, "Pediatric Emergencies").
   a. Very high incidence of poisonings in the toddler (and preschool) populations, including:
      i. Acute poisonings (e.g., medications, vitamins, and gasoline)
      ii. Chronic poisonings, primarily lead.
   b. Parents must have the poison control hotline and other emergency numbers visible by every telephone.
6. Near drownings (see Chapter 10, "Pediatric Emergencies").
   a. There is a high incidence of drownings in the toddler age group.
   b. Toddlers must never be left alone in or near water (e.g., bath water, pool, brook, or even a mop bucket).
   c. All supplies should be collected for a toddler's bath before immersing the child.
7. Personal safety: toddlers are much too young to protect themselves from sexual abuse. They need to be supervised around others at all times.

B. Health screenings: at each age level, children are assessed for possible diseases or illnesses. If the screenings are positive, an intervention is implemented. (See "Recommendations for Pediatric Preventive Health Care" for a complete list of procedures.)
1. By 18 months: autism screening should be performed.
2. 2 years.
   a. Lead and hemoglobin assessments: lead prevention principles are consistent with those cited in Chapter 2, "Normal Growth and Development: Infancy."
   b. Other, if indicated.
      i. Screening for hypercholesterolemia and/or tuberculosis.

C. Immunizations (see current Advisory Committee on Immunization Practices [ACIP] schedule).
1. 15 months.
   a. *Haemophilus influenzae* type B (Hib); measles, mumps, and rubella (MMR); varicella; and pneumococcal (if not given at 1 year).
   b. Hepatitis B (Hep B) (if not given earlier).
   c. Flu (every year).
2. 2 years.
   a. Catch up on any vaccines that have not yet been administered.
   b. Flu (every year).

D. Child abuse issues.
1. Shaken baby syndrome (SBS).
   a. Parents should be educated regarding actions that can lead to SBS.
2. Toilet training and other developmental issues.
   a. One of the most significant causes of child abuse in the toddler period is parental misunderstanding of normal child behavior.
   b. Nurses must educate parents regarding normal growth and development, including:
      i. Psychosocial norms.
      ii. Cognitive norms.
      iii. Readiness for toilet training.

CASE STUDY: Putting It All Together

2-year-old, Caucasian female child, father accompanying child for 2-year checkup

Subjective Data
- Father states,
  - "My wife didn't come today because she is home with the new addition. As you know, our new son is just a week old, and my wife felt it best to keep him away from the office just in case there were any sick children in the waiting room."
  - "Ever since the baby came, our daughter is a completely different child. She gave up the bottle months ago, but now she won't go to bed without it. Plus, she was always happy, and even when she said no, she usually meant yes. Now we have at least two tantrums a day and sometimes more!"
- When asked about toilet training, the father states, "My wife really wanted her trained before the baby came. This little girl won't go anywhere near a toilet."
- When asked about the child's diet, the father states, "She used to eat anything. Now she is picky, picky! Sometimes, we have to make her sit in her high chair for a long time just to get her to eat something!"
- When the nurse asks the father to take the child's clothes off for the examination, the child states, "No. No. Me do! Me do!"

Objective Data (examination performed while sitting in father's lap)

Nursing Assessment
- Child dressed in clothing appropriate to the weather
- One-year statistics
  - Weight: 21 lb
  - Length: 29 in.
  - Head circumference: 45 cm
- Current statistics
  - Weight: 26½lb
  - Height: 33¾ in.
  - Head circumference: 47½ cm

Vital Signs

Axillary temperature:	98.8°F
Apical heart rate:	100 bpm
Respiratory rate:	25 rpm

- Other current data
  - Dentition: 16 teeth, dental cavity noted in two premolars
  - Hematocrit: 40%, hemoglobin: 13.5%
  - Blood lead level: 2 mcg/dL
  - Remainder of physical assessment: within normal limits
  - Immunizations: up to date
- DDST-II results: child shakes her head and refuses to respond verbally for the nurse.
  - Gross motor—father reports that the child:
    - Throws a ball overhand.
    - Kicks balls.
    - Jumps up and down.
  - Fine motor: father states,
    - "She doesn't really like to play with blocks. I'm not sure how many she could stack."
    - "She does like to put stickers on to paper, and her nursery school teacher says she's the first one to go to the painting table."
  - Language: father states,
    - "She knows all her animals, and she knows circles and squares."
    - "She talks all the time."
  - Personal-social: nurse observed child when in the waiting room and when in the examining room.
    - Child pretended to feed her doll with a pretend bottle.
    - Child pulled down her shorts.

Health-Care Provider's Orders
- Refer child for dental check
- Provide needed education and anticipatory guidance

CASE STUDY: Putting It All Together *cont'd*

Case Study Questions

A. Which *subjective* assessments are important in this scenario?

1. ___
2. ___
3. ___
4. ___
5. ___

B. Which *objective* assessments are important in this scenario?

1. ___
2. ___
3. ___
4. ___
5. ___

C. After analyzing the data that has been collected, what **primary** nursing diagnoses should the nurse assign to this client?

1. ___
2. ___

D. What interventions should the nurse plan and/or implement to meet this child's and her family's needs?

1. ___
2. ___
3. ___
4. ___
5. ___
6. ___
7. ___
8. ___
9. ___

E. What client outcomes should the nurse evaluate regarding the effectiveness of the nursing interventions?

1. ___
2. ___
3. ___
4. ___

F. What physiological characteristics should the child exhibit before being discharged home?

1. ___
2. ___
3. ___

REVIEW QUESTIONS

1. The school nurse is observing an 18-month-old child during lunchtime in the nursery school cafeteria. Which of the following behaviors would the nurse expect to see?
  1. The child eats everything with her fingers. Picks up a bottle with 2 hands and drinks.
  2. The child uses a spoon but drops quite a bit. Picks up a sippy cup with 2 hands and drinks.
  3. The child uses a spoon and drops very little. Picks up a regular cup with 2 hands and drinks with some spillage.
  4. The child uses a fork and drops very little. Picks up a regular cup with 1 hand and drinks with no spillage.

2. The nurse is interviewing a parent of a 2½-year-old child. The parent states, "We are very careful about what our child eats and drinks. For example, we always give our child bottled water to drink." Which of the following responses is most appropriate for the nurse to make?
  1. "That is an excellent practice. It is so important for children to learn to drink water."
  2. "I am so glad to hear that. Many children consume drinks that contain empty calories."
  3. "Many parents give their children bottled water, but unless you have been told that your water is dangerous, it is fine to serve water from the tap."
  4. "It is your choice to serve your child bottled water, but it is important to check the bottle to see what substances may have been added to the water."

3. The parents of a 2-year-old child state that their child begins nursery school in one week. Which of the following actions should the nurse advise the parents to perform on the child's first day of school?
  1. When dropping the child off at school, quickly leave the classroom when the child is not looking.
  2. When preparing the child for the first day of school, tell the child that teachers do not like bad boys and girls.
  3. Tell the child that big boys and girls never cry on their first day of school.
  4. Make sure to let the child take to school any special object the child is attached to.

4. A nurse advises the parent of a 2-year-old that the child will have blood drawn during that day's well-child checkup. The nurse should advise the parents that the child's blood levels are being checked for which of the following substances?
  1. Calcium
  2. Mercury
  3. Lead
  4. Fluoride

5. A nurse in a day-care center is observing a 2-year-old child during recess. Which of the following actions would the nurse expect the child to perform?
  1. Ride a tricycle
  2. Kick a ball
  3. Climb the rungs of a ladder
  4. Build a sand castle

6. A mother asks which toy the nurse would suggest she purchase for her 15-month-old child. Which of the following would be appropriate for the nurse to recommend?
  1. Model kit
  2. Rattle
  3. Toy shopping cart
  4. Board game

7. A mother asks the nursery school nurse, "Whenever she is playing with other children in the playground, my 2½-year-old keeps throwing sand in other kids' faces. What am I to do?" Which of the following disciplinary methods would be most appropriate for the nurse to recommend?
  1. Inform the child that she will be grounded from going to the playground for 7 days.
  2. Spank the child on her buttocks.
  3. Throw sand in the child's face.
  4. Make the child sit on a bench away from the playground for 2 to 3 minutes.

8. A 2½-year-old boy is being seen by the primary health-care provider for a well-child checkup. Which of the following statements by the mother would indicate a need for teaching?
  1. "I bought a potty seat and put it into the bathroom next to the toilet. Johnny sits in it sometimes."
  2. "I worry that Johnny will get too close to the hot oven, so I put him in his playroom and have him play by himself with his toys while I'm making dinner."
  3. "When Johnny has a bottle with him in his crib, he goes to bed so much more easily. He drinks the water, and it helps him to go to sleep."
  4. "My husband and I converted Johnny's crib into a toddler bed because he climbed out of the crib twice last week."

9. An 18-month-old boy is being seen by the primary health-care provider for a well-child checkup. Refer to the growth charts in Appendix A. Which of the following assessments would indicate a need for further investigation?
  1. Head circumference of 18¾ in.
  2. Height of 32¼ in.
  3. Weight of 31¼ lb.

10. A 15-month-old child, who is being dropped off at nursery school, throws himself onto the floor, kicks, and screams, "No! No!" Which of the responses by the mother should the nursery school nurse recommend the mother change in the future?
1. The mother turns her back on the child while he is kicking and screaming.
2. The mother bends during the tantrum and states, "Honey, why are you so upset? We need to discuss your behavior."
3. After the tantrum is over, the mother turns around and states, "I am so proud of you when you act like a big boy."
4. After the tantrum is over, the mother bends down and gives her son a hug.

11. A mother reports to the nurse that she administers a vitamin to her toddler every morning. The nurse should praise the mother for using which of the following methods of administration?
1. Mother gives her child a vitamin each morning. When doing so, she states, "Here's your medicine. It tastes just like candy."
2. Mother leaves the vitamin pill bottle on the kitchen table. In the morning, mother states, "Take out your vitamin, and chew it up good."
3. Mother locks the vitamins in the medicine cabinet. When giving her child the vitamin, mother states, "Remember, only Mommy is able to give you the medicine."
4. Mother keeps the vitamins on top of the refrigerator. When giving the child the vitamin, mother states, "Remember, you must never climb on the counter to get your vitamins."

12. A mother of a 2½-year-old calls the health-care provider and states, "I don't know what to do. My son keeps taking off his diaper in public and playing with his penis." Which of the following responses by the nurse is appropriate?
1. "Slap his hand, and tell him that that behavior is unacceptable."
2. "He should be given a time out every time he does that."
3. "Laugh at him, and say that you understand that it feels good to play with his penis."
4. "Simply put his diaper back on, and tell him that he should do that in his own bedroom."

13. A nurse is providing education to the parents of a toddler. Which of the following information should the nurse include? **Select all that apply.**
1. The child should receive an influenza vaccination every year.
2. The child should brush his or her teeth with toothpaste every morning and night.
3. The child should consume foods from all food groups every day.
4. The child should continue to drink formula until he or she is two years old.
5. The child should be allowed to take his or her special object to nursery school.

14. The parents of a toddler, who is toilet trained and no longer drinks from a bottle, are expecting a new baby. The nurse should advise the parents that the toddler may respond in which of the following ways? **Select all that apply.**
1. Kiss the baby whenever the baby is near.
2. Repeatedly have temper tantrums.
3. Ask to drink milk from a bottle.
4. Have a number of toileting accidents.
5. Hit the baby on the head.

15. The nurse is providing anticipatory guidance to the parents of a 12-month-old child regarding bedtime issues. Which of the following statements is appropriate for the nurse to include?
1. "Don't put your child to bed each night until he appears to be really sleepy."
2. "Make sure to keep blankets, pillows, and stuffed toys out of your child's bed."
3. "Forewarn your child a few minutes before that it is time to go to bed. In other words, tell him when it is ten minutes before and then five minutes before bedtime."
4. "Make bedtime different and special every night. Some nights you could read him a story, other nights play a game with him, and other nights sing a song with him."

REVIEW ANSWERS

1. ANSWER: 2

Rationale:

1. This is an illustration of 1-year-old child's behavior.

2. The 18-month-old child tries to use a spoon but often tips it upside down on its way to the mouth.

3. The 2-year-old child is adept with the spoon but still needs two hands to pick up a cup.

4. Preschool children use forks and are able to pick up and drink from a cup steadily.

TEST-TAKING TIP: Children do develop at their own paces. Some will be more advanced than others at 18 months of age, but the behavior cited in the question is what is expected of children who are 1½ years of age.

Content Area: *Pediatrics—Toddlers*

Integrated Processes: *Nursing Process: Assessment*

Client Need: *Health Promotion and Maintenance: Developmental Stages and Transitions*

Cognitive Level: *Application*

2. ANSWER: 4

Rationale:

1. Water is an excellent fluid source for children, but this is not the best response.

2. Water is an excellent fluid source for children, but this is not the best response.

3. Tap water is usually appropriate for children to consume, but this is not the best response.

4. This is the best response. Parents should check to see which nutrients are in the water.

TEST-TAKING TIP: There are a number of waters on the market that contain substances (e.g., vitamins, electrolytes, flavorings, caffeine, and sweeteners). Alkaline water has a higher pH level than does plain tap water. In addition, most bottled water does not contain fluoride. Toddlers should consume only plain water, and they do need fluoride for the health promotion of their teeth.

Content Area: *Pediatrics—Toddlers*

Integrated Processes: *Nursing Process: Implementation*

Client Need: *Health Promotion and Maintenance: Health Promotion/Disease Prevention*

Cognitive Level: *Application*

3. ANSWER: 4

Rationale:

1. This action would be inappropriate.

2. This action would be inappropriate.

3. This action would be inappropriate.

4. The nurse should advise the parents to allow the child to take his or her transition object to school.

TEST-TAKING TIP: Toddlers are engaged in the Eriksonian stage of autonomy versus shame and doubt. Although they strive for independence, the process can be very stressful for them. Holding a transition object during a new experience can help them to make the transition from the safe environment of home to a new environment.

Content Area: *Pediatrics—Toddlers*

Integrated Processes: *Nursing Process: Implementation*

Client Need: *Health Promotion and Maintenance: Health Promotion/Disease Prevention*

Cognitive Level: *Application*

4. ANSWER: 3

Rationale:

1. Two-year-old children are assessed for elevated levels of lead.

2. Two-year-old children are assessed for elevated levels of lead.

3. Two-year-old children are assessed for elevated levels of lead.

4. Two-year-old children are assessed for elevated levels of lead.

TEST-TAKING TIP: Nurses should be familiar with routine assessments that are performed at well-child checkups (see Chapter 10, "Pediatric Emergencies," for additional information related to lead poisoning in children).

Content Area: *Pediatrics—Toddlers*

Integrated Processes: *Nursing Process: Implementation*

Client Need: *Health Promotion and Maintenance: Health Promotion/Disease Prevention*

Cognitive Level: *Application*

5. ANSWER: 2

Rationale:

1. Most children are unable to pedal a tricycle until they are 3 years of age.

2. 2-year-old children should be able to kick a ball.

3. Unless assisted by an adult, 2-year-old children are too young to be able to climb the rungs of a ladder.

4. Although most 2-year-old children love to play in the sand, they do not build sand castles.

TEST-TAKING TIP: Understanding normal growth and development is very important. Only when normal growth and development are understood is it possible for health-care providers to know when children are not developing normally and in need of early intervention.

Content Area: *Pediatrics—Toddlers*

Integrated Processes: *Nursing Process: Assessment*

Client Need: *Health Promotion and Maintenance: Developmental Stages and Transitions*

Cognitive Level: *Application*

6. ANSWER: 3

Rationale:

1. Model kits are appropriate for school-age children.

2. Rattles are appropriate for an infant.

3. Toy shopping carts are appropriate.

4. Board games are appropriate for preschool- and school-age children.

TEST-TAKING TIP: Children who are 15 months old are mastering the act of walking. They can practice walking while pushing a toy shopping cart.

Content Area: *Pediatrics—Toddlers*

Integrated Processes: *Nursing Process: Assessment*

Client Need: *Health Promotion and Maintenance: Developmental Stages and Transitions*

Cognitive Level: *Application*

7. ANSWER: 3

Rationale:

1. Grounding a child for a short period of time is an appropriate discipline for a school-aged child but not for a toddler.
2. Children learn by example. If a parent strikes a child, the child may believe that it is appropriate for him to strike the parent.
3. Children learn by example. If a parent throws sand at a child, the child may believe that it is appropriate for him to throw sand at the parent.
4. **Time out is an appropriate form of discipline for toddlers.**

TEST-TAKING TIP: Because they are so active, a 2- to 3-minute time out is hard for toddlers to experience. It is an appropriate disciplinary strategy for toddlers who have misbehaved.

Content Area: *Pediatrics—Toddlers*
Integrated Processes: *Nursing Process: Implementation*
Client Need: *Health Promotion and Maintenance: Health Promotion/Disease Prevention*
Cognitive Level: *Application*

8. ANSWER: 2

Rationale:

1. The parent's action is appropriate.
2. **This action should be questioned. Because toddlers are immature and inquisitive, it is inappropriate to leave them unsupervised.**
3. Although this child is relatively old to take a bottle to bed, the parent states that the bottle contains water.
4. To prevent serious injuries, it is recommended that toddlers be moved out of cribs once they are able to climb out of them.

TEST-TAKING TIP: Parents must be reminded that toddlers' cognitive skills are not advanced enough to know when something is dangerous and when it is not. They should be supervised at all times.

Content Area: *Pediatrics—Toddlers*
Integrated Processes: *Nursing Process: Analysis*
Client Need: *Health Promotion and Maintenance: Health Promotion/Disease Prevention*
Cognitive Level: *Application*

9. ANSWER: 3

Rationale:

1. The child's head circumference places his growth at approximately the 50th percentile.
2. The child's length places his growth at approximately the 50th percentile.
3. **The child's weight places his growth between the 90th and the 95th percentiles. The child is overweight.**

TEST-TAKING TIP: Growth values should be graphed onto growth charts. A weight over the 85th percentile, unless consistent with the child's height, places the child in the overweight category.

Content Area: *Pediatrics—Toddlers*
Integrated Processes: *Nursing Process: Analysis*
Client Need: *Health Promotion and Maintenance: Health Screening*
Cognitive Level: *Application*

10. ANSWER: 2

Rationale:

1. An excellent way to respond to a temper tantrum is to remain close by but to ignore the behavior.
2. **A parent who appears sympathetic during the tantrum is reinforcing the negative behavior.**
3. A parent is reinforcing appropriate behavior when he or she praises the child after the child's tantrum is over.
4. A parent is reinforcing appropriate behavior when he or she hugs the child after the child's tantrum is over.

TEST-TAKING TIP: Temper tantrums are relatively common in toddlers. Their egocentrism makes them expect that they will always get their way, and they often have difficulty clearly and unemotionally verbalizing their anger. An excellent parental response to a toddler's temper tantrums is to ignore the poor behavior and quickly reinforce the appropriate behavior after the tantrum stops.

Content Area: *Pediatrics—Toddlers*
Integrated Processes: *Nursing Process: Implementation*
Client Need: *Health Promotion and Maintenance: Health Promotion/Disease Prevention*
Cognitive Level: *Application*

11. ANSWER: 3

Rationale:

1. These actions are inappropriate. Children should never be told that medicine, including vitamins, is candy.
2. These actions are inappropriate. All medicine should be locked up and should be administered only by a parent.
3. **These actions are appropriate.**
4. These actions are inappropriate. All medicine should be locked up and should be administered only by a parent.

TEST-TAKING TIP: Parents may believe that toddlers are unable to access medicines and other unsafe items from high places, though that may not be the case. With determination, toddlers could climb up on a chair to a counter and then to the top of the refrigerator.

Content Area: *Pediatrics—Toddlers*
Integrated Processes: *Nursing Process: Implementation*
Client Need: *Health Promotion and Maintenance: Health Promotion/Disease Prevention*
Cognitive Level: *Application*

12. ANSWER: 4

Rationale:

1. This response is not recommended.
2. This response is not recommended.
3. This response is not recommended.
4. **This is an appropriate response.**

TEST-TAKING TIP: The Eriksonian stage of the toddler period is autonomy versus shame and doubt. The child who is able to remove his diaper and masturbate is exhibiting autonomous behavior that, to him, is pleasurable. When reprimanded and disciplined, the child believes that the action is wrong and he may develop feelings of guilt or shame. Masturbating in public is not socially acceptable; however, parents should simply advise the child that it is something that one does in private.

Content Area: *Pediatrics—Toddlers*
Integrated Processes: *Nursing Process: Implementation*

Client Need: *Health Promotion and Maintenance: Health Promotion/Disease Prevention*
Cognitive Level: *Application*

13. ANSWER: 1 and 5
Rationale:
1. Children should receive the influenza vaccine every year.
2. This statement is not correct. Parents should brush children's teeth until the children have the dexterity, at about 6 years of age, to brush their teeth themselves. Toothpaste should only be used when the child is able to spit out voluntarily.
3. This statement is not correct. Toddlers go on food fads, although they usually consume a balanced diet after about a week.
4. This statement is not correct. Children are physically able to consume unaltered cow's milk after they turn 1 year of age.
5. This statement is correct. Transition objects should accompany toddlers during new experiences.
TEST-TAKING TIP: Educating parents regarding health-care practices is an important role of the nurse. It is important that the nurse provide accurate information.
Content Area: *Pediatrics—Toddlers*
Integrated Processes: *Nursing Process: Implementation; Teaching/Learning*
Client Need: *Health Promotion and Maintenance: Health Promotion/Disease Prevention*
Cognitive Level: *Application*

14. ANSWER: 2, 3, 4, and 5
Rationale:
1. It is unlikely that the toddler will kiss the baby whenever the baby is near.
2. It is possible that the toddler will have temper tantrums.
3. It is possible that the child will regress and ask to drink from the bottle again.
4. It is possible that the child will have toileting accidents.
5. It is possible that the child may hit the baby on the head.
TEST-TAKING TIP: Because parents are excited and in love with the new baby as well as their older child, they often do not realize that the toddler may not have the same feelings. Indeed, the new baby is taking his or her parents' time and attention away from him or her. As a result, toddlers often regress and become angry.
Content Area: *Pediatrics—Toddlers*
Integrated Processes: *Nursing Process: Implementation*
Client Need: *Health Promotion and Maintenance: Health Promotion/Disease Prevention*
Cognitive Level: *Application*

15. ANSWER: 3
Rationale:
1. This statement is inappropriate. Rituals and consistency are best for toddlers.
2. This statement is incorrect. The threat of SIDS is past once a healthy child reaches 1 year of age.
3. This statement is appropriate. Toddlers accept change much easier when they are forewarned of the change.
4. This statement is inappropriate. Rituals and consistency are best for toddlers.
TEST-TAKING TIP: Bedtime rarely is difficult when parents establish a set prebedtime routine and follow the routine consistently.
Content Area: *Pediatrics—Toddlers*
Integrated Processes: *Nursing Process: Implementation; Teaching/Learning*
Client Need: *Health Promotion and Maintenance: Health Promotion/Disease Prevention*
Cognitive Level: *Application*

Normal Growth and Development: Preschooler

KEY TERMS

Associative play—A type of play in which children play with one another in an activity that is not directed toward a goal.

Magical thinking—a preschool-age child's conception that his or her thoughts can cause something to happen.

Nightmare—A frightening dream that awakens a child.

Night terror—Crying, screaming, or other physical unrest during sleep.

I. Description

The preschool period, often referred to as the age of the magical thinker, is defined as the time between 3 and 5 years of age. Preschool children truly believe that their thoughts have power. When serious illnesses or accidents occur, even if they are not involved, they often feel guilty for having wished harm on others. In addition, the vast majority of preschool children are verbally and physically capable of giving parents the impression that their child is knowledgeable about dangers and, therefore, no longer in need of constant supervision. Unfortunately, that is often not the case. Indeed, poisonings and accidental injuries are quite prevalent in this age group because the children continue to be inquisitive beings, often becoming entangled in precarious situations.

II. Biological Development

A. Growth: preschoolers are slimming down, losing the "baby fat" of toddlerhood.

1. Weight: preschoolers exhibit the same growth pattern as toddlers.
   a. Increase of 2.25 kg/year (5 lb/year).
2. Height: most of preschoolers' growth is in their legs.
   a. Increase of 5 to 7.5 cm/year (2 to 3 in./year).
3. BMI.
   a. BMI assessment criteria are the same from toddlerhood through to the end of adolescence.
   b. The following criteria should be used to interpret BMIs:
      i. BMI less than the 5th percentile: child is defined as underweight.
      ii. BMI between the 5th and the 85th percentiles: healthy weight for the child's height.
      iii. BMI greater than the 85th percentile: child is defined as overweight.
      iv. BMI greater than the 95th percentile: child is defined as obese.

4. By the time children reach the preschool period, head circumference is no longer measured.
   a. If head growth is a problem, it will have been identified by age 3.

B. Vital signs: all vital signs are consistent with those of the toddler.
1. Temperature.
   a. 98.6°F (36°C).
   b. Any method is acceptable (e.g., axillary, aural, temporal artery).
      i. Rectal temperature should be taken in preschoolers only when absolutely necessary.
2. Heart rate may be taken either apically or radially.
   a. 65 to 110 bpm.
3. Respiratory rate.
   a. 20 to 25 rpm.
4. Blood pressure: always using an appropriately sized cuff.

DID YOU KNOW?

An easy method that can be used to calculate the lowest safe blood pressure of preschool-age children is: 70 mm Hg plus two times the child's age in years.

C. Dentition.
1. Children should have a full set of 20 primary teeth at start of the preschool period.
2. Many preschoolers will start losing their primary teeth when they are 4½ or 5 years of age.
3. Parent education.
   a. Preschool children should be allowed to practice brushing their teeth, but a complete brushing should be performed by their parents.
   b. Parents should also floss their children's teeth.
   c. If a child is able to keep substances in his/her mouth without swallowing, toothpaste may be used.

D. Senses.
1. Hearing, smell, and touch are fully developed.
2. Vision—the normal visual acuity:
   a. Of 3- to 4-year-old children is 20/50 to 20/40.
   b. By age 5 should be 20/30.
3. Taste.
   a. Preschool children are often more adventurous eaters than they were as toddlers.

E. Motor development.
1. Gross motor development.
   a. At 3 years of age, preschoolers should be able to:
      i. Ride a tricycle.
      ii. Perform the broad jump.
      iii. Walk on tip toes.
   b. By 4 years of age, preschoolers should be able to:
      i. Hop on one foot.
      ii. Balance on one foot for a few seconds.
   c. By 5 years of age, preschoolers should be able to:
      i. Walk heel to toe.
      ii. Skip.
      iii. Jump rope.
2. Fine motor development.
   a. At 3 to 4 years of age, preschoolers begin using a fork.
   b. By 4 years of age, preschoolers are able to copy a circle.
   c. By 4½ years of age, they are able to copy a cross.
   d. By 5 years of age, they:
      i. Begin to use a dull knife for cutting.
      ii. Can draw a person with at least six anatomical parts that are drawn in their correct locations.

III. Language and Social Development

A. Language development.
1. 3-year-old children:
   a. Still use telegraphic speech.
   b. Talk nonstop to whomever will listen, including toys.
   c. Ask many questions, often beginning with "Why?"
2. 4- to 5-year-old children:
   a. Have a vocabulary that is becoming quite large.
   b. Speak using all parts of speech.
   c. Frequently use irregular verbs incorrectly (e.g., "I seed a kitten," rather than "I saw a kitten.").
   d. Have vivid imaginations, making up and telling very elaborate tales.
   e. Sometimes use "bad" language and look for a response from their parents.
      i. If parents ignore the comments, the children often stop using the inappropriate language.
      ii. If parents laugh or act appalled, children often continue using them as a means of getting attention.

B. Psychosocial development.
1. Preschoolers have entered into Erikson's developmental stage of initiative versus guilt.
   a. The major goal of the stage is the development of behavior that is appropriate and self-directed, while the potential problem associated with the stage is a child who is guilt ridden.

i. Because of "**magical thinking**" (see the section "Cognitive Development"), preschool children believe that they are bad or have caused bad things to happen simply because they have had bad thoughts.

ii. When punished for inappropriate behaviors, preschoolers think to themselves, "I am bad," rather than "I have acted inappropriately."

iii. Children often masturbate at this age. If reprimanded or punished, they may develop feelings of guilt.

2. Parent education.
   a. Because of the potential for guilt, when disciplining a preschooler, it is important to explain clearly that his or her action is bad, NOT that the child is bad.
   b. If a sibling or a parent becomes ill, it is important to explain to the child that he or she did not cause the condition.
   c. If the child did have a role in an accident, the parent must explain that he or she is not angry with the child.
   d. If a child masturbates, the parent should be advised:
      i. Not to reprimand or punish the child.
      ii. Simply to inform the child that the behavior should be performed in private, not in public.

C. Cognitive development.

1. Piaget's stage of preoperational thought continues throughout the preschool period to the age of 7 (see Chapter 3, "Normal Growth and Development: Toddlerhood," for characteristics of the stage and for suggestions of parent education).
2. Magical thinking.
   a. Preschoolers believe that inanimate objects (e.g., toys and chairs) are sentient and are able to think and act.
      i. This behavior is exhibited in their play, for example, the child may communicate that:
         (1) A tricycle is bad if the child fell from the trike.
         (2) A doll house is mad if it falls over during play.
   b. Preschoolers believe that whatever they think is real and will happen. They cannot distinguish between reality and fantasy.
   c. Just as in toddlerhood, preschoolers understand terms very literally, for example:
      i. Rather than hearing and understanding that "Mommy dyed her hair," the preschooler hears, "Mommy died her hair."
   d. Preschoolers' fears are often unrelated to reality, for example:
      i. When they have an injection, they often fear that their insides will fall out through the injection site.
      ii. They fear that they will go down the drain when the water in the bathtub is let out.
3. Parent education.
   a. Parents of preschoolers should continue to reinforce learning and language through:
      i. Reading to their children each night.
      ii. Talking with their children.
      iii. Restricting the children's time spent watching television and, when television is watched, primarily allowing the children to view educational programing.
      iv. Playing simple games with the children, such as:
         (1) Naming shapes, colors, and letters will help the child to be prepared to enter school.
         (2) Putting together jigsaw puzzles help preschoolers to develop spatial relationships and logical reasoning.
   b. Preschoolers begin to learn about reality by pretending to perform behaviors that they see their parents perform. To assist with that learning, parents can provide children with imaginary play materials (e.g., dress-up clothes, play kitchen utensils, and food items).
   c. Parents of preschoolers should be advised that their children may make some unusual requests or may act in unusual ways, for example:
      (1) A child may refuse to take a bath in the bathtub for fear of being washed down the drain.
      (2) A child may mandate that adhesive bandages be placed on all injuries to prevent their insides from leaking out.

D. Moral development: Kohlberg's first stage of premorality.

1. The preschooler is still egocentric in his or her moral behavior.
   a. Preschoolers primarily follow rules in order to stay out of trouble.

IV. Nursing Considerations: Health Promotion/Parent Education

A. Nutrition.

1. The food fads and anorexia of the toddler period eventually subside.
   a. The less attention paid to eating problems, the easier mealtime usually becomes.

2. Parent education: parents should be advised:
   a. To continue to provide healthful snacks and meals from a variety of foods.
   b. That vitamin supplements, if administered, must still be treated like medicine and kept in safe locations, ideally in a locked cabinet.

B. Sleep.
1. Maintaining rituals, especially at night, is still important.
   a. If a preschooler is not ready for sleep at his or her bedtime, the child should be encouraged to engage in a solitary activity while in bed, for example, read a book, complete a jigsaw puzzle, or make a Lego sculpture.
      i. It is not appropriate for preschool children to have distractions, like computers and televisions, in their bedrooms that can interfere with their sleep.
2. Preschoolers have difficulty differentiating between reality and fantasy.
   a. They may think (and truly believe) that there are monsters under the bed or in the closet.
   b. Preschoolers often become afraid of the dark.
3. **Nightmares** (child awakens from a scary dream) and **night terrors** (child is crying, screaming, physically restless in his or her sleep) are commonly experienced by preschoolers.
4. Parent education.
   a. Regarding preschool fears.
      i. Parents must not make light of such fears.
         (1) Before going to bed, parents may need to check in closets and under beds for ghosts or monsters.
         (2) Parents can be advised to provide the child with a night light or, in extreme cases, the main light in the room may need to remain lit all night.
         (3) Children often respond positively when books about children overcoming their fears are read to them (e.g., *There's An Alligator Under My Bed*, by Mercer Mayer, or *Where the Wild Things Are*, by Maurice Sendak).
   b. Nightmares.
      i. When preschool children have nightmares, parents should be advised to:
         (1) Reassure the child by acknowledging the fear because it is real to the child.
         (2) Sit with the child and provide comfort until the child is ready to settle back to sleep.
   c. Night terrors.
      i. Children experiencing night terrors often become more agitated when held or restrained, therefore it is best to advise parents:
         (1) Not to waken the child.
         (2) To stay close by the child but not to touch or speak with the child unless he or she awakens.
         (3) That terrors usually pass in a short period of time.
         (4) That children rarely remember what frightened them when they awaken in the morning.

C. Speech: stuttering.
1. Fairly common in preschoolers.
   a. Their verbal ability is less advanced than are their thought processes.
      i. Stuttering usually disappears once the child conquers language.
2. Parent education: parents should be advised:
   a. To allow their children time to complete their thoughts.
   b. To try not to complete the child's sentences.
   c. When interacting with the child, to:
      i. Respond to the thoughts, not to the child's speech patterns.
      ii. Try not to bring attention to the stuttering.
      iii. Slow down their speech to match the child's language ability.

D. Play and toys.
1. Because they are less apt to put toys in their mouths, preschoolers are more reliable than toddlers.
2. Preschoolers engage in dramatic or **associative play** (i.e., they play with each other in an activity that is not directed toward a goal).
   a. Play dress up and act like Mommy and Daddy.
   b. Play house.
   c. Pretend to work at an adult job (e.g., doctor, carpenter).
3. Preschoolers enjoy many kinds of play, such as:
   a. Building with blocks, especially Legos and other blocks that connect together.
   b. Physical play at the playground or at day care.
   c. Water play and sand play, both of which should be well supervised.
4. Many preschoolers have imaginary friends.
   a. The friends are common and real to the child. Playing with an imaginary friend is a form of pretend play.
   b. There is no need to contradict the child, unless everything that the child has done wrong has been done by the imaginary friend.
      i. It is fine, for example, to set a place at the dinner table for an imaginary friend or to invite an imaginary friend to go to the movies with the child.

ii. It is not appropriate to allow the child to blame all poor behavior on his or her imaginary friend.

5. Parent education.
   a. Supervision.
      i. Even though preschoolers are verbal and try hard to be good boys and girls, they may still engage in unsafe behavior.
      ii. They should be supervised during all playtime, especially if playing with a friend.
         (1) During pretend play, preschoolers often attempt to emulate a behavior of a parent or other adult, and the behavior may be dangerous (e.g., cleaning with bleach, shaving with father's razor, taking medicines).
   b. Appropriate toys that the nurse can recommend parents give to their preschool children include:
      i. Riding toys (e.g., tricycles).
      ii. Pretend materials (e.g., kitchens, houses, dolls, cars and trucks, dress-up clothes).
      iii. Art supplies (e.g., crayons, paints, safety scissors, stickers).
      iv. Building blocks.

V. Nursing Considerations: Disease Prevention/Parent Education

A. Safety.

1. In cars.
   a. Forward-facing car seats.
      i. Preschoolers should travel in forward-facing seats, in the rear of the car, until they reach the weight or height limit on that seat.
      ii. Once they reach the height or weight limit, they should be placed in a booster seat in the back seat of the car.
   b. Child-safety car door latches should be in place at all times.

(!) Children should NEVER be left unattended in a car, even for a few minutes. They may be abducted or may be locked in the car by mistake. Children left in a car may die from overheating or freezing.

2. As pedestrians.
   a. Preschoolers must be supervised at all times and, if anywhere near traffic, must always hold hands.
   b. Young children can dart quickly behind and/or in front of a moving vehicle.
3. In airplanes.
   a. Both the Federal Aviation Administration and the American Academy of Pediatrics recommend that children be in a child restraint system on airplanes until they are 4 years of age.
   b. Not all car seats are compatible with airline seats.
   c. Once a child is 5 years of age, he or she should be seated in the same airline harness system as the adult.
4. Burn safety and sun exposure (see also Chapter 3, "Normal Growth and Development: Toddlerhood").
   a. Preschoolers are especially at high risk for accidental burns because they are physically very capable and are often less well supervised than are toddlers.
   b. Prevention is key.
5. Poisonings (see also Chapter 10, "Pediatric Emergencies").
   a. Very high incidence of poisonings in the preschool population.
      i. Acute poisonings (e.g., medications, vitamins, gasoline).
      ii. Chronic poisonings, primarily lead.
   b. Parents should have the poison control hotline and other emergency numbers visible by every telephone.
6. Personal safety (see also Chapter 23, "Nursing Care of the Child With Psychosocial Disorders").
   a. At risk for personal and sexual abuse.
      i. Preschoolers are vulnerable to being enticed by promises of candy or presents from strangers.
      ii. Often play at a distance from adults on school or private play areas.
   b. Parent education.
      i. Educate child never to go with a stranger unless stranger uses safety word.
         (1) Safety word is a special word that the parents and child share.
         (2) Advise child never to divulge the safety word to anyone.

MAKING THE CONNECTION

Children should be taught about appropriate touching and inappropriate touching, and the child should be told to report any inappropriate touching to a parent or another adult. Parents should know that child sexual abuse is more frequently committed by someone the child knows than by a stranger.

ii. Teach child how to call 911 and how to respond appropriately when he or she calls 911.
(1) Preschoolers should know their full names, parents' names, address, and telephone number.

B. Preschool behavior and discipline.
1. Preschool behavior and discipline.
a. Preschoolers understand rules, although they will misbehave occasionally.
b. The tantrums of the toddler period fade rapidly in the preschool period.
c. Parent education.
i. Periods of time out usually work as well in the preschool period as they did in the toddler period.
ii. The period of time for time out can be extended to 4 or 5 minutes.

C. Health screenings: at each age level, children are assessed for possible diseases or illnesses. If the screenings are positive, an intervention is implemented. (See "Recommendations for Pediatric Preventive Health Care" for a complete list of procedures.)
1. Hearing.
a. Audiometric testing should be performed.
2. Vision.
a. Eye test should be performed using animal figures or tumbling E charts.
b. Glasses should be provided for any deviations from normal.
3. Lead.
a. If child's behavior indicates, blood lead levels should be assessed (see Chapter 10, "Pediatric Emergencies," for additional information on lead exposure).
4. Cholesterol and tuberculosis screenings should be performed, if indicated.

D. Immunizations.
1. Vaccines due for administration between 4 and 6 years of age are:
a. Fifth dose of DTaP (diphtheria, tetanus, and acellular pertussis).
b. Fourth dose of IPV (inactivated polio vaccine).
c. Second dose of MMR (measles, mumps, and rubella vaccine).
d. Second dose of VAR (varicella vaccine).
e. Yearly influenza vaccine.
2. Any recommended vaccines that the child has yet to receive should be administered per the Advisory Committee on Immunization Practices' catch-up vaccine schedule (www.cdc.gov/vaccines/schedules/hcp/index.html).

E. Childproofing issues: preschool children are at especially high risk for accidental injury (see Chapter 10, "Pediatric Emergencies," for an in-depth discussion).
1. Poisoning: steps that can prevent the accidental poisoning of preschool children include:
a. Plants should be kept out of children's reach.
b. All medicines, including vitamins, should be kept out of reach and in a locked cabinet.
c. All caustic powders and liquids, including cleaning supplies and gasoline, should be kept out of reach and in a locked cabinet.
d. The home should be kept clean of dust and dirt and other potential sources of lead, including paint chips.
2. Drowning and near drowning is another possible cause of injury and death in preschool children (see also Chapter 10, "Pediatric Emergencies").
a. High incidence of accidental drownings in preschoolers. They must never be left unattended around water. Preschool children should still be supervised at all times while in the bathtub and near a pool or any other large body of water.
b. Preschool children can and do drown in "kiddy" pools and other shallow bodies of water.

(!) Childproofing must continue in the preschooler's household. Even though preschool children appear much more reliable than infants and toddlers, they often are not. Parents may supervise their preschoolers less well than they did when the children were younger because they feel the children are more responsible. When childproofing is abandoned, however, many children do become injured.

3. Burn threats.
a. Electrical sockets: safety plugs should be inserted into all sockets.
b. Electrical cords should still be kept out of children's reach.
c. Because preschoolers' dexterity enables them to light matches, candles, and lighters, those items must be kept locked up and out of the children's reach.
4. Falls.
a. Preschoolers are much more capable than toddlers. As a result, they may fall from high places if unsupervised.
b. Preschoolers should be watched carefully during play on playgrounds and when around such things as ladders.
5. Choking hazards.
a. Preschool children should still have high-risk foods cut into manageable pieces.
b. Preschoolers should be discouraged from playing while eating.
6. If they have not already done so, parents should be encouraged to learn or be recertified in

emergency action skills for choking, infant and child CPR, and first aid.

F. Child abuse issues.
1. Stemming from developmental issues.
   a. Nurses must reinforce the need for parents to understand normal child behavior.
   b. Even though most children will be toilet trained by the time they are preschoolers, many still have daytime accidents, and a number will yet to be fully trained at night.
      i. Physically or emotionally abusing a child who has yet to be trained can adversely affect the child's current and future self-image.
   c. Nurses must educate parents regarding normal growth and development, including:
      i. Psychosocial norms.
      ii. Cognitive norms.
      iii. Physiological norms.

CASE STUDY: Putting It All Together

4-year-old, African American girl

Subjective Data
- Mother accompanies child for a sick visit at the child's primary health-care provider's office
- Mother states,
  - "My daughter's temperature has been between 100° and 101°F since yesterday."
- During the preliminary assessment, the nurse asks the mother, "Has your child had any additional symptoms besides the temperature?"
  - Mother replies, "Not really, although her nose has been running a little bit."
- Nurse asks, "How is she drinking?"
  - Child replies, "I been drinking good. I had all my juice this morning and a glass of water right before we comed."
  - After a few seconds, the child adds, "I know why I'm sick. I was bad yesterday. I hit my sister!"
  - Nurse responds, "You think you got sick because you were mean to your sister?"
  - Child replies, "Yup!! That's why!"

Vital Signs	
Temperature:	100°F
Pulse:	94 bpm
Respirations:	24 rpm
Blood pressure:	78/54 mm Hg

Objective Data (examination performed while sitting in mother's lap)

Nursing Assessments
- Weight: 38 lb
- Slightly enlarged cervical lymph nodes
- Slight rhinorrhea

Health-Care Provider's Orders
- Diagnosis: cold syndrome
- Keep home from preschool for next 3 to 4 days
- Increase fluids
- Acetaminophen 240 mg q 6 hr for temperature over 100.4°F
  - Child states, "Oh goody! I LOVE that medicine!"
- Call if child's symptoms worsen

Case Study Questions

A. What *subjective* assessments are important in this scenario?

1. ______________________
2. ______________________
3. ______________________
4. ______________________
5. ______________________

B. What *objective* assessments are important in this scenario?

1. ______________________
2. ______________________
3. ______________________
4. ______________________

Continued

CASE STUDY: Putting It All Together *cont'd*

Case Study Questions

C. After analyzing the data that has been collected, what **primary** nursing diagnosis should the nurse assign to this mother/daughter dyad?

1. ______________________________

D. What interventions should the nurse plan and/or implement to meet this child's and her family's needs?

1. ______________________________
2. ______________________________
3. ______________________________
4. ______________________________
5. ______________________________

E. What client outcomes should the nurse evaluate regarding the effectiveness of the nursing interventions?

1. ______________________________
2. ______________________________

F. What physiological characteristics should the child exhibit after treatment?

1. ______________________________

REVIEW QUESTIONS

1. A 4-year-old child, who is hospitalized with pneumonia, tells the nurse, "I got sick because I was bad. I yelled at my little sister yesterday." The nurse determines that which of the following is an accurate explanation for the child's comment? The child is:
1. Trying to get sympathy from the nurse.
2. Exhibiting an example of magical thinking.
3. Making up stories to entertain the nurse.
4. Expressing remorse for having yelled at her sister.

2. A kindergarten child, who has developed a fever since arriving at school, is resting in the school nurse's office. It is 11:30 a.m. The child asks, "When is my mommy going to get me?" The nurse knows that the mother will arrive in approximately 30 minutes. Which is the best response for the nurse to give to the child? "Your mommy should get here:
1. in about a half hour."
2. when both hands on the clock reach 12."
3. when lunch time begins for everyone."
4. at 12 o'clock noon."

3. The nurse is giving a 5-year-old child a vaccine injection. The child cries loudly during the procedure. Which of the following interventions would be appropriate for the nurse to perform after the injection?
1. Advise the child that big children are quiet during injections.
2. Explain to the child why vaccinations are administered.
3. Inform the child that the vaccine was ordered by the primary health-care provider.
4. Comfort the child and give the child a sticker as a present.

4. A nurse is preparing to give a 5-year-old child preoperative teaching for abdominal surgery. Which of the nurse's actions is most appropriate?
1. Explain the procedures that the child will experience.
2. Allow the child to dress up in surgical attire.
3. Tell the child why the surgery will make the child healthier.
4. Have the child meet another child who has had surgery.

5. A nurse is having difficulty communicating with a hospitalized 5-year-old child. Which of the following techniques is appropriate for the nurse to use to improve communication?
1. Have the child keep a diary of his or her feelings.
2. Read a fairy tale about scary adventures to the child.
3. Ask the mother to interpret the child's feelings.
4. Interact with the child through nurse and patient puppets.

6. A mother tells the nurse that it is difficult to get her 4-year-old child to bed at night. Which of the following should the nurse suggest that the mother do?
1. Give the child a small present if he goes to bed when he is asked to.
2. Play a running game with the child right before bedtime.
3. Develop a bedtime routine that is followed every night.
4. Let the child stay up late on weekends if he goes to bed on time on weeknights.

7. Parents inform the nurse that their 4½-year-old daughter "stutters a lot." The nurse should advise the parents to do which of the following? **Select all that apply.**
1. Wait patiently for the child to complete her sentences.
2. Give the child a treat whenever she speaks clearly.
3. Look directly at the child while she is speaking.
4. Respond to the child by speaking slowly and clearly.
5. Refrain from making any comments about the stuttering.

8. A parent asks the nurse the following question: "My son plays with his penis all the time. What should I do?" Which of the following responses is appropriate for the nurse to give the parent? "Advise your child that:
1. he should touch his penis only when he is urinating."
2. the behavior is appropriate when he is alone in a private place."
3. only boys who are old enough to have sex should touch their penises."
4. bad men may try to hurt him if they see him playing with his penis."

9. A parent telephones the nurse in the primary health-care provider's office and states, "My 4½-year-old child was screaming and kicking in her sleep. She really scared me, but by the time I got into her bedroom, she seemed to be quiet again. What should I do if that happens again?" Which of the following responses by the nurse is appropriate?
1. "The best way to stop night terrors is to have your child talk about her fears during the day."
2. "The best way to deal with nightmares is to keep a night light lit in your child's room all night."
3. "Night terrors usually go away on their own just like your daughter's did. It is best not to awaken the child."
4. "Nightmares are very common in children your daughter's age. Next time wake her up, and tell her that she is safe."

10. The mother of a 5½-year-old child who is 36 inches tall and who weighs 42 pounds states that the child complains every time she attempts to strap her child into the car seat. The nurse searches the Internet and finds the specifications of the child's car seat are as follows:
- Maximum weight forward facing: 40 lb
- Minimum weight forward facing: 22 lb
- Maximum weight rear facing: 40 lb
- Minimum weight rear facing: 5 lb
- Maximum height forward facing: 40 in.
- Minimum height forward facing: 28 in.

Which of the following statements would be appropriate for the nurse to make at this time?
1. "Because your child is not yet 40 inches tall, the child should still sit in the car seat."
2. "Because your child is over 40 pounds, the child should now be sitting in a booster seat."
3. "The minimum height of 28 inches means that your child would be safer if the child were sitting in a booster seat."
4. "The minimum weight for forward facing is 22 pounds, so your child may now sit in a booster seat in the car."

11. A nurse is educating the parents of a 4½-year-old child regarding personal safety issues. Which of the following statements should the nurse include in the teaching? **Select all that apply.** The parents should:
1. Choose a safety word for the child to remember in cases of an emergency.
2. Warn the child to report any unfamiliar adult who offers the child candy or toys.
3. Inform the child that it is safe to be alone with any of the parents' friends or neighbors.
4. Advise the child to report any adult who attempts to touch the child's shoulders and back.
5. Instruct the child regarding the information that should be given when a 911 call is made.

12. A nurse is educating a group of parents regarding disciplinary actions that they can take if their preschool child disobeys. Which of the following recommendations should the nurse make?
1. "Up to a 5-minute time out is often very effective when a preschooler disobeys."
2. "At this age, it is appropriate and effective to spank the child lightly on the behind."
3. "When preschool children disobey, it is very effective to send them to their rooms without supper."
4. "An excellent form of punishment when a preschooler disobeys is to take away the child's favorite toy for a few days."

REVIEW ANSWERS

1. ANSWER: 2
Rationale:
1. This explanation is unlikely.
2. This is the likely explanation. The child is exhibiting an example of magical thinking.
3. Preschool children do make up stories, but the statement is consistent with a child who is expressing a form of magical thinking.
4. The child may feel bad about yelling at her sister, but the child likely truly believes that the sister became ill because the child was yelling at her sister.
TEST-TAKING TIP: The Eriksonian psychosocial development stage of the preschool child is initiative versus guilt. Children during this stage of development often believe that their thoughts are powerful (i.e., that they can cause injury simply by having angry thoughts or expressing angry words and, unless they are told otherwise, they can become guilt-ridden).
Content Area: *Pediatrics—Preschool*
Integrated Processes: *Nursing Process: Assessment*
Client Need: *Health Promotion and Maintenance: Developmental Stages and Transitions*
Cognitive Level: *Application*

2. ANSWER: 3
Rationale:
1. Kindergarten children do not have the conceptual ability to understand how long either 30 minutes or a half hour will last.
2. Many kindergarten children have yet to learn their numbers. Also, because many clocks are digital, children are unfamiliar with analogue clocks.
3. It is best to advise the child that his or her mother will return when lunch is served.
4. Kindergarten children do not have the conceptual ability to understand the abstract concept of time.
TEST-TAKING TIP: As defined by Piaget, preschool children's cognitive stage is at the preoperational level. They view their world directly, unable to conceptualize things or events. Connecting a new event to the time of a known event will help the child to understand when the new event will occur.
Content Area: *Pediatrics—Preschool*
Integrated Processes: *Nursing Process: Implementation*
Client Need: *Health Promotion and Maintenance: Developmental Stages and Transitions*
Cognitive Level: *Analysis*

3. ANSWER: 4
Rationale:
1. Children should not be made to feel ashamed or believe that they are misbehaving by crying during painful procedures.
2. Preschool children are unable to conceptualize why causing pain will ultimately benefit them.
3. Although the primary health-care provider did order the vaccine, it is inappropriate to blame him or her for the child's painful experience.
4. Injections are painful, violent experiences for young children. They should be comforted and rewarded after the procedures.
TEST-TAKING TIP: Preschoolers may view injections as a form of punishment for poor behavior or for bad thoughts. To counter those misunderstandings, the nurse should comfort and praise the child for having successfully undergone the painful procedure.
Content Area: *Pediatrics—Preschool*
Integrated Processes: *Nursing Process: Implementation*
Client Need: *Health Promotion and Maintenance: Developmental Stages and Transitions*
Cognitive Level: *Application*

4. ANSWER: 2
Rationale:
1. Preschoolers do not possess the conceptual ability to understand from an explanation what procedure will be performed.
2. The nurse should allow the child to dress up in surgical attire.
3. Preschoolers do not possess the conceptual ability to understand from an explanation why a procedure is being performed.
4. Meeting another child who has had surgery would be appropriate for an older, school-age child or teenager.
TEST-TAKING TIP: Because preschoolers are in the preoperational stage of cognitive development, they are unable to understand explanations and rationalizations. The best way to enable young children to understand what actions will take place is to allow them to perform the actions themselves. They then have a clear understanding of what will happen.
Content Area: *Pediatrics—Preschool*
Integrated Processes: *Nursing Process: Implementation*
Client Need: *Health Promotion and Maintenance: Developmental Stages and Transitions*
Cognitive Level: *Analysis*

5. ANSWER: 4
Rationale:
1. Preschool children are unable to keep diaries. They have yet to learn how to express themselves using the written word.
2. Reading a scary fairy tale to the child is not appropriate.
3. Although the mother knows her child well, she may be unable to interpret the child's feelings completely.
4. Interacting with the child through nurse and patient puppets can be an effective way to improve communication with a preschool child.
TEST-TAKING TIP: Although preschool children are able to use all forms of speech, they are often unable clearly to put their feelings into words. Preschool children use imagination and play in their everyday lives. Puppetry can be an excellent means of utilizing play to foster communication.
Content Area: *Pediatrics—Preschool*
Integrated Processes: *Nursing Process: Implementation*

Client Need: Health Promotion and Maintenance: Developmental Stages and Transitions
Cognitive Level: Application

6. ANSWER: 3
Rationale:
1. The nurse should not suggest that the mother give the child a small present if he goes to bed when he is asked to.
2. The nurse should suggest that the child engage in quiet play before bedtime.
3. The nurse should suggest that she develop a bedtime routine that is followed every night.
4. The nurse should not suggest that the mother let the child stay up late on weekends if he goes to bed on time on weeknights.

TEST-TAKING TIP: Just as in the toddler period, routines help preschool children to know what is expected of them. Children then are more able to meet those expectations. If the child is not always able to go to sleep at bedtime, he or she can look at books in bed. Children should not have major distractions in their rooms, such as televisions or computers.
Content Area: Pediatrics—Preschool
Integrated Processes: Nursing Process: Implementation
Client Need: Health Promotion and Maintenance: Developmental Stages and Transitions
Cognitive Level: Application

7. ANSWER: 1, 3, 4, and 5
Rationale:
1. The parents should wait patiently for the child to complete her sentences.
2. The parents should not give the child a treat whenever she speaks clearly.
3. The parents should look directly at the child while she is speaking.
4. The parents should respond to the child by speaking slowly and clearly.
5. The parents should refrain from making any comments about the stuttering.

TEST-TAKING TIP: Parents frequently state that their preschoolers stutter. However, if the parents respond appropriately, the behavior rarely becomes a lifelong problem. The best way to respond to the child is to bring as little attention, either verbally or nonverbally, to the problem as possible. When parents patiently wait for the child to speak, the child will be able to organize his or her thoughts and communicate them to the parents. Parents who speak slowly and clearly to their child are role modeling a proper speech pattern for the child.
Content Area: Pediatrics—Preschool
Integrated Processes: Nursing Process: Implementation; Teaching/Learning
Client Need: Health Promotion and Maintenance: Developmental Stages and Transitions
Cognitive Level: Application

8. ANSWER: 2
Rationale:
1. This statement is inappropriate. Masturbation is a normal, natural act.
2. This response is appropriate. The behavior is normal and natural, but it is not appropriate to perform in public.
3. This statement is inappropriate. Masturbation is a normal, natural act.
4. This statement is inappropriate. Masturbation is a normal, natural act.

TEST-TAKING TIP: Masturbation is a normal, natural act that is evident throughout childhood and adulthood. It is inappropriate to scold a child or to frighten a child when he or she masturbates. It is appropriate, however, to remind a child that private acts should be performed in private places (i.e., in one's bedroom).
Content Area: Pediatrics—Preschool
Integrated Processes: Nursing Process: Implementation
Client Need: Health Promotion and Maintenance: Developmental Stages and Transitions
Cognitive Level: Application

9. ANSWER: 3
Rationale:
1. Children rarely remember their night terrors.
2. Night terrors and nightmares are common problems of the preschool period. Night lights can reduce children's fear of the dark, but they do not prevent night terrors or nightmares.
3. This statement is true. Night terrors usually go away on their own. It is recommended that parents be available to their child if he or she does awaken but not to wake the child up themselves.
4. This child is experiencing a night terror. Children usually awaken themselves if they are having a nightmare.

TEST-TAKING TIP: Nightmares and night terrors are slightly different phenomena. When children have a nightmare, they wake up frightened. Parents should comfort their child and sit close by until the child settles back to sleep. In contrast, night terrors are characterized by crying and agitation while still asleep. Children usually remain asleep and calm down spontaneously. It is best not to awaken children from night terrors.
Content Area: Pediatrics—Preschool
Integrated Processes: Nursing Process: Implementation
Client Need: Health Promotion and Maintenance: Developmental Stages and Transitions
Cognitive Level: Application

10. ANSWER: 2
Rationale:
1. This statement is incorrect. The child has exceeded the weight limit for the car seat.
2. This statement is correct. The child has exceeded the weight limit for the car seat.
3. This statement is incorrect. The minimum height is not relevant at this time.
4. This statement is incorrect. The minimum weight is not relevant at this time.

TEST-TAKING TIP: The National Highway Traffic Safety Administration recommends that once preschool children exceed the height and weight limits of their car restraint systems, they should be seated in the back seat

of cars in booster seats until shoulder and lap belts fit correctly.
Content Area: *Child Health*
Integrated Processes: *Nursing Process: Evaluation*
Client Need: *Health Promotion and Maintenance: Health Promotion/Disease Prevention*
Cognitive Level: *Application*

11. ANSWER: 1, 2, and 5
Rationale:
1. This statement is correct. The parents should choose a safety word for the child to remember in case of an emergency.
2. This statement is correct. The parents should warn the child to report any unfamiliar adult who offers the child candy or toys.
3. This statement is incorrect. Although it would be inappropriate to advise the child that friends and/or neighbors are dangerous, parents should remember that sexual abuse of children is most commonly performed by persons known to the child rather than by strangers.
4. This statement is incorrect. The child should be advised to report any adult who attempts to touch the child's "private parts."
5. This statement is correct. The parents should instruct the child regarding the information that should be given when a 911 call is made.
TEST-TAKING TIP: Preschool children should be taught, in a matter of fact way, regarding personal safety. They should be advised to report unwanted touching and strangers who try to entice them with candy, toys, and the like. They should be taught a safety word that only they and their parents know in case an emergency requires that someone other than their parents must care for them. They also should be taught when and how to call 911 and how to respond to the emergency operator who answers.
Content Area: *Child Health*
Integrated Processes: *Nursing Process: Implementation*
Client Need: *Health Promotion and Maintenance: Health Promotion/Disease Prevention*
Cognitive Level: *Application*

12. ANSWER: 1
Rationale:
1. This response is correct. Time out is often effective with preschoolers as well as with toddlers.
2. It is inappropriate to deprive a child of his or her supper.
3. Spanking is not the best disciplinary action to use with children.
4. Because preschoolers are still in Piaget's preoperational stage of cognitive development, this form of discipline is not recommended.
TEST-TAKING TIP: Preschool children are unable to conceptualize the meaning behind depriving them of a favorite toy for a number of days. It is much more effective to discipline the child immediately after the infraction by giving the child a time out for a few minutes.
Content Area: *Pediatrics—Preschool*
Integrated Processes: *Nursing Process: Implementation*
Client Need: *Health Promotion and Maintenance: Health Promotion/Disease Prevention*
Cognitive Level: *Application*

Normal Growth and Development: The School-Age Child

KEY TERMS

Concrete operational stage—Piaget's stage of cognitive development for the school-age child, characterized by sophisticated thinking that relies heavily on the need to see and feel in order to internalize new information.

Conservation—In Piaget's stage of concrete operations, a child develops the understanding that even when an object changes shape, it still is the same object (i.e., the inherent properties of the object are unchanged).

Conventional role development—Kohlberg's stage of moral development during which children become aware of actions that are right and wrong.

Industry versus inferiority—Erikson's stage of psychosocial development in which children may excel at a task, experiencing achievement, or develop a feeling of inferiority when he or she performs poorly.

Menarche—A girl's first menstruation, usually occurring between the ages of 9 and 15.

Precocious development—The early onset of sexual development.

Reversibility—In Piaget's concrete operational stage, a child's understanding that numbers and objects can be changed and later returned to their original state.

School refusal—Avoidance of school through vague symptoms (e.g., stomachache) caused by boredom, fear of the teacher, bullying, or other factors.

Tanner scale—A scale for assessing the sexual development of children.

I. Description

The school-age period, between 6 and 12 years of age, usually is referenced in one of two ways: the age of the "good kids" and/or the age of the "loose tooth." Beginning at about 6 years of age, children begin to lose their primary teeth and replace them with their permanent, adult teeth. During this time, children are in elementary school, working hard to learn and to please both their teachers and their parents. When children are unable to learn easily or to excel in any other area that they may endeavor to try they can become frustrated and develop a feeling of inferiority. It is important for adults to listen to children's desires and to provide positive feedback whenever possible.

II. Biological Development

A. Growth: when eating healthily and engaging in an appropriate amount of exercise, the nurse will note that school-age children exhibit a slow and steady growth.

1. Weight.
   a. Increase of 2.5 kg/year (5½ lb/year).
   b. Growth spurts.
      i. At age 12 or shortly before, the nurse may note a growth spurt in females.
      ii. Boys rarely exhibit their growth spurt until they are about 2 years older.
2. Height.
   a. Increase of 5.5 cm/year (2 in./year).
3. BMI assessment: same parameters as previously noted.
   a. BMI less than 5%: child is defined as underweight.
   b. BMI 5% to 85%: healthy weight for the child.
   c. BMI greater than 85%: child is defined as overweight.
   d. BMI greater than 95%: child is defined as obese.
4. Maturity of bodily systems.
   a. Brain growth is complete by about age 10.
   b. Other body systems.
      i. All organ systems are mature by about the age of 12.

B. Vital signs.
1. Temperature.
   a. 98.6°F (36°C).
   b. Any method is acceptable (e.g., axillary, aural, temporal artery).
      i. Rectal temperature should be taken only when absolutely necessary.
2. Heart rate may be taken either apically or radially.
   a. 60 to 100 bpm.
3. Respiratory rate.
   a. 18 to 22 rpm.
4. Blood pressure.
   a. The nurse should make sure to use an appropriately sized cuff.
   b. The same method that was used to calculate the lowest safe systolic blood pressure of preschool-age children is also used to determine the lowest safe systolic blood pressure of school-age children: 70 mm Hg plus two times the child's age in years.

C. Dentition and hygiene.
1. Tooth development (see Fig. 7.1).
   a. Beginning at age 6, children slowly lose all 20 primary teeth in approximately the same order and time frame as they appeared in infancy.
   b. By the end of the school-age period, most children will have acquired 28 secondary teeth, including:
      i. Central incisors: two upper and two lower at 6 to 8 years.
      ii. Lateral incisors: two upper and two lower at 7 to 9 years.
      iii. Canines: two upper and two lower at 9 to 12 years.
      iv. First bicuspids: two upper and two lower at 10 to 12 years.
      v. Second bicuspids: two upper and two lower at 10 to 12 years.
      vi. First molars: two upper and two lower at 6 to 7 years.
      vii. Second molars: two upper and two lower at 11 to 13 years.
2. Parent education.
   a. School-age children often try to skip dental care and baths.
      i. Parents should be counseled to monitor children's dental and hygiene activities.
   b. Dental health is especially critical.
      i. Secondary teeth must last for the rest of the child's life.
      ii. Children should receive biyearly dental care from a reputable dental health-care provider.
         (1) Dental caries are completely preventable.
         (2) Once children are able to retain fluids in their mouths without swallowing:
            (a) Daily use of a fluoride-containing tooth paste and
            (b) Topical fluoride treatments by a dental professional should begin.
      iii. By end of the school-age period: orthodonture work, if needed, may be started.
      iv. Parents should be counseled regarding food items that place children at high risk of dental caries.
         (1) Those that are quickly consumed and swallowed pose the least threat, such as:
            (a) Soda, chocolate, and cookies.
         (2) Those that stick to the teeth after chewing pose the greatest threat, such as:
            (a) Caramel, jelly beans, and raisins.

D. Senses.
1. Smell, hearing, touch, and taste are fully developed.
2. Vision.
   a. Should be assessed using the traditional Snellen chart at a 20-ft distance.
      i. At that distance, children should be able to see all letters on the 20-ft line of the chart.
   b. Any child who fails to see the 20-ft line clearly should be seen by an ophthalmic professional.

E. Motor development.
1. Gross motor development.
   a. Although actions are not yet refined, school-age children are capable of fairly sophisticated movements.
   b. During physical education classes and recess, school-age children should be exposed to a variety of physical activities.
   c. Depending on the child's interest, a school-age child is physically ready for a variety of activities. In each case, parents should make sure that the child is learning to perform the activities safely, including the wearing of safety helmets when head injuries are possible. Examples of the activities are:
      i. Dance classes.
      ii. Sports teams.
         (1) Contact sports, if not performed in a safe manner, can result in severe injuries, including fractures and concussion.
      iii. Two-wheeled bicycles.
      iv. Roller boarding.
      v. Skiing.
   d. Active play is important to maintain a healthy weight and to promote large muscle development.
2. Fine motor development.
   a. Again, although actions are not yet refined, school-age children are capable of fairly sophisticated movements.
   b. During the elementary period, school-age children are expected to master a number of small motor skills, including, but not limited to:
      i. Computer keyboarding.
      ii. Manuscript and cursive writing.
   c. Depending on the child's interest, a school-age child is physically ready for:
      i. Knitting, crocheting, and sewing.
      ii. Playing musical instruments.
      iii. Model building.
      iv. Completing studio art projects.

F. Sexual development.
1. Beginning at or slightly before age 12, children, especially young women, begin to exhibit signs of sexual development.
   a. The timing of sexual development is individual.
      i. Average age of **menarche** (first menstruation) is age 12, with a range from age 9 to age 15.
      ii. Male sexual maturation usually occurs approximately 2 years after female maturation.
   b. **Precocious development**, or pubertal changes occurring at an unexpectedly young age, can be seen as early as 6 years of age.
      i. Although some children do exhibit precocious physiological development, it is important to remember that psychologically they are rarely as precocious.
2. The **Tanner scale** (Figs. 6.1, 6.2, and 6.3) is employed as an objective method for assessing the sexual development of children (see Chapter 6, "Normal Growth and Development: Adolescence").
   a. Separate Tanner scales have been developed for males and females.
3. Parent education: parents must be included in any discussion about sex education for their children (*National Sexual Education Standards,* 2012).
   a. Highly controversial subject. Two issues debated about the subject are:
      i. Should sex education be formally provided in schools or houses of worship or informally provided by parents or health-care providers?
      ii. If sex education is to be provided, at what age should it begin?
   b. Depending on the location where the nurse provides care, sex education may begin in the elementary school years.
   c. Content, if provided, that may be included in the classes.
      i. Early elementary grades.
         (1) Appropriate physical contact versus inappropriate contact.
         (2) Appropriate names of external genitalia of boys and girls.
      ii. Later elementary grades.
         (1) Human reproduction.
         (2) Physiological changes that occur during puberty.
         (3) Infectious disease transmission, including sexually transmitted infections.
      iii. In later years, information regarding sexual changes, sexual preference, consensual sex versus forced intercourse, oral sex versus genital versus anal intercourse, and contraception choices.

III. Language and Social Development

A. Language development.
1. Vocabulary expands dramatically.
2. Through leisure reading and during language arts classes, children are exposed to and are

increasingly expected to use more and more sophisticated language.

B. Psychosocial development.

1. School-age children are in Erik Erikson's stage of **industry versus inferiority**.
2. Major goal: Achievement in school and in other activities, including playing cooperatively with others.
   a. School-age children thoroughly enjoy succeeding at activities.
      i. Every child succeeds at something.
   b. Socializing.
      i. Parents are still the most important people in the lives of school-age children, however:
      ii. Same sex peers and other adults become more and more important.
         (1) Group activities (e.g., girl scouts, boy scouts, little league) are excellent activities for children in this age group.
3. Potential problem: feelings of inferiority.
   a. Develop when a child is unable to achieve or is criticized for poor performance.
   b. Children must receive some positive reinforcement for their actions or they will feel inferior.
   c. When children feel inferior, they seek attention in less acceptable ways, for example, by acting out in school and/or in social situations.
4. Parent education.
   a. Parents should be encouraged to support their children's interests, as long as they are constructive and physically appropriate, for example:
      i. Same-sex group memberships.
      ii. Team sports.
      iii. Solitary activities, such as reading and painting.
   b. Parents should be forewarned that their children may try a number of activities before they find the one(s) that they are most interested in pursuing.
      i. Although economic considerations may preclude children from becoming too choosy, children should not be reprimanded unnecessarily for changing their minds.
      ii. Parents should encourage their children to pursue at least one or two aerobic activities.
   c. Because of the potential for children to develop inferior self-concepts, it is important for parents to:
      i. Provide appropriate positive reinforcement when their child is successful in whatever constructive endeavor the child may engage whether that activity be, for example:
         (1) In an academic setting.
         (2) As an athlete.
         (3) As a musician.
   d. It is especially important for parents to work to develop and maintain a strong bond with their school-age children.
      i. The adolescent years can provide a challenge for any parent-child relationship.
      ii. When parents and children have strong relationships during the school-age period, they will more likely be able to endure the difficult times that lie ahead when the children become adolescents.

C. Cognitive development.

1. Piaget's **concrete operational stage** is reflected in the cognitive development of the school-age child.
   a. School-age children's thinking is fairly sophisticated, but they need to see and feel when they are learning about new information in order to truly internalize the information, for example:
      i. When learning multiplication, they will more quickly understand that $10 \times 10 = 100$ when they see 10 groups of 10 blocks and are able to count, touch, and work with the objects.
      ii. Similarly, when teaching school-age children about an illness in their body, they will more clearly understand the process if they are provided with pictures, videos, or replicas of the organs that are adversely affected.
   b. During this period, children develop the ability to understand the concepts of **reversibility** and **conservation**, for example, they will learn that:
      i. $3 + 4 = 7$ and $4 + 3 = 7$ are the same and that $7 - 3 = 4$ and $7 - 4 = 3$ are similarly related.
      ii. When an equivalent amount of water is poured into two glasses, one tall and skinny and one short and wide, even though they appear to have different quantities of water in them, the amount of water in each is truly the same.
   c. School-age children can organize items into groups, see the logic of jokes, and deduce information from a scenario.

2. Because of their increasingly sophisticated thought processes, children are exposed to and are expected to learn more and more complex information in school.
3. Parent education.
   a. Encourage parents to provide their children with an environment conducive to learning, including access to books for leisure reading as well as academic study, computer access for research, and quiet space for the completion of homework.
   b. Encourage parents to assist their children to understand what is required of their homework but not to complete the child's homework themselves.
      i. If the child is being asked to perform at an unrealistic level, the parent should ask to meet with the teacher, principal, and/or others at the child's school.
   c. Encourage parents to use their local libraries as important adjuncts to their child's learning.

D. Moral development.

1. The school-age period is characterized by level II of Kohlberg's theoretical framework entitled **conventional role development** (good kid/law and order).
   a. During this stage, children become aware of actions that are right and those that are wrong.
   b. School-age children believe in rules and are inclined to follow rules explicitly whether in school, at home, or during play, for example:
      i. When left to play without adult involvement, school-age children create their own games, with strict rules, and often reprimand children who do not follow the rules.
   c. School-age children feel pressured to conform to the norms of the group.
      i. This can be difficult for children who engage in activities that are outside the norm (e.g., children who prefer classical music to popular music may be chastised for their choice).
2. Parent education.
   a. Because of school-age children's inclination to conform to rules, they have difficulty when parents and other adults do not follow rules.
      i. It is, therefore, important for parents and others in authority to set an excellent example by engaging in appropriate, lawful behavior.
   b. The school-age period is an excellent time for children to begin religious/spiritual instruction.

IV. Nursing Considerations: Health Promotion/Parent Education

A. Nutrition.

1. Promoting healthy eating can be challenging because the child eats many meals away from home.
2. To promote as healthy eating as possible:
   a. Snacks and meals at home must be healthy and tasty.
   b. Packed lunches and snacks must include favored foods and healthy items.
      i. Healthful food suggestions include fresh fruit, fresh vegetables, cheese chunks, whole grain crackers and baked goods, nuts, and peanut butter sandwiches.
   c. Prevention is the key to enabling children to maintain a healthy weight.
      i. To prevent children from becoming obese, parents must provide their children with foods that are attractive but that do not contain empty, innutritious calories.
3. Parent education: the nurse should encourage parents to:
   a. Choose rewards for their children's positive behavior that do not include innutritious foods that contain empty calories.
   b. Foster lively family mealtimes at which active communication takes place and healthful items are served.
   c. Serve fresh fruits and vegetables rather than canned fruits and vegetables or fruit juices.
   d. Serve foods made from scratch rather than prepared and/or processed foods.
   e. Encourage active exercise.
      i. Because of their sedentary nature, restrictions should be placed on the amount of television viewing and computer time in which children are permitted to engage.
   f. Vitamin or mineral supplements usually are recommended only if a child fails to consume an adequate diet.

B. Sleep.

1. School-age children need 9 to 12 hours of sleep each night.
   a. The longer sleep times are for the younger children.
2. An adequate quantity of sleep is essential for learning to take place.
3. Parent education.
   a. To meet the child's sleep needs, a consistent bedtime (e.g., 8:30 p.m.) should be enforced to enable the child to get an adequate amount of sleep for optimal school performance.

b. It is important to remove televisions, computers, and other electronic distractions from children's bedrooms.
   i. If a child is not yet ready for sleep at the stated bedtime, he or she should be encouraged to read in bed; they should not be allowed to stay up later than the established bedtime or to watch television or play on their electronic gadgets.

C. Play, toys, and leisure activities: play is still part of a school-age child's "work" and should reflect the child's growth and development.

1. School-age children engage in all forms of play, including:
   a. Solitary play, such as video gaming and puzzle solving.
   b. Associative play, such as building with blocks without a definite goal in mind.
   c. Cooperative play, such as playing a board game with another child or playing a competitive team sport.
2. A variety of toys and activities are appropriate for this age group.
   a. Riding toys, such as bikes, skateboards, and scooters.
   b. Sports equipment.
   c. Action figures.
   d. Books for leisure reading.
   e. Board games.
   f. Computer games.
3. Parent education.
   a. When choosing toys and activities for children from 6 to 12 years of age, parents must consider the abilities and interests of the child.
      i. To prevent a feeling of inferiority, parents should not provide items that are too far beyond the ability of the child.
      ii. To prevent an expression of disinterest, parents should query their children about which items and activities to which they are most attracted.
   b. When providing children with activities and toys, the children's safety must always be considered (see "Safety").

V. Nursing Considerations: Disease Prevention/Parent Education

A. Safety.

1. In cars.
   a. School-age children should continue to travel in forward-facing seats, in the rear of the car, until they reach the weight or height limit on that seat.
   b. Once they reach the height or weight limit, they should be placed in a booster seat in the backseat of the car.
   c. If they outgrow the booster seat, they should continue to sit in the backseat of the car but in the adult restraint system.
2. In and around school buses.
   a. Parents must always wait until the bus is fully stopped before allowing their children to approach the school bus.
   b. Parents must urge their children to follow the guidance of the school bus driver at all times, including:
      i. Crossing the street well in front of the bus after the bus has come to a full stop and the driver has given the child permission.
      ii. Remaining seated at all times while the bus is moving.
      iii. Fastening their seat belts, if required.
      iv. Speaking in an acceptable tone of voice while on the bus.
      v. Speaking in a polite manner to the driver as well as to all other children.
3. As pedestrians.
   a. Young, school-age children should be supervised when walking as pedestrians.
   b. Once the children are reliable when walking alone, or when they have reached an appropriate age, they must be reminded always to:
      i. Walk on the sidewalk or on the left-hand side of the road facing traffic.
      ii. Cross the road at the crosswalk.
      iii. Look both ways before crossing.
4. In airplanes.
   a. School-age children should be restrained in the same seat belt system as the adults.
5. On bicycles.
   a. The bicycle should:
      i. Be sized properly for the child.
      ii. Have reflectors on the front and back of the bike.
   b. The child should wear a properly sized safety helmet at all times.
   c. The bicycle should be ridden on the same side of the road as the rest of traffic.
   d. The child should be taught the proper use of hand signals in order to signal his or her intentions when riding on the road.
6. On in-line skates, skateboards, and scooters.
   a. The child should wear reflective clothing when riding the device.

b. The item should be ridden in a safe location (e.g., many communities have created skateboard and skating parks).
c. The child should wear a properly sized safety helmet, as well as knee, elbow, and wrist pads, at all times.

7. Burn safety and sun exposure (see also Chapter 3, "Normal Growth and Development: Toddlerhood").
   a. Sun exposure.
      i. Children must be reminded to reapply sunscreen at least every 2 hours and more frequently if they become wet.
   b. Fire and burns.
      i. Because of their increasing abilities, school-age children, especially those who are older, often are asked to assist in such activities as lighting fires and food preparation.
         (1) Children must be taught regarding appropriate safe use of matches, stoves, ovens, and grills.
      ii. Fireworks.
         (1) The misuse of fireworks can be dangerous.
         (2) Fireworks, if lawful, should only be used in the presence and guidance of an adult.
8. Poisonings (see also Chapter 10, "Pediatric Emergencies").
   a. The poison control hotline and other emergency numbers should still be available by every telephone.
   b. The intentional ingestion of poisons, including alcohol and prescribed and illicit drugs, becomes a problem starting in the school-age population.
   c. Parent education.
      i. Educate parents to communicate clearly to their children that such things as alcohol and medications are not to be ingested by the children.
      ii. If needed, all potentially hazardous items that may be ingested should be kept in locked cabinets.
9. Near drownings (see also Chapter 10, "Pediatric Emergencies").
   a. All children, by the time they are of school age, should be registered in swim lessons until they are capable swimmers.
   b. Parent education.
      i. Parents should admonish children never to swim when alone or where there is no lifeguard.
      ii. Children must be warned never to dive into shallow water.
         (1) Can result in severe head and/or neck injuries that can result in paralysis.
10. Personal safety.
   a. School-age children are at risk of personal and sexual abuse because:
      i. They are often separated from their parents while traveling to and from school, at sports practice, at music lessons, and at many other times.
   b. Parent education.
      i. Educate the child about appropriate physical touching and inappropriate touching.
      ii. Advise child to report any inappropriate touch to a parent or other trusted adult.
         (1) Child should be reminded that he or she will not be blamed for the inappropriate behavior of the adult.
      iii. Educate the child never to go with a stranger unless the stranger uses a predefined safety word.
         (1) Remind the child never to divulge the safety word to anyone.
11. Self-care: children.
   a. In many states, there is no law regarding the age when a child is old enough to be left alone.
   b. Because of parents' work obligations and financial constraints, many children, even as young as 6 years of age, return from school to an empty home.
   c. There are many potential consequences resulting from children who are home alone.
      i. Potential positive result.
         (1) Many children learn to be independent and to problem solve.
      ii. Potential negative results.
         (1) Children can develop a number of fears and can become anxious.
         (2) Because of the lack of supervision, they can develop a number of maladaptive behaviors, such as smoking, alcohol and drug use, and poor school performance.
   d. Parent education.
      i. When it is necessary to leave their children home unattended, parents should be encouraged to develop specific strategies to promote positive outcomes, including:
         (1) Being in frequent contact with the child, such as via telephone and text.

(2) Insisting that the child complete as much of his or her homework as possible while waiting for the parents' return.
(3) Insisting that the child never answer the door while alone.
(4) Insisting that the child have no friends in the home while alone.

12. Childproofing issues.
    a. If they have not already done so, parents should be encouraged to learn or be recertified in emergency action skills for choking, child CPR, and first aid.
13. Child abuse issues.
    a. See child abuse information included in chapters related to children at earlier ages.
14. School phobias and bullying.
    a. Parents should be forewarned that even though school is usually a positive experience for the child, fostering children's psychosocial, cognitive, and moral development, some children find the school experience difficult.
    b. **School refusal:** also called school phobia or school avoidance.
       i. When children complain of vague symptoms (e.g., stomachaches and headaches that resolve once the parents allow the children to stay home from school), school refusal should be suspected.
       ii. Etiologies of school refusal.
          (1) Bullying by another student.
          (2) Poor school performance.
          (3) Boredom.
          (4) Fear of teacher.
          (5) Embarrassment, for example, over how he or she is dressed.
    c. Parent education.
       i. When school refusal is suspected, parents should be encouraged to:
          (1) Solicit the assistance of school personnel to determine the specific problem that is leading to the refusal.
          (2) Deal with bullying or other potentially dangerous issues as quickly as possible, if necessary (see "Bullying").
          (3) Inform the child that the parent understands the child's discomfort.
          (4) Gently, but firmly, require the child to attend school.
    d. Bullying.
       i. Children may be victims of bullying by others who they are in face-to-face contact with or, because of the many electronic communication devices now available, via the Internet.
       ii. Parent education.
          (1) Parents should be encouraged to query their children periodically regarding the children's relationships, both positive and negative.
          (2) If a child does report being a victim of bullying, the parent should:
             (a) Immediately report the problem to the school and/or legal authorities, if appropriate.
             (b) Educate the child regarding actions that he or she can take in response to the bullying (e.g., reporting the episodes to an appropriate adult, avoiding contact with the bully when possible, clearly telling the bully that the behavior is inappropriate).

B. Behavior and discipline.
1. All children expect and want limits, but they will misbehave.
2. Common improper behaviors seen in school-aged children are disobeying and/or ignoring rules, stealing, and lying.
3. Parent education.
   a. When a school-age child misbehaves, the parent must impose a consequence that is equal to the infraction.
   b. If the parent imposes no consequence, the child becomes confused and never truly learns right and wrong.
   c. Discipline should be directed at the child's action, not at the child, to prevent the child from developing feelings of inferiority.

C. Health screenings. (See "Recommendations for Pediatric Preventive Health Care" for a complete list of procedures.)
1. As discussed in previous chapters, if screenings are positive, an intervention should be implemented.

MAKING THE CONNECTION

Examples of disciplinary actions that are equal to the infractions.

- Child steals from a store: parent accompanies the child to the store and requires the child to return the article to a store employee.
- Child lies about his or her action: parent requires the child to apologize to the individual to whom he or she lied and to tell the individual the truth.
- Child ignores a rule: parent requires the child to go without video game playing for 1 full day.

DID YOU KNOW?

Many developmental screening tests are valid only through part of the school-age period. For example, the Denver Developmental Screening Test II is valid through age 6, and the Ages and Stages Questionnaire is valid through the age of 10.

2. Hearing.
   a. Audiometric testing should continue to be assessed each year.
3. Vision.
   a. When children have vision problems, they rarely realize it.
      i. The nurse should monitor the child for signs of poor vision, including squinting and moving his or her head when viewing a specific object.
   b. Their vision should be checked by their pediatric health-care provider every year.
   c. If any evidence of poor vision is noted, the child should be referred to an ophthalmic specialist.
4. Other.
   a. Yearly complete blood count and urinalysis.
   b. Cholesterol and tuberculosis assessments, if the child is at high risk.
   c. Yearly scoliosis assessments, especially important for girls who are exhibiting pubertal changes (see Fig. 6.4).

D. Immunizations.
1. Vaccinations recommended to be administered between age 7 and 12 years.
   a. Throughout childhood: yearly influenza vaccines.
   b. From 11 to 12 years of age.
      i. Tdap (tetanus, diphtheria, acellular pertussis).
      ii. Three-dose series of human papillomavirus vaccines.
      iii. First dose of meningococcal vaccine.

Any recommended vaccines that the child has yet to receive should be administered per the Advisory Committee on Immunization Practices catch-up vaccine schedule.

CASE STUDY: Putting It All Together

An 8-year-old girl, Asian (Chinese) immigrant

Subjective Data
- The mother telephones the school nurse at the child's school. (Parent speaks English, but the family speaks Chinese in the home.)
- Mother states,
  - "I have kept my daughter home from school the last 3 days because she has had a headache and stomachache. Are other children sick with the same thing?"
- The nurse informs the mother that no other children have complained of the same illness.
- The school nurse then queries the mother about other symptoms the child is exhibiting. The mother states,
  - "No, she doesn't seem to have any serious symptoms. Her temperature is normal, and she hasn't vomited or had any diarrhea."
- When queried by the school nurse regarding the child's behavior once school is over, the mother states,
  - "That is interesting. She seems to feel much better in the late afternoon and evening."
- When queried by the school nurse regarding the child's school experiences, the mother states,
  - "A couple times last week, my daughter complained about being placed by her teacher into the bottom reading group in her classroom. She said that some of the children in the top reading group said something to her in the playground."
  - "She also said something about being the only Chinese student in the class."

Objective Data
- None obtained: child is at home

Health-Care Provider's Orders
- None made: child is at home

Continued

CASE STUDY: Putting It All Together

cont'd

Case Study Questions

A. Which *subjective* assessments are important in this scenario?

1. ______
2. ______
3. ______
4. ______
5. ______
6. ______

B. Which *objective* assessments are important in this scenario?

1. ______

C. After analyzing the data that has been collected, what **primary** nursing diagnosis should the nurse assign to this client?

1. ______

D. What interventions should the nurse plan and/or implement to meet this child's and her family's needs?

1. ______
2. ______
3. ______
4. ______
5. ______
6. ______
7. ______

E. What client outcomes should the nurse evaluate regarding the effectiveness of the nursing interventions?

1. ______
2. ______
3. ______
4. ______

F. What physiological characteristics should the child exhibit before being discharged home?

1. ______

REVIEW QUESTIONS

1. The nurse is assessing a 12 year-old boy during a well-child clinic visit. Which of the following findings would the nurse expect to see?
1. Weight gain of 2¼ lb (1 kg) since the last visit 1 year previously
2. Height increase of 2 in. (5.5 cm) since the last visit 1 year previously
3. 20 secondary teeth
4. Heart rate 124

2. A nurse is providing health promotion education to a 10-year-old child during a well-child clinic visit. Which of the following is an appropriate patient-care goal for the teaching session?

The child will:
1. Brush teeth using a fluoride toothpaste at least twice each day.
2. Receive the first dose of the meningococcal vaccine before leaving the clinic.
3. Begin to take swimming lessons before becoming an adolescent.
4. Always ride a bicycle on the left-hand side of the road.

3. A nurse is providing health promotion education to the parent of a 6-year-old child during a well-child clinic visit. Which of the following statements by the parent would indicate that further teaching is needed?
1. "Eating raisins and jelly beans is worse for my child's teeth than is drinking sugary soft drinks."
2. "My child loves to kick balls around the yard, so I think I will enroll my child in a soccer camp."
3. "I let my child watch television for a half hour in bed after bedtime when my child has been really good."
4. "My child took a pack of gum from the local store the other day, so I made my child give it back to the manager."

4. The parent of a 7-year-old child telephones the nurse at the child's school and states, "My child has had a stomachache and headache every morning this week. Is there a virus going around the school?" Which of the following responses would be appropriate for the nurse to make at this time? **Select all that apply.**
1. "Has your child ever expressed any concerns about school?"
2. "Does your child seem to feel better once your child has missed school?"
3. "Has your child had any problems with any of the other children in school?"
4. "I would recommend taking your child to the child's primary health-care provider for a complete assessment."
5. "Unless your child is exhibiting additional symptoms like a fever or a rash, I would recommend that the child return to school."

5. The nurse has confirmed that a 9-year-old child understands the concept of conservation when the child makes which of the following statements?
1. "There is the same amount of clay in a snake made out of a ball of clay than there was when it was a ball."
2. "I don't get as tired when I ride up in an elevator than I do when I walk up a whole flight of stairs."
3. "I'd rather read books and play video games than to play baseball or soccer."
4. "I try to get my homework done as soon as I get home from school."

6. A nurse is interviewing a group of 4th grade children. It would be appropriate for the nurse to diagnose the child who made which of the following statements as at "Risk for Altered Coping related to poor psychosocial development"?
1. "My teacher put the picture I drew up on the board."
2. "I made a goal during our soccer game yesterday."
3. "I strike out every time I bat when we play softball in gym class."
4. "My teacher let me read out loud last week and again this week."

7. A child's 3rd grade teacher informs the parents, "Your child's handwriting is quite poor. It is important that your child practice skills that might improve the handwriting." Which of the following activities could the parents encourage the child to perform? **Select all that apply.**
   1. Throw a ball back and forth
   2. Begin to play a musical instrument
   3. Build a model of a favorite structure
   4. Learn a new and popular dance
   5. Draw or paint a colorful picture

8. The nurse working in a local school district is developing the curriculum for a new sex education program for the 2nd grade students. Which of the following content would be appropriate to include in the class?
   1. External genitalia of males and females
   2. List of names of the registered sex offenders living in the school district
   3. Difference between heterosexual contact and homosexual contact
   4. Etiology of human immunodeficiency virus

9. The nurse is providing prehospital admission education to a 9-year-old child and family. Which of the following methods would be most appropriate for the nurse to utilize during the teaching session?
   1. Have the child speak with another child who was recently discharged from the hospital.
   2. Verbally explain to the child what the child will experience while in the hospital.
   3. Play a board game about hospitals and medical procedures with the child.
   4. Take the child on a tour of the pediatric unit, and introduce the child to the nurses.

10. During a well-child visit, the nurse asks the parents and their 11-year-old child about safety issues. In which of the following situations should the nurse provide disease prevention education?
   1. When playing in the sun, the child applies sunscreen every 4 hours.
   2. When riding in the car, the child sits in the backseat in a car restraint system.
   3. When rollerblading on the driveway, the child wears body and head protection.
   4. When baking something in the oven, the child wears 2 oven mitts and is assisted by a parent.

REVIEW ANSWERS

1. ANSWER: 2

Rationale:

1. On average, school-age children gain approximately 5½ lb, or 2½ kg, each year.
2. This statement is correct. On average, school-age boys grow about 2 in., or 5.5 cm, each year.
3. By the age of 12, the majority of children will have 24 to 28 secondary teeth. Twenty is the total number of primary teeth that erupt.
4. A 12-year-old child's heart rate will average between 60 and 100 bpm.

TEST-TAKING TIP: If the child had been a 12-year-old girl, the growth figures may have been quite different because girls often experience their pubertal growth spurts when they are 11 or 12.
Content Area: *Child Health*
Integrated Processes: *Nursing Process: Assessment*
Client Need: *Health Promotion and Maintenance: Health Screening*
Cognitive Level: *Application*

2. ANSWER: 1

Rationale:

1. This statement is correct. An appropriate patient-care goal is that the child will brush his or her teeth using a fluoride toothpaste at least twice each day.
2. The first dose of the meningococcal vaccine should be administered at either 11 or 12 years of age.
3. Children should be proficient swimmers by the time they reach 10 years of age.
4. Bicycles should be ridden with traffic on the right-hand side of the road.

TEST-TAKING TIP: Because the secondary teeth must support the child throughout the child's life, it is critically important for the child to perform proper dental care each day.
Content Area: *Child Health*
Integrated Processes: *Nursing Process: Planning*
Client Need: *Health Promotion and Maintenance: Health Promotion/Disease Prevention*
Cognitive Level: *Application*

3. ANSWER: 3

Rationale:

1. This statement is correct. Eating raisins and jelly beans is worse for a child's teeth than is drinking sugary soft drinks.
2. This is an appropriate statement for the parent to make. Soccer may be an excellent activity for this child.
3. This parent needs further education. If a child is unable to go directly to sleep, he or she should be encouraged to read in bed rather than to engage in such activities as watching television, playing video games, and playing on the computer.
4. Having a child return a stolen item to the person from whom it was stolen is an excellent form of discipline.

TEST-TAKING TIP: School-age children need 9 to 12 hours of sleep each night. They also need and respond well to consistent rules. In addition, solitary reading is an excellent means of increasing one's vocabulary and knowledge. The best action for a parent to make when a child is having difficulty falling asleep is to encourage the child to read in bed until he or she is able to sleep.
Content Area: *Child Health*
Integrated Processes: *Nursing Process: Evaluation*
Client Need: *Health Promotion and Maintenance: Health Promotion/Disease Prevention*
Cognitive Level: *Application*

4. ANSWER: 1, 2, 3, and 5

Rationale:

1. "Has your child ever expressed any concerns about school?" would be an appropriate question to ask.
2. "Does your child seem to feel better once your child has missed school?" would be an appropriate question to ask.
3. "Has your child had any problems with any of the other children in school?" would be an appropriate question to ask.
4. This would not be appropriate because it is unlikely that this child is suffering from a serious illness. Unless the preceding questions are all answered in the affirmative, the child will likely not need a complete physical assessment.
5. This would be an appropriate statement for the nurse to make.

TEST-TAKING TIP: School refusal is a relatively common problem of the school-age period. The symptoms that the child exhibits are vague and subjective and frequently disappear once the parent permits the child to remain at home for the day.
Content Area: *Pediatrics—School Age*
Integrated Processes: *Nursing Process: Implementation*
Client Need: *Health Promotion and Maintenance: Health Promotion/Disease Prevention*
Cognitive Level: *Application*

5. ANSWER: 1

Rationale:

1. This statement confirms that the child understands the concept of conservation.
2. This statement is unrelated to the concept of conservation.
3. This statement is unrelated to the concept of conservation.
4. This statement is unrelated to the concept of conservation.

TEST-TAKING TIP: A child understands the concept of conservation when he or she understands that when an object changes shape, it retains the properties that it had before its shape was changed.
Content Area: *Pediatrics—School Age*
Integrated Processes: *Nursing Process: Evaluation*
Client Need: *Health Promotion and Maintenance: Developmental Stages and Transitions*
Cognitive Level: *Application*

6. ANSWER: 3

Rationale:

1. This child is exhibiting positive psychosocial development.
2. This child is exhibiting positive psychosocial development.
3. **This child may be at risk of poor psychosocial development.**
4. This child is exhibiting positive psychosocial development.

TEST-TAKING TIP: The Eriksonian stage of the school-age period is called industry versus inferiority. Children try hard to succeed, but when they repeatedly are unable to achieve what they consider to be a successful result, they may develop a feeling of inferiority. It is important to note that it is a rare child who is successful in all that he or she endeavors. Rather, he or she should feel capable in at least one aspect of life. Parents who praise their children's achievements are fostering a belief in their children that if they work hard, they will perform their best.

Content Area: *Pediatrics—School Age*
Integrated Processes: *Nursing Process: Analysis*
Client Need: *Health Promotion and Maintenance: Developmental Stages and Transitions*
Cognitive Level: *Application*

7. ANSWER: 2, 3, and 5

Rationale:

1. Throwing a ball back and forth is a gross motor skill.
2. **Playing a musical instrument is a fine motor skill.**
3. **Building a model is a fine motor skill.**
4. Learning a new and popular dance is a gross motor skill.
5. **Drawing and painting are fine motor skills.**

TEST-TAKING TIP: Handwriting is a fine motor skill. To improve the handwriting, it would be appropriate for the child to be encouraged to practice other fine motor skills, including playing a musical instrument, building a model, and/or creating a piece of studio art.

Content Area: *Pediatrics—School Age*
Integrated Processes: *Nursing Process: Implementation*
Client Need: *Health Promotion and Maintenance: Developmental Stages and Transitions*
Cognitive Level: *Application*

8. ANSWER: 1

Rationale:

1. **External genitalia of males and females would be appropriate to include in the content of a sex education class for second-grade students.**
2. It would be inappropriate to include a list of names of the registered sex offenders living in the school district in a sex education class for second grade students.
3. It would be inappropriate to include the difference between heterosexual contact and homosexual contact in a sex education class for second grade students.
4. It would be inappropriate to include the etiology of HIV in a sex education class for second grade students.

TEST-TAKING TIP: Including sex education in young children's school curriculum is a controversial subject. If it is decided to include it in the children's education, a recommendation has been made regarding the content that should be included at each age level (*National Sexual Education Standards,* 2012).

Content Area: *Pediatrics—School Age*
Integrated Processes: *Nursing Process: Implementation*
Client Need: *Health Promotion and Maintenance: Developmental Stages and Transitions*
Cognitive Level: *Application*

9. ANSWER: 4

Rationale:

1. Having the child speak with another child who was recently discharged from the hospital is not the best option.
2. Verbally explaining to the child what the child will experience while in the hospital is not the best option.
3. Playing a board game about hospitals and medical procedures with the child is not the best option.
4. **It would be best to take the child on a tour of the pediatric unit and introduce the child to the nurses.**

TEST-TAKING TIP: School-age children are in Piaget's stage of concrete operations. They learn best by experiencing the information to be learned directly. Taking the child on a tour of the hospital would provide the child with that direct experience.

Content Area: *Pediatrics—School Age; Teaching/Learning*
Integrated Processes: *Nursing Process: Implementation*
Client Need: *Health Promotion and Maintenance: Developmental Stages and Transitions*
Cognitive Level: *Analysis*

10. ANSWER: 1

Rationale:

1. **When playing in the sun, the child should apply sunscreen at least every 2 hours.**
2. This statement is correct. When riding in the car, the child should sit in the backseat in a car restraint system.
3. This statement is correct. When rollerblading on the driveway, the child should wear body and head protection.
4. This statement is correct. When baking something in the oven, the child should wear two oven mitts and should be assisted by a parent.

TEST-TAKING TIP: By 11 years of age, children are performing many sophisticated skills independently. This independence places the children at risk for injury. The children should be reminded to apply sunscreen at least every 2 hours while playing in the sun.

Content Area: *Child Health*
Integrated Processes: *Nursing Process: Evaluation*
Client Need: *Health Promotion and Maintenance: Health Promotion/Disease Prevention*
Cognitive Level: *Application*

Chapter 6

Normal Growth and Development: Adolescence

KEY TERMS

Tanner scale—A scale of physical maturity from prepuberty to adult stages.

I. Description

Adolescence is the final growth and development stage of childhood. It is a transition period between dependency and self-sufficiency. Many teenagers move from being totally dependent on their parents financially to earning an income while working after school or during summer breaks. With money comes the ability to make adult-like decisions regarding where and how to spend that money. Many adolescents acquire independence after successfully passing a driving test. The ability to drive enables teenagers to determine where they wish to go and enables them to transport themselves to that location. In addition, the teen years are the time when most adolescents develop close relationships with members of the opposite sex, necessitating them to make decisions regarding how intimate those relationships will become.

II. Normal Growth

A. Biological development: outside of the infancy period, puberty is the most dramatic growth period of childhood. In a relatively brief period, males' and females' bodies change from the nubile appearance of the child to the mature appearance of the adult.
   1. Pubertal changes often begin during the latter school-age years.
      a. Growth spurt begins about 2 years earlier in girls than boys.
         i. Stimulated by hormonal secretions.
            (1) Estrogen in girls.
            (2) Testosterone in boys.
      b. Ends about 2 years after menarche in girls and between the ages of 18 and 20 in boys.
      c. Teens will attain their adult height during adolescence.
         i. That height is determined by a combination of many factors, including genetics, nutritional intake, and activity level.
   2. Bodily changes: the **Tanner scale** depicts the sequential development of male and female secondary sex characteristics (Figs. 6.1–6.3). Biological development is individualized but, in general, Tanner stage 1 is seen in young children and is characterized by the absence of secondary

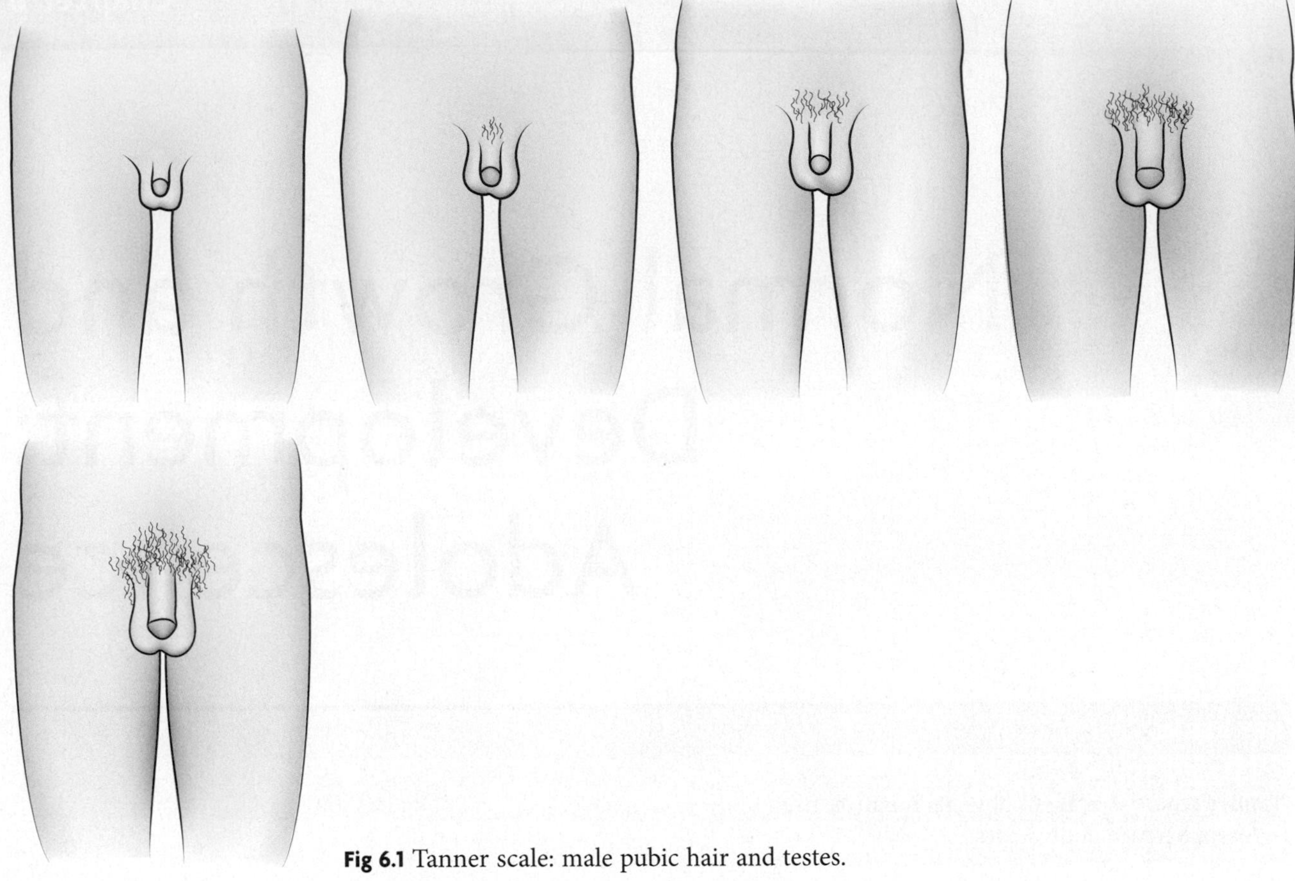

Fig 6.1 Tanner scale: male pubic hair and testes.

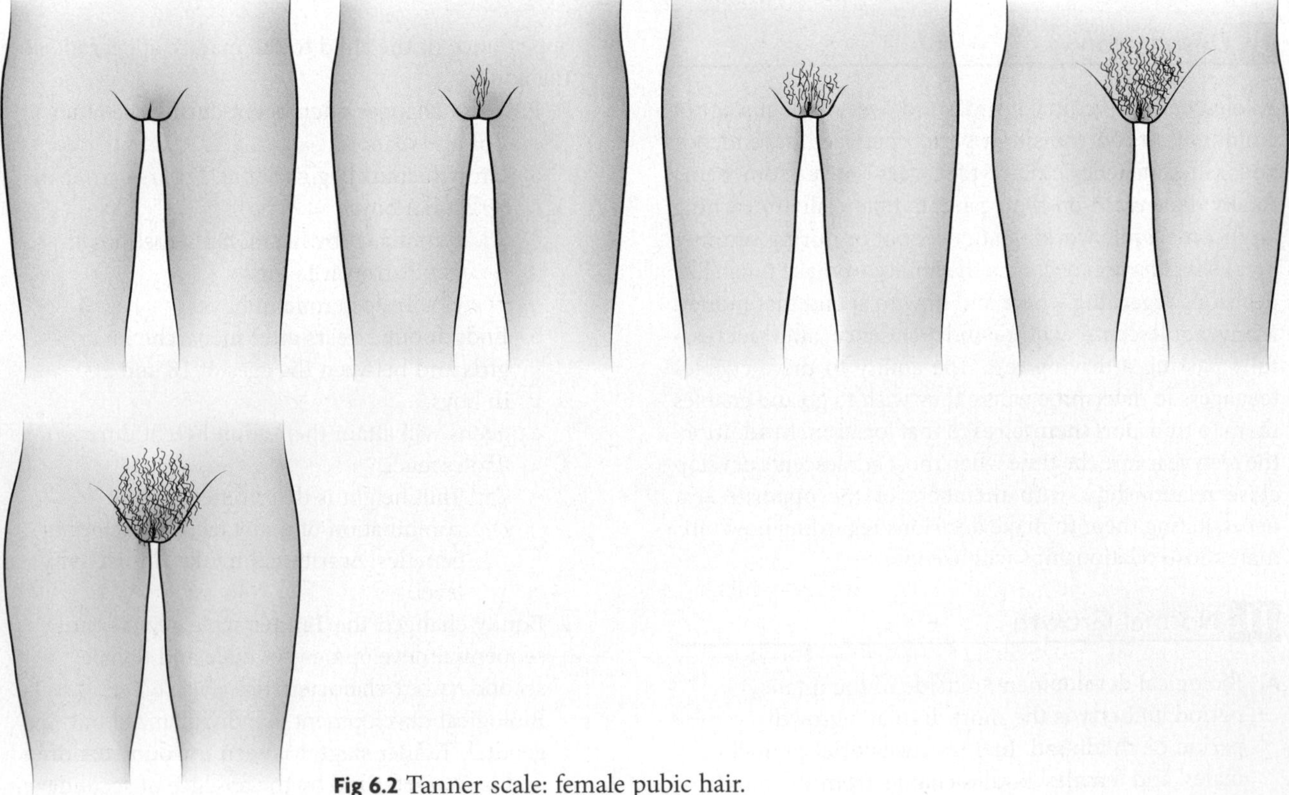

Fig 6.2 Tanner scale: female pubic hair.

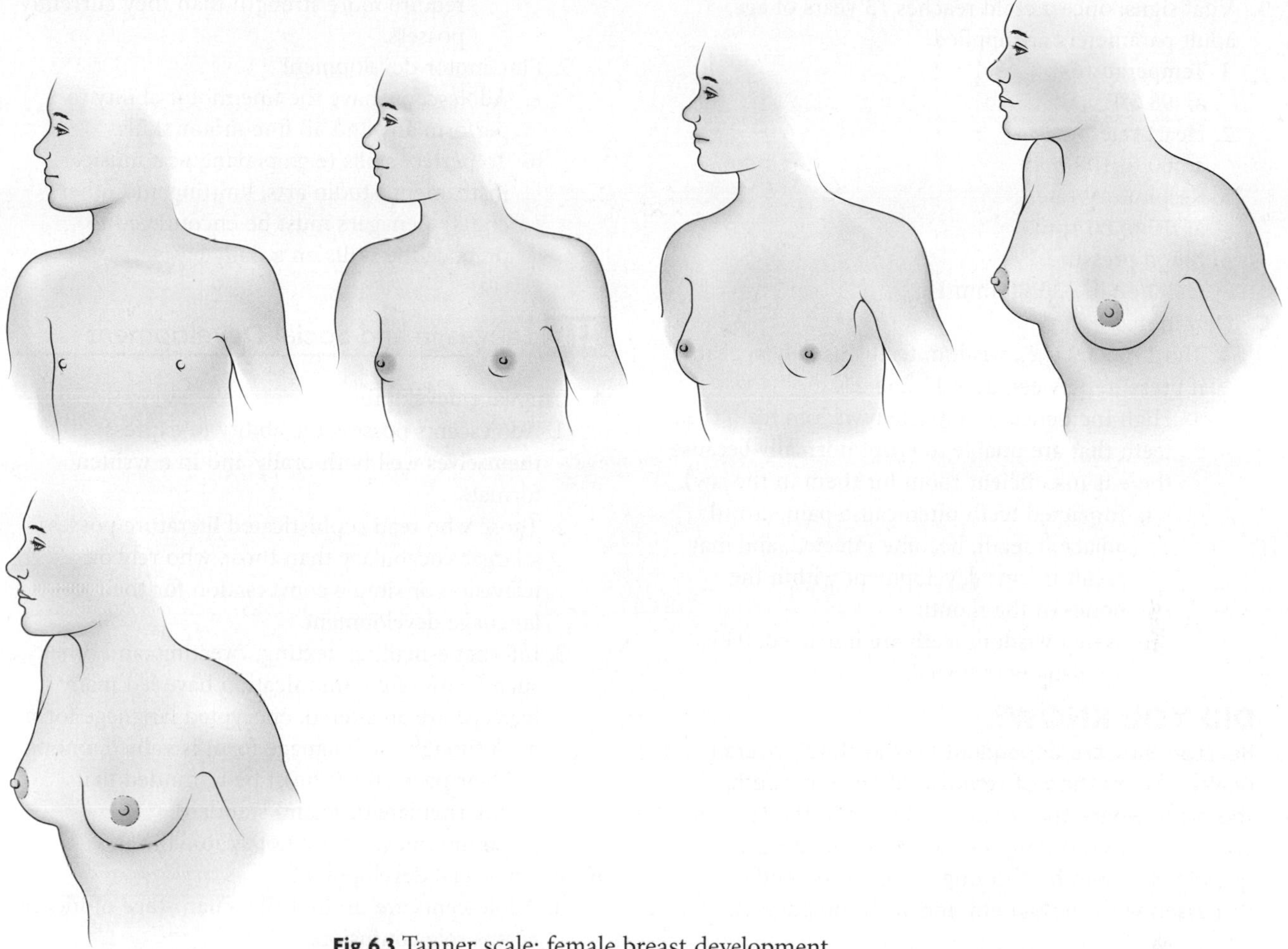

Fig 6.3 Tanner scale: female breast development.

sex characteristics. In the last year or two of the school-age period, many children will enter Tanner stage 2 and, as the child becomes more mature, he or she progresses through the remaining Tanner stages.

a. Stage 1: the pre-pubertal stage.
b. Stage 2:
    i. Females begin to exhibit breast budding.
    ii. Males.
        (1) Testicular enlargement begins.
        (2) In addition, breast enlargement may occur.
            (a) Boys must be advised that the breast changes will recede.
c. Stages 3 to 5:
    i. Females: stage 5 culminates with ovulation and menarche.
        (1) Most females grow up to 2 inches after menarche.
    ii. Males.
        (1) Stages 3 to 4: occur at the same time that boys' voices change.
        (2) Stage 5: culminates with appearance of facial hair and ejaculation (wet dreams).

3. Growth charts (see Appendix B).
    a. Accelerated height and weight changes are depicted on growth charts.
    b. Teens usually maintain the same growth patterns that they established when they were younger.
4. BMI assessments: growth charts (see Appendix B).
    a. The same BMI criteria are employed throughout the adolescent period as are employed for younger children.
        i. BMI less than 5%: child is defined as underweight.
        ii. BMI 5% to 85%: healthy weight for the child.
        iii. BMI greater than 85%: child is defined as overweight.
        iv. BMI greater than 95%: child is defined as obese.

B. Vital signs: once a child reaches 13 years of age, adult parameters are applied.
  1. Temperature.
    a. 98.6°F.
  2. Heart rate.
    a. 60 to 100 bpm.
  3. Respiratory rate.
    a. 15 to 20 rpm.
  4. Blood pressure.
    a. 90/60 to 120/80 mm Hg.

C. Dentition.
  1. Third molars (i.e., wisdom teeth) usually appear, if present, between ages 17 and 21.
    a. High incidence of impacted wisdom teeth (i.e., teeth that are unable to erupt normally because there is insufficient room for them in the jaw).
      i. Impacted teeth often cause pain, crowd adjacent teeth, become infected, and may result in cyst development within the bones of the mouth.
      ii. When wisdom teeth are impacted, they are usually removed.

DID YOU KNOW?

Because they are dependent on the child's overall health, the method of removal of wisdom teeth, the place where the removal will occur, the type of anesthesia used during the extraction, and other questions should be thoroughly reviewed and discussed with the patient and with the parents.

    b. Even when wisdom teeth erupt normally, there is a high incidence of dental caries in the teeth because of the difficulty in reaching the area with a toothbrush.
  2. Orthodontic work may continue from the school-age period.
  3. Parent/teen education.
    a. Parents and teens must be reminded that dental hygiene continues to be important.
    b. When adolescents participate in contact sports, they and their parents must be advised to have the teens' teeth protected by wearing a well-fitting mouth guard.

D. Senses.
  1. All senses are fully developed.

E. Motor development.
  1. Gross motor development.
    a. With the acquisition of increased muscle mass, especially in young men, adolescents are able to perform virtually all gross motor skills, including playing contact sports.
      i. Teens must be monitored carefully because they are at high risk for soft tissue and orthopedic injuries when they engage in repetitive actions and/or activities that require more strength than they currently possess.
  2. Fine motor development.
    a. Adolescents have the fine motor ability to perform any and all fine motor skills.
    b. To perfect skills (e.g., playing of a musical instrument, studio arts, knitting and other crafts) teenagers must be encouraged to practice the skills on a daily basis.

III. Language and Social Development

A. Language development.
  1. Adolescents possess the ability to express themselves well both orally and in a written format.
  2. Those who read sophisticated literature possess a larger vocabulary than those who rely on television or simple conversation for their language development.
  3. Internet e-mailing, texting, tweeting, and other such forms of communication have led many teens to use an altered, encrypted language form.
    a. Although the language form is valued among their peers, teens must be reminded that Internet language and standard communication are not synonymous.

B. Psychosocial development.
  1. Adolescents are in the Eriksonian stage of identity versus role confusion.
    a. During this stage, it is expected that teenagers will develop a true sense of themselves as separate and independent from people such as friends and parents.
      i. Peers are important in the process (e.g., adolescents compare and contrast themselves to their peers).
      ii. Body image is of particular import to teenagers.
    b. The adolescent period often is divided into three phases.
      i. Early adolescence: period of conformity.
        (1) When conformity with peers is a goal:
          (a) Young teens do such things as dress alike and wear their hair in similar styles.

! It can be traumatic for teens who feel that they are unable to conform because they believe that everyone is looking at them and judging them. An inability to conform may be related to a lack of money to purchase the latest style clothes, an inability to style one's hair like his or her friends' hair, or as significant as the inability of a gay teen to be attracted to the opposite sex.

ii. Middle adolescence: period of challenge.
(1) Teens most frequently challenge parental authority by challenging rules and curfews.
(2) This is the period when risk taking most frequently occurs.
(3) Parents often complain that their teens are lazy and unfocused during this period.
iii. Later adolescence: period of individuality.
(1) Begin to show their individuality.
(2) Successful completion of this phase is contingent on the ability to learn from experiences as a means of transitioning into an emotionally and financially independent adult.

2. Potential problems can arise during the teen years if an adolescent makes one or more poor choices (e.g., drug use, alcohol use, sexual encounters).
   a. Teens often take risks because they live in the moment, believing that "nothing can happen to me."
3. Relationships.
   a. Peers are important, but parents still are the most important people in adolescents' lives.
      i. Parents must be reminded of their influence, of the importance of maintaining the parental role, and of providing positive role modeling.
   b. This is a time for teens to develop one-on-one relationships.
      i. Often engage in serial relationships as a means of learning about which type of person he or she relates with the best.
      ii. Because heterosexuality is the norm, this can be a difficult time for adolescents who do not view themselves as heterosexual.
         (1) Depending on family and/or community acceptance, gay, lesbian, bisexual, and transsexual teens may be abused, shunned, and/or ridiculed.

C. Cognitive development.
1. Adolescence is defined by Piaget's stage of formal operations.
   a. Adolescents are capable of:
      i. Abstract thinking and logical reasoning.
      ii. Developing and analyzing new ideas.
   b. By the end of this period, adolescents are looking toward and planning for the future.
2. It is important to note that the brain is still vulnerable to injury because it is continuing to develop during this period, for example:
   a. Alcohol and illicit drug use can adversely affect brain development.
   b. Accidents and sports injuries can result in severe trauma to the brain.
3. Parent/teen education.
   a. Risk-taking behavior.
      i. Even though teens are becoming future thinkers, they are still unable to envision themselves as vulnerable.

MAKING THE CONNECTION

Often, the best way to dissuade teens from engaging in potentially destructive behavior is to remind them of the immediate consequences of their behavior. For example, to deter them from:

- Smoking, advise them that their breath will smell or that their teeth will stain.
- Drinking, remind them of the consequences of the behavior (e.g., the parent will take away their car keys).
- Using drugs, advise them that they will be banned from all extracurricular activities by the school authorities.

D. Moral development.
1. Although many teens remain in level II, conventional morality, during the adolescent period, many move into the early stage of postconventional morality, which is labeled by Kohlberg as the social contract.
   a. During this stage, teens understand and acknowledge that laws and rules are meant to protect everyone.
   b. But they also believe that challenging rules is acceptable, if there is a logical reason to do so.
      i. What a teen may determine as a logical reason is often, however, inconsistent with the beliefs of his or her parents.
2. Parent education.
   a. Parents must be strongly encouraged to practice what they preach.

DID YOU KNOW?

Adults must remember that teens are watching them and are noting the conflicts in people's behaviors. For example, a teen might think, "Why should I follow the rules when my parents cheat on their taxes?" or "when my parent has an affair?" or "when adults drink while driving?"

IV. Nursing Considerations: Health Promotion/Parent Education

A. Nutrition: adolescents consume much of their food with friends rather than with family. As a result, it becomes more and more difficult for parents to control their children's dietary intake.

1. Dietary needs do increase along with rapid growth and development.
   a. To promote healthy bone growth, teens have increased vitamin D and calcium needs.
      i. Ideally, they should consume at least three dairy servings each day.
   b. To maintain adequate iron supplies, especially in young women who are beginning to menstruate, teens have increased iron and folic acid needs.
      i. Ideally, foods high in iron and a minimum of 400 mcg of folic acid should be consumed each day.
   c. To maintain growth, caloric needs markedly increase to a recommended:
      i. 1600 to 1800 calories for adolescent girls.
      ii. 1800 to 2200 calories for adolescent boys.
2. Adolescents may try fad diets and/or develop poor eating habits, especially if their peer group eats poorly.
   a. Although not inherently unhealthy, vegetarian and vegan diets, which are common among adolescents, if not followed appropriately, can result in nutritional deficits.
   b. Teens who become vegetarians must be educated regarding the importance of eating a variety of foods in order to consume complete proteins.
      i. Ovolactovegetarians will likely meet their nutritional needs, including their calcium and protein needs.
      ii. Vegan dieters may consume insufficient quantities of calcium and proteins as well as essential vitamins (e.g., vitamin B_{12}).
   c. Teens, especially young women, frequently engage in weight-loss dieting in order to achieve an "ideal" figure (e.g., they want to look like a favorite model or movie star).
      i. Dieting may result in eating disorders when dieting becomes an obsession (see Chapter 24, "Nursing Care of the Child With Psychosocial Disorders").
   d. Energy drinks and soda are popular among many teens.
      i. These drinks are high in caffeine, sugar, and empty calories.
   e. Fast foods, including hamburgers, pizza, and french fries.
      i. Fast foods tend to be high in fat, cholesterol, and sodium.
3. It is especially difficult for teens with chronic illnesses (e.g., diabetes, phenylketonuria, celiac disease) to follow their diet restrictions.
4. Parent/adolescent education.
   a. Basic dietary information should be included in health classes.
      i. Especially important for students engaged in energy-draining sports, for young women who are menstruating, and for those following special diets.
   b. Keep the refrigerator and cupboards stocked with healthy, appealing snack foods (e.g., fruits, fresh vegetables, granola bars).
   c. Sell high-quality foods during lunch periods and in commercial machines for after-school snacks in all middle and high schools.
   d. Suggest that teens consume the more nourishing foods found at fast food restaurants, for example:
      i. In place of a soda, the teen may opt for a milk shake.
      ii. In place of a plain hamburger, the teen may opt for a cheeseburger with lettuce and tomato.
      iii. In addition to a hamburger, the teen may opt to add a side salad.

B. Sleep.

1. With the rapid growth and development of adolescence, teenagers need a great deal of sleep.
   a. Many teenagers are sleep deprived because of the time needed to complete their school requirements and to engage in their extracurricular, social, and other activities.
2. Teenagers' sleep patterns can be challenging for parents as well as for school officials.
   a. On average, teens should sleep at least 8 hours each night, but in reality, their sleep varies markedly.
      i. They often stay up late on school nights but must arise early during the school week.
         (1) Teachers often complain that students are dozing during many of their classes.
   b. To catch up on their sleep, teens often sleep for long hours on weekends when parents may expect them to participate in family activities.
3. Sleep is essential for learning, but school schedules often conflict with the normal rhythms of adolescence (i.e., most school days begin early in the morning, often by 7:30 a.m., when teens ideally should still be sleeping).
4. Parent/adolescent education.
   a. Sleep is essential for health, and a sleep pattern must be developed that will meet the teen's needs.
   b. Some school systems are reviewing the possibility of altering their schedules in order to better meet the needs of the students.

c. Parents should be encouraged to allow their teenagers to "sleep in" on the weekends in order to recoup sleep lost during the school week.

C. Physical activity.
1. Adolescence is an excellent time for children to engage in physical activities that they may continue to pursue throughout their lives, for example:
   a. Team sports, such as baseball and basketball.
   b. Swimming.
   c. Golf.
   d. Tennis.
2. Parent/adolescent education.
   a. Adolescents and parents must be reminded of the importance of seeking medical attention whenever an injury occurs.

V. Nursing Considerations: Disease Prevention/Parent Education

A. Safety.
1. Car safety.
   a. As a driver.
      i. Even if not required by law, all teens should pass a driver's education program as a means of encouraging safe driving practices.
      ii. Seat belts should be worn at all times.
      iii. It is important to note that:
         (1) The younger the driver, the more high risk the teen is of having a car accident.
         (2) Whenever there is a passenger in the car with an adolescent, the incidence of accidents rises.
   b. As a passenger.
      i. Teens must be taught to refrain from distracting the driver.
      ii. Again, safety restraints are important.
   c. Parent/adolescent education.
      i. If the teen is under the influence of alcohol or drugs, the child should know that the parent would be willing to pick the child up.
         (1) This is not the time to teach the teen a lesson. The child must be transported home safely.
         (2) Once the child is sober and both the child and parents are in a better state of mind, a discussion of the child's behavior must take place.
2. Poisonings: see Chapter 24, "Nursing Care of the Child With Psychosocial Disorders."
   a. During adolescence, accidental poisonings are replaced by purposeful ingestion of poisons (i.e., alcohol, illicit drugs, prescription medications).
3. Swimming and diving accidents.
   a. Often occur when alcohol or drugs have been ingested.
   b. May occur when teens swim in locations where there is no lifeguard.
   c. Diving into shallow places can result in severe head and neck trauma.
   d. Parent/adolescent education.
      i. Teens must repeatedly be forewarned regarding the perils of swimming and/or diving in places where there is no supervision.
      ii. Teens must be counseled that engaging in water play when under the influence of substances is especially dangerous.
4. Sun exposure.
   a. Tanning beds and tanning studios are quite popular among adolescents because many teens believe that a tan improves one's appearance.
   b. Parent/adolescent education.
      i. Frequent application of sunscreen while swimming or sunbathing must strongly be encouraged.
      ii. Teens must be counseled regarding the dangers of tanning beds and tanning studios.
5. Personal injury.
   a. Violence is one of the leading causes of death in teens.
   b. The media, including movies, television, and video games, expose teens to a great deal of violence, and that violence is often portrayed as transient.
   c. Gang membership, which increases markedly during the teen years, places adolescents in situations that escalate the likelihood of their being victims of violence.
   d. Suicide is especially prevalent in the teen population (see Chapter 24, "Nursing Care of the Child With Psychosocial Disorders.")
   e. Parent/adolescent education.
      i. Firearms must be locked up, with ammunition locked in a separate location, to prevent teens from accessing their parents' weapons.
      ii. Peer mediation programs are an important method of educating teens how to control their behavior and prevent violent interactions.

iii. Parents and educators must be aware of behaviors that place children at high risk of personal injury.

B. Tattoos (tats) and piercings: tats and piercings are popular among adolescents.

1. Piercings.
   a. Teens are having many locations of their bodies pierced, including the clitoris, breast, nipple, penis, and scrotum.
   b. If performed under unsanitary conditions, the potential exists for the teen to contract blood-borne diseases and infections.
   c. Unlike tattoos, piercings are removable.
   d. Parent/adolescent education.
      i. Piercings should be performed only by a reputable practitioner who uses sterile equipment.
      ii. Adolescents must be advised that piercings take a long time to heal.
         (1) Teen must be taught how to cleanse the piercing using aseptic techniques.
2. Tats: the forced injection of ink into the skin via a needle.
   a. Teens are tattooing their bodies in multiple locations.
   b. There are many possible complications that are associated with tattoos, including infections, allergies to the dyes, granulomas developing at the site of the tattoos, and scarring.
   c. Tats are impossible to remove completely, even with new laser techniques.
      i. The laser therapy, as well as the tattooing procedure, can be very painful.
   d. If the teen gains or loses weight, the shape of the tat will change.
   e. Parent/adolescent education.
      i. Tattooing should be performed only by a reputable practitioner who uses sterile equipment.
      ii. It is usually required that a person must wait a minimum of 1 year to donate blood after being tattooed.
      iii. If iron oxide is used as a tattooing agent, it can cause serious injury during an MRI.

C. Sexual activity: a full discussion of reproductive health is beyond the scope of this book. Please refer to a text on women's health and maternity for a comprehensive discussion of the topic.

1. The incidence of sexual activity in adolescents is on the decline but is still an important health issue.
2. Parent/adolescent education.
   a. By adolescence, children must receive education regarding their own bodily functions and on reproduction.
   b. Adolescents must be taught regarding all aspects of sexual health, including:
      i. Safe sex practices, including the use of infection control measures.
      ii. Contraceptive choices.
      iii. Hazards of oral and rectal intercourse as well as genital penetration.
   c. All adolescents should be encouraged to receive the full three-dose vaccination series to prevent the transmission of human papillomavirus.

D. Adolescent behavior and discipline.

1. Teens are risk takers, and they will misbehave, but even adolescents expect to have limits placed on their behavior.
2. Disciplinary practices must be employed in light of the fact that teens are developing a sense of morality as well as their independence.
3. Parents, as well as all other adults who are taking responsibility for teens' behaviors, must continually counsel teens about the potential consequences of poor choices.
   a. One of the best places to have in-depth discussions with teens is while driving in a car.
      i. Teens feel less threatened because the discussion is not taking place face to face. Rather, both the adult and the teen are facing forward.
      ii. Teen is unable to leave the discussion because he or she is in a moving automobile.
   b. Adults must advise teens that there will be consequences if they misbehave.
      i. But, only realistic and enforceable punishments should be established, for example:
         (1) Realistic and enforceable punishments: the teen may not drive the car for 1 week or may not go to the party on Friday night.
         (2) Unrealistic and punitive punishments: the teen is grounded for the rest of the year or never allowed to associate with a friend again.
   c. One expert on adolescent behavior, Michael Nerney (2014), often includes an excellent framework for monitoring teenagers' behavior called the five A's of parenting teens into his lectures (Box 6.1).

E. Health maintenance. (See "Recommendations for Pediatric Preventive Health Care" for a complete list of procedures.)

Box 6.1 The Five A's of Parenting Teens

Aware: parents must know where their child is at all times.
Parents must know what the teen is planning to do and where the teen will be (e.g., movie, dance). The teen should be expected to call in periodically, especially whenever he or she is moving to a new location.

Alert to change: parents must attend to any significant changes in their child.
Parents must monitor their child for behavioral changes that may indicate that they are engaging in risk-taking behavior, for example, the child:

- *Wears sunglasses all the time.*
- *Wears hats covering his or her eyes.*
- *Is completely disrespectful when speaking to his or her parents.*
- *Stops doing homework.*
- *Stops participating in extracurricular activities.*
- *Hangs out with a new group, but he or she refuses to let the parents meet them.*
- *Locks his or her bedroom door.*

Awake: parents must have meaningful interchanges with their child.
Parents should always meet and have a short conversation with their child when the child returns home after a date or another activity. During the conversation, the parent can determine whether the child is slurring his or her words, the child's breath smells like alcohol, the child's pupils are dilated, or other signs of substance abuse are present.

Assertive: parents must fulfill the parenting role, not act as a buddy to their child.
Parents should develop rules that the child must follow and stick to them. There should be realistic consequences for infractions, and parents must inform the child of those consequences. If the rules have been violated, once the child has slept and is coherent, advise them that the consequence will be applied.

Affirmation: parents must communicate their love for their child.
Even when children misbehave, they must be told that they are still loved and valued. Parents must let their child know that it is the behavior that is a problem and not the child. It is essential that children know that their parents are still there for them.

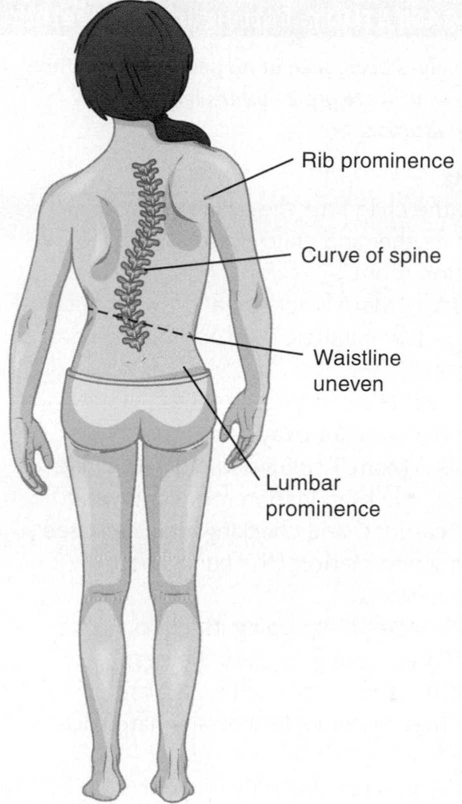

Fig 6.4 Scoliosis assessment.

1. Standard yearly lab testing.
   a. CBC, urinalysis, vitals.
   b. Cholesterol and tuberculosis testing, if indicated.
2. Yearly hearing and vision testing.
   a. Should be counseled regarding potential for hearing damage from loud music (e.g., from MP3 players, radio speakers, concerts).
3. Scoliosis screening (Fig. 6.4).
4. Teens must be asked whether or not they are sexually active.
   a. If a teen is sexually active, he or she should be screened for sexually transmitted infections, and females should have Pap or HPV smears.
5. Stress and depression assessments.
   i. Because depression and suicide are so prevalent in the teen population, they should be routinely assessed for signs of stress and/or depression.

F. Immunizations.
1. Vaccinations recommended to be administered between 13 and 18 years of age.
   a. Throughout childhood: yearly influenza vaccines.
   b. Second dosage of meningococcal vaccine as long as 8 weeks have passed from the first dosage.
2. Any recommended vaccines that the child has yet to receive should be administered per the Advisory Committee on Immunization Practices' catch-up vaccine schedule.

CASE STUDY: Putting It All Together

A 13-year-old male is being seen at his pediatrician's office for a camp physical. There are 2 months left of school before summer vacation.

Subjective Data

- Nurse calls the child into the examining room.
  - Both the mother and child rise to enter the examination room.
  - Nurse states, "Mom, your son and I will go it alone for a few minutes. I will ask you to come in a little later."
  - Mother looks at her son and replies, "Honey, are you sure that you are okay?"
  - Son replies, "Mom, I'm 13 years old. I'll be fine."
- After entering the examination room and while weighing, measuring, and checking vital signs (see the following information), the nurse and the patient converse.
  - Nurse: "How are things going in school?"
  - Patient: "Okay. I like gym class the best."
  - Nurse: "What about your other classes?"
  - Patient: "They're dumb. I especially hate social studies."
  - Nurse: "Are you keeping up with your homework?"
  - Patient: "Yeah, sometimes, but most times I blow it off. Mom and Dad get pretty mad when I do."
  - Nurse: "What happens when you don't do well in school?"
  - Patient: "Oh. I get yelled at, but that's about it."
  - Nurse: "What do you do instead of your homework?"
  - Patient: "I have the BEST video games ever. I either play with them or I watch TV. Either way, I'm having a lot more fun than learning about science or some other dumb subject."

Objective Data

Nursing Assessments

- Weight 98 lb: 50th percentile
- Height 61.5 in.: 50th percentile

Vital Signs	
Blood pressure:	100/60 mm Hg
Temperature:	98.6°F
Heart rate:	90 bpm
Respiratory rate:	18 rpm

Physical examination by primary health-care practitioner: WNL. After physical examination is complete, mother is escorted into examination room with child, primary health-care provider, and nurse.

- Primary health-care provider asks, "Your son's examination went very well. He is a healthy young man. Do you have any concerns about your child's health?"
- Mother replies, "No, he seems like a normal 13-year-old boy. Growing a lot and eating a lot."
- Nurse states, "He tells me that he hasn't been doing his homework like he should."
- Mother replies, "I know. We keep telling him that he has to do better in school or he won't be able to go to camp this summer."
- Nurse states, "It sounds like he often plays video games or watches TV when he should be doing his homework."
- Mother replies, "He does enjoy those things."
- Nurse states, "Have you considered requiring your son to complete his homework before he is allowed to watch TV or play the games? That may be a way to encourage him to do better in school. Camp is a long way away. It's hard to think about that when it is 2 months away."
- Mother replies, "That might work. We can try it."

Health-Care Provider's Orders

- Normal physical examination
- Child is physically able to attend camp

CASE STUDY: Putting It All Together *cont'd*

Case Study Questions

A. What *subjective* assessments indicate that the client is experiencing a health alteration?

1. ______________________________
2. ______________________________
3. ______________________________

B. What *objective* assessments indicate that the client is experiencing a health alteration?

1. ______________________________
2. ______________________________
3. ______________________________

C. After analyzing the data that has been collected, what **primary** nursing diagnosis should the nurse assign to this client?

1. ______________________________

D. What interventions should the nurse plan and/or implement to meet this child's and his family's needs?

1. ______________________________
2. ______________________________
3. ______________________________
4. ______________________________

E. What client outcomes should the nurse evaluate regarding the effectiveness of the nursing interventions?

1. ______________________________

F. What physiological characteristics should the child exhibit before leaving the clinic?

1. ______________________________

REVIEW QUESTIONS

1. A 13-year-old girl, 61 inches tall, is seen for a yearly checkup. She tells the nurse, "I'm the shortest one of my friends. Do you think that I'll grow anymore?" In which of the following situations is it most likely that the young woman will continue to grow?
   1. Her growth spurt began when she was 9 years old.
   2. She started to menstruate 3 months earlier.
   3. She is at the 75th percentile for weight.
   4. Her parents are both average for height and weight.

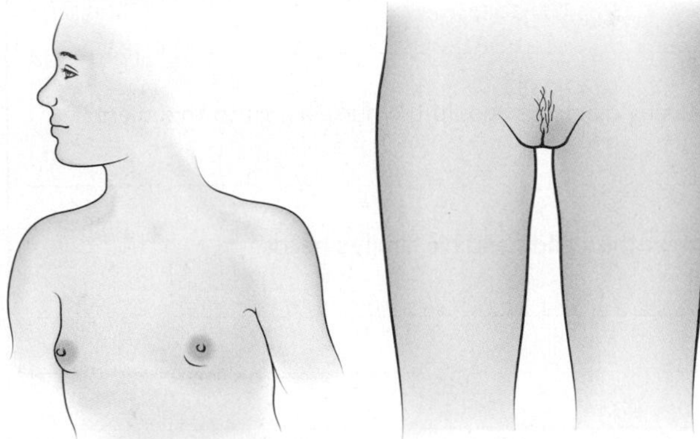

2. A nurse, who is performing the preliminary physical examination of a female patient, notes the physical changes shown in the figures above. The nurse should interview the child about which of the following information at this time? The young woman's:
   1. Readiness for menstruation to begin.
   2. Sexual activity.
   3. Menstrual cycle.
   4. Feelings about her bodily changes.

3. A nurse is providing anticipatory guidance to a young man who is at Tanner stage 2. Which of the following information should the nurse discuss with the young man?
   1. Voice changes
   2. Sexually transmitted infections
   3. Condom use
   4. Nocturnal emissions

4. An 18-year-old, who is being seen for a routine dental examination, is told that 2 wisdom teeth are impacted. Which of the following complications should the adolescent and his parents be advised may develop? **Select all that apply.**
   1. Pain
   2. Cysts
   3. Infections
   4. Tooth misalignment
   5. Mandibular osteopenia

5. To promote language development in the adolescent, parents, educators, and health-care professionals should encourage teenagers to perform which of the following activities?
   1. Surf the Internet
   2. Read a variety of literature
   3. Engage in public speaking
   4. Write letters

6. A school nurse determines that a group of young women is in early adolescence based on which of the following observations? All of the young women:
   1. Have decided on which career they wish to pursue.
   2. Are dressed in the same style clothes and wear the same hairdos.
   3. Broke curfew by staying late at a party they all went to.
   4. Brag about drinking beer when their parents are at work.

7. A school nurse is providing an educational session for parents of high school students. Which of the following actions should the nurse encourage parents to perform in relation to the moral development of their teenagers?
   1. Threaten a severe consequence if their child breaks any rules.
   2. Role-model ethical and moral behavior in their everyday lives.
   3. Take their child on a trip to the local jail to show what happens when adults break the law.
   4. Require their child to sign an honor pledge never to break house rules or to break the law.

8. The school nurse is providing nutrition education to a group of high school students. Which of the following information should be included in the teaching session? **Select all that apply.**
   1. Energy drinks are high in sugar and caffeine.
   2. Vegan diets are low in complete proteins.
   3. Fast foods are low in fat and cholesterol.
   4. Sodas are high in sugar and empty calories.
   5. Adolescents often need to limit their intake of calories.

9. A school nurse is providing an education session for parents of high school students. Which of the following information should be included in the teaching session?
1. It is important for teens to catch up on their sleep on weekends.
2. Teens are less likely to get into an automobile accident if others are in the car with them.
3. Adolescents are especially at high risk for accidental poisonings.
4. Tanning beds are safe as long as the adolescent reapplies sunscreen every ten minutes.

10. A student informs the school nurse that she is planning to get a tattoo. Which of the following information should the nurse teach the student about tattoos?
1. Tattoos are easily removed with lasers and bleach.
2. The student should request that only blue and red dye be used.
3. Infections are rare because tattoo needles and inks are kept hot.
4. Skin lesions may develop where tattoos are placed.

11. A school nurse is providing an educational session regarding actions parents can take to assess whether or not their child is engaging in risk-taking behavior. Which of the following actions should the nurse recommend? **Select all that apply.**
1. Periodically search their child's room for illicit substances.
2. The morning after a party, ask their child what drinks and foods were served.
3. Have a conversation with their child when the child returns home from a date.
4. Before allowing their child to leave for the evening, know where the child will be.
5. Be alert for changes in the child's usual behavior, including a change in friendship groups.

REVIEW ANSWERS

1. ANSWER: 2

Rationale:

1. The fact that her growth spurt began when she was 9 years old may or may not mean that the young woman will continue to grow.
2. Young women usually continue to grow for approximately 2 years after menarche.
3. The fact that she is at the 75th percentile for weight may or may not mean that the young woman will continue to grow.
4. The fact that her parents are both average for height and weight may or may not mean that the young woman will continue to grow.

TEST-TAKING TIP: The nurse is able to state that the child will likely continue to grow because young women usually continue to grow past their menarche. The young woman's menarche occurred 3 months earlier.

Content Area: *Adolescent*
Integrated Processes: *Nursing Process: Assessment*
Client Need: *Health Promotion and Maintenance: Health Screening*
Cognitive Level: *Application*

2. ANSWER: 4

Rationale:

1. It would be inappropriate for the nurse to interview the child about her readiness for menstruation to begin.
2. It would be inappropriate for the nurse to interview the child about her sexual activity.
3. It would be inappropriate for the nurse to interview the child about her menstrual cycle.
4. It would be appropriate for the nurse to interview the child about her feelings about her bodily changes.

TEST-TAKING TIP: The child is in Tanner stage 2. She has minimal breast and pubic hair changes. She will not reach sexual maturation until she is in Tanner stage 5.

Content Area: *Adolescent*
Integrated Processes: *Nursing Process: Implementation*
Client Need: *Health Promotion and Maintenance: Health Screening*
Cognitive Level: *Application*

3. ANSWER: 1

Rationale:

1. The nurse should discuss voice changes with the young man.
2. It would be inappropriate to discuss sexually transmitted infections with the young man.
3. It would be inappropriate to discuss condom use with the young man.
4. It would be inappropriate to discuss nocturnal emissions with the young man.

TEST-TAKING TIP: The child is in Tanner stage 2. He will not reach sexual maturation until he is in Tanner stage 5. He will, however, begin to experience vocal changes. The nurse should forewarn him of those changes.

Content Area: *Adolescent*
Integrated Processes: *Nursing Process: Implementation*
Client Need: *Health Promotion and Maintenance: Health Screening*
Cognitive Level: *Application*

4. ANSWER: 1, 2, 3, and 4

Rationale:

1. Pain is a common complication of impacted wisdom teeth.
2. Cysts may develop where the wisdom teeth erupt.
3. Infections of the gums or other structures may develop as a result of wisdom tooth impaction.
4. Tooth misalignment is a common complication of impacted wisdom teeth.
5. Mandibular osteopenia is unrelated to tooth impaction.

TEST-TAKING TIP: Third molars, or wisdom teeth, usually erupt in late adolescence. Unfortunately, they are frequently impacted, resulting in a number of complications.

Content Area: *Adolescent*
Integrated Processes: *Nursing Process: Implementation*
Client Need: *Physiological Integrity: Physiological Adaptation: Alterations in Body Systems*
Cognitive Level: *Application*

5. ANSWER: 2

Rationale:

1. Surfing the Internet is not recommended as a means of promoting language development in adolescents.
2. Reading a variety of literature is recommended as a means of promoting language development in adolescents.
3. Conversing with friends is not recommended as a means of promoting language development in adolescents.
4. Writing letters is not recommended as a means of promoting language development in adolescents.

TEST-TAKING TIP: By the school-age period, children have acquired the ability to engage in conversation and to use all parts of speech. Reading a variety of literature is recommended to enhance their vocabularies and to improve their scholarly writing during their adolescent years.

Content Area: *Adolescent*
Integrated Processes: *Nursing Process: Implementation*
Client Need: *Health Promotion and Maintenance: Developmental Stages and Transitions*
Cognitive Level: *Application*

6. ANSWER: 2

Rationale:

1. Deciding on which career to pursue is a characteristic of late adolescence.
2. Dressing in the same style clothes and wearing the same hairdos are characteristic of early adolescence.
3. Breaking curfew by staying late at a party is consistent with behavior of middle adolescents.
4. Bragging about drinking beer when their parents are at work is consistent with behavior of middle adolescents.

TEST-TAKING TIP: Erik Erikson's psychosocial stage of the teen years, identity versus role confusion, is often broken

down into three phases: early, middle, and late. Early adolescence is considered the phase of conformity, middle adolescence as the phase of challenge, and late adolescence as the phase of individuality.
Content Area: *Adolescent*
Integrated Processes: *Nursing Process: Diagnosis*
Client Need: *Health Promotion and Maintenance: Developmental Stages and Transitions*
Cognitive Level: *Application*

7. ANSWER: 2
Rationale:
1. The nurse should encourage parents to develop consequences that are reasonable and that are enforceable.
2. The nurse should encourage parents to role model ethical and moral behavior in their everyday lives.
3. It is not recommended that parents take their child on a trip to the local jail to show what happens when adults break the law.
4. It is not recommended that parents require their child to sign an honor pledge never to break house rules or to break the law.
TEST-TAKING TIP: Adolescents are aware of rules and laws and know that they are expected to abide by those restrictions. They challenge those expectations, however, when they observe their parents and other adults failing to comply with legal restrictions. When parents role model appropriate behavior, they are reinforcing the expectations that they are placing on their children.
Content Area: *Adolescent*
Integrated Processes: *Nursing Process: Implementation*
Client Need: *Health Promotion and Maintenance: Developmental Stages and Transitions*
Cognitive Level: *Application*

8. ANSWER: 1, 2, and 4
Rationale:
1. Energy drinks are high in sugar and caffeine. It is recommended that teens limit their intake of energy drinks.
2. Vegan diets are low in complete proteins. If teens choose to follow a vegan diet, they will need professional assistance to make sure that they consume adequate quantities of protein and other nutrients.
3. Fast foods are high in fat and cholesterol. It is recommended that teens limit their intake of fast foods.
4. Sodas are high in sugar and empty calories. It is recommended that teens limit their intake of soft drinks.
5. Adolescence is a period of rapid growth. Although they need to consume calories for growth, some teens engage in weight-loss dieting, often because they wish to emulate a favored model or actor. .
TEST-TAKING TIP: Because of the rapid growth during adolescence, teenagers need to maintain an excellent dietary intake. Unfortunately, many teenagers eat poorly. It is important for nurses to encourage parents to provide their children with easily accessible, nutritious foods and snacks.
Content Area: *Adolescent*
Integrated Processes: *Nursing Process: Implementation; Teaching/Learning*
Client Need: *Health Promotion and Maintenance: Health Promotion/Disease Prevention*
Cognitive Level: *Application*

9. ANSWER: 1
Rationale:
1. This statement is true. Adolescents are often sleep deprived during the school week.
2. Teens are more likely to get into an automobile accident if others are in the car with them.
3. Adolescents are at less risk for accidental poisonings than are younger children. They are, however, at high risk for intentional ingestion of substances (e.g., alcohol, illicit drugs, prescription drugs).
4. It is recommended that sun and ultraviolet light exposure be minimized.
TEST-TAKING TIP: Teens often stay up late at night but must rise early for school. As a result, they sleep many fewer hours than the recommended 8 or more hours each weeknight. To make up for the lack of sleep, teens need to "catch up" on weekends, often sleeping 10 to 12 hours each night. Unfortunately, parents often perceive the long sleep periods as laziness.
Content Area: *Adolescent*
Integrated Processes: *Nursing Process: Implementation; Teaching/Learning*
Client Need: *Health Promotion and Maintenance: Health Promotion/Disease Prevention*
Cognitive Level: *Application*

10. ANSWER: 4
Rationale:
1. Tattoos are difficult to remove, even with lasers.
2. It is not necessary for teens to request that only blue and red dye be used, but they should be aware that iron oxide can cause serious injury during an MRI.
3. Infections are a common complication from tattooing.
4. Granulomas do sometimes develop where tattoos are placed.
TEST-TAKING TIP: Tattooing and piercing are popular among adolescents. Teens should be thoroughly educated regarding the pros and cons of the actions so that they can make informed decisions regarding whether or not to have them placed.
Content Area: *Adolescent*
Integrated Processes: *Nursing Process: Implementation; Teaching/Learning*
Client Need: *Health Promotion and Maintenance: Health Promotion/Disease Prevention*
Cognitive Level: *Application*

11. ANSWER: 3, 4, and 5
Rationale:
1. Unless the parents have reason to believe that their child is engaging in risk-taking behavior, it is not recommended that parents search their child's room for illicit substances.

2. The parent can ask regarding the drinks and foods that were served at a party, but the conversation should take place when the child returns home, not the morning after the party.
3. It is recommended that parents have a conversation with their child when the child returns home from a date.
4. It is recommended that parents know where the child will be before allowing their child to leave for the evening.
5. It is recommended that parents be alert for changes in the child's usual behavior, including a change in friendship groups.

TEST-TAKING TIP: Michael Nerney has developed the five A's of parenting: aware, alert, awake, assertive, and affirmation. The first four actions increase parents' attentiveness to their teenagers' actions. The last action, repeatedly telling their children that they are loved, helps parents to maintain a bridge between them and their child during the turbulent period of adolescence.
Content Area: *Adolescent*
Integrated Processes: *Nursing Process: Implementation; Teaching/Learning*
Client Need: *Health Promotion and Maintenance: Health Promotion/Disease Prevention*
Cognitive Level: *Application*

Physical Assessment of Children: From Infancy to Adolescence

KEY TERMS

Apex beat—Also called the point of maximum impulse (PMI). The location on the chest where the left ventricular beat is felt most strongly.
Crepitus—A cracking or popping sound from the joints caused by trapped air.
Head lag—In infants, the drooping of the head forward or backward from the trunk of the body.
Hirsutism—Excessive hair growth.
Hypotelorism—Narrowly spaced eyes.
Hypertelorism—Widely spaced eyes.
Inspiratory stridor—A high-pitched wheezing sound resulting from a blockage in the upper airway.
Kyphosis—Curvature of the spine resulting in a slouched or hunchback position.
Lordosis—Inward curvature of the lower spine.
Normotensive—Normal blood pressure.
Nystagmus—Fast, involuntary eye movements.
Patency—The quality of being unblocked or open.
Philtrum—The indented segment between the upper lip and the nose.
Prehypertensive—A condition of elevated blood pressure that may lead to hypertension.
Red reflex—The reddish reflection that occurs when light is shined into the retina.
Scoliosis—Condition in which there is lateral curvature of the spine.
Thrill—Palpable vibration of the heart.

I. Description

Traditionally, in physical assessment class, students are taught to identify subjective and objective findings via oral communication with the patient and while performing head-to-toe assessments. Those techniques, however, are not necessarily appropriate, especially for the very young. First, infants, toddlers, and even some preschoolers are either incapable or unwilling to communicate with a stranger, namely the nurse. In addition, the nurse is often able to obtain more accurate physical data if he or she assesses the child using a less structured, hands-on approach. Adaptations to the standard processes are, therefore, often required.

II. Examination

A. Techniques.
1. Inspection, palpation, percussion, and auscultation.
   a. Essentially performed on children in the same manner as with adults.
   b. As with the adult, the order of the abdominal assessment is changed slightly—inspection,

auscultation, percussion, and palpation—to prevent a disruption of bowel sounds.

2. Communication.
   a. It is essential to speak slowly and clearly when assessing children.
   b. Plain language, especially when assessing young children, is critical.
      i. Many words are unfamiliar to children even, for example, "inspection," "palpation," "percussion," and "auscultation."
      ii. Many words are interpreted differently by children than by adults.
         (1) For example, telling a child that he or she will feel a stick when a blood test is being performed may be understood as a stick from a tree, or telling a child that dye will be infused intravenously for an x-ray image may be understood as to die from a disease.
3. Other principles to follow. The nurse should:
   a. Warm his or her hands and instruments (e.g., stethoscope) to make the experience as pleasant as possible.
   b. Try to be at the same height as the child so that the nurse is talking on the same plane as the child.
   c. Offer the child choices only when they are possible, for example:
      i. The nurse should not ask a child whether he or she wants to receive a vaccination because the child has no choice. Rather, the nurse could ask whether the child wants a pretzel or a cracker as a treat after the painful procedure.
   d. Be honest with the child. If a procedure is going to hurt, the child should be told.
   e. Use play as a means of acquiring information and/or cooperation from a child, for example:
      i. Have the child tell a story about another child in a similar situation.
      ii. Have the child talk through a puppet
      iii. Give the child three wishes, and ask him or her to describe what they are.
      iv. Read a book to the child about the problem, and ask the child to discuss the book.
      v. Have the child draw a picture and describe what the picture means.

B. Age differences.

1. Infants.
   a. Subjective data.
      i. Usually provided by the parents, except when the child cries in response to an intervention (see "History").
   b. Objective data.
      i. To obtain the cooperation of the child, it often is best to perform the majority of the physical assessment while the child is being held by the parents. If this is not feasible, the parent should at least be close by to support the child.
      ii. If the child is quiet or sleeping, in order to obtain as accurate data as possible, the nurse should auscultate the respiratory and cardiac systems and the abdomen first.
      iii. It often is best to touch the child's feet first and work up the body because the feet are often viewed as less intrusive by the child.
      iv. Areas of pain or areas that may elicit crying should always be assessed last (e.g., site of injury, inspection of the ear, palpation of the abdomen).
      v. Using toys or songs to distract the child often is helpful.
2. Toddlers.
   a. See the sections on subjective and objective data of infants from earlier.
   b. Toddlers are often fearful and uncooperative.
      i. The nurse should begin the examination by focusing attention on the caregiver for a few minutes. He or she will answer the nurse's questions. This helps the child to see that the parent trusts the nurse and, as a result, the child may become more cooperative.
      ii. Distraction with toys, lights, or books may help to elicit the child's cooperation.
      iii. Again, moving from the least invasive areas to areas that may elicit discomfort (and/or from feet to head) is recommended.
3. Preschoolers.
   a. See the sections on subjective and objective data of infants and toddlers from earlier.
   b. Preschoolers often are more cooperative than are younger children. The head-to-toe assessment may be possible, but waiting to perform invasive procedures should still be followed.
4. School-age children.
   a. Subjective data.
      i. School-age children usually will respond readily to age-appropriate questions (e.g., related to school, homework, after-school activities, the family pet).
      ii. However, the nurse must supplement that information by asking the parent.

b. Objective data.
   i. Usually, a traditional head-to-toe assessment is possible.
   ii. The nurse must remember that the school-age child is likely becoming sensitive about his or her body, so a cover should be provided to the child.

5. Adolescents.
   a. Subjective data.
      i. In general, the teen should be queried in private. Sensitive information may be asked, and the teen will likely be unwilling to share responses if the parent is present.
      ii. The parent, too, should be provided the opportunity to discuss issues with the nurse. The discussion may be in the presence of the teen or independent of the child.
   b. Objective data.
      i. The physical examination should be conducted without the presence of the parent.
      ii. The teen should be given the same gowning that an adult would be given.

C. Prior to the examination.

1. Before actually performing the examination, the nurse should make some initial observations. The observations are often best performed while the child, especially the young child, is in the waiting room with the parents.
2. Observing the child's skin color, activity level, play activity, posturing, child-to-child interactions, and parent-to-child interactions provide the nurse with baseline information regarding the child's health and well-being (Table 7.1).

D. History.

1. First visit to the health-care practitioner.
   a. The initial history should include information from birth onward, for example:
      i. The child's health up to the current age.
      ii. Perinatal history, especially if the child is under 3 years of age.
   b. Additional important information that should be obtained includes, but is not limited to:
      i. Family health history, including at least a three-generation pedigree.
      ii. Ethnicity, religious preferences, as well as country of origin, if appropriate.
      iii. Previous illnesses and surgeries.
      iv. Vaccination history.
      v. Dietary patterns.
      vi. Current medications, including vitamins.
      vii. Allergy history.
      viii. Pain issues, including coping strategies.
      ix. School performance, social interactions, and extracurricular activities.
      x. Use of cultural/family remedies, if appropriate.
      xi. Environmental factors (e.g., pet ownership, cigarette smoking, alcohol, and/or illicit drug use by the child or someone in his or her environment, location of the child's home).
2. Well-child visits.
   a. Once the child is known to the health-care practitioner, information regarding important facts or changes that have occurred since the preceding visit should be elicited.
3. Sick-child visits.
   a. Whenever the child is seen for an episodic illness or injury, specific facts related to that illness or injury should be obtained.

Table 7.1 Initial Observation of the Child

	Healthy	Ill
Skin Color	• Pink	• Dusky (i.e., grayish coloration, indicates oxygen depletion) • Cyanosis indicates marked hypoxemia
Activity Level or Responsiveness	• Usually consistent with growth and development: *Infant: eye contact, attracted by colors, moves extremities with vigor* *Toddler and older child: actively playing, talking with parents and/or other children, reading a book, etc.*	• Often see behavioral regression, disinterest in toys or other activities, lying still, unexpectedly napping, etc. • **If unresponsive to painful stimulus:** serious finding that may indicate: *Serious cardiorespiratory function and neurological deterioration*
Posturing	• Sitting up • Normal posture or other comfortable position	• Lying down, hugging parent, etc. (especially if toddler or preschooler) • Tripod posturing or refusing to lie down often indicates respiratory distress

III. Physiological Findings

A. Overall growth and development.
1. In children up to age 6, fine and gross motor development should be assessed objectively using standardized scales (e.g., Denver Development Screening Test II, Ages and Stages Questionnaire).
2. Older children's development can be assessed with relative accuracy during the examination.

B. Vital signs.
1. Temperature.
   a. Methods.
      i. Any age-appropriate method (rectal, oral, tympanic, or axillary) may be used.
         (1) Oral thermometers should not be used with infants or toddlers.
      ii. Type of method should be documented, including which ear if tympanic.
      iii. Parents are often encouraged not to perform rectal readings because of the potential for physical and/or psychological trauma.
         (1) Rectal route is especially traumatic for toddlers and preschoolers.
   b. Normal: 97.7° to 99°F (36.5°C to 37°C).
2. Heart rate.
   a. Method.
      i. Apical rate should be assessed for a full minute in the following situations
         (1) Infants and children up to at least 2 years of age.
         (2) Any child with a known cardiac arrhythmia.
         (3) Sick children.
      ii. Radial method for well-child checks after age 2.
      iii. Quality of femoral pulses and pedal pulses should be assessed bilaterally, and pulsation in the fontanel, if still open, should be assessed.
   b. Normal rate drops slowly over time from a high of 110 to 160 bpm in infancy to 60 to 80 bpm in adolescents.
      i. Tachycardia.
         (1) Unless there is a clear explanation for an increase in a child's heart rate, nurses should carefully assess for the cause of the tachycardia.
         (2) Tachycardia often is a dangerous sign in children because children are unable to increase cardiac output by changing their stroke volume.
            (a) To increase stroke volume, therefore, they increase their heart rates.
      ii. Bradycardia.
         (1) If bradycardia is present, it is often an ominous sign.
         (2) Cardiac arrest often is imminent.
   c. Children's pulses often fluctuate:
      i. In relation to inhalation and exhalation.
      ii. In relation to exercise, crying, and other activities.
   d. Auscultations: especially in toddlers, preschoolers, and school-age children.
      i. Allowing children to play with the stethoscope and listen to their own or their parent's hearts and lungs often will facilitate the assessment.
      ii. Distraction with a puppet or toy may help to calm an anxious child.
      iii. If the child is crying, assess the sounds between sobs.
      iv. A pause that may be heard during S2 (i.e., "dub" sounds) is considered normal in children.
      v. Assessing for murmurs and other excess heart sounds is important, especially in infants and young children.
         (1) Many murmurs are considered functional or nonpathological but must be assessed by an expert in the field.
         (2) Location and characteristics of any abnormal heart sounds should be documented (see Chapter 17, "Nursing Care of the Child With Cardiovascular Illnesses").
3. Respirations.
   a. Method.
      i. Respirations should be assessed for a full minute in the following situations.
         (1) Infants and children up to at least 2 years of age.
         (2) Any child with a known cardiac arrhythmia.
         (3) Sick children.
      ii. To obtain as accurate a rate as possible, the nurse should count the respirations while performing another action (e.g., while assessing pulse) because the child is less likely to alter his or her breathing patterns.
   b. Normal rate drops slowly over time from high of 30 to 60 rpm in infancy to 15 to 20 rpm in adolescents.
      i. Like children's pulses, children's respiratory status often fluctuates in relation to exercise, crying, and other activities.

ii. Pulse oximetry should be at least 93% and ideally greater than 98%.

c. Auscultations: especially in toddlers, preschoolers, and school-age children.

i. Allowing them to play with the stethoscope and listen to their own or their parent's hearts and lungs often facilitates the assessment.

ii. Distraction with a puppet or toy may help to calm an anxious child.

iii. Having the child blow bubbles or blow on a pinwheel often helps the practitioner to hear inhalations and exhalations.

iv. If the child is crying, assess the sounds between sobs. Listen for adventitious sounds (e.g., assess for rales, rhonchi, coughing, inspiratory stridor). **Inspiratory stridor** is a high-pitched wheezing sound resulting from a blockage in the upper airway.

(1) Location and characteristics of any abnormal breath sounds should be documented (see Chapter 16, "Nursing Care of the Child With Respiratory Illnesses").

4. Blood pressure (BP).

a. Method.

i. BP is not routinely assessed until children are 3 years of age.

(1) If infant or toddler BP is needed, an electronic BP machine should be utilized, and the pressure should be assessed in all four limbs.

ii. The correct size cuff should always be used.

(1) Width: should cover approximately 40% of the upper arm.

(2) Length: should cover between 80% and 100% of the upper arm without overlapping.

iii. It is important to forewarn the child regarding the pressure that they will feel when the cuff is inflated.

b. Normal: 50th percentile values rise slowly from a low of 65/30 mm Hg in infants to 111/66 mm Hg in teenage girls and 116/65 mm Hg in teenage boys.

i. Children whose BP is above the 90th percentile should be evaluated for hypertension.

ii. Adolescents whose BP is above 120/80 mm Hg should be diagnosed as **prehypertensive**, an elevated level that may lead to hypertension.

MAKING THE CONNECTION

Although there is debate in the literature, the following formula may be used to determine a dangerously low systolic BP in children—usually suggested to be at the 5th percentile: multiply the child's age in years by two and add 70 (some sources say to add 65). For example, the calculation for a 5-year-old is:

$$5 \times 2 + 65 \text{ (or 70)} = 75 \text{ to } 80 \text{ mm Hg}$$

A systolic blood pressure of 75 to 80, therefore, would indicate significant hypotension in the child.

iii. Subtle changes in BP may indicate marked changes in mean arterial pressure and perfusion.

(1) **Normotension** (normal BP) in a child does not mean that he or she is well.

(2) Hypotension is a late sign of shock in the pediatric patient.

(a) The etiology of hypotension in a child should be determined as soon as possible so that appropriate intervention(s) can be implemented.

5. Pain assessment (see Chapter 8, "Nursing Care of the Child in the Health-Care Setting").

a. Method.

i. An age-appropriate pain assessment tool should always be used to assess pain in the child. Examples:

(1) Infant: CRIES pain scale.

(2) Infants and toddlers: FLACC (face, legs, activity, cry, consolability) scale.

(3) Preschoolers and young school-age children: Wong-Baker FACES Pain Rating Scale and Oucher Pain Scale.

(4) Older school-age children and adolescents: Numeric pain scales and visual analog scales.

C. Growth.

1. Measurements should be assessed at each well-child check and during episodic illnesses, if appropriate.

a. Head circumference.

i. Measured from birth until 36 months of age.

ii. Until 12 months of age, circumference usually grows about one-half inch each month.

b. Chest circumference.

i. Until 12 months of age, the head circumference is slightly larger than the chest circumference.

ii. After 12 months of age, the head and chest circumferences are approximately the same.

c. Height.

i. Until the child is able to stand still (usually by 2 years of age) the height is measured while the child is lying down.

d. Weight.

i. Infants and toddlers who are still in diapers.

(1) All clothing should be removed.

(2) Child lies or sits on a pediatric scale.

ii. Older children.

(1) Underpants are usually left on.

(2) Child stands on a floor scale.

e. Body mass index (BMI).

i. Calculated using the following formula:

(1) $\text{BMI} = \dfrac{\text{child's weight in kg}}{\text{child's height in m}^2}$

or $\dfrac{\text{child's weight in lb} \times 703}{\text{child's height in in.}^2}$

2. Growth charts.

a. All measurements should be plotted on growth charts (see Alert below.).

b. Deviations from the child's normal growth curves should be evaluated further.

c. Measurements above the 97th or below the 3rd percentiles may indicate alterations from normal and should be assessed further.

d. BMIs above the 85th percentile indicate a child whose weight is above normal.

All measurements—height; weight; BMI; and, if appropriate, head circumferences—should be plotted on growth charts. (See Appendices for growth charts recommended by the Centers for Disease Control and Prevention. All of the charts are available online at www.cdc.gov/growthcharts/clinical_charts.htm.)

D. Body structures.

1. Skin.

a. The skin should initially be inspected for:

i. Cleanliness versus signs indicating a lack of parental or self-care.

ii. Color (i.e., pink versus dusky versus cyanotic).

iii. Moles or other incidental discolorations.

iv. Signs of injury.

v. Dryness or flaking of the mucous membranes.

b. The skin should be palpated for altered:

i. Temperature.

ii. Turgor.

iii. Edema.

2. Nails.

a. The nails should be inspected for:

i. Cleanliness versus signs of lack of parental or self-care.

ii. Strong versus brittle nails.

(1) Brittle nails may indicate altered nutritional status.

b. The nails should be palpated for:

i. Capillary refill time.

ii. Clubbing.

3. Head.

a. Head should be inspected for:

i. Symmetry of features.

ii. Symmetry of movements.

iii. Movement ability, for example:

(1) **head lag,** drooping of the head forward or backward from the body, which should not last past 6 months of age.

b. Head should be palpated for:

i. Symmetry of the skull.

ii. Size and quality of fontanels in infants.

(1) Bulging fontanel is a symptom of increased intracranial pressure.

(2) Sunken fontanel is a symptom of dehydration.

(3) Posterior fontanel usually closes between 6 and 8 weeks of age.

(4) Anterior fontanel closes between 12 and 18 months of age.

4. Hair.

a. Hair should be inspected for:

i. Cleanliness versus signs of lack of parental or self-care.

ii. Signs of lice.

iii. Alopecia.

iv. **Hirsutism** (i.e., excessive hair growth).

5. Face.

a. Should be inspected for:

i. Symmetry and location of structures (Box 7.1).

6. Eyes.

a. During inspection.

i. Ophthalmoscopic assessment should be performed:

(1) Presence of **red reflex,** the reddish reflection when light is shined in the retina.

(2) Retina and other internal structures should be inspected, if nurse is skilled in the technique.

ii. Vision testing (often conducted at the conclusion of the examination).

(1) First test should be performed by age 3 using age-appropriate eye charts (e.g., symbols, pictures).

Box 7.1 Examination of Facial Characteristics

- *Low-set ears: a sign present in some genetic/chromosomal disorders*
- *Eye spacing (i.e., widely spaced [**hypertelorism**] or narrowly spaced [**hypotelorism**] eyes): signs seen in some genetic/ chromosomal and/or congenital disorders*
- *Size and shape of nose and nasal bridge: deviations of which are seen in some genetic or chromosomal disorders*
- ***Philtrum**, the indented segment between the upper lip and the nose, absent or minimal in children with fetal alcohol effects*
- *Lips: should be pink, moist, and without cracking. Thin lips are seen in children with fetal alcohol effects*
- *Symmetry of movements: provides an assessment of cranial nerve function*

(2) School-age and older children can use the Snellen chart.
(3) Child's peripheral vision should also be assessed.

DID YOU KNOW?

Vision improves from the neonatal period through preschool age. As infants, children see clearly about 8 to 12 in. away from an object. Young children normally are hyperopic, or farsighted. Normal 20/20 vision should be present by age 5.

iii. Color vision.
(1) Usually tested when the child is in early elementary years using specially created color images.
(2) If unable to see the requisite images, the child likely has inherited a recessive gene on the X-chromosome. Boys are, therefore, more frequently affected than are girls.

iv. Binocular vision.
(1) In early infancy, pseudostrabismus (i.e., the false appearance of crossed eyes resulting from the baby's weak musculature) may be present.
(2) By 6 months of age, binocular vision should be intact, as evidenced by:
(a) The light appearing at the same spot in both eyes when the ophthalmoscope light is shined into the eyes.
(3) Older children should be able to track a finger, puppet, or other object through all fields of vision with no signs of **nystagmus** (i.e., involuntary eye movement) or other deviations.

v. All structures of the eye should be inspected.
(1) Lids, tear ducts, eyebrows, and eyelids for symmetry and appearance.
(2) Conjunctiva.
(a) Should appear pink.
(b) If reddened or with exudate, infection is likely present.
(3) Sclerae.
(a) Should be whitish in color.
(b) Yellow appearance may indicate liver dysfunction.
(4) Iris and pupils.
(a) Should be the same size when not manipulated. If the pupil size is unequal, central nervous system assessment should be conducted.
(b) Both pupils should contract and expand in concert with each other when the light from the ophthalmoscipe is shined into the eye.
(c) The pupils should accommodate when a moving object (e.g., finger, puppet, toy) is moved from far away to within close proximity of the eyes.

7. Nose.
a. Should be inspected for:
i. Open and unblocked nostrils (i.e., **patency** of nostrils).
ii. Presence and characteristics of discharge, if present.
(1) Glove should be worn for protection.
(2) A child who repeatedly wipes the base of the nose could indicate the presence of a discharge.
iii. Sense of smell:
(1) To assess, the child's eyes should be covered and the child should then be asked to sniff and identify a familiar substance (e.g., spice).
iv. Characteristics of the nasal passages should be examined with an otoscope.
(1) May need to be deferred to the end of the exam because of the intrusive nature of the action.
b. Inspect and palpate sinuses.
i. Inflammation may be present when:
(1) Puffiness and/or redness are present.
(2) There are dark circles under the child's eyes.

8. Mouth and throat.
a. May need to be deferred to the end of the exam because of the intrusive nature of the action.
b. The structures should be inspected for:
i. Frenulum for tongue-tie or injury.

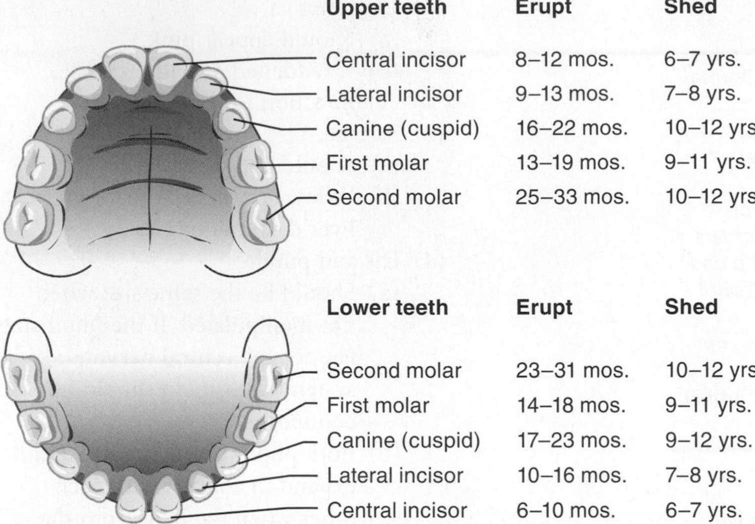

Fig 7.1 Primary and secondary tooth development.

ii. Buccal mucosa for color, injury, or signs of dehydration.

iii. Mouth for presence of odors.

iv. Teeth for number and quality.

(1) Number of teeth should be consistent with the child's age and overall development (Fig. 7.1).

(2) Cavities may be present, especially if a young child is put to bed with a bottle of formula.

v. Gums.

(1) Should be inspected for:

(a) Color: they should be pink. For an accurate assessment, blanching may be needed in children of color.

(b) Any ulcerations, abrasions, or other unusual appearance (e.g., Koplik spots in a child with rubeola) (see Chapter 11, "Nursing Care of the Child With Infectious Diseases").

(2) Palpate: gums should feel firm.

vi. Tongue (and structures under the tongue).

(1) Inspect both the upper and lower aspects for:

(a) Color: should be pink with slight whitish surface.

(b) Intact papillae of the tongue.

(c) Any ulcerations or abrasions.

(d) Symmetry: by having child stick out his or her tongue.

(2) Palpate the tongue for hard or rigid areas

When examining the tongue, it is wise for the nurse to hold the child's cheeks with the fingers and thumb of one hand to prevent being bitten.

vii. Hard and soft palates.

(1) Should be inspected for:

(a) Color.

(i) Hard palate: should be whitish pink with ridges.

(ii) Soft palate: usually appears pinker than the hard palate.

(b) Shape: should be arched but not peaked.

(c) Intact hard and soft palate: especially important at delivery.

(i) Both the hard and soft palate should be palpated at birth to verify that they are both intact.

(d) Uvula: should move freely and elevate slightly when the child says, "ah."

viii. Throat and tonsils.

(1) Should be inspected with a tongue blade.

(a) The tongue blade should be carefully inserted along the side of the tongue until the nurse is able to depress the back of the tongue. At that time, the gag reflex should be elicited.

(b) The size and shape of the tonsils should be noted. Enlarged tonsils are relatively common in young children.

(i) Enlarged tonsils frequently result in snoring while asleep.

(c) If exudate is present, a throat infection is likely and a culture should be taken.

9. Ears.
   a. The ears should be inspected for:
      i. Symmetry of the external structures.
      ii. Presence of discharge.
   b. The bony prominence behind the ear should be palpated for tenderness.
   c. Child's hearing should be assessed.
      i. Neonate and infant.
         (1) The presence of nerve conduction should be assessed while in the hospital in the newborn nursery prior to discharge.
         (2) When a bell is rung or other noisy toy is rattled behind the infant, he or she should move in an attempt to see the object.
      ii. Preschool and school-age children should undergo audiometry testing to assess for overall hearing ability and/or precise frequencies of the child's hearing.
      iii. A whisper test should be conducted on all children from preschool age through adolescence:
         (1) To perform the test, the nurse should stand behind the child, whisper a command, and watch to see if the child carries out the action. For example, whisper for the child to wave his or her hand.
         (2) The child should be warned before attempting the test in order not to confuse the child.
      iv. Bone and/or air conduction hearing tests may also be performed.
   d. Otoscopic assessment.
      i. May need to be deferred to the end of the exam because of the intrusive nature of the action.
      ii. Method (Fig. 7.2).
         (1) Infants and toddlers: the practitioner should pull the pinnae of the ear down and back while inserting the otoscope into ear.
         (2) Children 3 years and older: the practitioner should pull the pinnae of the ear up and back while inserting the otoscope into ear.

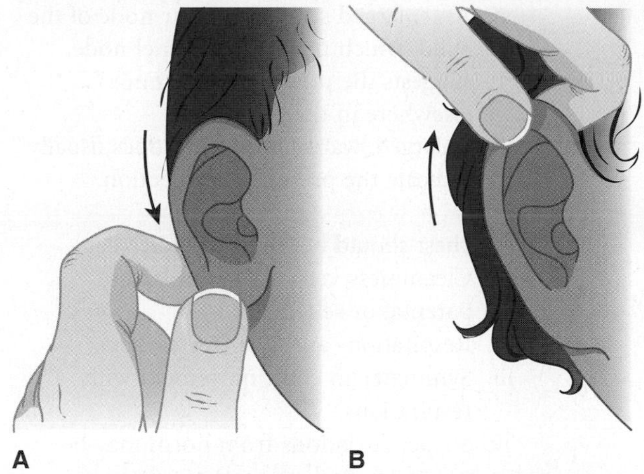

Fig 7.2 Otoscopic assessment of children. (A) Infant exam, pulling the pinnae down and back. (B) Children 3 years and older, pulling the pinnae up and back.

      iii. Inspect the tympanic membrane.
         (1) The membrane should appear pale gray in color, and the practitioner should be able to discern some of the ear's internal structures. When a puff of air is inserted into the ear canal, the membrane usually moves slightly.
         (2) Abnormal findings include (see Chapter 16, "Nursing Care of the Child With Respiratory Illnesses"):
            (a) A red and enflamed membrane indicative of a middle-ear infection.
            (b) A membrane that is dull and bulging that is consistent with a middle ear that is filled with fluid.

10. Neck.
    a. The nurse should inspect for:
       i. Cleanliness versus signs of lack of parental or self-care.
       ii. Symmetry, shape, and size.
          (1) The neck usually is short in infants and slowly elongates as the child ages.
       iii. Presence of webbing: seen in some chromosomal syndromes.
    b. The neck should be palpated for:
       i. Symmetry and mobility.
       ii. Thyroid gland enlargement.

11. Lymph nodes.
    a. The nurse should palpate the child's superficial lymph nodes.
       i. Small, firm nodes in the young child are within normal limits.

ii. An enlarged supraclavicular node of the child, which may be a sentinel node, suggests the presence of a tumor elsewhere in the body.
iii. Enlarged, warm, and firm nodes usually indicate the presence of infection.

12. Chest.
  a. The chest should be inspected for:
    i. Cleanliness versus signs of lack of parental or self-care.
    ii. Respirations and size (see earlier).
    iii. Symmetry in chest movement with respirations.
    iv. Shape: deviations from norm may be pigeon, funnel, or scoliotic chest.
    v. Breasts:
      (1) Should be assessed for symmetry.
      (2) The appearance should be assessed in relation to the child's age and development.
        (a) Neonates and young infants may have engorged breasts from maternal hormonal stimulation.
        (b) In young children, the breast appears flat, with a pigmented nipple and flat areola.
        (c) During puberty, both boys and girls exhibit breast changes (see the Tanner scale in Chapter 6, "Normal Growth and Development: Adolescence").
          (i) Breast development often occurs asymmetrically.
          (ii) Changes often begin as early as 7 to 9 years of age in both males and females.
      (3) Breast self-examination is an excellent self-care technique to teach the older school-age child or teen.
  b. Starting on the child's back to minimize fear, the chest should be palpated for:
    i. Pain, vibrations during respirations, areas of edema, or masses.
    ii. Abnormal breast changes.
  c. Lungs: see the previous "Respirations" section.
  d. Heart: see the previous "Heart rate" section.
    i. The nurse should palpate for:
      (1) **Apex beat** (also called the point of maximum impulse [PMI]): the location on the chest at which the left ventricular beat is felt most strongly.
        (a) From infancy until about 7 years of age, the apex beat is usually located at the fourth intercostal space lateral to the midclavicular line.
        (b) In older children, the apex beat is located at the fifth intercostal space at the midclavicular line.
      (2) The nurse should also assess for **thrills**, or palpable vibrations.
    ii. Auscultation: see the previous "Vital signs" section.

13. Abdomen: during the assessment of the abdomen, the child should lie supine with his or her head on a pillow and his or her knees bent.
  a. The abdomen should be inspected for:
    i. Cleanliness versus signs of lack of parental or self-care.
    ii. Signs of injury.
    iii. Characteristics of the umbilicus, including possible presence of herniations or other abnormalities.
    iv. Size and shape of abdomen: may indicate either insufficient or excess dietary intake.
      (1) Toddlers normally have distended abdomens due to large abdominal contents.
    v. Aortic pulsations may be visible through the abdominal wall in thin children.
  b. The abdomen should be auscultated for:
    i. Bowel sounds in all four quadrants.

DID YOU KNOW?

Only after 5 full minutes of no sound in any quadrant may the nurse declare that the child has no bowel sounds.

    ii. May also assess for arterial bruits, which are sounds that are heard when a vessel is obstructed.
  c. Percussion: should be performed only by advanced practitioners who are skilled at assessing for organ margins.
  d. The abdomen should be palpated for (palpation may need to be deferred to the end of the exam because of the nature of the action, especially if the practitioner is expecting that the procedure will be painful):
    i. Masses and painful areas.
      (1) Should be performed initially using light palpation followed by deep palpation.
    ii. A rigid abdomen, which may be related to the tension of the child or may be related to pathology, should be documented.
    iii. Liver margin is felt 1 to 3 cm below the costal margin in infants and toddlers but should not extend past the costal margin in an older child.

14. Buttocks and spine.
    a. After the abdominal examination, the child is turned over to reveal the buttocks and lower spine.
    b. The buttocks and spine should be inspected for:
        i. Cleanliness versus signs of lack of parental or self-care.
        ii. Signs of injury.
        iii. Masses.
        iv. Patency of the anus at the time of delivery (gloves should be worn for the exam).
        v. Tufts of hair or deep dimples at the base of the spine may indicate the presence of a neural tube defect (see Chapter 22, "Nursing Care of the Child with Neurological Problems").
        vi. Deviations from midline of the spine.
            (1) **Kyphosis:** spine curvature resulting in a slouching or hunchback posture.
            (2) **Lordosis:** inward curvature of the lower spine, or swayback posture.
            (3) **Scoliosis:** lateral curvature of the spine (see Chapter 20, "Nursing Care of the Child with Musculoskeletal Disorders").
                (a) When able, the child should stand on one leg. Hip heights should remain stable.
                (b) The child should be asked to bend at the waist and dangle his or her arms freely. The hip heights and ribs should be symmetrical, and the spine should be straight.

15. Genitourinary.

DID YOU KNOW?

The genitourinary examination can be upsetting to both parents and older children. In young children, the parents should be forewarned prior to the examination. In school-age and adolescent children, the intent of the practitioner should be communicated to the child in a matter-of-fact manner, and the child should be draped appropriately.

    a. Male.
        i. Inspection.
            (1) Gloves should be worn during the exam.
            (2) The Tanner scale should be used as reference for all developmental staging (see Chapter 6, "Normal Growth and Development: Adolescence").
            (3) Examine circumcised versus uncircumcised penis.
                (a) In children of all ages: For lesions and injuries (e.g., abrasions, lacerations, or other injuries that may be evidence of sexually transmitted infections or child sexual abuse).
                (b) By the preschool period, the uncircumcised glans should be retractable and the glans carefully examined.
                (c) Meatus should be pink, at the middle of the glans, and devoid of discharge.
            (4) Examine the scrotum for the presence of rugae and expected maturation in relation to the child's age and overall level of development.
        ii. The scrotum should be palpated:
            (1) In neonates and infants:
                (a) For the presence of normal testes bilaterally (i.e., smooth and slightly barrel shaped).
                (b) For the presence of masses in the older child.
        iii. The child's urinary output should be assessed.
            (1) This assessment is of particular importance if the child is exhibiting signs of fluid overload or dehydration (i.e., changes in weight, mucous membranes, skin turgor, and, if an infant, fontanel status).
            (2) See minimum urinary outputs in Table 7.2.
            (3) Normal special gravity values are between 1.000 and 1.030.
                (a) Because they concentrate their urine poorly, infants rarely have a specific gravity above 1.006.
    b. Female.
        i. Inspection.
            (1) Gloves should be worn during the exam.
            (2) All external structures should be identified and examined.
                (a) The hymen may be intact, or may be partially open. If lesions or injuries are present, there may be evidence of sexually transmitted infection or child sexual abuse.
                (b) Labia majora are often wide spread in the young child.

Table 7.2 Minimum Urinary Outputs

Age	Urinary Output
Infant and young child	2–4 mL/kg/hr
School-age child	1–2 mL/kg/hr
Adolescent	0.5–1 mL/kg/hr

(c) Any evidence of vaginal discharge should be without odor. Malodorous discharge may be related to the presence of a sexually transmitted infection.

(3) If indicated, speculum exams of internal structures should be performed by experienced practitioners only.

ii. Palpation.

(1) While carefully spreading the labia, the clitoris, urethra, and vagina are assessed.

(a) If lesions or injuries are present, they must be carefully examined. They may be evidence of sexually transmitted infection or child sexual abuse.

(b) All structures should be pink, moist, and soft to the touch.

16. Extremities.

a. The extremities should be inspected for:

i. Cleanliness versus signs of lack of parental or self-care.

ii. Signs of injury.

(1) Bruising is common in young children but should still be viewed carefully.

(2) Queries should be asked regarding possible overuse and/or stress injuries.

iii. Signs of peripheral circulation: capillary refill should occur in less than 2 seconds.

iv. Signs of inflammation: redness, warmth, pain, swelling may indicate injury or a presence of disease.

v. Flat footedness: normal until approximately 2 years of age.

vi. Bow-leggedness: normal in children who walk until approximately 3 years of age.

vii. Gait: should be inspected for symmetry and age-appropriate ability.

(1) To enhance their stability, toddlers walk with a wide, often waddling gait.

b. Palpate for:

i. Full range of motion of all joints (both active and passive) in all ages with the addition of the following important additions:

(1) In infants (see Chapter 20, "Nursing Care of the Child With Musculoskeletal Disorders"):

(a) Developmental dysplasia of the hip, including Ortolani's, Allis', and Barlow's signs as well as gluteal and thigh fold symmetry.

(i) These signs should be assessed at each well-child visit during the infancy period.

(b) Club foot: both feet should be able to be moved to normal positioning without any resistance.

ii. Muscle strength by having the child resist movement when the practitioner pushes the extremity, shoulder, or joint. If differences are noted, muscle measurements should be performed to assess for symmetry.

iii. Areas of tenderness.

iv. Masses or the presence of edema.

v. **Crepitus** (i.e., cracking or popping sound when the joints are bent).

17. Neurological system.

a. Age-appropriate reflex assessments should be performed, especially:

i. Neonatal reflexes, most importantly Babinski; grasp, palmar, and pedal; Moro; rooting; suck; tonic neck; and trunk incurvation (see Table 7.3).

ii. Patellar, biceps, and triceps reflexes in all children.

IV. Psychological and Intellectual Assessment

A. Cognitive and psychological testing.

1. Assessments, using normed assessment tools, should be performed by trained practitioners.

2. Theories developed by Erik Erikson, Jean Piaget, and Lawrence Kohlberg may be used to determine normal growth patterns in children (see "Growth and Development" in Chapters 2–6).

Table 7.3 Reflexes

Reflex	How the Reflex Is Elicited	Age Changes	Illustration
Babinski	When the sole of the outer aspect of the baby's foot is stroked from heel upward, the baby's toes will flare.	Fades after about 1 year of age. When the reflex is elicited in the toddler through adulthood, the toes curl rather than flare.	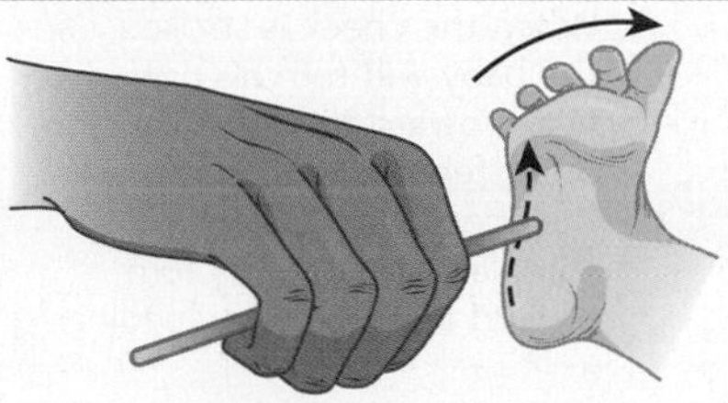
Grasp: Palmar	When the base of the fingers of a baby's hand are compressed, the baby's fingers will curl.	Fades after 3 months of age and is replaced by a voluntary grasp at approximately 5 months of age.	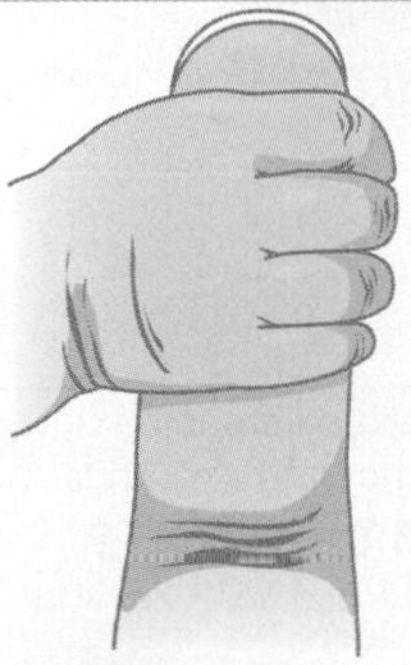
Grasp: Pedal	When the base of the toes of a baby's foot are compressed, the baby's toes will curl.	Fades completely by approximately 8 months of age.	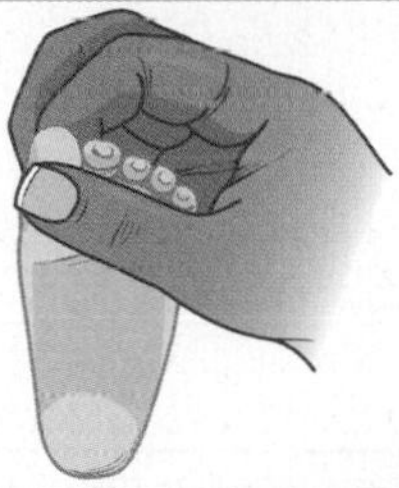
Moro	When a sudden loud noise is produced or the baby's crib is suddenly jarred, the baby will exhibit a full-body response, validating the fact that the child's central nervous system is intact. Arms, legs, hands, and fingers extend, followed by flexion of all of the extremities. Simultaneously, babies often cry.	Fades after 3 or 4 months of age.	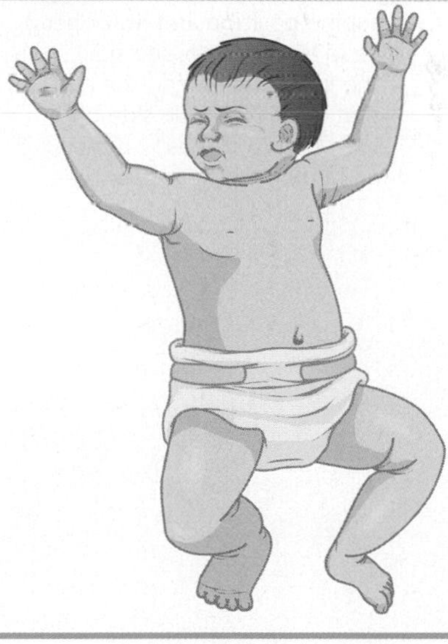

Continued

Table 7.3 Reflexes *cont'd*

Reflex	How the Reflex Is Elicited	Age Changes	Illustration
Rooting	When the cheek is stroked, the baby will turn his or her head toward that direction. Breastfeeding mothers stroke the cheek with the breast to stimulate the baby to turn toward the breast for feeding.	Usually fades after 3 to 4 months but may persist, especially in breast-fed babies.	
Suck	When the hard palate is stimulated, the baby responds with a strong suck. They also often suck spontaneously, even during sleep.	Fades only after the child stops breast or bottle feeding.	
Tonic Neck	When a baby is placed in the supine position and his or her head is turned to one side, the baby will extend the arm that is on the same side of the body as the baby is facing and flex the opposite arm.	Usually fades after 3 to 4 months when the baby will lie symmetrically.	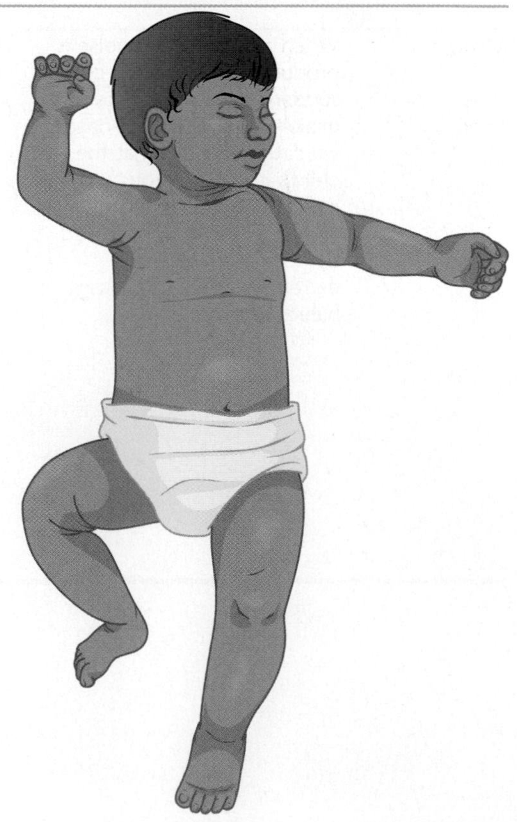

Table 7.3 Reflexes *cont'd*

Reflex	How the Reflex Is Elicited	Age Changes	Illustration
Trunk Incurvation	When a baby is placed in the prone position and his or her back is stroked along one side of the spine, the baby's body will turn toward the side of the body that was stroked.	Usually fades at about 1 month of age.	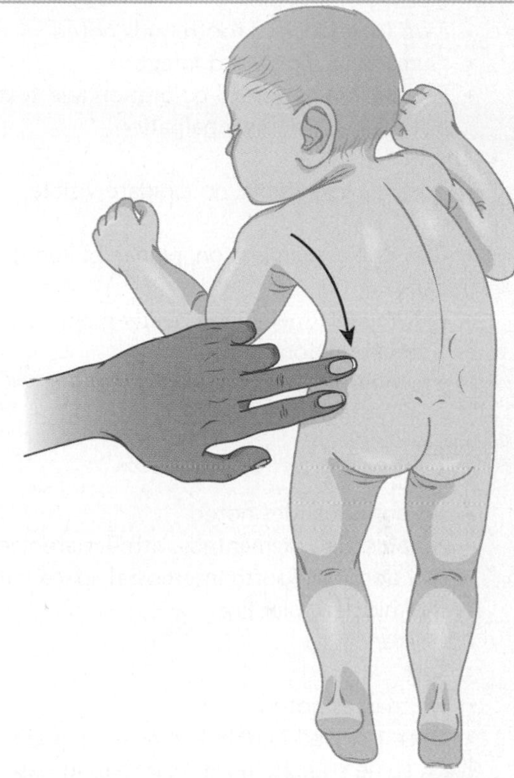

CASE STUDY: Putting It All Together

Mother brings baby girl, age 6 months old, to the primary health-care provider for a well baby checkup

Subjective Data

- The child is sleeping in her mother's arms when the nurse enters the examination room.
- Mother states,
  - "She's such an angel when she's sleeping. And she is great fun when she is playing."

Objective Data

Nursing Assessment, performed head to toe as child sleeps in mother's arms (in order of completion)

- Assessment:
- Nail beds pink, capillary refill less than 2 sec

Vital Signs

Apical heart rate for 60 seconds: 124 bpm, no murmurs noted

Respiratory rate for 60 seconds: 30 rpm

Bowel sounds: present in all four quadrants

- Head: symmetrical
  - Circumference: 42.4 cm, 50th percentile
  - Anterior fontanel: flat
  - Posterior fontanel: closed
- All facial structures symmetrical
  - Top of ears 1 cm above an imaginary line from the inner canthus through the outer canthus of the eyes
- Hair: minimal but symmetrically placed, fine, blond
- Nose: patent as seen via otoscope

Child wakes up, baby undressed completely. Remainder of examination performed with child crying in mother's arms

- Skin: pink throughout; no visible moles or other blemishes
- Eyes
  - Symmetrical
  - Sclerae white
  - Ophthalmoscopic Examination
    - Red reflex present
    - Light seen at same location in both eyes
    - Pupils equal and react equally to light

Continued

CASE STUDY: Putting It All Together *cont'd*

- Mouth
  - Lips moist and pink
  - Two lower incisor tooth buds noted
  - Gums pink, moist, and intact
  - Palates intact, normal coloration and texture; both visually and via palpation
- Throat
  - Tonsils pink; visible; no exudate visible
- Ears
  - Otoscopic examination, pinnae pulled down and back
    - Tympanic membrane pearly gray, no signs of inflammation or effusion
- Neck: moving spontaneously while crying
- Lymph nodes: palpable but not inflamed
- Chest
  - Symmetrical
  - No abnormalities noted
  - Nipples: flat, pigmented, with flat areolae
  - PMI noted at fourth intercostal space lateral to the midclavicular line
- Abdomen
  - Soft
  - No masses noted
  - Liver assessed 1 cm below costal margin
- Back: spine straight; no tufts of hair at base of spine
- Buttocks and rectum: gloves on
  - Anus patent; no fissures noted
  - When asked, mother states that child's stools are "bright yellow and loose. She stools about three or four times a day. I'm still exclusively breastfeeding her."
- Genitalia assessed after advising mother
  - Hymen visible
  - Labia majora wide spread
  - Clitoris, urethra, and vagina assessed; all pink and moist
  - No vaginal discharge noted
  - When asked, mother states that the child "has about six really, really wet diapers a day. And when she wakes up, her pajamas are sometimes even wet."
- Extremities and joints
  - No head lag noted when raised from the supine by her arms
  - Arm and leg lengths equal and of normal appearance
  - Ortolani's, Allis', and Barlow's signs negative
  - Thigh and gluteal folds equal
  - No crepitus noted
  - When raised to a standing position with support under the arms:
    - Legs dangle in parallel
    - When placed on her feet, she holds her weight momentarily
  - When placed in the sitting position, tripods and falls over after 10 seconds
- Neurological assessment
  - Babinski reflex present
  - Voluntary grasp: spontaneously grasps nurse's stethoscope
  - Moves toward the sound of a bell
- Other
  - While crying, repeatedly says, "Da, da, da, da, da!!"
  - *Placed supine on scale covered with exam paper:* weight 7.2 kg, 50th percentile
  - *Measured lying supine on examination table covered with exam paper:* length 65 cm, 50th percentile

Health-Care Provider's Orders

- Healthy 6-month-old female
- Begin solid foods: cereal with iron followed by meats, vegetables, and fruits
- Provide stimulation (e.g., auditory, visual, movement)
- Return for follow-up visit in 3 months
- Administer 6-month vaccines
  - DTaP (diphtheria, tetanus, acellular pertussis)
  - IPV (inactivated polio virus)
  - Hib (*hemophilus influenzae* type b)
  - PCV13 (pneumococcal conjugate)
  - RV-5 (rotavirus)
  - Hep B (hepatitis B)
  - IIV (inactivated influenza vaccine)

CASE STUDY: Putting It All Together *cont'd*

Case Study Questions

A. What *subjective* assessments indicate that the client is a healthy child?

1. ______
2. ______
3. ______
4. ______

B. What *objective* assessments indicate that the client is a healthy child?

1. ______
2. ______
3. ______
4. ______
5. ______
6. ______

C. After analyzing the data that has been collected, what **primary** nursing diagnosis should the nurse assign to this client?

1. ______

D. What interventions should the nurse plan and/or implement to meet this child's and her family's needs?

1. ______
2. ______
3. ______
4. ______

E. What client outcomes should the nurse evaluate regarding the effectiveness of the nursing interventions?

1. ______
2. ______
3. ______
4. ______
5. ______

F. What physiological characteristics should the child exhibit before being discharged home?

1. ______

G. What subjective characteristics should the child exhibit before being discharged home?

1. ______

REVIEW QUESTIONS

1. A 4½-year-old child is being assessed after sustaining an injury. The child is reluctant to tell the nurse exactly how the injury occurred. Which of the following statements made to the child by the nurse would likely result in the child communicating with the nurse? **Select all that apply.**
1. "Would you please draw me a picture of what happened to you?"
2. "Would you please write me a story about what happened to you?"
3. "Here is a puppet friend of mine. Could he tell me what happened to you?"
4. "What if your friend were hurt in the same way. What would have happened to him?"
5. "I can't help you if I don't know what happened. Would you please tell me how you got hurt?"

2. A nurse is attempting to get a 5-year-old child's cooperation when auscultating heart sounds. Which of the following comments is most likely to elicit the child's cooperation?
1. "It's time for me to listen to your heart go boom boom."
2. "Did you know that your heart beats in your chest?"
3. "Would you like to listen to the sounds your heart makes?"
4. "Let me show you a picture of a heart and where I want to listen."

3. The nurse enters the examination room of a mother and her 8-month-old. The baby is asleep in the mother's arms. Which of the following actions would be best for the nurse to perform at this time?
1. Ask the baby's mother for an updated history since the last well-child check.
2. Auscultate the baby's heart, lung, and bowel sounds.
3. Begin a full body assessment, starting with the baby's head and neck.
4. Wake the baby by playing with the baby's toes and feet.

4. The nurse is preparing to perform an examination of a 2-year-old boy. The child's mother is present. At the start of the examination, which of the following actions by the nurse may help to prevent a negative response from the child?
1. Refrain from touching the child, and speak directly to the child's mother.
2. Gently touch the child's hair while looking directly into his eyes.
3. Smile broadly while placing the bell of the stethoscope on the child's chest.
4. Ask the child to describe his favorite television show or favorite toy.

5. The nurse is obtaining a health history of a 6-year-old child who is being seen at the clinic for the first time. Which of the following questions should the nurse ask the child during the interview? **Select all that apply.**
1. "Do you have any pets at home?"
2. "Can you tell me how many 1 plus 1 makes?"
3. "Can you tell me the name of one of your school friends?"
4. "Can you tell me the names of any medicines that you take?"
5. "What kinds of things do you like to play during recess at school?"

6. A 9-year-old child is being seen in the pediatrician's office after experiencing a head injury. The nurse assesses the child's vital signs as: TPR – 98.0°F, HR: 52 bpm, RR: 12 rpm, and BP: 88/50 mm Hg. The child's capillary refill is 2 sec. Which of the following actions would be appropriate for the nurse to take?
1. Immediately notify the primary health-care practitioner of the findings.
2. Ask the child to describe how the head injury occurred.
3. Immediately administer two rescue breaths.
4. Carefully examine the child's head for signs of fracture.

7. The nurse is assessing a 5-year-old child with a possible fractured leg following a bicycle accident. Which of the following actions would best determine the child's pain level?
1. Observe the child's behavior.
2. Ask the child, "How bad does your leg hurt?"
3. Provide the child with a pain rating scale.
4. Ask the parent, "How much pain do you think he is in?"

Boys — birth to 36 months of age

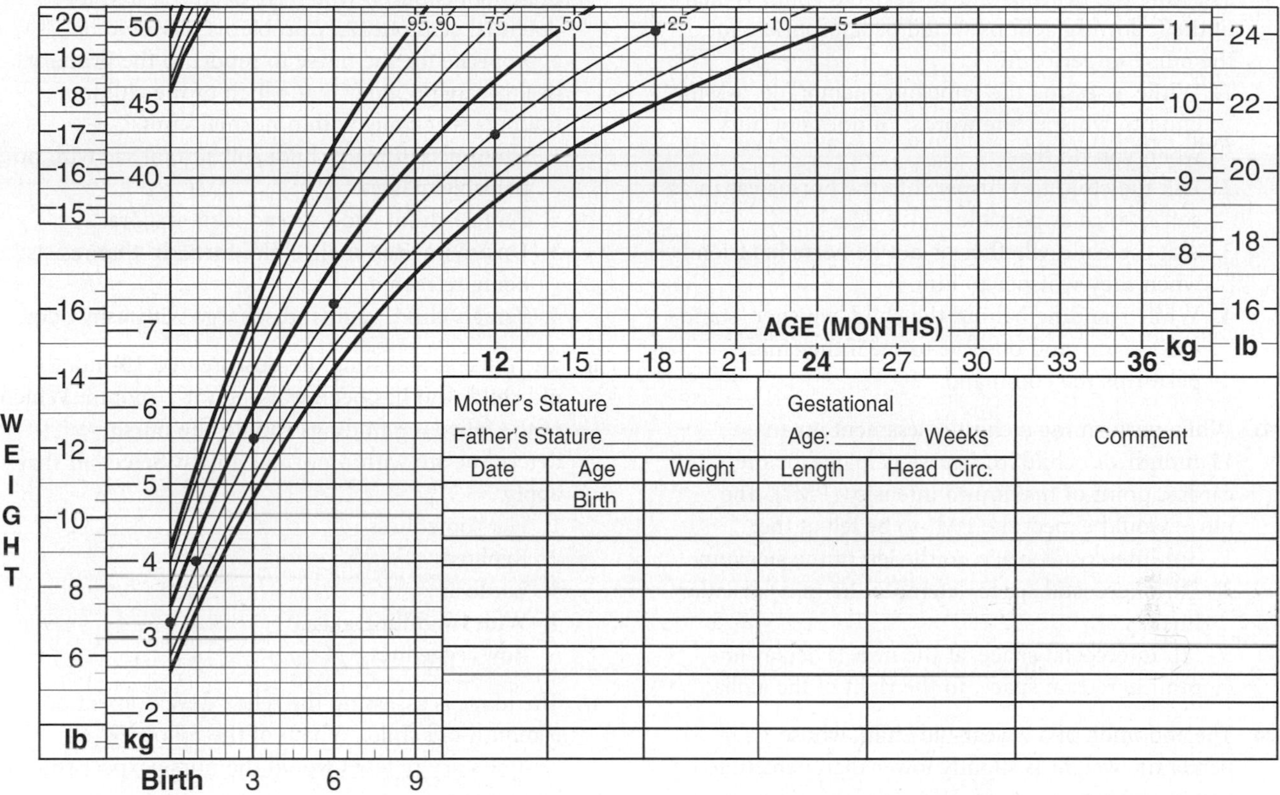

8. A nurse is assessing the weight chart of a boy 18 months of age (above). Which of the following conclusions should the nurse make based on the child's growth pattern?
   1. The child's weight has been consistently below normal. A complete diet history should be obtained.
   2. The child's weight is consistent and within normal limits.
   3. The child's weight is increasing rapidly. A nutrition consult is warranted.
   4. The child's weight has dropped slightly but is still within normal range.

9. The nurse is assessing the accommodation of a child's eyes. Which of the following techniques would be appropriate for the nurse to perform?
   1. Ask the child to follow the nurse's fingers in all six quadrants.
   2. Have the child cover one eye and read from a vision chart.
   3. Use an ophthalmoscope to assess for the red reflex.
   4. Move a puppet away from and close into the child's field of vision.

10. The nurse is assessing the dental development of a 7-month-old child. Which of the following findings would the nurse expect to see?
    1. No teeth: drooling and chewing behavior
    2. Two teeth: lower incisors
    3. Two teeth: upper incisors
    4. Four teeth: both upper and lower incisors

11. The nurse is preparing to palpate a 2-year-old girl's tongue during a physical examination. Which of the following actions would help to prevent the nurse from being bitten?
    1. Have the parent open the girl's mouth.
    2. Ask the child to open her mouth big and wide.
    3. Hold the toddler's cheeks with the fingers of one hand.
    4. Place a tongue blade in the middle of the tongue.

12. The nurse is performing a whisper test when assessing the hearing of a 10-year-old child. Which of the following actions would be appropriate for the nurse to perform?
1. While assessing the tympanic membrane, ask the child to whisper the words, "It does not hurt when you do that."
2. Ask the child to whisper into the nurse's ear in as soft a voice as possible.
3. Ask the child whether or not he hears his friends when they whisper to him.
4. While standing behind the child, whisper "stand on one leg" and observe to see if the child performs the command.

13. While performing a chest assessment on an 11-month-old child, the nurse palpates for the cardiac point of maximum intensity (PMI). The nurse would expect the PMI to be felt at the:
1. 3rd intercostal space, to the left of the sternum.
2. 4th intercostal space, lateral to the midclavicular line.
3. 5th intercostal space, at the midclavicular line.
4. 6th intercostal space, to the right of the axilla.

14. The abdomen of a 7-year-old child, whose percentile weight is slightly lower than percentile height, is being assessed. Which of the following findings would the nurse expect to see?
1. Umbilical hernia on inspection
2. Liver below the right costal margin on palpation
3. Aortic pulsations on inspection
4. Spleen below the left costal margin on palpation

15. The nurse has performed physical assessments on 4 preschool children who have been referred for potential genitourinary problems. It would be appropriate for the nurse to report to the primary health-care provider that which of the children's findings is actually within normal limits?
1. Circumcised male child: soft scrotal sac with no palpable masses.
2. Female child: wide-spread labia majora.
3. Uncircumcised male child: foreskin that resists being retracted.
4. Female child: vaginal discharge with fishy odor.

16. The nurse is assessing the posture of a 13-month-old child who has been walking for 1 month. Which of the following findings should the nurse determine are within normal limits? **Select all that apply.**
1. Flat-footedness
2. Kyphosis
3. Lordosis
4. Wide, waddling gait
5. Bow-leggedness

17. The nurse is assessing the reflex development of a 5-month-old child. Which of the following rudimentary reflexes would the nurse expect still to be present?
1. Moro
2. Trunk incurvation
3. Babinski
4. Grasping

REVIEW ANSWERS

1. **ANSWER: 1, 3, and 4**

Rationale:

1. Children often communicate by drawing pictures.

2. A 4½-year-old is too young to be able to write a story.

3. Children often communicate while playing with puppets.

4. Children often communicate when they are pretending to be speaking about someone else.

5. Such directed questioning is unlikely to elicit a response in a young child.

TEST-TAKING TIP: Young children are wary of communicating with adults they do not know or trust. Using forms of play, including drawing, puppetry, and verbal storytelling, can often elicit responses in children.

Content Area: *Child Health*

Integrated Processes: *Nursing Process: Implementation; Communication and Documentation*

Client Need: *Psychosocial Integrity: Therapeutic Communication*

Cognitive Level: *Application*

2. **ANSWER: 3**

Rationale:

1. Although this statement might elicit a child's cooperation, it is not the best statement for the nurse to make.

2. Although this statement might elicit a child's cooperation, it is not the best statement for the nurse to make.

3. Asking the child whether he or she would like to hear his or her own heart is an excellent way to get the child's cooperation.

4. Although this statement might elicit a child's cooperation, it is not the best statement for the nurse to make.

TEST-TAKING TIP: Although no action is foolproof, preschool children often want to play with the equipment that the nurse is using. Giving the child the option of listening to his or her own heart with the stethoscope would provide that opportunity.

Content Area: *Child Health*

Integrated Processes: *Nursing Process: Assessment*

Client Need: *Health Promotion and Maintenance: Techniques of Physical Assessment*

Cognitive Level: *Application*

3. **ANSWER: 2**

Rationale:

1. Obtaining an updated history can wait.

2. The nurse should take the opportunity to auscultate the baby's heart, lungs, and bowel sounds.

3. The full assessment should wait.

4. The nurse should take the opportunity to auscultate the baby's heart, lungs, and bowel sounds.

TEST-TAKING TIP: An 8-month-old is likely to be exhibiting signs of stranger anxiety. Once awake, therefore, he or she will likely cry when touched by the nurse. It is best to auscultate the heart, lungs, and bowel sounds while the child is quiet and sleeping.

Content Area: *Child Health*

Integrated Processes: *Nursing Process: Assessment*

Client Need: *Health Promotion and Maintenance: Techniques of Physical Assessment*

Cognitive Level: *Application*

4. **ANSWER: 1**

Rationale:

1. When the nurse waits to touch the toddler and speaks directly to the child's mother, the toddler begins to see that the mother trusts the nurse and, therefore, is more likely to begin to trust the nurse.

2. Children are often protective of their heads and may be wary of the nurse making direct eye contact immediately on entering the examination room.

3. Even though the nurse is smiling broadly, he or she is making direct contact with the child immediately on entering the examination room.

4. The verbal skills of a 2-year-old usually are not developed enough to be able to describe a favorite television show or favorite toy. Also, the nurse is questioning the child directly on entering the examination room.

TEST-TAKING TIP: Toddlers often are the least cooperative during physical examinations. They are protective of their bodies and wary of strangers. The nurse allows the child to become familiar with the surroundings and with the nurse as the nurse has a conversation with the parent, asking questions regarding the child's health. In this way, the nurse is more likely to elicit the child's cooperation.

Content Area: *Child Health*

Integrated Processes: *Nursing Process: Implementation*

Client Need: *Health Promotion and Maintenance: Techniques of Physical Assessment*

Cognitive Level: *Application*

5. **ANSWER: 1, 2, 3, and 5**

Rationale:

1. "Do you have any pets at home?" should be asked.

2. "Can you tell me how many 1 plus 1 makes?" should be asked.

3. "Can you tell me the name of 1 of your school friends?" should be asked.

4. "Can you tell me the names of any medicines that you take?" should be a question directed to the parents.

5. "What kinds of things do you like to play during recess at school?" should be asked.

TEST-TAKING TIP: The questions that the nurse is asking the child will provide information regarding the child's progress in school, the child's environment, the child's social interactions, and the child's activity level. The parent, however, is responsible for medication administration.

Content Area: *Child Health*

Integrated Processes: *Nursing Process: Implementation; Communication and Documentation*

Client Need: Health Promotion and Maintenance: Techniques of Physical Assessment
Cognitive Level: Application

6. ANSWER: 1
Rationale:
1. The nurse should immediately notify the primary health-care practitioner of the findings.
2. The nurse should immediately notify the primary health-care practitioner of the findings.
3. The nurse should immediately notify the primary health-care practitioner of the findings.
4. The nurse should immediately notify the primary health-care practitioner of the findings.
TEST-TAKING TIP: Bradycardia is an ominous sign in children. A heart rate of less than 60 bpm with poor perfusion would warrant the beginning of chest compressions. In addition, although this child is exhibiting satisfactory perfusion, the child's blood pressure is low: $9 \times 2 + 70$ (or 65) = a minimal systolic pressure of 88 (or 83). The primary health-care provider should be notified of the child's condition.
Content Area: Pediatrics
Integrated Processes: Nursing Process: Implementation
Client Need: Physiological Integrity: Physiological Adaptation: Medical Emergencies
Cognitive Level: Application

7. ANSWER: 3
Rationale:
1. A child's behavior is not the best method to determine his or her pain level.
2. Asking a child a general question regarding the severity of the pain is not the best method to determine his or her pain level.
3. Providing a child with an age-appropriate pain rating scale is the best method to determine his or her pain level.
4. Asking the parent of a child regarding the child's pain is not the best method to determine his or her pain level.
TEST-TAKING TIP: Just as when working with adults, when children use pain scales to rate their pain, the nurse obtains an objective determination of the severity of the child's pain. There are pain scales for all age patients, from nonverbal neonates through to adults.
Content Area: Pediatrics
Integrated Processes: Nursing Process: Implementation
Client Need: Health Promotion and Maintenance: Techniques of Physical Assessment
Cognitive Level: Application

8. ANSWER: 3
Rationale:
1. The child's weight is within normal limits. No special intervention is needed.
2. The child's weight is within normal limits. No special intervention is needed.
3. The child's weight is within normal limits. No special intervention is needed.
4. The child's weight is within normal limits. No special intervention is needed.
TEST-TAKING TIP: This child's weight is consistently at the 25th percentile. Although the child's weight is not average, it is consistent over time.
Content Area: Child Health
Integrated Processes: Nursing Process: Analysis
Client Need: Health Promotion and Maintenance: Techniques of Physical Assessment
Cognitive Level: Application

9. ANSWER: 4
Rationale:
1. Asking a child to follow fingers in all six quadrants enables the nurse to assess the child's binocular vision.
2. Having the child cover one eye and read from a vision chart enables the nurse to assess the child's ability to see distances.
3. Using an ophthalmoscope and assessing for the red reflex enables the nurse to assess the health of the retina.
4. Moving a puppet away from and close into the child's field of vision enables the nurse to assess visual accommodation.
TEST-TAKING TIP: The muscles of the iris change when the eye accommodates from distance to close vision. The nurse can assess that change when a child looks at an object that is moving from close up to far from the child.
Content Area: Child Health
Integrated Processes: Nursing Process: Assessment
Client Need: Health Promotion and Maintenance: Techniques of Physical Assessment
Cognitive Level: Application

10. ANSWER: 2
Rationale:
1. No teeth, and drooling and chewing behavior usually are noted in 5- to 6-month-old babies.
2. Two teeth: lower incisors are usually seen at 7 months of age.
3. Two teeth: upper incisors usually appear at about 9 months of age.
4. Four teeth: both upper and lower incisors usually are present at 9 months of age.
TEST-TAKING TIP: Although tooth development may be slightly early or slightly delayed, the progression of tooth eruption is usually consistent. Also, it is important for the nurse to educate the parents that once the child begins to have teeth, they should be cleaned each day.
Content Area: Child Health
Integrated Processes: Nursing Process: Assessment
Client Need: Health Promotion and Maintenance: Developmental Stages and Transitions
Cognitive Level: Application

11. ANSWER: 3
Rationale:
1. Having the parent open the child's mouth is not the best method.
2. Asking the child to open her mouth big and wide is not the best method.
3. Holding the child's cheeks with one hand is the best method. The jaw is kept open by gentle pressure exerted through the cheeks.
4. Placing a tongue blade in the middle of the tongue may elicit a gag reflex and is not the best method.
TEST-TAKING TIP: Young children are unpredictable. The nurse must protect him or herself from potential injury because a toddler may bite the examiner.
Content Area: *Child Health*
Integrated Processes: *Nursing Process: Assessment*
Client Need: *Health Promotion and Maintenance: Techniques of Physical Assessment*
Cognitive Level: *Application*

12. ANSWER: 4
Rationale:
1. The whisper test is performed to assess whether or not the child can hear the practitioner when he or she whispers.
2. The whisper test is performed to assess whether or not the child can hear the practitioner when he or she whispers.
3. Asking the child whether he hears his friends when they whisper to him provides only subjective information.
4. It would be appropriate for the nurse to stand behind the child, to whisper "stand on one leg," and to observe to see if the child performs the command.
TEST-TAKING TIP: To make certain that the child does not become startled by the nurse's actions, the child should be forewarned of the whisper test. To make sure that the child is not lip reading, the nurse should stand behind the child while conducting the test.
Content Area: *Child Health*
Integrated Processes: *Nursing Process: Assessment*
Client Need: *Health Promotion and Maintenance: Techniques of Physical Assessment*
Cognitive Level: *Application*

13. ANSWER: 2
Rationale:
1. The PMI is never found at the third intercostal space to the left of the sternum.
2. Until a child reaches about 7 years of age, the PMI is found at the fourth intercostal space lateral to the midclavicular line.
3. After the age of 7, the PMI is found at the fifth intercostal space at the midclavicular line.
4. The PMI is never found at the sixth intercostal space to the right of the axilla.
TEST-TAKING TIP: It is important to note that not only do children's vital signs change as they grow, but also the physiological landmarks change as children grow.
Content Area: *Child Health*
Integrated Processes: *Nursing Process: Assessment*
Client Need: *Health Promotion and Maintenance: Techniques of Physical Assessment*
Cognitive Level: *Application*

14. ANSWER: 3
Rationale:
1. The nurse would not expect to note an umbilical hernia in a 7-year-old child.
2. The nurse would not expect to find the child's liver below the right costal margin on palpation of a 7-year-old child.
3. The nurse would expect to see aortic pulsations on inspection.
4. The nurse would not expect to find the spleen below the left costal margin on palpation.
TEST-TAKING TIP: Umbilical hernias sometimes are seen in neonates. As the abdominal musculature improves, they often resolve on their own. The liver is felt below the right costal margin in neonates but not in school-aged children. Unless markedly enlarged, the spleen is not felt below the costal margin.
Content Area: *Child Health*
Integrated Processes: *Nursing Process: Assessment*
Client Need: *Health Promotion and Maintenance: Techniques of Physical Assessment*
Cognitive Level: *Application*

15. ANSWER: 4
Rationale:
1. The testes should be felt in the scrotal sacs of both circumcised and uncircumcised males. Further investigation is warranted.
2. The labia majora of a preschool female is usually wide spread.
3. The foreskin of the uncircumcised preschool male child should be easily retractable. Further investigation is warranted.
4. The vaginal discharge should have no odor. Further investigation is warranted.
TEST-TAKING TIP: Just as a reminder, prior to performing an examination of a child's genitalia, both the parent and the child should be forewarned. In addition, the procedure should be performed in a matter of fact way in order not to embarrass or frighten the child.
Content Area: *Child Health*
Integrated Processes: *Nursing Process: Assessment*
Client Need: *Health Promotion and Maintenance: Developmental Stages and Transitions*
Cognitive Level: *Application*

16. ANSWER: 1, 3, 4, and 5
Rationale:
1. Toddlers usually are flat-footed until about 2 years of age.
2. Kyphosis is not an expected posture of the toddler.
3. Lordosis often is seen in toddlers.
4. Toddlers usually walk with a wide, waddling gait.
5. Bow-leggedness is normally seen in the toddler.

TEST-TAKING TIP: If the test-taker remembers that the toddler has weak abdominal muscles and large abdominal organs, it is understandable that the toddler would be lordotic. The wide, waddling gait helps toddlers to lower their center of gravity and, therefore, better enable them to walk on two feet.
Content Area: *Child Health*
Integrated Processes: *Nursing Process: Assessment*
Client Need: *Health Promotion and Maintenance: Developmental Stages and Transitions*
Cognitive Level: *Application*

17. **ANSWER: 3**
Rationale:
1. By 5 months of age, the Moro reflex has disappeared.
2. By 5 months of age, the trunk incurvation reflex has disappeared.
3. The Babinski reflex usually disappears at 1 year of age.
4. By 5 months of age, the grasp reflex has disappeared.

TEST-TAKING TIP: When reflexes last longer than expected, especially the grasp reflex, the child should be assessed for possible illness (e.g., cerebral palsy).
Content Area: *Child Health*
Integrated Processes: *Nursing Process: Assessment*
Client Need: *Health Promotion and Maintenance: Developmental Stages and Transitions*
Cognitive Level: *Application*

Chapter 8

Nursing Care of the Child in the Health-Care Setting

KEY TERMS

Assent—An implicit or explicit statement that a treatment may be performed.

Despair—One of the three stages of separation in which the child is sad and withdrawn.

Detachment—One of the three stages of separation in which the child becomes emotionally separated from family and friends and becomes resigned to the separation.

Protest—One of the three stages of separation in which the child exhibits anger, physically and verbally.

Therapeutic holding—A form of physical restraint in which one or more nurses hold a child during a painful or scary procedure.

I. Description

Because of the changing health-care climate, the vast majority of sick children will be cared for in outpatient facilities or in the home, while surgical and other significant illnesses will require hospitalization.

A child who is ill and/or hospitalized responds much differently from an adult who is sick. When caring for a sick child, the nurse must first consider the child's chronological age because his or her physiological assessments will be evaluated in reference to the child's age. Next, the nurse must determine whether the child's developmental level is in synchrony with the child's age because the behaviors and characteristics the child are expected to exhibit for that period will be evaluated in relation to the child's developmental level. In addition, many interventions will be tailored to the child's development. The nurse must also consider other factors that may affect the child's responses (e.g., the child's family constellation, including siblings and pets; classmates from whom the child will be separated during a hospitalization; favorite toys or other items cherished by the child; nicknames used by the child).

II. Hospitalization

A. Child.

1. Nursing history and physical assessment (see Chapter 7, "Physical Assessment of Children: From Infancy to Adolescence").
   a. It is important for the nurse first to conduct a thorough history and physical assessment of the sick child.
2. Major stressors experienced by sick children, especially those who are hospitalized, must be considered by the nurse.

a. Children are both emotionally and cognitively immature. The stress of illness can be as taxing to the child—both emotionally and developmentally—as the illness itself.
   i. To minimize the stressors of hospitalization as much as possible, both the child and the family members should be carefully prepared for the experience.
   ii. The comprehensiveness and method of the preparation is dependent on the severity of the illness, seriousness of the interventions that the child will experience, and the developmental level of the child (see the "Growth and Development" sections for each age level).
      (1) Information must be accurate but geared to the cognitive level of the recipient.
         (a) Parents often will need much more comprehensive education than is appropriate for the child.

b. Separation: when a child must be hospitalized, he or she is being cared for in an unfamiliar environment. The separation from home can be frightening.
   i. Stages of separation.
      (1) Occur when children must be cared for at a location far from family and friends.
      (2) The longer the separation, the more pronounced the responses seen in children.
         (a) Stages of separation (Box 8.1) are seen less frequently today than in the past because of the multiple means of communication that are available (e.g., telephone, Skype, FaceTime, Twitter).

Box 8.1 Stages of Separation

1. ***Protest:*** *child is angry and exhibits that anger both physically and verbally. For example, the child cries, kicks, resists being consoled, pulls off bandages, and exhibits other temper tantrum–like behaviors. This protest is most dramatically seen in older infants and toddlers.*
2. ***Despair:*** *child is sad and withdrawn. He or she cries infrequently, exhibits little interest in play or any activities, is listless, and appears dispirited.*
3. ***Detachment:*** *child becomes emotionally separated from family and friends and resigned to the separation. The child plays with staff, forms relationships with those in the health-care facility, and pays little attention to family and/or friends who do visit the child.*

   ii. Age issues: separation is most difficult for older infants and toddlers, but all children—even adolescents—are stressed when separated from family and friends.
   iii. Nursing considerations: risk for altered coping.
      (1) Encourage important individuals in the child's life, such as parents, family members, close friends, classmates, and others (e.g., pets), to stay with and visit the child as much as possible.
         (a) Adolescents often find it difficult to ask their parents to stay in the hospital with them. Nurses can help teenagers to communicate their need for parental support.
         (b) When it is impossible for the child to have family or friends with him or her at all times, it is important for the nurse to reassure family members that the child will receive the care and comfort needed while he or she is alone.
         (c) When important individuals must leave the child, instruct them never to sneak out while the child is sleeping or to tell the child that they will return when they are unable or unwilling to do so.
            (i) The child may feel betrayed by a parent who disappears while the child is asleep.
         (d) Encourage parents to provide the child with his or her cherished, transition objects.
            (i) Encourage parents and others to bring in objects to remind the child of home and friends.
            (ii) Encourage parents and others to communicate frequently with the child using any and all forms of communication, including, but not limited to, pictures, videos, Skype, phone calls, and texts.
      (2) Place the child with a roommate of a similar developmental level and with a similar illness, for example:
         (a) If the child is a preschooler who is bedbound, the roommate should also be a preschooler who is bedbound.

(3) Assign the same nurse to take care of the child each day as much as possible.

c. Loss of control: because the child is in an unfamiliar setting and he or she must follow unfamiliar rules and be subjected to prescribed treatments and procedures, the child will experience a loss of control.

i. Children's responses to the loss of control during illnesses usually are directly related to their developmental levels (Table 8.1).

d. Bodily injury and pain: Rarely are children hospitalized and not subjected to painful procedures.

i. Lack of effective pain management has crucial consequences for the child.

ii. Nursing considerations: pain/risk for altered coping.

(1) Based on their weight and recommended dosage levels, children at all age levels, including infants, should receive adequate pain medication, for example:

(a) Children who are postoperative, in sickle cell crisis, immediately postfracture, or in similar situations should receive narcotic medications, as indicated by the rating noted on an age-appropriate pain rating scale.

(b) The nurse must anticipate a child's pain needs because:

(i) Children fear injections and, therefore, often fail to ask for pain medication.

(ii) Children think adults know when they are in pain and, therefore, may not ask for pain medication.

(2) Pharmacological pain management.

(a) Age: nurses should respond to children in relation to their developmental and chronological age.

(b) Source of the pain: procedural versus physiological in origin.

(i) If procedural (i.e., pain is occurring because of a medical procedure):

(I) The child must be told beforehand that the procedure will be painful.

Table 8.1 Characteristics of Loss of Control by Developmental Stage

Stage of Development	Characteristics	Nursing Considerations (Risk for Altered Coping)
Infants	Because of their immaturity, infants show little to no response to loss of control	N/A
Toddlers	Developmentally, toddlers are seeking autonomy When restrained or bedbound, toddlers often become angry and verbally and physically resist the confinement	Allow child to make choices, when appropriate Daily routines are comforting Try to continue home rituals and provide the child with his or her security object
Preschoolers	Preschoolers may think they are being punished for bad behavior Preschoolers often misunderstand language used by doctors and nurses	Clearly communicate to the child that he or she is not bad and not being punished but rather that care is needed to help him or her to get better Be sure to speak in clear, unambiguous language
School-Agers	School-age children often express anger that their school routine and beginning independence is being taken away	Give them some decision-making ability (e.g., "Would you like the dressing changed at 3 p.m. or 4 p.m.?") Encourage them to participate in their care (e.g., "Would you please give me strips of tape while I change your bandage?")
Adolescents	Teenagers are often most affected by the loss of control. They resent being treated like a "kid."	Must be provided choices in their care and, when appropriate, opportunities to provide their own care. However, because they often have difficulty asking for help, always ask them if they need assistance Provide them with space where they can engage in private conversations

MAKING THE CONNECTION

There are a number of myths—believed by health-care professionals—surrounding pain management in children.

Myth—Children are at high risk of becoming addicted to narcotics.

Correction—Children are no higher risk than are adults.

Myth—Children are at high risk of developing respiratory depression if given narcotics.

Correction—If a safe dosage of a narcotic is administered, the incidence of respiratory depression is rare. In addition, if respiratory depression does occur, Narcan (naloxone), a narcotic antagonist, may be administered.

Myth—Infants do not feel pain as much as older children and adults.

Correction—Infants do feel pain. Objective infant pain assessment scales should always be used to assess infants' pain levels (e.g., Neonatal Infant Pain Scale; Postoperative Pain Score; CRIES scale).

Myth—Children tolerate pain better than adults.

Correction—Young children rate procedural pain higher than older children and adults. Age-appropriate pain scales should always be used to assess the pain level of children at all ages (e.g., Infant pain scales [see earlier], Wong-Baker scale, the Oucher scale).

Myth—Children cannot tell you where they hurt.

Correction—By 3 years of age, children can effectively use pain scales and point to areas of pain.

Myth—Children become accustomed to pain or painful procedures.

Correction—Children often exhibit increasingly intense responses to repeated painful procedures. It is essential that adequate levels of pain medications be administered for all painful procedures, especially if the procedures will be repeated in the future.

Myth—Children's behaviors reflect their pain intensity.

Correction—Children often rate their pain higher than would be indicated by their behavior. Children's pain should be medicated as indicated by the rating scale, not by their behavior.

Myth—Narcotics are more dangerous for children than they are for adults.

Correction—By early infancy, children can metabolize opioids as well as older children and have no higher incidence of addiction and respiratory depression than older children and adults.

(II) The nurse should learn how the child has dealt with painful experiences in the past and try to incorporate those coping skills into the treatment plan.

(III) The child should be pretreated with an adequate dosage of medication.

(IV) Parents should be encouraged to be present during the procedure. When sick, even teenagers want their parents present.

(V) Nurses should incorporate age-based principles into their care (Table 8.2).

(c) Important principles related to the administration of pain medication (see also Chapter 9, "Pediatric Medication Administration").

(i) Right drug.

(I) NSAIDS should be administered for mild pain, but opioids should be administered for moderate to severe pain.

(II) Morphine is often the narcotic of choice.

(ii) Right dose: The nurse must calculate the safe dosage for each child based on the pediatric dosage recommendations in a reliable medication text.

(iii) Right route.

(I) The nurse must remember that intramuscular administration produces pain even though ultimately it will relieve pain.

(II) Patient-controlled anesthesia can be used by older school-age children and above.

(III) The epidural or intrathecal route may also be used in some cases.

Table 8.2 Age-Based Considerations in Procedural Pain Management

Developmental Stage	Considerations
Infants	Infants rarely anticipate procedures; nurses should perform the procedures quickly then provide comfort and reassurance to the child
Toddlers and Preschoolers	Nurses must be truthful, use clear language, and give the young child choices, if appropriate
School-Agers	School-age children often feel they need to be brave, but they must be allowed to cry and should never be reprimanded for not being a "big" boy or girl
Adolescents	Nurses must be honest and nonjudgmental because adolescents often fear being perceived as weak. Teens are acutely aware of their bodies. Often they are as concerned about bodily injury as they are of the pain itself.

(iv) Right time: Pain medications may be ordered as a standing order to avoid the need for the child to request a pain medication.

(v) Right patient: The nurse must always employ safe administration principles set forth by the Joint Commission.

(3) Nonpharmacological pain management.

(a) Nonpharmacological interventions may be employed alone or in conjunction with pharmacological methods.

(b) Because children engage in play and fantasy in their daily lives, nonpharmacological pain management techniques are often effective.

(c) Examples of nonpharmacological methods that may be used are:

(i) Distracting the child (e.g., reading a book to a child, having the child blow bubbles, listening or singing to music, watching a video, playing with favored toys/games).

(ii) Conducting a guided imagery session with the child.

(iii) Repositioning and/or swaddling the child.

(iv) Holding and cuddling the child with his or her transitional object.

(v) Applying hot packs and/or cold packs to the painful site.

(vi) Employing powers of positive thinking by advising the child how well medications and other interventions help to reduce pain.

3. Suggested process to follow when caring for children who are in pain: QUESTION (Box 8.2).

Box 8.2 QUESTION Process for Caring for Children Who Are in Pain

QUESTION

Q: question *the child*
- *Learn what word the child uses for pain*
- *Ask the child to point where the pain is, but if the child is reluctant to speak:*
  - *Ask the child to tell the parent because he or she may not feel comfortable telling a stranger*
  - *Have the child tell a puppet where the pain is*

U: use *an age-appropriate pain scale*

E: evaluate *behavioral and physiological changes*
- *If behavior differs from pain rating, believe the pain rating*
- *Although not completely reliable, especially if the child experiences chronic pain, physiological changes may be present (e.g., flushing; sweating; rise in blood pressure and heart and respiratory rate; restlessness)*

S: secure *the parents' involvement*
- *Ask the parents whether the child's behavior is consistent with past experiences with pain*
- *Ask the parents regarding suggestions for nonpharmacological pain management methods that have worked in the past.*

T: take *a nursing history to determine the source and/or cause of the pain*

I: intervene
- *To assess and not to take action is unprofessional.*
- *Both pharmacological and nonpharmacological interventions are often appropriate*

O: ongoing *assessment is essential to determine whether or not the intervention has been effective.*

N: new intervention
- *If a child's pain is not being treated effectively, report to the child's primary health-care provider that additional medication or a different medication is needed.*

4. Regression.
   a. Children who recently have reached developmental milestones will almost always regress when they are sick, whether they are being cared for at home or in a health-care setting.
   b. Parents should be advised that:
      i. Regression is expected and normal.
      ii. Children should not be punished or made to feel ashamed of the regression.
      iii. Children usually regain the lost milestones in a short period of time once they are well.
   c. Examples of regression.
      i. Infant who has started to drink out of a cup may revert to using a bottle.
      ii. Toddler who has become fully toilet trained may wet the bed.
      iii. School-age child who normally dresses him or herself may ask to have assistance from parents.
5. Play.
   a. Play is a child's work, even while he or she is in the hospital.
      i. Play is comforting and a means of diverting the child's attention away from his or her illness.

Although play is important, the nurse must remember that all prescribed medical interventions must take precedence over play because the main goal of the interventions is to improve the child's health.

   b. Toys and games provided to the child must be kept clean and safe.
      i. Any broken items should be thrown away or repaired.
      ii. Only items that can easily be cleaned should be given to sick children.
   c. Location and type of play must be appropriate to the child's physical and emotional well-being, for example:
      i. If child is bedbound, toys and games should be provided that are easily enjoyed in bed.
      ii. If child is receiving oxygen, toys and games that produce no sparks should be provided.
   d. Playroom.
      i. The majority of pediatric units have at least one room on the unit that is devoted to play.
         (1) Ideally, two rooms are set aside for sick children—one for infants, toddlers, preschoolers, and young school-age children and one for older school-age children and adolescents.
      ii. Children should know that the playroom is a safe haven in which no treatments or procedures are performed.
         (1) If a child must have a treatment administered or procedure performed, the nurse should escort the child to a treatment room where the procedure is performed and then, if appropriate, escort the child back to the playroom.
   e. Play as therapy: play can be employed in a variety of therapeutic ways.
      i. To help children to express their feelings.
         (1) Children's drawings often convey emotions that they may be feeling but find difficult to speak about.
         (2) Pretend play through puppets or other imaginary experiences can enable children to convey their feelings in indirect ways.
      ii. To release their frustrations.
         (1) Throwing bean bags at a target can help children to release their anger over being ill.
         (2) Changing a pretend dressing or giving an injection with a pretend syringe to a teddy bear can help children to express their frustrations with painful procedures and injections.
      iii. To educate them about their illnesses.
         (1) Computer programs can be used to educate diabetic children about insulin, dietary restrictions, and other aspects of their illness.
         (2) Allowing children to play with surgical hats, gowns, masks, and booties can help them to see what the surgeons and nurses will look like when they are in the surgical suite.
6. Limit setting and discipline.
   a. Children expect to have limits set for them.
   b. Although rules may be eased when children are ill, they often become anxious when all rules are abolished.
      i. They may ask themselves, "Am I sicker than I thought I was?"
   c. Examples of limits that should be retained as much as possible.
      i. School work must be done.
         (a) Tutors or school representatives will provide children with their schoolwork.
         (b) Although it may not be as time consuming or difficult as it was when they were well, the children should still know that they are expected to

complete at least some of the work required.

ii. Child must go to bed at a certain hour.

(1) Although the child may be allowed to watch a favored television program before bedtime that he or she is not usually allowed to watch, the child should be expected to go to bed at approximately the same time as he or she does at home.

iii. Child must act in a respectful manner.

(1) Even though a child is ill and uncomfortable, the child is still expected to speak respectfully to his or her parents and health-care providers.

B. Family (see also Chapter 1, "The Child as a Member of the Family").

1. The nurse must consider the entire family when admitting a child to the health-care setting.
   a. The nurse may find that parents, siblings, grandparents, and other family members accompany the child to the hospital.
   b. Every member of the family is stressed and concerned.

DID YOU KNOW?

The nurse should be especially attuned to the developmental levels and needs of the child's siblings because, for example, preschool siblings often feel responsible for causing their brother's or sister's illness.

2. To provide holistic care, the nurse must communicate acceptance and compassion to all present in relation to the unique needs of the family

C. The dying child.

1. Nurse.
   a. First, the nurse must assess his or her own feelings regarding the death of a child.
      i. If needed, the nurse should seek guidance and/or counseling from a social worker or other health-care professional.
   b. Compassion and caring are critical.
   c. When a patient dies, it is important for the nurse to grieve the loss.
      i. To provide caregivers who have cared for clients who have died with an opportunity to express their grief, many clinical units conduct debriefing/therapy sessions.
2. Child.
   a. The child should receive unconditional love and understanding.
      i. The child must be allowed to communicate his or her feelings in a nonjudgmental environment.

MAKING THE CONNECTION

Should a Dying Child Be Told That He or She Is Dying?

There are conflicting views regarding whether or not a child should be advised that he or she is dying. Although the child's parents may feel one way or the other, one of the best recommendations for the nurse to make is for the parents and others to respond to the needs of the child. Children often question the severity of their illnesses. They respond to the nonverbal behaviors of their parents and other important people in their lives as well as to the behaviors of the health-care professionals who are caring for them. Although a declaration of the child's imminent death may be too harsh, when a child begins to ask questions about death and about his or her own mortality, the child needs an honest response by those caring for him. Avoiding the issue will negatively affect the relationship that the nurse has developed with the child. If the parents are especially adamant that the nurse not tell the child of his or her diagnosis, the nurse can simply tell the parent that he or she will not bring the subject up but, if the child broaches the subject, that the nurse will provide an empathic, honest response.

ii. Presence.

(1) Often, the most comforting and compassionate care that a nurse can provide a dying child is simply to be quietly present.

(2) No child should be allowed to die alone.

b. Pain control.

i. As in any situation, sufficient pain medication should be provided to the child who is dying (see earlier).

c. Guilt.

i. The child must be reminded that he or she did not do anything to warrant contracting such a devastating illness.

ii. Preschool-age children especially are high risk for feeling guilty for becoming so ill.

d. Age-related concept of death: children's understanding of death and the permanency of death develop over time (Table 8.3).

D. Safety: because children are at high risk for accidental injury, the nurse must be especially aware of potential dangers that are present in the hospital setting.

1. Name bands.
   a. Name bands must always be checked.
      i. The nurse must not assume that the child will give his or her name if asked.

Table 8.3 Understanding of Death by Developmental Age

Developmental Stage	Conceptions
Infants and Toddlers	Have no cognitive understanding of death Experience death as a loss of comfort and caring • *Parents often respond differently to their dying child* • *The dying child often feels more pain and other discomforts as death approaches*
Preschoolers	See severe illness and death as a punishment View death as a temporary state
School-Agers	Begin to grasp the permanency of death; by 9 or 10 years of age, they begin to understand that they, themselves, are mortal Often express a fear of death and may ask questions about the process of dying
Adolescents	Fully understand the concept of death but see death as something that happens to older people Often experience a distancing from their peers because their friends are uncomfortable maintaining a relationship with someone their own age who is dying

ii. The nurse must not assume that because a child is in a bed that the child is in his or her bed.
(1) Children may be playing a game and switching beds.

2. Environmental factors that may pose a possibility of injury.
   a. Cribs present a distinct fall potential.
      i. Rails should always be kept up unless an adult is present who is willing and able to take responsibility for the child.
   b. Windows and elevator shafts pose fall potentials.
      i. They should always be kept closed.
      ii. Cribs should always be placed at a distance from all windows.
   c. Objects left on floors can cause injury.
      i. Children often walk barefoot.
3. Small children must have constant supervision because they often wander into dangerous areas or simply get lost.
4. Holding and transporting children.
   a. Infants.
      i. Ideally, infants should always be placed in a crib, stroller, or other safe location.
      ii. If the child is held, either the cradle or the football hold permits the nurse safely to utilize the other hand for child care.
   b. All children.
      i. When a child must be transported, he or she should always be placed in a crib with rails up, stroller with straps fastened, stretcher with straps fastened and side rails up, or wheel chair with straps fastened.
5. Physical restraint.
   a. To ensure safety of children, restraints are often used in the pediatric setting.
   b. Physical restraint must never be used as punishment or as a form of discipline.
   c. When a responsible adult is present, restraints are often not needed.
   d. Physical restraint is comprised of four main categories, all of which may be employed when caring for children.
      i. **Therapeutic holding.**
         (1) When a painful or scary procedure is being performed, children are often unable or unwilling to remain still.
         (2) One or more nurses or other health-care personnel will assist the child by holding him or her in position.
         (3) No order is required for this action.
         (4) The mummy hold is one example of therapeutic holding.
      ii. Transportation restraint systems.
         (1) As stated above, when transported, children should always have restraint straps fastened to prevent the child from injury.
         (2) No order is required for this action.
      iii. Procedure restraint systems.
         (1) When procedures are performed, health-care professionals often must act to protect the site from injury (e.g., arm boards and padding are applied to prevent infants and toddlers from removing or dislodging intravenous catheters).
         (2) No order is required for this action, but the nurse must assess the site regularly.
      iv. Physical restraint devices.
         (1) To prevent injury, physical restraint devices (e.g., elbow, jacket, wrist, or

other restraints) may be used in specific situations (e.g., elbow restraints may be applied to an infant who is immediately post-op cleft lip surgery [Fig. 8.1] and jacket restraints [Fig. 8.2] may be applied to a toddler who is in skeletal traction).

(2) The restraint device must be applied safely.

(3) An order with a rationale for the restraint and a time frame for restraint use is required.

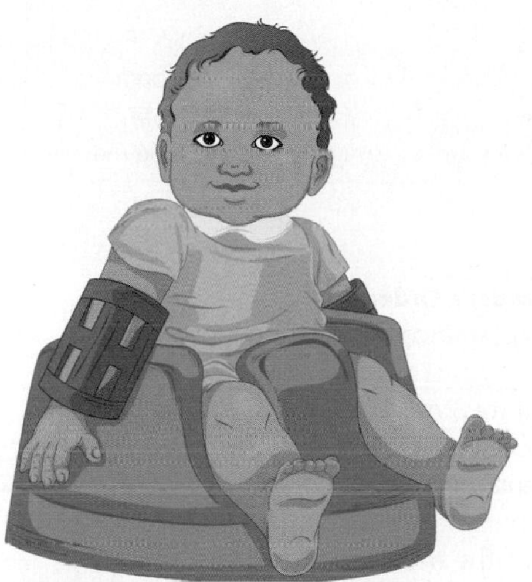

Fig 8.1 Elbow restraints.

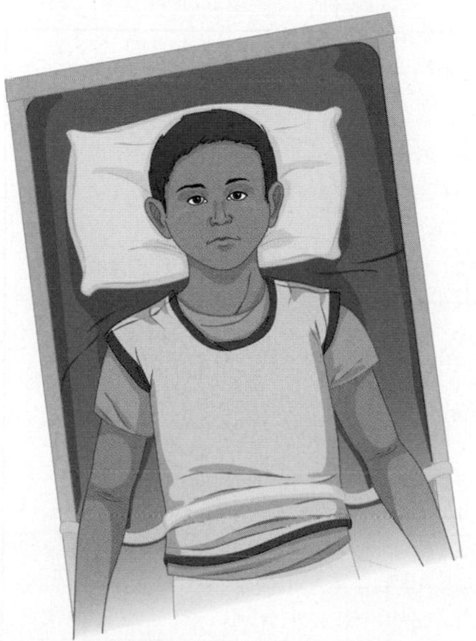

Fig 8.2 Jacket restraints.

(4) The nurse must assess the restraint site regularly.

(a) Check site distal to the restraint for circulatory compromise by assessing capillary refill, color, temperature, and movement.

(b) Assess under the restraint for signs of altered skin integrity (e.g., decubiti).

(c) Assess neurological status distal to the site by monitoring pain levels and movement.

E. Infection control.

1. Standard precautions: in general, nurses in the pediatric setting follow the same infectious disease procedures as nurses in other areas of the hospital.
2. Contact precautions: in some situations, because of the age of the child, nurses must use more restrictive precautions than are used in other hospital areas, for example:
   a. Toddler with diarrhea: although an adult with diarrhea may be maintained on contact isolation in a multibedded room, to keep a toddler from having physical contact with a roommate or a roommate's items would be difficult. As a result, it would be more appropriate to place the child on contact isolation in a private room.

III. Important Modifications in Procedures When Caring for a Pediatric Patient

A. Physical assessment (see Chapter 7, "Physical Assessment of Children: From Infancy to Adolescence").

B. Specimen collection and procedures.

1. Because of the small physical size as well as the developmental level of young children, changes often are needed in the way procedures are performed.
2. The nurse should consult a procedure manual on the clinical unit when asked to collect a specimen or to perform or to assist with a procedure.

C. Informed consent: before many invasive procedures can be performed (e.g., lumbar puncture) an informed consent must be obtained.

1. The health-care professional who will be performing the procedure must obtain the consent.
   a. When age appropriate, both the child and the parents should be informed of the benefits as well as the risks of the procedure.

i. **Assent:** once a child reaches approximately 7 years of age, it has become common practice to ask him or her to agree with procedures that are to be performed.

2. Nursing responsibilities.
   a. The nurse should refer to the laws and regulations regarding informed consent of the state in which he or she is employed.
   b. Prior to the procedure, the nurse should check that the consent has been signed and witnessed.
   c. Prior to the procedure, the nurse should make sure that the parents and child, when appropriate, have had all of their questions answered.

CASE STUDY: Putting It All Together

15-year-old girl in the emergency department accompanied by her parents

Subjective Data

- Mother informs the nurse,
  - "My daughter has a very high fever, and she isn't acting herself."
- Adolescent weakly states to the mother and nurse,
  - "Mother, I can talk for myself. I really feel awful."
- When queried by the nurse what the teen means by "I really feel awful," the young woman vomits.
- During nursing history, with mother not present, teenager admits to forcefully vomiting after meals in order to lose weight and states,
  - "Do NOT tell my mother!!"

Objective Data

Nursing Assessments

- During physical assessment, with mother not present, the teenager complains of epigastric pain of 5 out of 10 on a numeric pain rating scale.
- 250 mL of blood-tinged (bright-red) vomitus

Vital Signs

Temperature:	105.5 °F
Heart rate:	126 bpm
Respiratory rate:	32 rpm
Blood Pressure:	80/56 mm Hg

Health-Care Provider's Orders

- Administer acetaminophen 1,000 mg per rectum STAT
- Morphine sulfate 3 mg SC STAT
- IV Ringer's lactate at 150 mL/hr
- Prepare patient for STAT endoscopy
  - When the nurse advises the young woman about the route of the medication and the endoscopy, the teenager states, "Do you have to do all that? I'm really okay."

Case Study Questions

A. What *subjective* assessments indicate that the client is experiencing a health alteration?

1. ____________________
2. ____________________
3. ____________________
4. ____________________
5. ____________________

B. What *objective* assessments indicate that the client is experiencing a health alteration?

1. ____________________
2. ____________________
3. ____________________
4. ____________________

CASE STUDY: Putting It All Together

cont'd

Case Study Question

C. After analyzing the data that has been collected, what **primary** nursing diagnoses should the nurse assign to this client?

1. Physiological diagnosis ______
2. Psychosocial diagnosis ______

D. What interventions should the nurse plan and/or implement to meet this child's and her family's immediate needs?

1. ______
2. ______
3. ______
4. ______
5. ______
6. ______
7. ______
8. ______

E. What client outcomes should the nurse evaluate regarding the effectiveness of the nursing interventions?

1. ______
2. ______
3. ______
4. ______
5. ______

F. What physiological characteristics should the child exhibit before being discharged home?

1. ______
2. ______

G. What psychological characteristics should the child and family exhibit before being discharged home?

1. ______
2. ______

REVIEW QUESTIONS

1. The parents of a hospitalized 2½-year-old child tell the nurse and the child that they must leave the hospital to care for their children who are at home. Which of the following responses would the nurse expect the child to exhibit?
   1. Kicking and crying
   2. Waving goodbye
   3. Sucking a thumb
   4. Hugging a doll

2. The nurse is developing a plan of care to prevent separation behaviors in children who are hospitalized for long periods of time. Which of the following items should the nurse include in the plan of care? **Select all that apply.**
   1. Provide the child with the child's favorite transitional object.
   2. When possible, assign the same nurse to care for the child each day.
   3. Admit the child to the patient room that is closest to the nurse's station.
   4. Tape pictures of the child's friends and family members to the walls of the child's hospital room.
   5. Inform the parents that at least one person must stay with the child at all times during the hospitalization.

3. The nurse is caring for a 14-year-old adolescent after a serious injury. A twice-daily dressing change has been ordered by the child's primary health-care provider. When planning care with the patient, which of the following statements would be best for the nurse to make?
   1. "I'll be in to change your dressing twice today."
   2. "When do you think will be the best times for me to change your dressing?"
   3. "I'm going to have you help me when I change your dressing."
   4. "Can you help me to figure out how best to change your dressing?"

4. An 8-year-old child, who is post-op appendectomy, is playing with a set of building blocks. The child's pulse and blood pressure are slightly elevated above their presurgery levels. When asked what level the child would rate the postoperative pain on a numeric pain scale, the child states that the pain is "8 on a scale of 1 to 10." The child's primary health-care provider has ordered Tylenol (acetaminophen) and morphine sulfate for pain. Which of the following actions should the nurse perform at this time?
   1. Report the child's pain level to the child's primary health-care provider.
   2. Administer acetaminophen to the child based on the child's behavior.
   3. Administer morphine to the child based on the child's rating of the pain.
   4. Query the child about how the child is able to play with such severe pain.

5. To enhance the effectiveness of the pharmacological pain intervention administered to a 4-year-old child with an injured knee, the nurse plans to add a nonpharmacological pain intervention. Which of the following actions would be appropriate for the nurse to perform? **Select all that apply.**
   1. Read a book to the child.
   2. Hold and cuddle with the child.
   3. Put an ice pack on the child's knee.
   4. Have the child watch a favorite program on television.
   5. Perform passive range of motion exercises on the injured knee.

6. An 8-year-old child is in the playroom drawing a picture. The child's painful dressing change is due to be performed. Which of the following actions by the nurse is appropriate?
   1. Delay the dressing change until the child is finished playing in the playroom.
   2. Perform the dressing change in the playroom while the child finishes drawing the picture.
   3. Escort the child to the treatment room for the dressing change and back to the playroom once it is done.
   4. Ask the child whether the dressing change should be performed at that time or after the child has finished the drawing.

7. A nurse has been assigned to care for a 12-year-old child who will likely die from his illness. The child asks the nurse, "Do you think I am going to die?" Which of the following responses would be appropriate for the nurse to make?
   1. "Don't talk like that. You are going to get better very soon."
   2. "It would be best if you were to ask your doctor about that."
   3. "Some children who have been diagnosed with your illness do die."
   4. "It's hard for me to talk about death. It would be best if you were to ask your parents."

8. A 7-year-old child, who must have a lumbar puncture, begins to cry and squirm when the nurse advises him that he must lie curled on his side with his back facing the primary health-care provider. Which of the following actions should the nurse perform at this time?
   1. Advise the child that he must remain still during the procedure or else he will get injured.
   2. Question the parents regarding how to get the child's cooperation for the procedure.
   3. Request the assistance from another nurse to hold the child still during the procedure.
   4. Tell the child that children who are in elementary school are big enough to be still during procedures.

9. An 18-month-old child has just returned from the operating room with intravenous solution running into a vein in the right hand, a nasogastric tube in place, and a dressing covering the abdomen. Which of the following actions by the nurse would be appropriate? **Select all that apply.**
   1. Administer an NSAID per the health-care provider's orders.
   2. Place an intake and output sheet at the child's bedside.
   3. Request an order for an elbow restraint for the child's left arm.
   4. Assess the child's pain level using an age-appropriate pain rating scale.
   5. Compare the intravenous solution to the health-care provider's orders.

10. A 5-month-old girl's arms are encased in elbow restraints following facial surgery. Which of the following situations would warrant removal of the restraints?
    1. Narcotic medication has been administered, and the child's pain rating has dropped.
    2. Infant has been put to sleep for the night in her crib lying on her back.
    3. The infant's hands are pink with spontaneous movement and capillary refill of two seconds.
    4. A responsible adult is holding the baby and preventing her from touching the operative site.

11. A 13-year-old adolescent is in hospital for reconstructive surgery after a severe automobile accident. During rounds, the nurse notes that the teen is watching television and playing a video game. Which of the following should the nurse assess regarding the patient's well-being? **Select all that apply.**
    1. Teen's pain level
    2. How often friends visit the teen
    3. Level of healing of the teen's surgical site
    4. Teen's progress on daily homework assignments
    5. How well the teen is performing on the video games

12. The nurse is assessing whether or not an 8-year-old child has given assent for a scheduled painful procedure. Which of the following statements by the child would reflect that the child has given assent?
    1. "I know that the procedure is supposed to make me better."
    2. "The procedure is going to be done at 10 a.m. this morning."
    3. "Dr. Jones wants to perform the procedure on me."
    4. "My mother signed the form that the doctor brought in."

REVIEW ANSWERS

1. ANSWER: 1
Rationale:
1. The nurse would expect the child to kick and cry.
2. It is unlikely that the child will wave goodbye.
3. It is unlikely that the child will simply suck a thumb.
4. It is unlikely that the child will simply hug a doll.
TEST-TAKING TIP: The nurse would expect the child to exhibit the characteristic signs of the protest stage of separation. Toddlers tend to exhibit the most pronounced behaviors when they must be separated from their parents.
Content Area: *Pediatrics*
Integrated Processes: *Nursing Process: Evaluation*
Client Need: *Psychosocial Integrity: Coping Mechanisms*
Cognitive Level: *Application*

2. ANSWER: 1, 2, and 4
Rationale:
1. The nurse should provide the child with the child's favorite transitional object.
2. When possible, the same nurse should be assigned to care for the child each day.
3. The child need not be admitted to the patient room that is closest to the nurse's station.
4. The nurse should tape pictures of the child's friends and family members to the walls of the child's hospital room.
5. The nurse should not inform the parents that at least one person must stay with the child at all times during the hospitalization.
TEST-TAKING TIP: Although it is ideal for at least one parent to stay with a child during the child's hospitalization, it is not always possible. For example, the parents may have to work, they may live miles away from the hospital, or they may need to be at home to care for the child's siblings. To maintain a strong relationship between the child and his or her parents, the nurse should implement actions as stated above as well as encourage direct communication via a number of routes (e.g., via telephone, texting, video conferencing).
Content Area: *Pediatrics*
Integrated Processes: *Nursing Process: Implementation*
Client Need: *Psychosocial Integrity: Coping Mechanisms*
Cognitive Level: *Application*

3. ANSWER: 2
Rationale:
1. This is not the best statement for the nurse to make.
2. This is the best statement for the nurse to make.
3. This is not the best statement for the nurse to make.
4. This is not the best statement for the nurse to make.
TEST-TAKING TIP: During adolescence, teenagers are progressing through the Eriksonian psychosocial stage of identity versus role confusion. During this stage, adolescents are developing a sense of self as an independent individual. To become a unique individual, teens seek to become more and more independent. When the nurse solicits the teenager's help in determining when the dressing should be changed, the nurse is providing the teen with some independence.
Content Area: *Pediatrics*
Integrated Processes: *Nursing Process: Implementation*
Client Need: *Psychosocial Integrity: Therapeutic Communication*
Cognitive Level: *Analysis*

4. ANSWER: 3
Rationale:
1. It is not necessary to report the child's pain level to the child's primary health-care provider.
2. It would be inappropriate to administer acetaminophen to the child based on the child's behavior.
3. The nurse should administer morphine to the child based on the child's rating of the pain.
4. It is inappropriate for the nurse to question the child's veracity.
TEST-TAKING TIP: A child's rating on a pain rating scale is more accurate than a nurse's interpretation of the child's pain based on the child's behavior. The nurse should always believe the child's rating of the pain.
Content Area: *Pediatrics*
Integrated Processes: *Nursing Process: Implementation*
Client Need: *Caring; Physiological Integrity; Pharmacological and Parenteral Therapies: Pharmacological Pain Management*
Cognitive Level: *Application*

5. ANSWER: 1, 2, 3, and 4
Rationale:
1. Distraction is an excellent nonpharmacological intervention. The nurse could read a book to the child.
2. Holding and cuddling with a child can enhance the therapeutic action of a pain medication.
3. Putting an ice pack on the child's knee could enhance the therapeutic action of a pain medication.
4. Distraction is an excellent nonpharmacological intervention. The nurse could let the child watch a favorite program on television.
5. Passive range of motion exercises on the injured knee could enhance the child's pain rather than reduce it.
TEST-TAKING TIP: A number of nonpharmacological interventions are available to the nurse to reduce a pediatric patient's pain. The nurse should use all the methods that are available when caring for a child who is in pain.
Content Area: *Pediatrics*
Integrated Processes: *Nursing Process: Implementation*
Client Need: *Physiological Integrity: Basic Care and Comfort: Nonpharmacological Comfort Management*
Cognitive Level: *Application*

6. ANSWER: 3
Rationale:
1. This action is inappropriate. The child's medical care must take precedence over play.
2. This action is inappropriate. The playroom should be a sanctuary where no treatments are performed.
3. This action is appropriate. The nurse should escort the child to the treatment room for the dressing change and back to the playroom once it is done.

4. This action is inappropriate. The child's medical care must take precedence over play

TEST-TAKING TIP: Both play and medical interventions are critical to the health and well-being of children. In the hierarchy of care, however, medical managements must take precedence. However, because a child's play and emotional integrity are so important, no treatment should take place in the playroom or, if possible, in the child's hospital room. All treatments and procedures should be performed in a treatment room.

Content Area: *Pediatrics*

Integrated Processes: *Nursing Process: Implementation*

Client Need: *Safe and Effective Care Environment: Management of Care: Establishing Priorities*

Cognitive Level: *Application*

7. ANSWER: 3

Rationale:

1. It would be inappropriate for the nurse to make this reply.
2. It would be inappropriate for the nurse to make this reply.
3. **This is an appropriate response for the nurse to make.**
4. It would be inappropriate for the nurse to make this reply.

TEST-TAKING TIP: Children who are dying often sense that death is near. If they ask about death, it is important for the nurse to give an honest answer. If the nurse evades the question or gives a dishonest answer, the child will have difficulty trusting the nurse in the future.

Content Area: *Pediatrics*

Integrated Processes: *Nursing Process: Implementation*

Client Need: *Psychosocial Integrity: Therapeutic Communication; Psychosocial Integrity: End-of-Life Care*

Cognitive Level: *Analysis*

8. ANSWER: 3

Rationale:

1. It would be inappropriate for the nurse to advise the child that he will get injured if he does not remain still.
2. It would be inappropriate for the nurse merely to question the parents regarding how to get the child's cooperation for the procedure.
3. **The nurse should request the assistance from another nurse to hold the child still during the procedure.**
4. It would be inappropriate for the nurse to tell the child that children who are in elementary school are big enough to be still during procedures.

TEST-TAKING TIP: Young children are often unable to remain still during treatments and procedures. To assist them to remain still, the nurse should hold the child in the appropriate position. This action is called therapeutic holding. If the nurse is unable to hold the child by himself or herself, the assistance of one or more other health-care practitioners should be requested.

Content Area: *Pediatrics*

Integrated Processes: *Nursing Process: Implementation*

Client Need: *Safe and Effective Care Environment: Safety and Infection Control: Use of Restraints/Safety Devices*

Cognitive Level: *Analysis*

9. ANSWER: 2, 3, 4, and 5

Rationale:

1. It would be inappropriate for the nurse to administer an NSAID per the health-care provider's orders. If the child is in pain, he or she should receive a narcotic analgesic medication immediately postsurgery.
2. **Because the child has both an IV and an NG tube, it would be appropriate for the nurse to place an intake and output sheet at the child's bedside.**
3. **It would be appropriate for the nurse to request an order for an elbow restraint for the child's left arm.**
4. **It would be appropriate for the nurse to assess the child's pain level using an age-appropriate pain rating scale.**
5. **It would be appropriate for the nurse to compare the intravenous solution to the health-care provider's orders.**

TEST-TAKING TIP: The nurse must be prepared to provide patients with comprehensive care. Making certain that the patient is receiving the correct therapy is important as is assessing the intake and output of a patient who is receiving parenteral fluids and who has an NG tube. It is also important for the nurse to make sure that the child does not remove or displace the therapeutic objects. In the case of the scenario, an elbow restraint for the left arm would be appropriate.

Content Area: *Pediatrics*

Integrated Processes: *Nursing Process: Implementation*

Client Need: *Physiological Integrity: Physiological Adaptation: Illness Management; Safe and Effective Care Environment: Safety and Infection Control: Use of Restraints/Safety Devices*

Cognitive Level: *Application*

10. ANSWER: 4

Rationale:

1. Although the child's pain rating may have dropped, the child will still need elbow restraints.
2. Although the infant has been put to sleep for the night in her crib lying on her back, the child will still need elbow restraints.
3. When an infant's hands are pink with spontaneous movement and capillary refill of two seconds, the restraints are not adversely affecting the child's neurovascular status.
4. **If a responsible adult is holding the baby and preventing her from touching the operative site, the restraints may be removed.**

TEST-TAKING TIP: Restraints should only be used when necessary and never should be applied as punishment. If a responsible adult is able to monitor the child's actions and prevent injury to the therapeutic sites, restraints should be removed.

Content Area: *Pediatrics*

Integrated Processes: *Nursing Process: Implementation*

Client Need: *Physiological Integrity: Physiological Adaptation: Illness Management; Safe and Effective Care Environment: Safety and Infection Control: Use of Restraints/Safety Devices*

Cognitive Level: *Application*

11. ANSWER: 1, 2, 3, and 4

Rationale:

1. The teen's pain level should be assessed.

2. The nurse should assess how often friends visit the teen.

3. The nurse should assess the healing of the teen's surgical site.

4. The nurse should assess the teen's progress on daily homework assignments.

5. It is not important for the nurse to assess how well the teen is performing on the video games.

TEST-TAKING TIP: When a nurse is performing holistic nursing care in the pediatric setting, he or she must assess not only the physiological aspects of the child's well-being but also the psychosocial aspects. Completion of the child's homework is one of those aspects.

Content Area: *Pediatrics*

Integrated Processes: *Nursing Process: Implementation*

Client Need: *Physiological Integrity: Physiological Adaptation: Illness Management; Psychosocial Integrity: Behavioral Interventions*

Cognitive Level: *Application*

12. ANSWER: 2

Rationale:

1. This statement does not indicate that the child has given assent.

2. This statement indicates that the child has given assent.

3. This statement does not indicate that the child has given assent.

4. This statement does not indicate that the child has given assent.

TEST-TAKING TIP: When a child provides assent for a treatment or procedure to be performed, he or she is making an implicit or explicit statement that the treatment or procedure may be performed.

Content Area: *Pediatrics*

Integrated Processes: *Nursing Process: Assessment*

Client Need: *Safe and Effective Care Environment: Management of Care: Ethical Practice*

Cognitive Level: *Application*

Pediatric Medication Administration

KEY TERMS

Body surface area (BSA)—A measurement of body mass based on the relationship between height and weight.

Daily maintenance volume (DMV)—The minimum amount of fluid a child needs on a daily basis to maintain his or her optimal health.

Drop factor—The number of drops in one milliliter of fluid, labeled on the packaging of IV tubing.

EMLA cream—An anesthetic cream (lidocaine 2.5% and prilocaine 2.5%).

IV piggyback (IVPB)—A method of delivering medication into an existing IV line.

Metered dose inhaler (MDI)—A device used to deliver a measured amount of medication into the respiratory tract.

Nebulizer—A machine that aerosolizes medication so that the medication can be inhaled into the respiratory tract.

Nomogram—A tool used to calculate BSA based on the relationship between height and weight.

Phlebitis—An inflammation of the vein that can be a complication of IV therapy.

Spacer—A device used with an MDI that is employed when patients are unable to inhale their medication at exactly the same time that the MDI is compressed.

I. Description

Medication administration is a process that requires teamwork. Each practitioner—the primary health-care provider, the pharmacist, and the nurse—has a responsibility to ensure that pediatric medication administration is performed safely. Medication errors are preventable. Unless all steps are followed closely, however, a medication error may occur.

II. Primary Health-Care Provider's Medication Order

A. Required before administering a medication to any patient.

B. Order must include:

1. The name of the medication to be administered.
2. The dosage of the medication.
3. How often the medication is to be administered, including whether the order is a standing order or prn order.
4. The route of administration.

III. Preliminary Responsibilities of the Nurse

A. Safe dosages: when a medication is ordered for a pediatric patient, the nurse must determine whether the dosage is safe for the child.

1. Dosage units.
   a. The nurse must first determine whether the medication dose is ordered per kilogram (kg) or per **body surface area (BSA)**, which is a measurement of body mass based on the relationship between height and weight.
   b. The nurse must then calculate the dosage that the child can safely receive.
      i. The nurse must first consult a pharmacology reference to determine the recommended units per kilogram or BSA.
      ii. Second, the nurse must calculate the safe dose for the child.
      iii. Finally, the nurse must determine whether the primary health-care provider's order is safe or unsafe.

Even though the primary health-care provider prescribes medications, it is the nurse's responsibility, along with the pharmacist, to make sure that the order is safe. If the nurse were to administer an unsafe medication, he or she would be responsible for any untoward effects sustained by the child.

2. Factors related to safe medication dosages.
   a. Range of safety.
      i. When only a maximum safe dosage limit is cited in a reference text.
         (1) If a calculated safe dose is higher than the primary health-care provider's order, the order is safe.
         (2) If a calculated safe dose is lower than the primary health-care provider's order, the order is unsafe.
      ii. When a range of safety with both minimum and maximum dosage limits is cited in a reference text.
         (1) The primary health-care provider's order must be between the minimum and maximum calculated safe dosages.
   b. Time.
      i. Both the calculated dosage and the primary health-care provider's order must be in the same time units before they can be compared.
   c. Dosage units.
      i. Both the calculated dosage and the primary health-care provider's order must be in the same dosage units before they can be compared.
3. Method for calculating safe pediatric dosages. (For a full discussion on calculating safe pediatric dosages, please refer to a med math text.)
   a. Recommended dosages are cited in nursing drug handbooks, physicians' desk references, and other reliable medication references.

MAKING THE CONNECTION

To determine whether the BSA or the weight method of calculating safe pediatric dosages should be used, the nurse must carefully read the recommended pediatric dosage information in a reliable medication reference.

If, for example, the reference states:

pediatric dosage is: 20 mg/**m^2 (i.e., per meters squared)**

The nurse should determine the child's BSA and calculate the safe dosage using the BSA formula.

However, if, for example, the reference states:

pediatric dosage is: 20 mg/**kg (i.e., per kilogram)**

The nurse should determine the child's weight in kilograms and calculate the safe dosage using the weight formula.

   b. Children's medication dosages are calculated in one of two ways.
      i. Per kilogram (kg).
      ii. Per BSA (i.e., m^2).
   c. BSA calculations (see Making the Connection).
      i. BSAs are based on the relationship between the child's height and weight.
      ii. This method is used **only** when the drug reference states that the medication is administered per meters squared (i.e., per m^2).
      iii. A child's BSA is determined by using a **nomogram** (Fig. 9.1).
         (1) The nomogram is comprised of four columns (the second column from the left, with the rectangle surrounding it, should not be used).
            (a) Height column—On the far left, calibrated both in inches and in centimeters.
            (b) Weight column—On the far right, calibrated both in pounds and kilograms.
            (c) BSA column (labeled S.A. m^2) is the body surface area column.
      iv. Procedure (see Box 9.1 for examples).
         (1) Using the correct calibration, locate the child's height on the height column.
         (2) Using the correct calibration, locate the child's weight on the weight column.

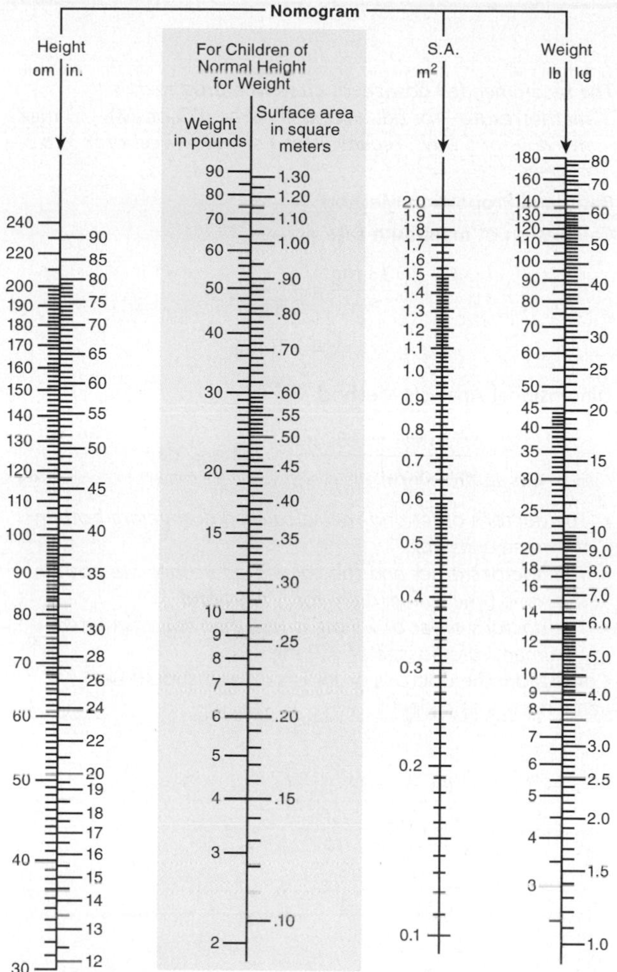

Fig 9.1 Nomogram.

(3) Carefully place a straight edge to connect the two points.

(4) Note where the straight edge crosses the S.A. m^2 column. This is the child's BSA.

(a) Note: BSA is always calculated to the nearest hundredth (i.e., two places to the right of the decimal point).

(5) Next, the safe dosage of the desired medication must be calculated. This can be done using one of two methods—ratio and proportion or dimensional analysis.

d. Weight calculations (see Making the Connection).

i. This method is used **only** when the drug reference states that the medication is administered per kilogram.

ii. Procedure (see Box 9.2 for examples).

MAKING THE CONNECTION

BSA Dosages May Be Calculated Using Either the Ratio and Proportion or the Dimensional Analysis Method

Basic formula for ratio and proportion method:

$$\frac{\text{recommended dosage}}{1\ \text{m}^2} = \frac{\text{safe pediatric dosage}}{\text{child's m}^2\ \text{(BSA)}}$$

Once the calculation has been performed, if the time and/or dosage units in the result are different from those in the order, the nurse must convert the results.

Formula for dimensional analysis method:

recommended dosage	child's BSA (m^2)	time conversion	unit conversion
per m^2/day		(if needed)	(if needed)

= safe pediatric dosage

MAKING THE CONNECTION

Weight Dosages May Be Calculated Using Either the Ratio and Proportion or the Dimensional Analysis Method

Using the ratio and proportion method, the nurse may need to complete a number of steps:

First, the child's weight (in kilograms) must be determined.

If the child's weight is cited in pounds (lb), the weight must be converted to kilograms.

$$\frac{1\ \text{kg}}{2.2\ \text{lb}} = \frac{x\ \text{kg}}{\text{child's weight in pounds}}$$

Then, the following formula should be used to calculate safe pediatric dosage:

$$\frac{\text{recommended dosage}}{1\ \text{kg}} = \frac{\text{safe pediatric dosage}}{\text{child's weight in kilograms}}$$

Once the calculation has been performed, if the time and/or dosage units in the result are different from those in the order, the nurse must convert the results.

The following formula should be used for the dimensional analysis method:

recommended dosage	child's weight	weight conversion	time conversion	unit conversion
per kg/day		(if needed)	(if needed)	(if needed)

= safe pediatric dosage

4. Volume.

a. Once the dosage has been determined, the nurse must calculate how much volume of the medication is equal to the dosage.

Box 9.1 Examples of BSA Dosage Calculation

Example 1

Doctor's order reads: administer methotrexate 2.5 mg PO daily for 5 days
Child's height is: 125 cm
Child's weight is: 20 kg
Nomogram: the child's BSA, as noted in the S.A. m^2 column, is 0.82

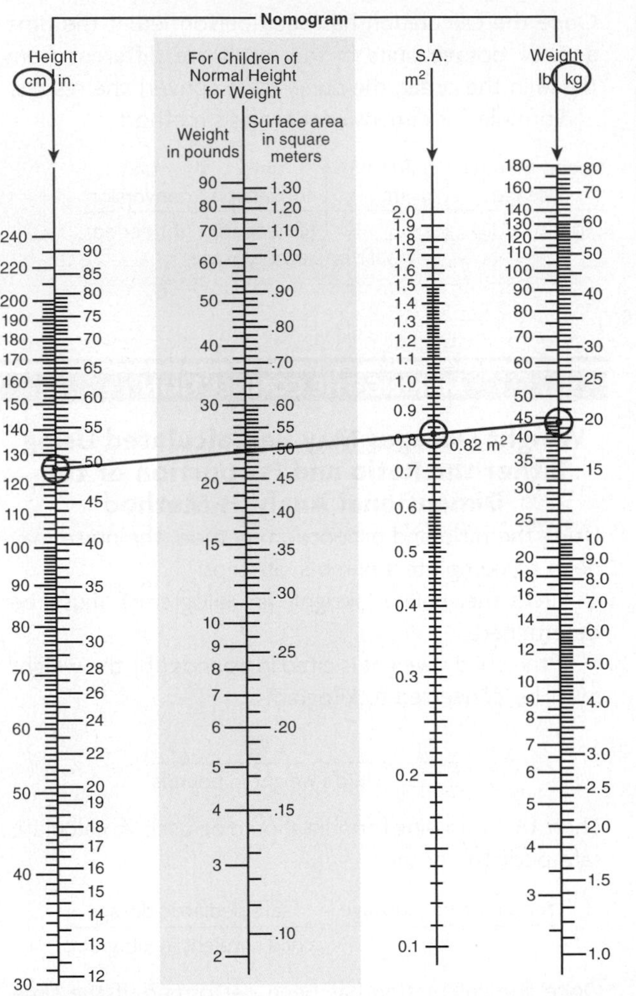

The recommended dosage, as cited in a drug text, is: methotrexate—for adults and children (PO or IM)—3.3 mg/m^2/day for 5 days, repeat after 1 or more weeks for 3 to 5 courses

Ratio and Proportion Method

Calculation of **maximum** safe dosage:

$$\frac{3.3 \text{ mg}}{1 \text{ m}^2} = \frac{x}{0.82 \text{ m}^2}$$

$$x = 2.71 \text{ mg}$$

Dimensional Analysis Method

$$\frac{3.3 \text{ mg}}{\text{m}^2/\text{day}} \Big| \frac{0.82 \text{ m}^2}{} = 2.71 \text{ mg/day}$$

- *The doctor's order and the calculated dosage are both in the same units: mg.*
- *The doctor's order and the calculated dosage are both in the same time frame: daily for 5 days* ***and***
- *The doctor's order of 2.5 mg is less than the calculated maximum safe dosage of 2.71 mg.*

Conclusion: the doctor's order is safe and should be administered as ordered.

Box 9.1 Examples of BSA Dosage Calculation—cont'd

Example 2

Doctor's order reads: administer Cytoxan 50 mg PO bid
Child's height is: 82 cm
Child's weight is: 8.6 kg
Nomogram: The child's BSA, as noted in the S.A. m^2 column, is 0.45

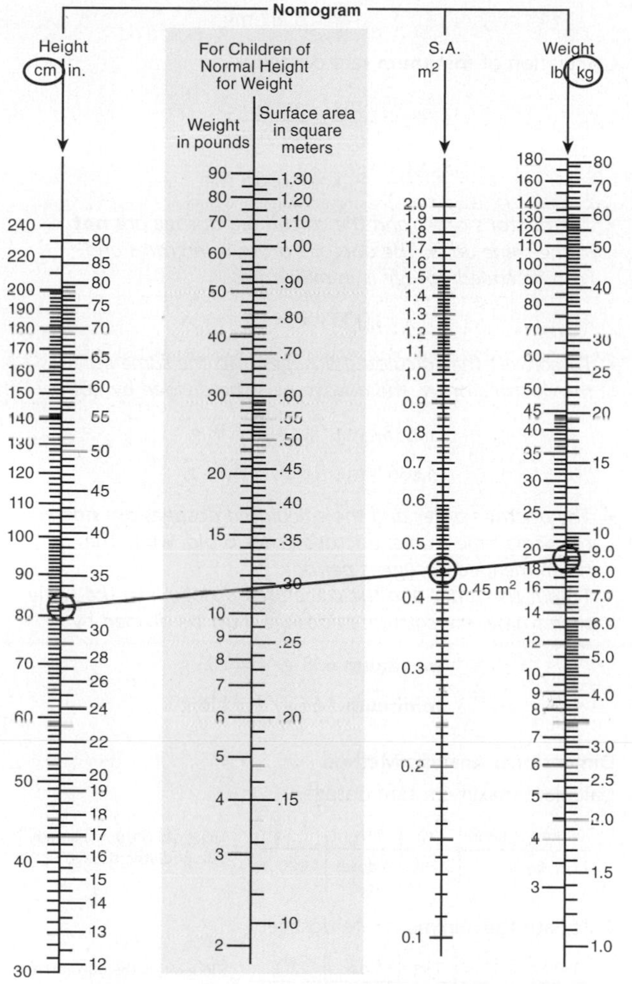

The recommended dosage, as cited in a drug text, is: Cytoxan PO, 60 to 250 mg/m²/day

Ratio and Proportion Method

Calculation of **maximum** safe dosage.

$$\frac{250 \text{ mg}}{1 \text{ m}^2} = \frac{x}{0.45 \text{ m}^2}$$

$$x = 112.5 \text{ mg}$$

Calculation of **minimum** safe dosage.

$$\frac{60 \text{ mg}}{1 \text{ m}^2} = \frac{x}{0.45 \text{ m}^2}$$

$$x = 27 \text{ mg}$$

- *The doctor's order and the calculated dosage are both in the same units: mg.*
- *The doctor's order and the calculated dosages are **not** in the same time frame: doctor's order is bid while the recommended dosage is per day.*
- *To put the order and the calculated dosage into the same time frame, the calculated dosages must be divided by two.*

maximum 112.5 mg/2 = 56.3 mg

minimum 27 mg/2 = 13.5 mg

Dimensional Analysis Method

Calculate maximum safe dosage.

$$\frac{250 \text{ mg}}{\text{m}^2/\text{day}} \Big| \frac{0.45 \text{ m}^2}{} \Big| \frac{1 \text{ day}}{2 \text{ doses bid}} = 56.3 \text{ mg bid}$$

Calculate minimum safe dosage.

$$\frac{60 \text{ mg}}{\text{m}^2/\text{day}} \Big| \frac{0.45 \text{ m}^2}{} \Big| \frac{1 \text{ day}}{2 \text{ doses bid}} = 13.5 \text{ mg bid}$$

- *The doctor's order of 50 mg is **between** the maximum of 56.3 mg and the minimum of 13.5 mg.*
- *Conclusion: the doctor's order is safe and should be administered as ordered.*

Box 9.2 Examples of Weight Dosage Calculation

Example 1

Doctor's order reads: Benadryl 50 mg PO every 6 hr
Childs' height: not needed—only the kilogram weight is needed
Child's weight: 23 kg
Nomogram: not needed—only the kilogram weight is needed
The recommended dosage, as cited in a drug text, is: Benadryl PO, 5 mg/kg/day

Ratio and Proportion Method

Calculation of **maximum** safe dosage.

$$\frac{5 \text{ mg}}{1 \text{ kg}} = \frac{x}{23 \text{ kg}}$$

$$x = 115 \text{ mg}$$

- *The doctor's order and the calculated dosage are both in the same units: mg.*
- *The doctor's order and the calculated dosages are **not** in the same time frame: doctor's order is every 6 hr, while the recommended dosage is per day.*
- *To put the order and the calculated dosage into the same time frame, the calculated dosage must be divided by four.*

maximum safe dosage 115 mg/4= 28.75 mg

Dimensional Analysis Method

5 mg	23 kg	1 day	= 28.75 mg every 6 hr is the maximum safe pediatric dosage
kg/day		4 doses (every 6 hr)	

- *The doctor's order of 50 mg is **more than** the calculated maximum safe dosage of 28.75 mg.*

Conclusion: the doctor's order is **not safe**. The doctor should be notified of the error, and a change of order should be requested.

Example 2

Doctor's order reads: Gantrisin 1.5 g PO qid
Child's height: not needed
Child's weight: 68 lb

Ratio and Proportion Method

Because the weight is given in pounds, a conversion must be calculated.

$$2.2 \text{ lb} = 1 \text{ kg, so:}$$

$$\frac{2.2 \text{ lb}}{1 \text{ kg}} = \frac{68 \text{ lb}}{x \text{ kg}}$$

$$2.2x = 68$$

$$x = 30.91 \text{ kg}$$

Nomogram: not needed
The recommended dosage, as cited in a drug text, is: Gantrisin PO, 150 to 200 mg/kg/day

Calculation of **maximum** safe dosage.

$$\frac{200 \text{ mg}}{1 \text{ kg}} = \frac{x}{30.91 \text{ kg}}$$

$$x = 6{,}182 \text{ mg}$$

Calculation of **minimum** safe dosage.

$$\frac{150 \text{ mg}}{1 \text{ kg}} = \frac{x}{30.91 \text{ kg}}$$

$$x = 4{,}636.5 \text{ mg}$$

- *The doctor's order and the calculated dosage are **not** in the same units: The doctor's order is in grams and recommended dosage is in milligrams.*

$$1{,}000 \text{ mg} = 1 \text{ g}$$

- *To convert the calculated dosages into the same units as the doctor's order, the dosage must be divided by 1,000.*

$$6{,}182 \text{ mg}/1{,}000 = 6.18 \text{ g}$$

$$4{,}636.5 \text{ mg}/1{,}000 = 4.64 \text{ g}$$

- *The doctor's order and the calculated dosages are **not** in the same time frame: doctor's order is qid, while the recommended dosage is per day.*
- *To put the order and the calculated dosage into the same time frame, the calculated dosage must be divided by 4.*

maximum 6.18 g/4 = 1.55 g

minimum 4.64 g/4 = 1.16 g

Dimensional Analysis Method

Calculate maximum safe dosage.

200 mg	68 lb	1 kg	1 day	1 g	= 1.55 g qid is the maximum safe pediatric dosage
1 kg/day		2.2 lb	4 doses (qid)	1,000 mg	

Calculate the minimum safe dosage.

150 mg	68 lb	1 kg	1 day	1 g	= 1.16 g qid is the maximum safe pediatric dosage
1 kg/day		2.2 lb	4 doses (qid)	1,000 mg	

- *The doctor's order of 1.5 g is **between** the maximum of 1.55 g and the minimum of 1.16 g.*

Conclusion: the doctor's order is safe and should be administered as ordered.

b. Depending on the route of administration and the form of the medication, the volume may be in a liquid measurement as numbers of milliliters (mL) or a solid measurement as numbers of tablets or capsules.

5. Finally, the nurse must establish confirmation of the accuracy of all calculations by:
   a. Having another nurse check the arithmetic or
   b. If another nurse is unavailable, the same nurse carefully rechecking his or her own arithmetic.

B. The five rights of medication administration: prior to administering any medication, a nurse must always check the order, the patient's medical record, and the patient to determine that the five patient rights have been met.

DID YOU KNOW?

The Institute of Medicine (IOM) has reported that adverse drug events are a leading cause of patient morbidity in the United States. Because nurses administer the majority of medications in hospitals, it is reasonable to say that nurses are responsible for many of the errors. If nurses faithfully follow the five rights, they will be much less likely to commit a medication error.

1. Is this the right patient?
    a. First, check the patient's name and hospital number on the order sheet and the medication record.
    b. Next, compare them to the name and hospital number on the patient's identification bracelet.
    c. Only if they are all the same may the medication may be administered.
2. Is this the right medication?
    a. First, check the name of the medication on the order sheet and the medication record.
    b. Next, compare them to the name on the medication label.
    c. Only if they are all the same may the medication be administered.
3. Is this the right dosage of the medication?
    a. First, perform necessary calculations to make sure that the dosage that is ordered is safe.
    b. Second, check the dosage of the medication on the order sheet and the medication record, and compare them to the dosage on the medication label.
    c. Only if the dosages are the same may the medication be administered.
    d. If the dosages are the not the same, additional calculations must be performed to determine how much of the medication should be administered, and that information must be communicated to the primary health-care provider.
4. Is this the right route?
    a. First, check the route stated on the order sheet and the medication record.
    b. Next, compare them to the form of the medication that is available.
    c. Only if the routes are the same may the medication be administered.
5. Is this the right time?
    a. First, check the time frame stated on the order sheet and the medication record.
    b. Next, compare them to the time when the medication is being poured.
    c. Only if the times are the same (within 30 minutes before or after the ordered time) may the medication be administered.

IV. General Guidelines Regarding Administering Medications to Children

A. Handwashing should always precede medication administration.

B. Medication effects.
1. Carefully monitor the child for the desired effects.
    a. Medications are given to treat a specific medical problem.
2. Carefully monitor the child for undesired effects.
    a. All medications cause side effects, and some may be life threatening.

C. Children are not small adults.
1. Medication dosages must be adjusted according to a child's size and metabolism (see earlier).
    a. This consideration is especially important when administering digoxin, insulin, and heparin.
2. What is the child's growth and development?
    a. Pediatric drug therapy is guided by the child's age, weight, and level of growth and development.
    b. When appropriate, children should be informed regarding why they are receiving medications.
    c. Give honest explanations using language based on the child's level of understanding.

V. Intravenous Infusions

A. Inserting intravenous (IV) catheters.
1. Sites where IVs may be inserted.
    a. Most common sites.
        i. Hand, wrist, and antecubital veins.
        ii. Dorsal foot: for infants who do not yet crawl or walk.
        iii. Scalp veins: for infants because there are no valves in the vessels, so the catheters can be inserted in either direction.
2. Catheter gauge: most commonly 20 to 24 gauge.
3. Procedure: nurses must be approved before inserting IVs in children.
    a. Check the five rights of medication administration **plus:**
    b. Insert IVs in the treatment room, not in the child's bed or in the playroom.
    c. Obtain all equipment before child enters the room.
        i. IV catheter.
        ii. IV solution.

iii. Infusion set.
iv. Extension tubing with a T-connector, if needed.
v. Sterile occlusive dressing.
vi. Padded arm board, if needed—especially important for infants and toddlers.
vii. Alcohol (or Betadine) pads.
viii. Tourniquet.
ix. Gloves.
x. Tubes for blood draws, if needed.

d. Using age-appropriate language, prepare the child and parents regarding:
   i. Where the IV will be placed.
   ii. Why it is being inserted.
   iii. About the infusion pump, or other equipment, if being used.
e. Wash hands and glove.
f. Use pain reduction techniques.
   i. Nonpharmacological methods: for example, guided imagery or distraction.
   ii. Pharmacological methods: ice or numbing meds, such as **EMLA cream.**
      (1) Check a reliable reference to determine the exact dosage of EMLA (lidocaine 2.5 mg/prilocaine 2.5 mg).
      (2) EMLA must be applied at least 1 hr before the insertion for adequate pain relief.
      (3) It would be appropriate to apply the cream well before the child is taken to the treatment room.
   iii. Determine the child's ability to remain still and restrain, if needed.
      (1) Encourage parents to stay with their child during the procedure, but do not expect them to restrain the child.
   iv. Identify the site.
   v. Keep the child and parents informed throughout the procedure.
   vi. Let the child know when the sharp pinch will occur.
   vii. Assess for blood return and IV fluid flow to confirm that the catheter is in the vein.
   viii. Secure the catheter with tape and occlusive dressing.
   ix. Secure the arm to the arm board with a clear shield (e.g., one-half medicine cup) to provide visual access.
   x. Praise both the child and the parents.
   xi. Document, including location and condition of the site, type and gauge of catheter and date and time of insertion.

B. IV fluids.
1. Children are at high risk for fluid volume overload.
2. Administer via infusion pump or, only if a pump is unavailable, via in-line volume control tubing (e.g., Soluset, Buretrol).
   a. If using a volume control device, clamp the tubing to prevent large quantities of fluid from entering the device—usually, the maximum amount is 100 mL.

C. Monitoring of IV infusions.
1. Assess the infusion at least every hour, even if an infusion pump is being used.
   a. Check the rate of infusion to make sure that it is accurate.
2. Monitor for signs and symptoms of infiltration and remove the IV if it is infiltrated.
   a. Swollen, taut skin: compare with the other extremity to determine whether or not the sign is related to the IV.
   b. Coolness and blanching of the skin.
   c. No backflow when the IV bag is placed below the extremity.
   d. Slowed or stopped infusion.
3. Monitor for signs and symptoms of **phlebitis** (inflammation) and remove the IV, if phlebitis is present.
   a. Redness, pain, edema, warmth, and induration.
4. Document the quantity infused on the intake and output record.

D. Changing IVs.
1. If either infiltration or phlebitis is present:
   a. Discontinue the IV.
   b. Report findings to the primary health-care provider.
2. To prevent infection:
   a. IV bags should be changed at least every 24 hr.
   b. IV sites are usually changed every 96 hr.

E. Infusion rates: nurses must carefully calculate rates to maintain safety.
1. Infusion rates are based on **daily maintenance volumes (DMV)** (i.e., the minimum amount of fluid a child needs on a daily basis to maintain his or her optimal health) (see Chapter 13, "Nursing Care of the Child With Fluid and Electrolyte Alterations").
   a. If the child weighs less than 10 kg: DMV = 100 mL/kg
   b. If the child weighs between 10 and 20 kg: DMV = 100 mL times 10 plus 50 mL for every kilogram between 10 and 20 kg.
   c. If child weighs over 20 kg: DMV = 100 mL times 10 plus 50 mL times 10 PLUS 20 mL for every kilogram above 20 kg.

2. A child's DMV will be higher if he or she is dehydrated or is losing fluids.

F. IV drip rate calculations.

1. Based on:
   a. The volume of fluid that is to be infused and
   b. The time during which the fluid is to be infused.
2. Only when no pump is available, the **drop factor** of the tubing must be known.
   a. Tubing.
      i. The drop factor is found on the packaging of all IV tubing.
      ii. Only microdrip tubing (60 gtt/mL) should be used when administering IVs to young children.
   b. Nurse must calculate drops per min (gtt/min).
   c. Two methods may be used to calculate drop infusion rates (examples in Box 9.3).
      i. Standard method formula.

$$\text{drip rate (gtt/min)} = \frac{\text{volume to be infused (mL)} \times \text{drop factor (gtt/min)}}{\text{time (in minutes)}}$$

      ii. Dimensional analysis method formula.

$$\frac{\text{volume ordered}}{\text{time for infusion}} \left| \frac{60\text{ gtt}}{1\text{ mL}} \right| \frac{\text{time conversion}}{\text{(if needed)}} \left| \frac{\text{volume conversion}}{\text{(if needed)}} \right. = \frac{\text{infusion rate}}{\text{gtt/min}}$$

3. If a pump is used, the nurse must calculate the pump setting (mL/hr).
   a. Two methods may be used to calculate pump infusion rates (examples in Box 9.4).
      i. Standard method.

$$\text{pump setting (mL/hr)} = \frac{\text{volume to be infused (mL)}}{\text{time (in hours)}}$$

      ii. Dimensional analysis method.

$$\frac{\text{volume ordered}}{\text{time for infusion}} \left| \frac{\text{time conversion}}{\text{(if needed)}} \right| \frac{\text{volume conversion}}{\text{(if needed)}} = \text{pump setting (mL/hr)}$$

DID YOU KNOW?

To prevent the possibility of causing fluid volume overload, it is recommended that all pediatric IV solutions be administered via IV pumps. Only if an IV pump is unavailable should IV solutions be administered via microdrip IV tubing.

G. Administering IV push medications.

1. Nurses must be approved before being allowed to administer medications via IV push.
2. Student nurses may never give IV push medications.
3. Important considerations.
   a. Type of IV solution: check health-care practitioner's order.
   b. Compatibility of medication with the IV solution: check published reference.
   c. Dilution volume of the medication: check published reference.
   d. Amount of flush needed: usually based on hospital protocol.
   e. Infusion rate: check published reference.
   f. Volume of medication: should be no more than 5 mL.
   g. Nurse should expect immediate responses to the medication.

Box 9.3 Example of No Pump IV Drip Rate Calculation

Doctor's order reads: infuse 800 mL normal saline over 24 hr. Infuse via microdrip.
Child weighs 8 kg.
Check safety of infusion volume.

$$\text{DMV} = 8\text{ kg} \times 100\text{ mL/day} = 800\text{ mL/day}$$

Infusion volume is safe.

Ratio and Proportion Method

Calculate infusion drip rate.

$$\text{gtt/min} = \frac{800\text{ mL} \times 60\text{ gtt/mL}}{60\text{ min/hr} \times 24\text{ hr}}$$

$$= 800/24 = 33.33 = 33\text{ gtt/min}$$

Dimensional Analysis Method

$$\frac{800\text{ mL}}{24\text{ hr}} \left| \frac{60\text{ gtt}}{1\text{ mL}} \right| \frac{1\text{ hr}}{60\text{ min}} = 33.33 = 33\text{ gtt/min}$$

Box 9.4 Example of Pump IV Drip Rate Calculation

Doctor's order reads: infuse 333 mL normal saline over 8 hr. Infuse via infusion pump.
Child weighs 10 kg.
First, check safety of infusion volume.

$$\text{DMV} = 10\text{ kg} \times 100\text{ mL/day} = 1{,}000\text{ mL/day}$$

$$1{,}000\text{ mL}/3 = 333.33\text{ mL}/8\text{ hr}$$

Infusion volume is safe.
Next, calculate the pump infusion rate.

Ratio and Proportion Method

$$\text{ordered pump infusion rate} = \frac{333\text{ mL}}{8\text{ hr}} = 41.63\text{ mL/hr}$$

Dimensional Analysis Method

$$\frac{333\text{ mL}}{8\text{ hr}} = 41.63\text{ mL/hr infusion rate}$$

The pump infusion rate is 41.63 mL/hr.

4. Procedure: check the five rights of medication administration plus:
   a. Check that the medication may be administered via IV push.
   b. Check compatibility of the medication with the IV solution.
   c. Calculate the safe dosage for the child and compare with the order.
   d. Wash hands.
   e. Assure the child that the procedure is painless.
   f. Assess the IV to make sure that the catheter is patent (or flush as per hospital protocol).
   g. Clamp the IV tubing above the injection port that lies closest to the child.
   h. Alcohol (or Betadine) the injection port.
   i. Attach the syringe to the port and administer at the recommended rate for that medication.
   j. After infusing, remove the syringe, and clean the port again with alcohol or Betadine.
   k. Document on both the medication administration record (MAR) and on the child's intake and output sheet.
   l. Monitor the child for physiological responses.

VI. Administering IV Piggyback Medications

A. **IV piggyback** medications are delivered into an existing IV line.

1. Check important considerations from earlier plus:
   a. Recommended dilution amounts and recommended infusion rates for the medications.
   b. Compare the dilution amounts and infusion rates with the fluid volume that the child can safely receive.
   c. Administer via pump, if at all possible.
      i. **Only** if no pump is available, administer via volume-controlled device (e.g., Soluset, Buretrol).
      ii. In some institutions, syringe pumps are used to administer IV medications.
2. Procedure: check the five rights of medication administration plus:
   a. Calculate safe dosage for child and compare with the order.
   b. Wash hands.
   c. Draw up the prescribed medication and assess compatibilities.
   d. Assure the child that the procedure is painless.
   e. Assess IV flow (or flush as per hospital protocol) to make sure that the catheter is patent.
   f. Alcohol (or Betadine) the injection port (or the saline lock).
   g. Attach the piggyback set to the primary line (or the saline lock).
   h. Gently mix the medication with the diluent (either in new IV bag or in a volume-control device).
   i. Either set the infusion pump to the rate for the infusion or manually adjust the rate for the piggyback infusion.
   j. After infusing, restart the IV infusion per protocol.
   k. Document on both the MAR and on the intake and output sheet.
   l. Monitor the child for physiological responses.

VII. Administering Blood Products

A. Important considerations.

1. Educate parents and child, using age-appropriate language, regarding the rationale for the transfusion.
2. Packed red blood cells usually are administered to children to prevent fluid overload.
3. Blood products should only be administered piggyback with normal saline and through a filter.
   a. Small clots are captured by the filter in the IV tubing.
   b. Dextrose solutions are contraindicated when infusing blood because blood hemolyzes when exposed to dextrose.
4. Infants under 4 months of age need only one type and cross match because they rarely develop antibodies.
5. Blood products should infuse over no more than 4 hr.

MAKING THE CONNECTION

The process of blood administration is even more sensitive than is medication administration. Because of the possibility of blood incompatibility, it is essential that two professionals—either two nurses, two doctors, or one nurse and one doctor—carefully check to make sure that the correct patient is receiving the correct blood product. In addition:

- Because of the potential for thrombi to be present in the blood, it is essential that only tubing with a filter be used for the transfusion, and,
- Because blood hemolyzes when exposed to dextrose, it is essential that only normal saline solutions be administered with blood products.

6. Because of the potential for serious transfusion reactions, all hospitals have protocols for identifying and verifying—with another RN or an MD—that the blood being administered is correct.
7. If the blood is very cold, it could affect the child's core temperature. A blood warmer may be needed.

B. Administration.

1. Procedure: check the five rights of medication administration plus:
   a. Identify the child, and verify the blood data per hospital protocol.
   b. Wash hands.
   c. Ideally begin infusing blood within 15 min of its arrival on the unit.
      i. The blood should not be infused if it has been over 30 min since its arrival on the unit.
   d. Vital signs.
      i. Assess before administration.
      ii. After the transfusion is begun, monitor vitals every 15 min for 2 hr and every 30 min until fully infused.
   e. Rate.
      i. Some pumps can injure the cells in the blood. Only infuse with an infusion pump if it is identified as safe for the administration of blood.
      ii. Infuse slowly for first 15 min and monitor carefully for transfusion reactions.
      iii. Then shift to ordered rate.
   f. Monitor child closely for transfusion reactions.
      i. Repeatedly assess lung fields of infants and toddlers throughout the transfusion period because of their poor communication skills.
      ii. Closely monitor the child's serum glucose levels.
         (1) Children may become hypoglycemic after the dextrose infusion is stopped.
   g. Advise parents and child, if appropriate, immediately to report:
      i. Chills.
      ii. Headache.
      iii. Nausea.
      iv. Pain, especially back or flank pain.
      v. Difficulty breathing.
      vi. Bloody urine.
   h. If a transfusion reaction occurs:
      i. Stop the transfusion **immediately**.
      ii. Notify the primary health-care provider, and continue to monitor vital signs.
      iii. Send samples of the child's urine and blood to the blood bank.
      iv. Monitor urine output hourly.
   i. After the transfusion, document per hospital protocol.
   j. Praise both the child and the parents.

VIII. Administering Oral Medications

A. The oral (PO) route is the preferred route for most pediatric medications, however:

1. It should not be used if the child is vomiting, has malabsorption syndrome, or refuses to swallow the medication.

B. Important considerations.

1. For children under 5 years of age, as well as some older children, who are unable to swallow tablets:
   a. Give liquid or a chewable form of the medication. The nurse should ask for an order change, if needed.
   b. Only well-calibrated instruments should be used to measure the medication, for example:
      i. Oral syringes and medication cups rather than household teaspoons or tablespoons.
   c. Divide scored tablets.
   d. Crush tablets only after a reliable source has been consulted to determine whether crushing is contraindicated or not.
   e. Empty and mix medication in capsules with food or liquid only after a reliable source has been consulted to determine whether emptying is contraindicated.
2. To dull the unpleasant taste of PO meds:
   a. Mix distasteful medications or crushed tablets with a **small** amount of applesauce, juice, or gelatin.
      i. Five to 10 mL only because larger quantities may be rejected.
      ii. Honey should never be given to children under 1 year of age because the child may develop infantile botulism.
      iii. It is important to avoid using essential foods, such as milk and formula, to disguise the flavor of a medication because the child may refuse to consume those items in the future.
   b. Or, give the child something such as a sip of fruit juice, a peppermint, or a few ice chips before and after the medication.
3. Be prepared for all types of reactions when administering medications.
   a. Children are unpredictable!
4. Never threaten a child with an injection if he or she refuses an oral medication.

5. Never tell a child that an oral medication is candy or tastes like candy.
6. Feeding tube.
   a. If a feeding tube is in place, oral medications may be administered through the tube.
      i. First, verify that the tube is in the stomach.
      ii. Before and after administering the medication, flush the tube with a small quantity of water to make sure that the medication has reached the stomach and that the tube remains patent.

C. Administering oral medications to infants.
1. Considerations.
   a. Only liquid medications are administered to infants.
   b. Only needleless syringes or well-calibrated droppers should be used to measure medications for infants.
2. Procedure: check five rights of medication administration plus:
   a. Wash hands.
   b. Carefully draw up the medication.
   c. Elevate the infant's head and shoulders, hold infant in a feeding position, and stabilize both arms.
   d. Depress the chin with the thumb to open the infant's mouth.
   e. Direct the medication toward the inner aspect of the infant's cheek.
   f. Slowly "inject" the medication, regulating the flow to the speed of the infant's swallowing.
   g. Release the thumb, and allow the infant to finish swallowing.
   h. Give the infant a hug.
3. Vomiting or spitting up the medication.
   a. Notify the primary health-care provider if the child vomits or spits up large quantities of the medication.
   b. A repeat dose may need to be administered.
   c. Keep in mind that if administering digoxin, vomiting is one of the first signs of dig toxicity (See Chapter 17, "Nursing Care of the Child With Cardiovascular Illnesses").
      i. An order for a dig level should be requested from the primary health-care provider.

D. Administering oral medications to toddlers/preschoolers.
1. Considerations.
   a. Needleless syringes, droppers, and medicine cups may be used to administer medications to toddlers.
   b. Some toddlers willingly take a chewable medication if the taste is not too unpleasant.
   c. Straws.
      i. Young children often take a medication if they are allowed to suck the medication through a straw.
      ii. The straw should be short to avoid large quantities of the medication adhering to the sides.
2. Procedure: check the five rights of medication administration plus:
   a. Wash hands.
   b. Carefully draw up the medication.
   c. Position the child.
      i. If the child is cooperative, allow the child to assume a comfortable position.
      ii. If the child is uncooperative, the nurse may need assistance or may need to restrain temporarily.
   d. Administer the medication.
      i. If by syringe, slowly "inject" the medication, directing it toward the inner aspect of the cheek.
      ii. If by cup or straw, allow the child to hold the medicine cup and drink it at his or her own pace.
3. Praise the child after the medicine has been taken.
4. Document.

E. Administering oral medications to school-age children and adolescents.
1. Considerations.
   a. Determine whether the child is able to swallow tablets or not.
      i. If unable to swallow tablets, either chewables or liquids may be appropriate.
2. Procedure: check the five rights of medication administration plus:
   a. If tablet or capsule, direct him or her to place the medicine near the back of the tongue and to immediately swallow with a fluid (i.e., water or juice).
   b. Offer praise after the medicine is taken and document.

IX. Administering Intramuscular (IM) Medications

A. Considerations.
1. Before administering, ask the child or parent what behaviors the child usually exhibits when receiving injections.
2. Using age-appropriate language, prepare the child for the injection (e.g., where the shot will be given, how the shot will feel, how long the feeling will last).

3. If needed, teach the child distraction techniques that he or she can use (e.g., deep breathing, counting, clenching fists, singing).
4. Numb the site: ice applied to the site can reduce the pain of an injection.
5. Tell the child the injection is not a punishment for being bad but is given to make him or her better.
6. Keep the child safe.
   a. This is as important as making sure that the child receives the medication.
   b. Swaddling and/or other methods of restraint often are required to help the child to stay still.
7. After administering an injection.
   a. Praise and cuddle the child after administering a painful injection, even if the child fought and yelled during the procedure.
   b. Dispose of the needle and syringe in an infection control sharps container.
   c. Document:
      i. Not only that the medication was administered but
      ii. Where the injection was given. Injection sites should be rotated to prevent injuring tissue.

B. Administering IM injections to infants.
1. Considerations.
   a. Until a baby is able to walk, IM injections should be given in the vastus lateralis—on the anterior surface of the midlateral thigh (Fig. 9.2).
   b. Being breast-fed or sucking on sucrose soothies has been shown to reduce the pain of injections in infants.
   c. Maximum amount to be administered.
      i. Neonates: 0.5 mL.
      ii. Infants: 1 mL.
   d. Maximum needle length.
      i. Neonates: one-half to five-eighths inch (1.3 to 2 cm).
      ii. Infants: 1 inch (2.5 cm).
   e. Needle gauge: should be appropriate to the medication being administered.
      i. Unless highly viscous, 22- to 25-gauge needles are best.
2. Procedure: check the five rights of medication administration plus:
   a. Wash hands and glove.
   b. Place the infant in the supine position.
   c. Divide the distance between the trochanter and the patella into thirds, and locate the middle third.
   d. Locate the anterolateral aspect of the middle third.
   e. Securely stabilize the child's leg.

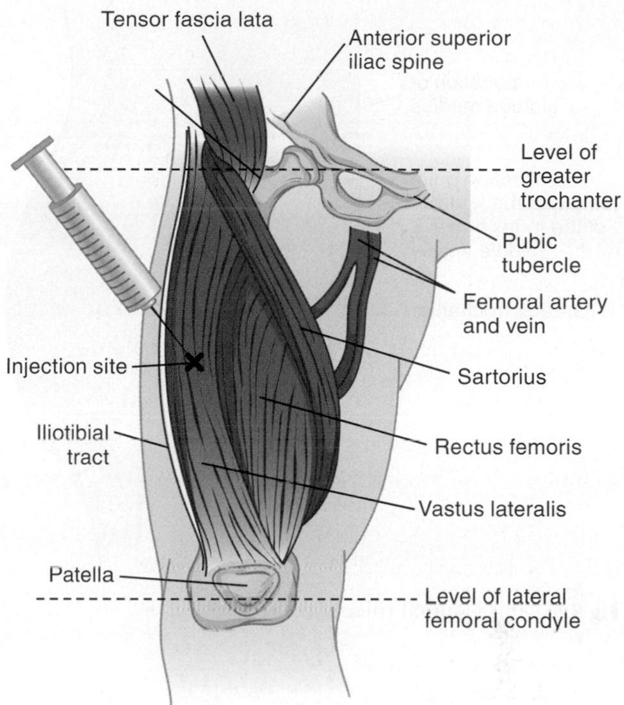

Fig 9.2 Vastus lateralis injection site in infants.

      i. Get a second person to secure the infant, if needed.
   f. Clean the site with alcohol and allow to dry.
   g. Insert the needle at a 90-degree angle.
   h. If immunization, inject.
   i. If medication:
      i. Aspirate for the presence of blood.
      ii. If no blood is aspirated, inject slowly.
   j. Remove the needle, and massage the site, if not contraindicated.
   k. Dispose of the needle and syringe in a sharps container.
   l. Hold, cuddle, and comfort the infant after the injection.
   m. Document.

C. Administering IM injections to toddlers, preschoolers, school-age children, and adolescents.
1. Considerations.
   a. Maximum amount: depends on muscle but, in general:
      i. Toddlers and preschoolers: 1.5 mL.
      ii. School-agers and adolescents: 2 mL.
   b. Needle length: approximately one-half the width of the muscle.
   c. Needle gauge.
      i. Should be appropriate to the medication being administered.
      ii. Unless highly viscous, 22- to 25-gauge needles are best.

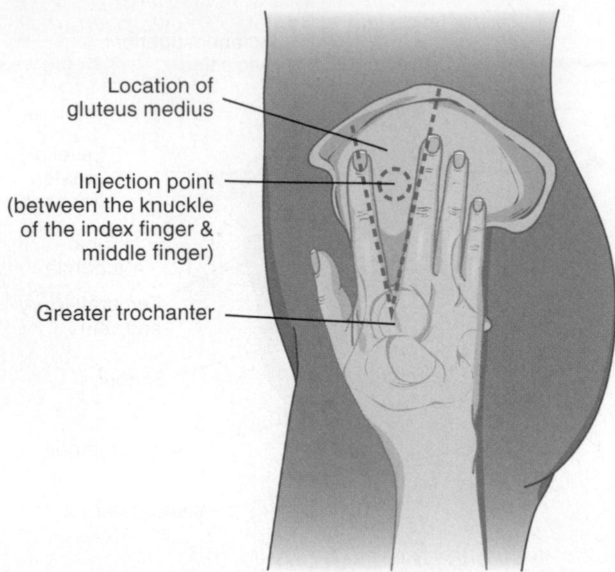

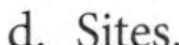

Fig 9.3 Ventrogluteal injection site.

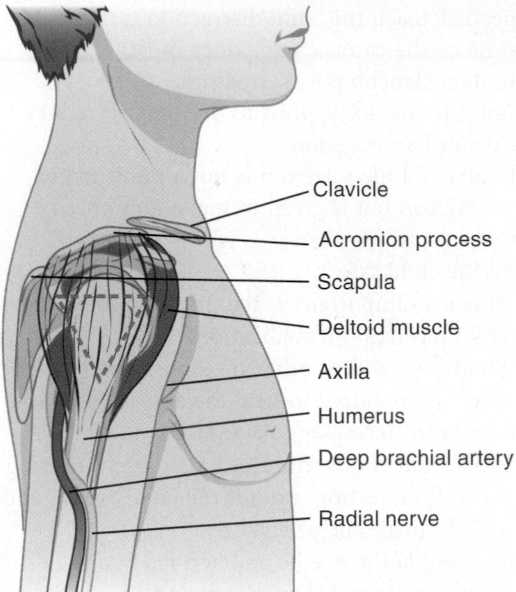

Fig 9.4 Deltoid injection site.

d. Sites.
   i. Vastus lateralis: excellent site. Devoid of large vessels and nerves and large muscle, but the site is visible to the child.
   ii. Ventrogluteal: excellent site after 18 months of age, but the site is visible to the child (Fig. 9.3).
      (1) To locate the site: with the thumb facing toward the child's anterior, the palm of the hand is placed on the trochanter. The index finger is then placed on the anterior superior iliac spine, and the middle finger is slid over the iliac crest toward the child's posterior. A "V" is then created between the index and middle fingers. The injection is given in the center of the "V."
   iii. The deltoid (Fig. 9.4) is the preferred site for immunizations **after** the child reaches 3 years of age.
      (1) For small quantities of medication only.
      (2) To locate the site: create an upside-down triangle with the base of the triangle formed below the acromion process and the point of the triangle at the level of the axilla. The injection should be administered in the center of the triangle.
   iv. Dorsogluteal (Fig. 9.5): rarely used in children because of safety concerns. This site should be used when **no other option** is available.

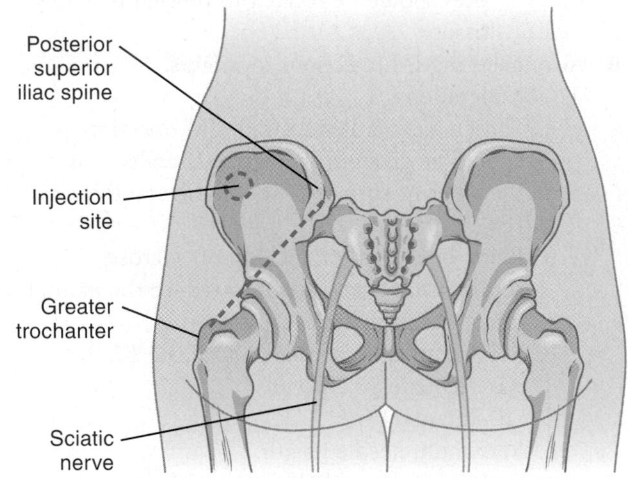

Fig 9.5 Dorsogluteal injection site.

      (1) Use **only** after the child reaches age 5.
      (2) To locate the site: the nurse should draw an imaginary line between the trochanter and the child's posterior superior iliac spine on the same side as the trochanter. The injection should be administered above and lateral to the line.

2. Procedure: check the five rights of medication administration plus:
   a. Wash hands and glove.
   b. Apply ice to the site, if requested.

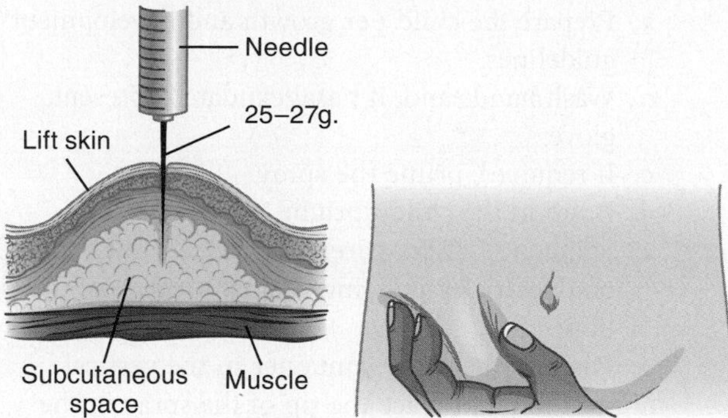

Fig 9.6 Subcutaneous injection.

c. Prepare the child.
   i. Be honest; never tell a child that a shot will not hurt.
d. Restrain the child obtaining assistance, if needed.
e. Keep the needle out of the child's field of vision.
f. Prepare the site, and inject the medication, as described earlier. Perform the procedure as quickly as possible.
g. Dispose of the needle and syringe in a sharps container.
h. Allow the child to express his or her feelings while praising and comforting the child.
i. Document.

X. Administering Subcutaneous (Subcu) Injections (Fig. 9.6)

A. Considerations.
1. Subcu injections are administered into fat pads located in:
   a. Hips; lateral upper arms; anterior thighs; stomach, excluding the area surrounding the navel and above the iliac crests.
   b. Sites should be rotated to prevent tissue damage.
2. A short needle must be used to prevent injecting into the muscle.
3. A small (25 to 27 gauge) needle usually is used.
4. See earlier for age-related issues.

B. Administering to any age child.
1. Procedure: check the five rights of medication administration plus:
   a. Wash hands and glove.
   b. Clean site with alcohol and allow to dry.
   c. Pinch the tissue to reveal the fat tissue.
   d. Insert the needle at a 45- to 90-degree angle.
   e. Inject the medication and then remove the needle.
   f. Massage the site, unless contraindicated.
   g. Dispose of the needle and syringe in a sharps container.
   h. Praise and comfort the child.
   i. Document.

XI. Administering Otic Medications

A. Considerations.
1. The drops should be allowed to warm to room temperature before administering to reduce pain during administration.
2. Clean the area outside the ear canal before instilling the drops.
3. Never insert the dropper into the ear canal.

B. Administration.
1. Procedure: check the five rights of medication administration plus:
   a. Wash hands.
   b. Prepare the child using developmentally appropriate language.
   c. Position the child so that the ear in which the drops are to be administered is up.
   d. Position the pinna of the ear, and instill the correct number of drops (see Fig. 7.2).
      i. For infants and children up to 3 years of age, pull the pinna of the ear back and down.
      ii. For children over 3 years of age, pull the pinna of the ear back and up.
   e. Rub the tissue immediately in front of the canal to make sure that the drops descend fully.
   f. Keep the child in the position for a few minutes—distraction will help.
   g. Praise and comfort the child.
   h. Document.

XII. Administering Ophthalmic Medications (Fig. 9.7)

A. Considerations.
1. The drops should be allowed to warm to room temperature to reduce pain during administration.
2. The dropper should never touch the eye. If the dropper touches the eye, the medication bottle is contaminated and should be disposed of.

B. Administration.
1. Procedure: check the five rights of medication administration plus:
   a. Wash hands and, if exudate is present, glove hands.

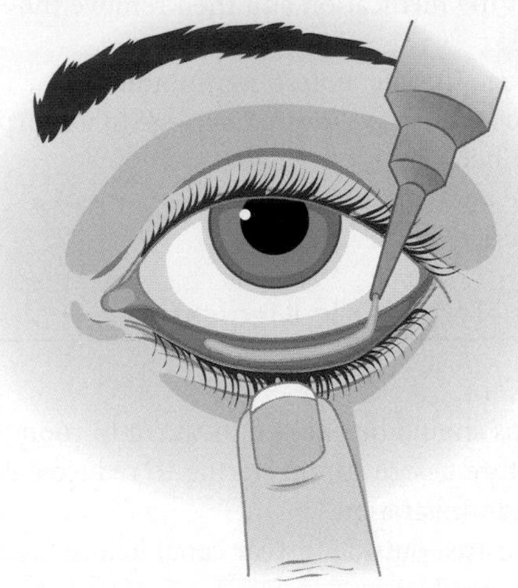

Fig 9.7 Administering ophthalmic medications.

b. Assist child into a position with the neck slightly hyperextended.
   i. For infants and toddlers, have an assistant restrain the child's arms, or wrap a towel around the child's arms.
   ii. For older children, ask the child to look up.
c. Depress the lower lid of the eye.
d. Place the medication into the lower conjunctival sac.
e. If both drops and ointment are ordered, insert drops first and ointment second.
f. Release the lid, and have the child close his or her eyes for a few seconds.
g. Wipe any excess medication away with a tissue.
h. Praise and comfort the child.
i. Document.

XIII. Administering Medications Into the Respiratory Tract

A. Considerations.
1. Administered in one of three ways.
   a. Via nasal sprays, **nebulizers,** or **metered dose inhalers (MDIs)**.
2. Child must carefully be monitored following administration for systemic effects, both therapeutic and adverse.
3. If the medication is to be administered at home, educating parents and child on their administration is critical.
4. Nebulizer medications usually are first diluted with normal saline.

B. Administering medications via nasal sprays.
1. Procedure: check the five rights of medication administration plus:
   a. Prepare the child per growth and development guidelines.
   b. Wash hands and, if nasal exudate is present, glove.
   c. If required, prime the spray.
   d. Position the child upright.
   e. Someone—child, parent, or nurse—must close one nostril by pressing against the side of the nose.
   f. Position the spray container in the vertical position and place the tip of the spray in the alternate nostril.
   g. Gently compress the container.
   h. Encourage the child to breathe in through his or her nose, although there is no need to breathe in forcefully.
   i. Repeat the procedure in the alternate nostril.
   j. Encourage the older child to refrain from blowing his or her nose immediately after the medication administration.
   k. If the child complains of an unpleasant taste in his or her mouth, provide the child with a sip of juice or water.
   l. Praise and comfort the child.
   m. Document.

C. Administering medications via nebulizer.
1. Procedure: check the five rights of medication administration plus:
   a. Wash hands.
   b. Dilute medication per instructions.
   c. Place diluted medication into nebulizer reservoir.
   d. Position child.
      i. For infants and toddlers, place mask over child's face.
      ii. For older children, have child place a plastic mouthpiece in his or her mouth, and have the child secure his or her lips around the mouthpiece.
   e. Encourage the child to breathe in and out slowly.
   f. Praise and comfort the child.
   g. Cleanse the nebulizer reservoir with mild soap and water.
   h. Document.

D. Administering medications via MDIs.
1. Considerations.
   a. Monitor usage.
      i. Parents and child must be reminded to monitor the MDI usage and replace the container, when needed.
         (1) Each MDI has a specific number of administrations per container.

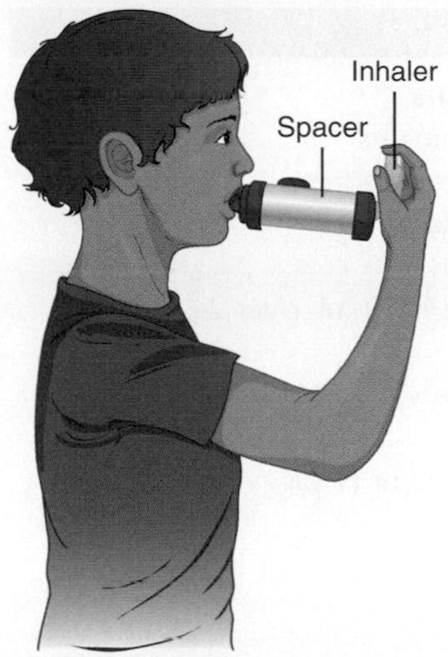

Fig 9.8 Spacer aid in use with MDI.

ii. Advise parents that MDIs should never be placed in water.

2. Procedure: check the five rights of medication administration plus:
   a. Prepare the child per growth and development guidelines.
   b. Wash hands.
   c. If more than one medication is ordered and one is a steroid, the steroid should be administered last.
   d. Prepare the child.
      i. For young children.
         (1) Place a **spacer** (Fig. 9.8) onto the MDI.
         (2) Have the child let out a "big breath."
         (3) *Before* the child inhales, have the child place the mouthpiece of the spacer in his or her mouth, and have the child secure his or her lips around the mouthpiece.
         (4) Compress the MDI, have the child inhale the medicine from the spacer and hold his or her breath while you count slowly to five.
         (5) If two puffs have been ordered, wait 2 min, have the child exhale again, and repeat the process.
         (6) Praise and comfort the child.
         (7) Clean the MDI and spacer with water.
         (8) Document.
      ii. For older children.
         (1) Have the child exhale.
         (2) Before he or she inhales, have the child place the mouthpiece of the MDI in his or her mouth.
         (3) *At the same time as the child inhales,* have the child compress the MDI.
         (4) Have the child hold his or her breath for about 10 sec.
         (5) If two puffs have been ordered, wait 2 min, have the child exhale again, and repeat the process.
         (6) Clean the MDI.
         (7) Praise the child.
         (8) Document.

DID YOU KNOW?

When respiratory medications are administered via an MDI, it is important that the child inhale at the same time that he or she compresses the MDI. Only when the two actions occur simultaneously will a therapeutic response occur when the medication reaches the lower respiratory tract. If the child compresses the MDI before or after inhaling, the medication will remain in the child's mouth, and no therapeutic response will occur. If a child is unable to compress the MDI and breathe in simultaneously, a spacer should be used.

E. Administering medications via the rectum.

1. Considerations.
   a. The rectal route should be used as infrequently as possible. If another route is available, especially the oral route, it should be used.
   b. Preparing a child for a rectal medication is important because children find penetration of the rectum frightening.
2. Procedure: check the five rights of medication administration plus:
   a. Wash hands and glove.
   b. While keeping the child as covered as possible, place the child on his or her left side with the upper leg bent, and expose the rectum.
   c. Lubricate the medication with a water-soluble lubricant.
   d. Encourage the child to breathe in and out.
   e. While the child is breathing in, insert the medication about 1 to 2 cm into the rectal cavity.
   f. Briefly hold the child's buttocks together.
   g. Praise and comfort the child.
   h. Document.

CASE STUDY: Putting It All Together

8-year-old male, Caucasian child admitted to the pediatric unit

Subjective Data

- Child crying, complaining of neck pain and of the bright lights
- Mother at child's bedside, stroking child's forehead
- Mother states,
  - "He's so sick. Please make him better."

Objective Data

Nursing Assessment

- Positive Kernig's sign
- Positive Brudzinski's sign
- Weight: 55 lb
- Height: 50 in.

Vital Signs

Temperature:	103.8 °F
Heart rate:	124 bpm
Respiratory rate:	26 rpm
Blood pressure:	98/58 mm Hg

Lab Results

Lumbar Puncture

Pressure:	23 cm H_2O (normal less than 20 cm H_2O)
Color:	cloudy (normal clear)
Blood:	none (normal none)
White blood cells:	15 cells/microliter (normal 0–5 cells/microliter)

- Predominantly neutrophils

Culture:	*N. meningitides* (normal none)
Protein:	80 mg/dL (normal up to 70 mg/dL)
Glucose:	18 mg/dL (normal 50–75 mg/dL)

Complete Blood Count

Red blood cell count:	5.5 million/mm^3
Hemoglobin:	14 g/dL
Hematocrit:	42%
White blood cell count:	25,000/mm^3
Platelet count	225,000/mm^3
Urine:	within normal limits

Health-Care Provider's Orders

- Diagnosis: Bacterial meningitis
- Admit to pediatric unit on bedrest
- Place on respiratory isolation
- Seizure precautions
- Start IV D5 ½ NS: infuse 1,750 mL over 24 hr via infusion pump
- Vancomycin 400 mg every 6 hr IV piggyback via infusion pump
- Ceftriaxone 1.25 g every 12 hr IV piggyback via infusion pump

CASE STUDY: Putting It All Together *cont'd*

Case Study Questions

A. What *subjective* assessments indicate that the client is experiencing a health alteration?

1.
2.
3.
4.

B. What *objective* assessments indicate that the client is experiencing a health alteration?

1.
2.
3.
4.
5.
6.

C. After analyzing the data that has been collected, what primary nursing diagnosis should the nurse assign to this client?

1.

D. What interventions should the nurse plan and/or implement to meet this child's and his family's needs?

1.
2.
3.
4.
5.
6.

E. What client outcomes should the nurse evaluate regarding the effectiveness of the nursing interventions?

1.
2.
3.
4.

F. What physiological characteristics should the child exhibit before being discharged home?

1.
2.
3.

G. What subjective characteristics should the child exhibit before being discharged home?

1.

REVIEW QUESTIONS

1. An order is written to administer 5 mL of an oral liquid medication to a toddler. The toddler says, "Me do it!!" Which of the following modes of administration would be appropriate for the nurse to perform?
   1. Draw up the medication in a needleless syringe, and inject the medication into the child's mouth.
   2. Pour the medication into a medicine cup, and hold the cup while the child drinks from the cup.
   3. Pour the medication into a teaspoon, hand the teaspoon to the child, and watch the child drink the medicine.
   4. Draw up the medication in a needleless syringe, hand the syringe to the child, and watch the child squirt and drink the medicine.

2. A nurse is to administer ear drops into the right ear of a 6-year-old child. Which of the following actions by the nurse is appropriate?
   1. Nurse warms the medication in the microwave.
   2. Nurse pulls the pinna of the ear up and back.
   3. Nurse rubs the area behind the ear after administering the medication.
   4. Nurse has the child lie supine for one-half hr after administering the medication.

3. A nurse is to administer 2 ophthalmic medications—an ointment and drops. Which of the following actions by the nurse is appropriate?
   1. Rest the medication containers on the lower lid of the eye.
   2. Administer the eye drop medication before administering the medicated ointment.
   3. Administer both medications into the lateral sclera of each eye.
   4. Squeeze the ointment into the sac created by raising the upper eyelid of the eye.

4. A nurse is to administer tablets to a 7-year-old child. The child begins to cry and states, "I can't. I'll choke." Which of the following actions by the nurse is appropriate for the nurse to perform?
   1. Gently tell the child, "I bet you can do it. Just try."
   2. Simply state, "Of course you can. You are a big kid."
   3. Crush the tablets and mix with a full glass of juice.
   4. Ask the doctor to order chewable tablets.

5. A nurse is to administer packed red blood cells to a severely anemic child. Which of the following actions should the nurse perform during the procedures? **Select all that apply.**
   1. Use intravenous tubing that contains a filter.
   2. Take a full set of vital signs every 15 minutes for 2 hours.
   3. Stop the infusion after the cells have been hanging for 2 hours.
   4. Identify the child, and verify the blood data with another nurse.
   5. Make sure that the main intravenous solution is a dextrose solution.

6. A 5-year-old child with a high fever is vomiting. The doctor orders acetaminophen 80 mg per rectum. Which of the following actions by the nurse is appropriate?
   1. Request that the health-care practitioner change the order to oral acetaminophen.
   2. Position the child on the right side with the upper leg bent.
   3. Insert the medication into the rectum, and place the child in semi-Fowler's position.
   4. After inserting the medication, hold the child's buttocks together.

7. A toddler admitted to the pediatric unit is to have an intravenous catheter inserted and an IV of D5 ½ NS infused. No pump is available for the infusion. Which of the following actions by the nurse is appropriate?
   1. Infuse the solution through macrodrip tubing.
   2. Cover the infusion site with opaque adhesive tape.
   3. Calculate the daily maintenance volume for the child.
   4. Change the intravenous bag every twelve hours.

8. The nurse is administering an oral medication to a school-age child. The medication is known to taste very bitter. Which of the following actions by the nurse would be most appropriate?
   1. Encourage the child to hold his or her nose while swallowing the medication.
   2. Have the child suck on ice chips immediately before swallowing the medication.
   3. Mix the medication with a small amount of the child's favorite flavor of gelatin.
   4. Request the primary health-care provider to change the order to an injection.

9. A toddler is to receive a medication to take at home that is administered via a metered dose inhaler (MDI). Which of the following information should the nurse include in the patient teaching regarding the medication?
1. The parent should attach a spacer onto the mouthpiece of the MDI.
2. The parent should position the child supine while the medication is administered.
3. The parent should have the child inhale right before the medication is administered.
4. The parent should place the face mask on the child and attach it to the MDI.

The following nomogram *is available to answer all relevant questions:*

10. A doctor is ordering a medication for a child who weighs 26 lb and who is 43 in. tall. A reliable medication reference states that the recommended pediatric dosage is 50 to 60 mg/kg/day in divided doses every 6 hr. Which of the following medication orders is safe for the child?
1. 100 mg every 6 hr
2. 150 mg every 6 hr
3. 200 mg every 6 hr
4. 250 mg every 6 hr

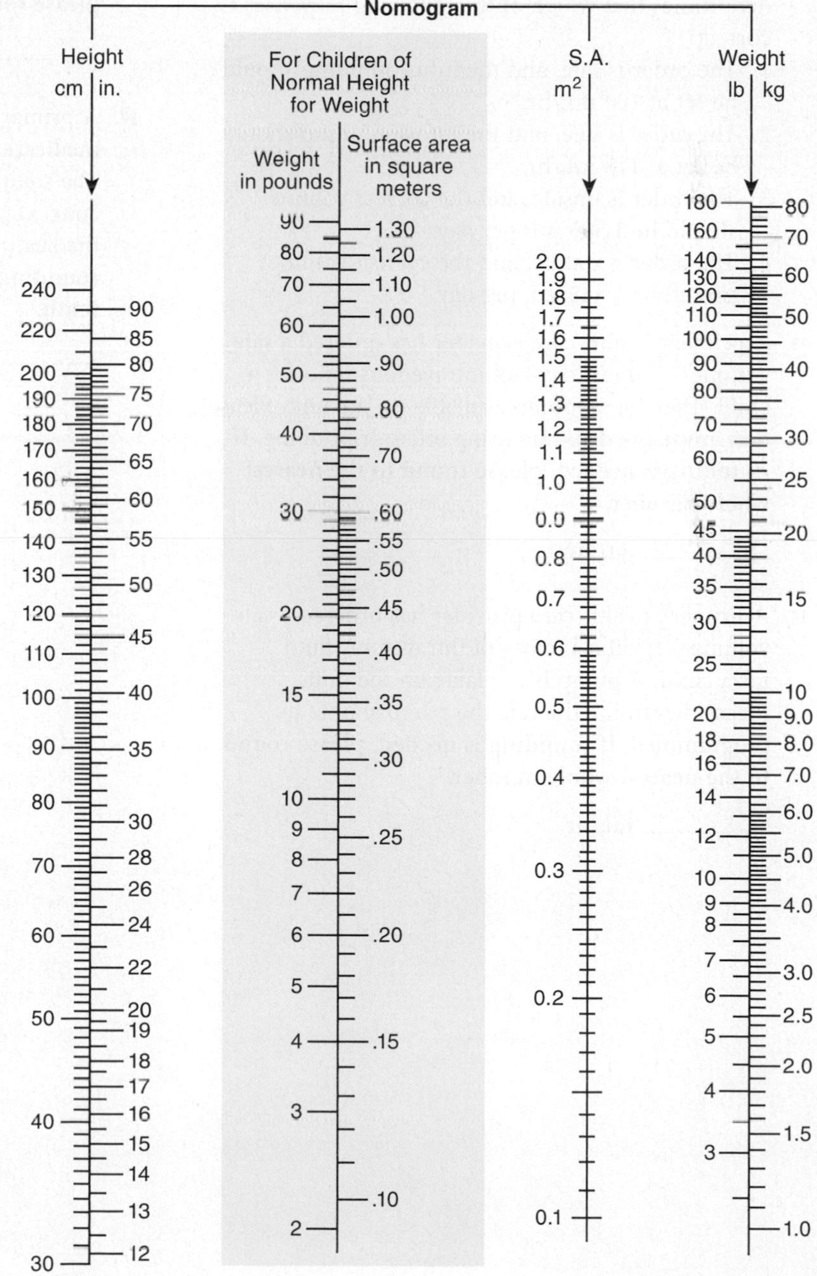

11. A doctor is ordering a medication for a child who weighs 15.2 kg and who is 112 cm tall. A reliable medication reference states the recommended pediatric dosage is 10 to 20 mg/m^2/day in 2 equal doses. Which of the following medication orders is safe for the child?
    1. 5 mg every 12 hr
    2. 8 mg every 12 hr
    3. 10 mg every 12 hr
    4. 13 mg every 12 hr

12. A primary health-care provider orders a maintenance intravenous fluid volume of 2,500 mL per day for a school-age child who weighs 82 lb and is 5 ft 2 in. tall. The nurse caring for the child determines that which of the following responses is correct?
    1. The order is safe, and the infusion pump should be set at 100 mL/hr.
    2. The order is safe, and the infusion pump should be set at 118 mL/hr.
    3. The order is unsafe, and the correct volume should be 1,575 mL per day.
    4. The order is unsafe, and the correct volume should be 1,845 mL per day.

13. A primary health-care provider has ordered a safe volume—720 mL/day—of intravenous fluid for a child. There is no pump available on the unit. Please determine the drip rate using microdrip tubing. **If rounding is needed, please round to the nearest whole number.**

    __________ gtt/min

14. A primary health-care provider has ordered a safe volume—1,460 mL/day—of intravenous fluid for a child. A pump is available on the unit. Please determine the rate the pump should be programmed. **If rounding is needed, please round to the nearest whole number.**

    __________ mL/hr

15. A primary health-care provider has ordered a medication for a child—16 kg and 132 cm. A reliable medication reference states the safe pediatric dosage is 250 mg/m^2/day divided every 8 hr. Please calculate the maximum safe dosage of the medication for this child. **If rounding is needed, please round to the nearest hundredth.**

    __________ mg every 8 hr

16. A primary health-care provider has ordered a medication for a child: 250 mcg PO every 4 hr. The medication is only available on the unit in scored tablets: 0.125 mg. How much medication should the nurse administer per dose? **If rounding is needed, please round to the nearest tenth.**

    __________ tablets every 4 hr

17. A primary health-care provider has ordered a medication for an infant: 250 mg PO every 4 hr. The solution is available on the unit in the following concentration: 500 mg/5 mL. How much medication should the nurse administer per dose? **If rounding is needed, please round to the nearest tenth.**

    __________ mL every 4 hr

REVIEW ANSWERS

1. **ANSWER: 4**
Rationale:
1. Although the medication would safely be administered, this does not meet the toddler's need for autonomy.
2. Although the medication would safely be administered, this does not meet the toddler's need for autonomy.
3. Although the nurse has met the toddler's need for autonomy, a teaspoon is not a reliable measurement instrument.
4. This method would meet the toddler's need for autonomy, and the measurement tool is reliable.
TEST-TAKING TIP: When administering medications, it is essential that the nurse use a reliable measurement instrument in order to provide the correct dosage. In addition, the nurse should consider the child's level of growth and development.
Content Area: *Pediatrics—Toddler*
Integrated Processes: *Nursing Process: Implementation*
Client Need: *Physiological Integrity: Pharmacological and Parenteral Therapies: Medication Administration*
Cognitive Level: *Application*

2. **ANSWER: 2**
Rationale:
1. The medication should be warmed to room temperature, but it would be unsafe to warm it in the microwave.
2. This statement is correct. The nurse should pull the pinna of the ear up and back.
3. The nurse should rub the area in front of the ear after administering the medication.
4. The child should lie on the unaffected side for a few minutes after administering the medication.
TEST-TAKING TIP: Because the anatomy of the ear changes as the child grows the nurse should pull the pinna of the ear down and back until the child reaches 3 years of age. When the child is over 3 years, the pinna of the ear should be pulled up and back.
Content Area: *Pediatrics—School Age*
Integrated Processes: *Nursing Process: Implementation*
Client Need: *Physiological Integrity: Pharmacological and Parenteral Therapies: Medication Administration*
Cognitive Level: *Application*

3. **ANSWER: 2**
Rationale:
1. An ophthalmic medication container should never touch the patient. If it does, it is considered contaminated.
2. This is a correct statement. Eye drop medication should be inserted before ophthalmic ointments.
3. The medications should be administered into the conjunctival pocket formed when the lower lid is depressed.
4. The medications should be administered into the conjunctival pocket formed when the lower lid is depressed.
TEST-TAKING TIP: The nurse could actually cause an eye infection if he or she administered an ophthalmic medication that had been contaminated during a previous administration.
Content Area: *Pediatrics*
Integrated Processes: *Nursing Process: Implementation*
Client Need: *Physiological Integrity: Pharmacological and Parenteral Therapies: Medication Administration*
Cognitive Level: *Application*

4. **ANSWER: 4**
Rationale:
1. This statement is not appropriate. The child has indicated that he or she is unable to swallow tablets.
2. This statement is not appropriate. Not only has the child indicated that he or she is unable to swallow tablets, but also the nurse is intimating that the child is not performing at his or her level of growth and development.
3. This action is not appropriate. Medications should not be mixed with large quantities of juice or other substances. The child will likely not finish all of the juice and, therefore, not receive the full dose of the medication.
4. This action is appropriate. School-age children who are unable to swallow medications would be able to consume a chewable tablet.
TEST-TAKING TIP: When administering medications to children, nurses should employ the procedure that will result in the safe administration of the medication while meeting the child's needs. Chewable medications enable children who are unable to swallow pills safely to take oral medications.
Content Area: *Pediatrics—School Age*
Integrated Processes: *Nursing Process: Implementation*
Client Need: *Physiological Integrity: Pharmacological and Parenteral Therapies: Medication Administration*
Cognitive Level: *Application*

5. **ANSWER: 1, 2, and 4**
Rationale:
1. Filtered tubing must be used when infusing a blood product.
2. A full set of vital signs should be taken every 15 min for 2 hr.
3. A blood infusion should be stopped after it has been hanging for 4 hr.
4. This statement is correct. The nurse should identify the child and verify the blood data either with another nurse or with a physician.
5. The main IV line should be normal saline with no dextrose.
TEST-TAKING TIP: It is critical that nurses follow all safety precautions when administering blood products. To ensure that the patient is receiving blood that is compatible to his or her blood type, protocols require that two professionals check all identifying indicators. Filtered tubing must be used to make sure that no thrombi enter into the patient's bloodstream. Vital signs are monitored carefully in order to detect a transfusion reaction as quickly as possible. Blood hemolyzes when exposed to a dextrose solution. Only normal saline should be used when hanging blood.

Content Area: *Pediatrics*
Integrated Processes: *Nursing Process: Implementation*
Client Need: *Physiological Integrity: Pharmacological and Parenteral Therapies: Blood and Blood Products*
Cognitive Level: *Application*

6. ANSWER: 4
Rationale:
1. This action is inappropriate. The child is vomiting, so an oral medication is contraindicated.
2. The child should be positioned on his or her left side with the upper leg bent.
3. The child should remain in the lateral position for a few minutes after the rectal medication has been inserted.
4. The nurse should hold the child's buttocks together for a short time after the medication has been inserted.
TEST-TAKING TIP: Children, especially toddlers and preschoolers, find rectal temperatures and medications traumatic. They should be used only when necessary (e.g., when a child is vomiting and an oral medication is contraindicated).
Content Area: *Pediatrics—Preschool*
Integrated Processes: *Nursing Process: Implementation*
Client Need: *Physiological Integrity: Pharmacological and Parenteral Therapies: Medication Administration*
Cognitive Level: *Application*

7. ANSWER: 3
Rationale:
1. Only tubing with microdrip chambers should be used when infusing IV solutions to children.
2. The nurse should be able easily to assess the infusion site. Covering it with a translucent material, such as a medication cup and clear tape, enables the nurse to assess the site.
3. The nurse should calculate the DMV for the child. If the volume ordered is markedly higher than the DMV, the nurse should question the order. (It is important to note, however, that if the child is febrile or is dehydrated, the order may be higher than the DMV.)
4. The IV bag should be changed every 24 hr.
TEST-TAKING TIP: To minimize the potential of fluid volume overload, the nurse should always calculate the DMV of any child on IV fluids. Similarly, if the child is receiving nothing by mouth, to minimize the potential for dehydration, the nurse should make sure that the child is receiving the DMV via IV each day. In addition, to reduce the potential for infection, IV bags and tubing should be changed every 24 hr and IV sites changed every 96 hr.
Content Area: *Pediatrics—Toddler*
Integrated Processes: *Nursing Process: Implementation*
Client Need: *Physiological Integrity: Pharmacological and Parenteral Therapies: Medication Administration*
Cognitive Level: *Application*

8. ANSWER: 2
Rationale:
1. This action is not the best action for the nurse to perform.
2. Having the child suck on ice chips immediately before swallowing the medication is the best action.
3. Mixing the medication into a favorite flavor of any substance may result in the child no longer liking the substance because the substance now is associated with the bitter taste of the medication.
4. Although this may be an option, it is not the best action for the nurse to perform. Injections are painful and traumatic. It would be best to have the child suck on ice chips immediately before taking the bitter medicine.
TEST-TAKING TIP: When administering medications to children, nurses should employ the procedure that will result in the safe administration of the medication while meeting the child's needs. Ice chips help to numb the taste buds. They could also be given to the child immediately after he or she finishes taking the bitter-tasting medicine.
Content Area: *Pediatrics—School Age*
Integrated Processes: *Nursing Process: Implementation*
Client Need: *Physiological Integrity: Pharmacological and Parenteral Therapies: Medication Administration*
Cognitive Level: *Analysis*

9. ANSWER: 1
Rationale:
1. The parent should attach a spacer onto the mouthpiece of the MDI.
2. The parent should position the child upright while the medication is administered.
3. The parent should have the child inhale after placing his or her mouth tightly around the mouthpiece and after the medication has been sprayed into the spacer.
4. Face masks are not used with MDIs. They should be used for infants and small toddlers when nebulizers are used for medication administration.
TEST-TAKING TIP: In order for the medication to reach the bronchi, it is essential that the child fully inhale the medication from the MDI. Older children are able to inhale at the same time that the medication container is compressed. Toddlers, however, are not. Spacers trap the medication enabling toddlers to breathe the medication in more slowly and in their own time.
Content Area: *Pediatrics—Toddler*
Integrated Processes: *Nursing Process: Implementation*
Client Need: *Physiological Integrity: Pharmacological and Parenteral Therapies: Medication Administration*
Cognitive Level: *Application*

10. ANSWER: 2
Rationale:
1. 100 mg every 6 hr is incorrect.
2. 150 mg every 6 hr is correct.
3. 200 mg every 6 hr is incorrect.
4. 250 mg every 6 hr is incorrect.
TEST-TAKING TIP: *Ratio and proportion method:* The recommended pediatric dosage is stated as per kilogram. The weight calculation formula must be used.

Convert 26 lb to kg: 26/2.2 = 11.82

Calculate the maximum safe dose per day.

60 mg/1 kg = x mg/11.82 kg

x = 709.2 mg

Calculate the maximum safe dose per 6 hr.

709.2/4 (4 doses per day) = 177.3 mg

Calculate the minimum safe dose per day.

50 mg/1 kg = x mg/11.82 kg

x = 591 mg

Calculate the minimum safe dose per 6 hr.

591/4 (4 doses per day) = 147.75 mg

Dimensional analysis method:
Calculate the maximum safe dosage.

60 mg	26 lb	1 kg	1 day	= 177.3 mg every 6 hr is the maximum safe dosage
kg/day		2.2/lb	4 doses (every 6 hr)	

Calculate the minimum safe dosage.

50 mg	26 lb	1 kg	1 day	= 147.75 mg every 6 hr is the minimum safe dosage
kg/day		2.2/lb	4 doses (every 6 hr)	

The doctor's order should be between 147.75 mg every 6 hr and 177.3 mg every 6 hr. The only order that meets the criteria is 150 mg every 6 hr.
Content Area: Pediatrics
Integrated Processes: Nursing Process: Dosage Calculation
Client Need: Physiological Integrity: Pharmacological and Parenteral Therapies: Medication Administration
Cognitive Level: Application

11. ANSWER: 1
Rationale:
1. **5 mg every 12 hr is correct.**
2. 8 mg every 12 hr is incorrect.
3. 10 mg every 12 hr is incorrect.
4. 13 mg every 12 hr is incorrect.

TEST-TAKING TIP: The recommended pediatric dosage is stated as per meters squared. The BSA calculation formula must be used.
Determine the BSA on the nomogram.
Connect a line between the child's weight (15.2 kg) and the child's height (112 cm.).

BSA = 0.68 m^2

Ratio and proportion method:
Calculate the maximum safe dose per day.

20 mg/1 m^2 = x mg/0.68 m^2

x = 13.6 mg

Calculate the maximum safe amount per dose.

13.6/2 (2 doses per day) = 6.8 mg

Calculate the minimum safe dose per day.

10 mg/1 m^2 = x mg/0.68 m^2

x = 6.8 mg

Calculate the minimum safe amount per dose.

6.8/2 (2 doses per day) = 3.4 mg

Dimensional analysis method:
Calculate the maximum safe dosage.

20 mg	0.68/m^2	1 day	= 6.8 mg bid is the maximum safe dosage
m^2/day		2 doses	

Calculate the minimum safe dosage.

10 mg	0.68/m^2	1 day	= 3.4 mg bid is the minimum safe dosage
m^2/day		2 doses	

The doctor's order should be between 3.4 mg every 12 hr and 6.8 mg every 12 hr. The only order that meets the criteria is 5 mg every 12 hr.
Content Area: Pediatrics
Integrated Processes: Nursing Process: Dosage Calculation
Client Need: Physiological Integrity: Pharmacological and Parenteral Therapies: Medication Administration
Cognitive Level: Application

12. ANSWER: 4
Rationale:
1. The order is unsafe, and the correct volume should be 1,845 mL per day.
2. The order is unsafe, and the correct volume should be 1,845 mL per day.
3. The order is unsafe, and the correct volume should be 1,845 mL per day.
4. **The order is unsafe, and the correct volume should be 1,845 mL per day.**

TEST-TAKING TIP: To calculate the daily maintenance fluid volume (DMV) for a child, the nurse must convert the child's weight to kg.

82/2.2 = 37.27 kg

Next, the nurse must remember the DMV formulas.
a. If child weighs less than 10 kg: DMV = 100 mL/kg
b. If child weighs between 10 and 20 kg: DMV = 100 mL times 10 PLUS 50 mL for every kilogram between 10 and 20 kg.
c. If child weighs over 20 kg: DMV = 100 mL times 10 PLUS 50 mL times 10 PLUS 20 mL for every kilogram above 20 kg.
Because this child weighs over 20 kg, the c. formula should be used.

$$DMV = 1.000 \text{ mL} + 500 \text{ mL} + 20 \text{ mL}$$

for every kilogram above 20 kg (37.27 − 20 = 17.27)

$$DMV = 1.500 \text{ mL} + (20 \times 17.27)$$

$$DMV = 1.500 \text{ mL} + 345.4 \text{ mL}$$

DMV = 1,845.4 mL or, to the nearest whole number, 1,845 mL

The doctor's order is 654.6 mL higher than the child's DMV. The nurse should question the physician's order.
Content Area: Pediatrics
Integrated Processes: Nursing Process: Dosage Calculation
Client Need: Physiological Integrity: Pharmacological and Parenteral Therapies: Medication Administration
Cognitive Level: Application

13. **ANSWER: 30 gtt/min**

TEST-TAKING TIP: There is no pump available. The no pump formula, therefore, must be used.

Standard method:

$$\text{drip rate (gtt/min)} = \frac{\text{volume to be infused (mL)} \times \text{drop factor (gtt/min)}}{\text{time (in minutes)}}$$

$$x \text{ gtt/min} = \frac{720 \text{ mL} \times 60 \text{ gtt/mL}}{24 \text{ hr} \times 60 \text{ min/hr}}$$

$$x = \frac{43{,}200 \text{ gtt}}{1{,}440 \text{ min}}$$

$$x = 30 \text{ gtt/min}$$

Dimensional analysis method:

$$\frac{720 \text{ mL}}{\text{day}} \left| \frac{60 \text{ gtt}}{1 \text{ mL}} \right| \frac{1 \text{ day}}{24 \text{ hr}} \left| \frac{1 \text{ hr}}{60 \text{ min}} \right. = \text{30 drops per minute (gtt/min)}$$

The drip rate should be regulated by the nurse to 30 gtt/min.
Content Area: Pediatrics
Integrated Processes: Nursing Process: Dosage Calculation
Client Need: Physiological Integrity: Pharmacological and Parenteral Therapies: Medication Administration
Cognitive Level: Synthesis

14. **ANSWER: 61 mL/hr**

TEST-TAKING TIP: There is a pump available. The pump formula, therefore, must be used.

Standard method:

$$\text{pump setting (mL/hr)} = \frac{\text{volume to be infused (mL)}}{\text{time (in hours)}}$$

$$\text{pump setting} = \frac{1{,}460 \text{ mL}}{24 \text{ hr}}$$

$$\text{pump setting} = 60.83 = 61 \text{ mL/hr}$$

Dimensional analysis method:

$$\frac{1{,}460 \text{ mL}}{\text{day}} \left| \frac{1 \text{ day}}{24 \text{ hr}} \right. = 60.83 = 61 \text{ mL/hr}$$

The pump should be set at 61 mL/hr.
Content Area: Pediatrics
Integrated Processes: Nursing Process: Dosage Calculation
Client Need: Physiological Integrity: Pharmacological and Parenteral Therapies: Medication Administration
Cognitive Level: Synthesis

15. **ANSWER: 61.67 mg every 8 hr**

TEST-TAKING TIP: The recommended pediatric dosage is stated as per meters squared. The BSA calculation formula must be used.
Determine the BSA on the nomogram.
Connect a line between the child's weight (16 kg) and the child's height (132 cm).

$$BSA = 0.74 \text{ m}^2$$

Ratio and proportion method:
Calculate the maximum safe dose per day.

$$250 \text{ mg/1 m}^2 = x \text{ mg/0.74 m}^2$$

$$x = 185 \text{ mg}$$

Calculate the maximum safe amount per dose.

185/3 (3 doses per day) = 61.6666 = 61.67 mg

Dimensional analysis method:

$$\frac{250 \text{ mg}}{\text{m}^2/\text{day}} \left| \frac{0.74 \text{ m}^2}{} \right| \frac{1 \text{ day}}{3 \text{ doses (every 8 hr)}} = \text{61.67 mg every 8 hr is the safe pediatric dosage}$$

The doctor's order should be below 61.67 mg every 8 hr.
Content Area: Pediatrics
Integrated Processes: Nursing Process: Dosage Calculation
Client Need: Physiological Integrity: Pharmacological and Parenteral Therapies: Medication Administration
Cognitive Level: Synthesis

16. **ANSWER: two tablets every 4 hr**

Rationale:

TEST-TAKING TIP:

Ratio and proportion method:
On hand: 0.125 mg/one tablet; needed: 250 mcg/x tablets
First, 250 mcg must be converted to mg.

$$1{,}000 \text{ mcg/1 mg} = 250 \text{ mcg/}x \text{ mg}$$

$$1{,}000x = 250$$

$$x = 0.25 \text{ mg}$$

Next, a ratio and proportion calculation must be performed to determine how many tablets are needed for the dosage.

$$0.125 \text{ mg/one tablet} = 0.25 \text{ mg/}x \text{ tablets}$$

$$0.125x = 0.25$$

$$x = \text{two tablets}$$

Dimensional analysis method:

$$\frac{250 \text{ mcg}}{\text{every 4 hr}} \bigg| \frac{1 \text{ mg}}{1{,}000 \text{ mcg}} \bigg| \frac{1 \text{ tablet}}{0.125 \text{ mcg}} = \text{two tablets every 4 hr}$$

Each time the medication is administered, the nurse should give the child two tablets.

Note: Although the last statement in the question is **"If rounding is needed, please round to the nearest tenth"** the answers do not include a trailing zero, or 2.0 tablets. The Joint Commission has noted, to prevent errors, trailing zeroes should not be included in medication orders or calculations.

Content Area: *Pediatrics*
Integrated Processes: *Nursing Process: Dosage Calculation*
Client Need: *Physiological Integrity: Pharmacological and Parenteral Therapies: Medication Administration*
Cognitive Level: *Synthesis*

17. **ANSWER: 2.5 mL every 4 hr**

Rationale:

TEST-TAKING TIP:

Ratio and proportion method:

On hand: 500 mg/5 mL = 250 mg/x mL

$$500x = 250 \times 5$$

$$500x = 1250$$

$$x = 2.5 \text{ mL}$$

Dimensional analysis method:

$$\frac{250 \text{ mg}}{\text{every 4 hr}} \bigg| \frac{5 \text{ mL}}{500 \text{ mg}} = 2.5 \text{ mL every 4 hr}$$

Each time the medication is administered, the nurse should give the child 2.5 mL of the medicine.

Content Area: *Pediatrics*
Integrated Processes: *Nursing Process: Dosage Calculation*
Client Need: *Physiological Integrity: Pharmacological and Parenteral Therapies: Medication Administration*
Cognitive Level: *Synthesis*

Pediatric Emergencies

KEY TERMS

Automated external defibrillator (AED)—A portable device used to diagnose arrhythmias and treat the patient with electrical therapy.

CAB—The acronym for CPR intervention, which stands for chest compression, airway, breathing.

Chelation therapy—The administration of a medication to remove heavy metals from the body.

Distributive shock—Reduced circulatory perfusion to the vital organs and the periphery, commonly caused by a massive infection, anaphylaxis, or drug overdose.

Extracorporeal membrane oxygenation (ECMO)—Treatment similar to cardiopulmonary bypass, usually only used as treatment for infants and young children.

Hypovolemic shock—A condition resulting from excessive blood or fluid loss, in which the heart is unable to pump enough blood to the body.

Pica—The ingestion of nonfood substances, such as dirt.

Trauma—A major, potentially life-threatening injury to the body.

Waddell's triad—Three distinct traumatic injuries sustained by pedestrian children who are hit by a car, consisting of abdominal injuries from the initial strike, injuries to the extremities from contact with the ground after being thrown into the air, and head injuries that occur when the child lands on his or her head after being thrown.

I. Description

Accidental injury is the number one cause of illness and death of children in the United States. In fact, over 9 million children are seen in emergency departments each year after such incidences as accidental or intentional consumption of poisons, traffic accidents, immersion in water, and falls. Of that number, well over 10,000 will die. In addition, children may need immediate intervention because of a disease process. The nurse must be prepared to intervene if he or she should be a witness to a child in immediate need of care. Figure 2.1 specifies the American Heart Association's protocol for pediatric basic life support.

II. Emergent Care

A. Initial assessment.

1. Check for safety.
   a. Before a nurse performs any intervention, he or she should make sure that there is nothing in the vicinity of the child that could injure the nurse. If the area is not safe, the nurse should contact emergency services immediately and report that a child is in distress but that the scene is unsafe.

DID YOU KNOW?

The most likely cause of cardiopulmonary arrest in a child is different from that of an adult. In infants, the most common causes of cardiopulmonary arrest are congenital heart disease, sudden infant death syndrome, and prematurity. For children over 1 year of age, the most common causes of cardiopulmonary arrest are accidental injury, as cited earlier, and respiratory failure resulting from an acute or chronic upper respiratory illness. Except during the infancy period, cardiopulmonary arrest rarely is caused by a cardiac event as it is in adults.

2. Awaken the child.
   a. If the environment is safe, the nurse should attempt to awaken the victim.

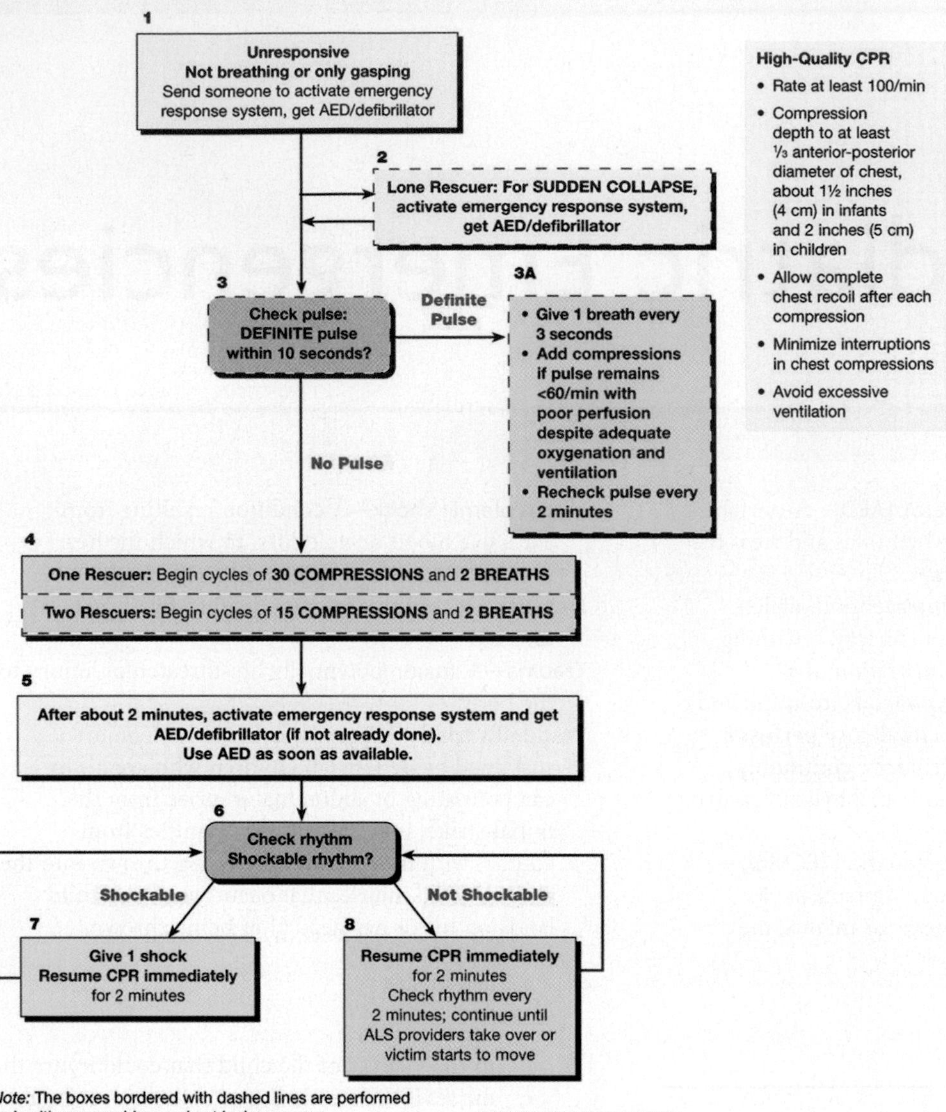

Fig 10.1 Pediatric basic life support algorithm.

   i. The nurse should pat the child and ask the child if he or she is okay. Adding the child's name, if it is known, may improve the possibility of the child responding.
   ii. When attempting to arouse the child, the nurse should be careful not to cause additional injury. In the case of a fall, for example, the neck should not be moved, if possible, to prevent injury to the spinal cord.

3. Get help.
   a. If the child fails to respond, the nurse should assume the worst and should shout "Help!" to attract the attention of others who can assist in the care of the child.
   b. If no one is available to assist, the nurse should care for the child for 2 full minutes, then leave the child and go to call for emergency personnel (e.g., call 911).
4. Assess for breathing.
   a. The nurse must next determine whether the child is breathing. A head tilt may need to be performed in order to open the child's airway.
      i. If the child is not breathing at all or is only gasping for breath, the nurse should assume that the child is in need of resuscitation.
5. Assess for a pulse: this procedure should take no longer than 10 sec.
   a. This procedure differs depending on the age of the child.

MAKING THE CONNECTION

Guidelines for emergency care of children are dependent on two important factors: the age of the child and the number of rescuers who are present.

To enable health-care practitioners to easily differentiate which age-specific guidelines to use in an emergency, the following criteria should be used:

- Infant criteria: except for those newly born, children during their 1st year of life. (See a maternal-newborn text for information related to the resuscitation guidelines for a newborn baby.)
- Child criteria: from 1 year of age to puberty, which is defined as:
  - Early breast development in girls.
  - Presence of axillary hair in boys.
- Adult criteria: from puberty throughout adolescence.

For the sake of simplicity, guidelines related to the number of rescuers are highlighted as "one rescuer" and "two rescuers."

i. Infants: because carotid and femoral pulses are difficult to assess, the brachial pulse is assessed.

ii. All children over 1 year of age: either the carotid or femoral pulses should be assessed.

b. If the pulse rate is greater than or equal to 60 bpm, rescue breaths should be administered at a rate of one every 3 to 5 sec (i.e., 12 to 20 per min).

c. If the pulse rate is less than 60 bpm, and the child is exhibiting signs of poor oxygenation (e.g., pale, cyanotic), cardiopulmonary resuscitation (CPR) should be begun.

6. Perform age-appropriate CPR.

a. The acronym **CAB** (chest compression, airway, breathing) should be used in order to remember the intervention sequence.

b. Infants.

i. The one rescuer procedure should be performed as follows:

(1) Thirty chest compressions followed by two rescue breaths through an open airway. Compressions should be performed:

(a) Using two fingers placed just below an imaginary line drawn between the nipples (i.e., on the lower one-third of the sternum).

(b) To an approximate depth of 1½ in.

(c) Rapidly at an average of 100 compressions per min.

(d) So that the thorax is allowed to return to its original height after each compression.

(2) CPR should be continued in the 30 to 2 pattern for 2 min. At that time, if it has not already been done, the rescuer should call for emergency assistance (i.e., call 911 in most areas of the United States). In addition, the nurse should obtain an **automated external defibrillator (AED)**, if available.

(3) The AED should be used as soon as it is acquired.

(a) CPR should be stopped after the compression phase.

(b) The machine should be turned on.

(c) The AED pads should be applied to the infant's chest, per machine instructions. (Adult pads may be used if the machine is not equipped with infant pads.)

(d) The AED prompts should be followed.

(e) After the AED sequence is complete, CPR should be resumed.

(f) An AED reanalysis and shock, if applicable, should be performed every 2 min or as prompted by the machine.

(4) The rescuer should continue CPR until emergency personnel arrive or until the child responds.

ii. Two rescuers.

(1) At the time the infant is discovered:

(a) Rescuer one should begin CPR, as detailed earlier.

(b) Rescuer two should immediately call for emergency assistance and obtain an AED, if available.

(2) Once rescuer two returns:

(a) Rescuer one should stop CPR, ending with the compression phase, and the AED procedure should be followed, as stated earlier.

(3) Following each AED intervention, rescuers one and two should alternate positions between performing chest compressions and rescue breaths.

(4) It is important to note that in two-rescuer CPR:

(a) A 15 compression to 2 rescue breath ratio and the two-thumb compression technique are recommended.
(b) Every 2 min, or as prompted by the machine, an AED analysis and intervention should be performed.
(5) CPR should be continued until emergency personnel arrive or until the child responds.

c. Child.
i. The infant CPR procedure should be followed for child CPR with the following minor changes:
(1) Chest compressions should be performed to a depth of 2 in.
(2) To achieve the desired depth, the rescuer should compress the lower one-third of the thorax using the palm of one (or two) hands.

d. Adolescent.
i. Adult CPR criteria should be employed when the victim is past the pubertal period.
ii. Although many of the actions of adolescent rescuers are similar to those stated earlier, there are some important differences. The adult CPR procedure should be performed as follows:
(1) Responsiveness assessed.
(2) Breathing assessed.
(3) Emergency personnel notified and an AED obtained as soon as the victim is found to be unresponsive and not breathing or gasping.
(4) Pulse assessed **for a maximum of 10 sec.**
(a) If a pulse is present, rescue breaths should be provided every 5 sec.
(b) If a pulse is absent, CPR procedure should be begun.
(c) Adult CPR procedure.
(i) AED procedure should be followed using adult-sized pads, as stated earlier.
(ii) Compressions and rescue breaths, whether by one or two rescuers, should be performed in a 30 to 2 ratio.
(iii) Compressions should be performed to a depth of 2 in.
(iv) To achieve the desired depth, the rescuer should compress the lower one-third of the thorax using the palms of two hands.

7. If available, masks and/or other airway barriers should be used to deliver rescue breaths.
8. If the child's airway is obstructed (see "Obstructed Airway"), additional actions that are determined by the age of the child should be performed.
i. Nursing actions that are performed are based on the age of the child.
(1) In infants (Fig. 10.2).
(a) Holding the infant in a head-down position, alternately provide the baby with five slaps on the back with the palm of the hand and five two-finger chest compressions until the item is dislodged.

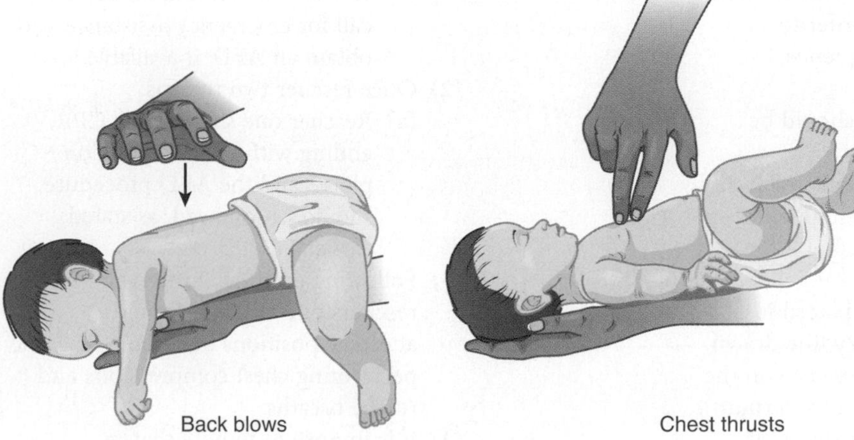

Fig 10.2 Back blows and chest thrusts.

(b) **Only if the item is seen in the mouth** should the nurse attempt to remove the item by inserting a pinky finger and using it to clear the object.
(c) Once the item appears to be dislodged, rescue breaths should be performed.
(d) If the infant should become unresponsive, CPR should be started.

(2) In all children over the age of 1, the Heimlich maneuver, or abdominal thrusts, should be performed (Fig. 10.3).
(a) The nurse should:
(i) Stand (or kneel) behind the child.
(ii) Make a fist with one hand.
(iii) Wrap his or her arms around the child and place the fist on the child's abdomen just below the rib cage.
(iv) Cover the fist with the second hand and repeatedly thrust upward in sets of five thrusts until the object is expelled or until the child becomes unresponsiveness and CPR is needed.

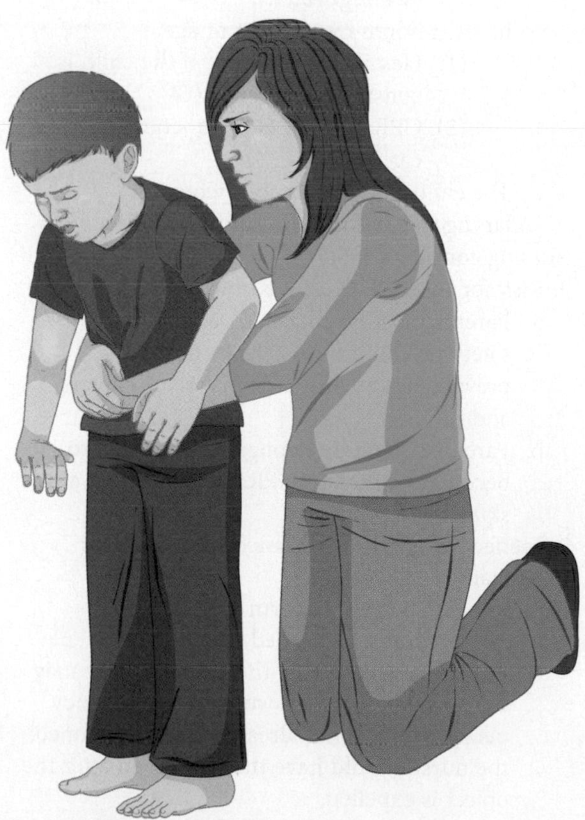

Fig 10.3 The Heimlich maneuver in children over age 1.

B. Secondary assessment: when the child is breathing and his or her heart is beating normally, the nurse should take a full history and perform a head-to-toe assessment, as needed.
1. To remember all items that should be covered in the secondary assessment, the acronym SAMPLE should be used (Box 10.1).

III. Obstructed Airway

It is not uncommon for children to experience an obstructed airway. Children, who already have narrow tracheas, frequently move and play while eating snacks and insert objects into their mouths that should not be placed there. Because it is essential that the airway be patent for gas exchange to take place, immediate intervention is needed.

A. Incidence.
1. Most commonly seen in children under 5 years of age (greater than 90% of cases).

Box 10.1 SAMPLE for Secondary Assessment

S—signs and symptoms: *the nurse should query the parents and/or child, if applicable, regarding what signs and symptoms the child is exhibiting.*
A—allergies: *the nurse should question whether the child has any allergies, especially medication allergies, and what reactions the child exhibits when exposed to the allergens. The nurse should check whether the child is wearing MedicAlert® identification.*
M—medications: *the nurse should ask what medications the child is taking, including vitamins, and what vaccines the child has received.*
P—point of injury: *if the child is injured, the parent and/or child, if applicable, should be asked regarding the location of the injury and the level of his or her pain.*
L—last meal: *the nurse should ask the parent and/or child, if applicable, when and what the child last ate.*
E—events surrounding the event: *finally, as a means of determining the extent of the injury, the nurse should query the parent and/or child, if applicable, regarding what the child was doing right before he or she was injured. For example:*
- *If the child had been playing in the garage, are cans of gasoline and lawnmowers stored there?*
- *If the child had been playing in the bathroom, are medicines or razor blades accessible?*
- *If the child had been playing in the back yard, might he or she have been climbing trees or been bitten by a snake?*

B. Etiology.
1. Objects that frequently lead to an obstructed airway in children are:
    a. Liquids, especially common choking item in infants.
    b. Food items (e.g., carrots, hot dogs, hard candies, grapes, bagels).
    c. Play items (e.g., uninflated balloons, small toys).
    d. Everyday items (e.g., coins, buttons).

C. Pathophysiology.
1. Children who are choking on objects usually present with sudden upper respiratory difficulty without any other symptoms.
2. When a mild obstruction is present, the airway is not completely occluded, and air exchange is occurring.
    a. Signs and symptoms.
        i. The child may begin to cough violently and/or appear to gag, but the child is able to cough effectively enough to be able to expel the object himself or herself.
3. When a moderate or severe obstruction is present, little to no gas exchange is taking place.
    a. Signs and symptoms.
        i. The conscious child will appear frightened and panicky with:
            (1) Inspiratory stridor and ineffective cough.
            (2) Little to no air exchange.
            (3) May wrap his or her hands around his or her own throat to indicate the presence of an obstruction (Fig. 10.4).
        ii. Unconscious child.
            (1) While attempting to perform rescue breaths, the nurse is unable to instill any air into the lungs.

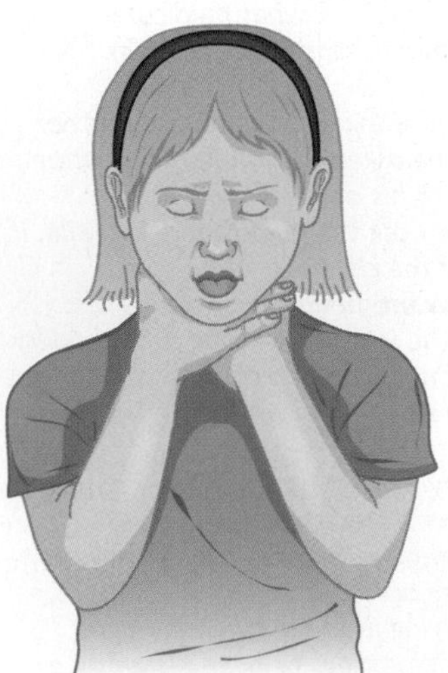

Fig 10.4 Obstruction of airway.

4. If the obstruction is not life threatening, it may not be diagnosed in a timely fashion and, therefore, may remain in place over time.
    a. Eventually, the child will develop pneumonitis with diminished breath sounds, wheezing, and coughing.

D. Diagnosis.
1. Clinical history and picture are most common.
2. X-ray, CT, MRI.

E. Treatment.
1. Prevention.
    a. Because many obstructions are caused by items that are unsafe for young children to eat, to play with, or have access to, the majority of airway obstructions are preventable.
    b. See "Growth and Development" in Chapters 2 and 3 for specific safety recommendations.
2. Treatment.
    a. Mild obstruction.
        i. Unless the obstruction should worsen, emotional support should be provided while the child coughs up the obstruction.
    b. Moderate to severe obstructions.
        i. In infants.
            (1) Back blows and chest compressions (see Fig. 10.3).
        ii. In children over 1 year of age.
            (1) Heimlich maneuver, if the child is conscious (see Fig. 10.4).
            (2) CPR, if the child is unconscious (see earlier).
    c. The child may require bronchoscopy or laryngoscopy for removal of the object.

F. Nursing considerations.
1. Risk for Injury/Deficient Knowledge.
    a. Parents must be educated regarding safety precautions to take in order to prevent airway obstructions (see Chapters 2 and 3).
    b. Parents should be strongly encouraged to become certified in CPR and other first aid skills.
2. Ineffective Airway Clearance/Impaired Gas Exchange.
    a. The nurse must perform emergency interventions, as needed (see earlier).
    b. Because the tissues in the child's airway may become dangerously swollen, if emergency personnel have not already been summoned, the nurse should have the child seen after the object is expelled.
3. If the child dies, Grieving/Risk for Complicated Grieving (Box 10.2).

Box 10.2 Nursing Considerations for Grieving and the Risk for Complicated Grieving

- *Provide the parents and others, if appropriate, with the opportunity to express their feelings.*
- *Allow the parents and others, if appropriate, time to be with and to say good-bye to their child.*
- *Educate the parents and others, if appropriate, regarding the five stages of grieving.*
- *Encourage the parents and others, if appropriate, to seek spiritual guidance from their clergyperson, if desired.*
- *Advise the parents and others, if appropriate, to seek grief counseling, if needed.*

IV. Shock

A. Incidence.
  1. Statistics are unavailable, but the younger the child, the more serious the diagnosis.

B. Etiology.
  1. **Hypovolemic shock,** caused by extensive loss of blood.
  2. **Distributive shock.**
    a. Most commonly caused by a massive infection (e.g., *Escherichia coli, Streptococcus pyogenes* (group A strep), *Neisseria meningitides*).
    b. Also may be caused by anaphylaxis or drug overdose.
  3. Cardiogenic shock, caused by severe injury to the heart muscle.

C. Pathophysiology.
  1. Regardless of the etiology, the resulting pathophysiology is characterized by markedly reduced circulatory perfusion to the vital organs and the periphery.
  2. Signs and symptoms.
    a. Initially, the body attempts to compensate for the inadequate perfusion by:
      i. Tachycardia, tachypnea, and vasoconstriction.
      ii. Infants' and young children's abilities to compensate are limited.
    b. If the cause of shock is not treated effectively, the physiological status rapidly deteriorates resulting in:
      i. Bradycardia, apnea, hypotension, and cardiac arrest.

D. Diagnosis.
  1. Clinical picture in conjunction with:
  2. X-rays and a variety of laboratory data, including blood cultures, complete blood counts (CBC), lumbar puncture, blood gases, and serum electrolytes.

E. Treatment: depends on the etiology of the shock.
  1. Emergency intervention (see earlier).
  2. Control bleeding, if present.
  3. Oxygen.
  4. Intravenous (IV) therapy.
  5. Blood transfusion.
  6. Identify pathogen and treat, if present.
  7. Medications (e.g., epinephrine).
  8. **Extracorporeal membrane oxygenation (ECMO):** treatment similar to cardiopulmonary bypass, usually only used as treatment for infants and young children.

F. Nursing considerations.
  1. Risk for Ineffective Airway Clearance/Risk for Impaired Gas Exchange/Risk for Decreased Cardiac Output/Risk for Ineffective Perfusion/ Risk for Deficient Fluid Volume.
    a. Perform emergency interventions, as needed (see earlier).
    b. Control source of shock (i.e., source of bleeding, infection).
    c. Assist with intubation, as needed.
    d. Administer oxygen, as needed.
    e. Carefully monitor vital signs.
    f. Keep child NPO (i.e., give the child nothing by mouth).
    g. Administer IV therapy, as ordered.
    h. Administer blood transfusion, as ordered.
    i. Maintain strict intake and output.
    j. Monitor laboratory values, including blood gases, serum electrolytes, complete blood count, glucose levels, and blood urea nitrogen.
  2. Risk for Altered Coping/Anxiety.
    a. Calmly provide the child and parents with information regarding trauma care, employing simple and concise language.
    b. Provide opportunities for the child and parents to express fears, concerns, and guilt.
    c. Encourage the parents to assist with the child's care, as able.
    d. Refer the family, as needed, to social services.
    e. Encourage the family, if appropriate, to seek spiritual guidance from a clergyperson.
    f. Assist the family to identify support systems and coping strategies.
  3. If the child dies, Grieving/Risk for Complicated Grieving (Box 10.2).

V. Trauma

The term **trauma** refers to a major, potentially life-threatening injury to the body.

A. Incidence.
  1. There are a number of ways that children may experience trauma up to and including gun

violence. The most common traumatic events in children of all ages, however, are caused by automobile accidents.

B. Etiology: the vast majority of traumatic events are preventable.
1. Automobile accidents.
   a. When the child is a passenger in the car.
   b. When the child is a pedestrian.
2. Falls.
3. Violence, especially common etiology of adolescent trauma.

C. Pathophysiology.
1. The precise nature and severity of the trauma is dependent on the type of injury sustained by the child.
2. **Waddell's triad,** which is important to highlight, refers to the traumatic injuries sustained by pedestrian children who are hit by a car. The children are injured in three distinctly serious ways.
   a. Abdominal injuries that occur during the initial strike.
   b. Injuries to the extremities that occur when the child lands on the ground after being thrown through the air.
   c. Head injuries that occur when the child lands on his or her head after being thrown through the air.
      i. Because children's heads are often the heaviest parts of their bodies, their heads frequently sustain serious injury.

D. Diagnosis.
1. Clinical picture in conjunction with:
2. X-rays and a variety of laboratory data, including blood cultures, CBCs, lumbar puncture, blood gases, and serum electrolytes.

E. Treatment.
1. Prevention.
   a. The parents and child must be educated regarding car and pedestrian safety practices (see the "Safety" headings in the "Growth and Development" chapters, 2–6).
   b. Infants and young children should be supervised whenever on elevated surfaces.
   c. All firearms and ammunition should be kept in separate, locked safes.
2. Treatment.
   a. Depends on the etiology of the trauma but will likely include:
      i. Emergency intervention (see earlier).
      ii. Control of bleeding, if present.
      iii. Oxygen therapy.
      iv. IV therapy.
      v. Surgery.

F. Nursing considerations.
1. Deficient Knowledge.
   a. Parents must be educated regarding safety precautions to take to prevent traumatic injury.
   b. Parents should strongly be encouraged to become certified in CPR and other first aid skills.
2. Injury/Risk for Ineffective Airway Clearance/Risk for Impaired Gas Exchange/Risk for Decreased Cardiac Output/Risk for Ineffective Perfusion/Risk for Deficient Fluid Volume.
   a. Carefully assess the child for traumatic injury, including the Glasgow assessment for possible central nervous system impairment.
   b. The nurse must perform emergency interventions, as needed (see earlier).
   c. Assist with intubation, as needed.
   d. Administer oxygen, as needed.
   e. Carefully monitor vital signs.
   f. Keep the child NPO.
   g. Administer IV therapy, as ordered.
   h. Maintain strict intake and output.
   i. Monitor laboratory values, including blood gases, serum electrolytes, CBCs, glucose levels, and blood urea nitrogen.
3. Risk for Infection.
   a. Employing the five rights of medication administration, administer safe dosages of antibiotics/antivirals/antifungals, as prescribed.
   b. Carefully monitor vital signs.
   c. Employing the five rights of medication administration, administer safe dosages of antipyretics, as prescribed.
   d. Provide hydration and nourishment, as prescribed.
4. Risk for Altered Coping/Anxiety.
   a. Calmly provide the child and parents with information regarding trauma care, employing simple and concise language.
   b. Provide opportunities for the child and parents to express fears, concerns, and guilt.
   c. Encourage the parents to assist with the child's care, as able.
   d. Refer the family, as needed, to social services.
   e. Encourage the family, if desired, to seek spiritual guidance from a clergyperson.
   f. Assist the family to identify support systems and coping strategies.
   g. Depending on the source of injury/emergency, the parents should be educated regarding prevention strategies to prevent future trauma.
5. Risk for Altered Parenting.
   a. Depending on the source of the injury/emergency, and if applicable, the nurse should notify child protective services of child abuse

or child neglect (see Chapter 23, "Nursing Care of the Child With Psychosocial Disorders").

6. If the child dies, Grieving/Risk for Complicated Grieving (see Box 10.2).

VI. Acute Poisonings

A. Incidence.
1. Accidental poisoning (e.g., from the ingestion of medications, cleaning products, or plants) most commonly is seen in the toddler and preschool populations.
2. Intentional poisoning (i.e., from the ingestion of alcohol and/or prescription medications) most commonly is seen in the adolescent population.

B. Etiology.
1. Medication ingestion.
   a. Tylenol (acetaminophen), aspirin (acetylsalicylic acid), and vitamins are the most common poisons in toddlers and preschoolers.
   b. Prescription medications (e.g., analgesics, narcotics, antidepressants, antianxiety medications, as well as illicit drugs) often are purposefully ingested by older school-age and adolescent children.
2. Other poisons that may be ingested.
   a. Cleaning products, gasoline, and kerosene most commonly are ingested by toddlers and preschoolers.
   b. Alcohol most commonly is ingested by older school-age and adolescent children.
3. Poisons may also be "ingested" via the respiratory system in the form of a gas or aerated particles or via the skin in the form of a topical substance.

C. Pathophysiology is dependent on the poison.
1. Acetaminophen.
   a. Ingestion of greater than 150 mg/kg is considered toxic.
      i. Therapeutic dose is 10 to 15 mg/kg every 6 to 8 hr.
   b. Hepatotoxicity can develop from the physiological metabolism of the medication.
   c. Signs and symptoms depend on the quantity ingested.
      i. Initially, nausea and vomiting and flu-like symptoms.
      ii. After 24 hours.
         (1) Elevated liver enzymes.
         (2) Elevated bilirubin.
         (3) Right upper quadrant pain.
      iii. In 3 to 7 days, the child may develop liver failure.
      iv. After 1 week, either the child will recover or the child's health will deteriorate further.
2. Aspirin.
   a. Ingestion of greater than 150 mg/kg is considered toxic.
      i. Therapeutic dose is 10 to 15 mg/kg every 4 to 6 hr.
   b. Many organ systems may be adversely affected.
      i. Initially, the child will exhibit respiratory alkalosis in an attempt to compensate for the ingestion.
      ii. The alkalosis quickly shifts to metabolic acidosis with hypokalemia and dehydration when the salicylic acidemia overwhelms the compensatory response.
   c. Signs and symptoms.
      i. Initially, nausea and vomiting with hyperpnea.
      ii. Followed by:
         (1) Central nervous system changes (i.e., confusion, seizures, coma)
         (2) Renal failure.
         (3) Bleeding.
         (4) Hyponatremia, hypokalemia, hypoglycemia.
         (5) Dehydration.
         (6) Tinnitus or deafness.
3. Cleaning supplies, gasoline, and other such substances.
   a. Severe damage to the mouth, esophagus, and stomach.
   b. Respiratory compromise.
   c. Blood chemistry disruptions.
4. Alcohol: a physiological depressant.
   a. Signs and symptoms.
      i. Confusion.
      ii. Vomiting.
      iii. Stupor.
      iv. Respiratory compromise.

D. Diagnosis.
1. Clinical picture and clinical evidence.
2. Serum assays and nomogram evaluation.
   a. Nomogram analyses (see *Interactive Rumack-Matthew Nomogram for Acetaminophen Toxicity* at www.ars-informatica.ca/toxicitynomogram.php?calc=acetamin and *Interactive Done Nomogram for Salicylate Toxicity* at www.ars-informatica.ca/toxicitynomogram.php?calc=salic).
      i. The blood level of acetaminophen and salicylate, respectively, and the time since the ingestion of the drug are inputted into the appropriate nomogram.
      ii. The potential for toxicity is calculated, and the recommended treatments are reported.
   b. Blood alcohol levels.

3. Laryngoscopy.
4. X-ray, MRI, CT.

DID YOU KNOW?

For many years, parents were told to keep a bottle of syrup of ipecac at home and to administer it to stimulate vomiting if a child swallowed a poison. This is no longer recommended primarily for two reasons: (1) Waiting for the child to vomit at home resulted in a delay in providing care at the emergency department and (2) vomiting can seriously injure a child's gastrointestinal and respiratory systems if the poison the child swallowed is a corrosive substance.

E. Treatment.
1. Immediate care at the scene.
   a. Assess the child.
      i. The child must be assessed for responsiveness and for the need of emergency intervention.
         (1) The child's immediate, physiological needs must be met (see the previous "Emergent Care" section).
   b. Terminate the exposure: depending on the situation, for the safety of the child and/or the nurse, this action may take precedence over the assessment of the child.
      i. If possible, exposure to the poison should be terminated.
         (1) Medications or alcohol: if safe to perform, remove all of the residual substance from the child's mouth.
         (2) Gas or topical: if safe to perform, the child must immediately be removed from the area where the gas or topical is being emitted, the source of the gas or topical must be shut off, and/or contaminated clothing must be removed.
   c. Identify the poison.
      i. The exact identity of the poison must be determined.
         (1) The victim and/or witnesses should be queried.
         (2) Any empty containers should be located, inspected, and saved.
   d. Call the poison control center (PCC).
      i. PCC should be called and notified of the identity of the substance.
      ii. Any actions recommended by the PCC should be implemented (e.g., drinking a full glass of water or milk, flushing the eyes and/or skin with water).
   e. Seek emergency medical assistance.
      i. Following immediate intervention and if recommended by PCC, the child should be seen and evaluated in an emergency department.
2. Follow-up treatment.
   a. All evidence of the exposure should be taken to the emergency department for analysis, such as:
      i. Vomitus, urine, empty bottles, and containers.
   b. Specific treatment is dependent on the exact poison. Examples of care are listed in Table 10.1.

F. Nursing considerations.
1. Risk for Injury/Risk for Deficient Fluid Volume.
   a. Perform CPR, as needed.
   b. Take excellent history, including examining any evidence that parents and/or friends took to the emergency department.
   c. Assist with gastric lavage, if needed.
   d. Reference *Rumack-Matthew Nomogram* or *Done Nomogram,* as needed (see the previous "Diagnosis" section).
   e. Administer IV solution, as ordered.
   f. Monitor intake and output.
   g. Monitor bowel function if activated charcoal has been administered.
      i. Activated charcoal, a tasteless powder, is mixed with a clear liquid and the resulting slurry is drunk.
      ii. Children are more likely to drink the slurry if a cap is placed on the cup to hide the liquid and the child is advised to drink it through a straw.
      iii. Because activated charcoal is desiccated, it acts by absorbing the poison from the gastrointestinal system.
         (1) Common side effects of the medication are dehydration and constipation.
   h. Administer safe dosages of antidotes, as ordered.
   i. Administer oxygen, as ordered.
2. Deficient Knowledge/Anxiety/Risk for Altered Coping/Risk for Future Poisoning.
   a. Allow the parents to express feelings/fears regarding the injury and future health of the child.
   b. Carefully explain, in an understandable language, all interventions, with rationales for each.
   c. Explore reasons for poisonings, and offer advice regarding means of preventing poisonings in the future, including locking

Table 10.1 Care for Ingestion of Common Poisons

Poison	Immediate Care (after resuscitation)	Long-Term Care
Tylenol (acetaminophen)	*Lavage: performed if within 1 hr of ingestion* *Activated charcoal: administered if within 2 hr of ingestion and child is alert* *Mucomyst (acetylcysteine), PO or IV: administration dependent on likelihood of liver toxicity*	*Monitor hepatic function* *Liver transplant, if needed* *Educate family regarding safety issues*
Aspirin (acetylsalicylic acid)	*Lavage: performed if within 1 hr of ingestion* *Activated charcoal: performed if within 2 hr of ingestion and child is alert* *Dextrose and electrolytes via IV infusion with sodium bicarbonate to reverse acidosis* *Vitamin K to reverse bleeding disorder*	*Hemodialysis, if needed* *Educate family regarding safety issues*
Corrosives and hydrocarbons	*Vomiting should **never** be induced* *Lavage: performed carefully to prevent additional injury to tissues of the gastrointestinal tract* *Nothing by mouth* *IV fluids*	*Reconstruct trachea and/or esophagus, if needed* *Educate family regarding safety issues*
Alcohol	*Lavage: performed if within 1 hr of ingestion* *Supportive care must be provided until the alcohol is fully metabolized*	*Psychological and/or substance abuse counseling* *Educate students, family, and/or friends regarding safety issues*

away medications and poisonous substances and the use of Mr. Yuk stickers.

DID YOU KNOW?

The Mr. Yuk symbol is used to warn children and adults about poisoning hazards. Parents may be advised that Mr. Yuk stickers can be requested at no charge. Each sticker lists the toll-free number for the nearest poison center. For more information, visit the Children's Hospital of Pittsburgh's Web site at www.chp.edu/CHP/mryuk.

VII. Chronic Heavy Metal Poisoning

The most common heavy metals ingested by children are lead and iron.

A. Incidence.

1. Infants, especially breast-fed infants, and young children are the most vulnerable to chronic heavy metal poisoning because:
   a. Of their behaviors.
      i. They explore their environment through their hands and mouth (e.g., chew painted furniture, put dirt in their mouths, eat with their hands, put toys in their mouths).
      ii. They assist fathers/mothers with home repairs.
   b. Their brains are not fully developed.
2. Fetuses are vulnerable if their mothers ingest heavy metals.

B. Etiology.

1. Lead is internalized via two routes: oral ingestion and respiratory inhalation.
   a. Many indoor paints contained lead until 1978.
      i. Paint chipping from furniture, walls, antique toys, and other objects can be ingested.
      ii. Paint sanded during renovations can be aerosolized and breathed in.
   b. The plumbing in many old homes is comprised of lead pipes and/or lead soldering.
      i. Lead leaches into the water and is consumed.
   c. Automotive gasoline contained lead until the 1970s. The exhaust from automobiles contaminated the soil throughout the United States.
      i. The contaminated dirt and dust surrounding homes can be ingested on hands that are washed infrequently.
2. Iron is usually ingested through accidental ingestion most frequently by toddlers and preschoolers.

C. Pathophysiology.

1. Multiple systems are affected adversely by lead.
   a. Hematological system: adverse effects are reversible.
      i. Anemia develops because lead interferes with the biosynthesis of the heme portion of the hemoglobin molecule.

b. Gastrointestinal system: adverse effects are reversible.
    i. Nausea and vomiting, constipation, and anorexia.
    ii. Lead in the GI tract can be seen on an x-ray.
c. Renal system: adverse effects are reversible unless there has been continued ingestion over a long period of time.
    i. Lead damages the tubules of the kidney, leading to abnormal excretion of glucose and proteins.
d. Skeletal system.
    i. If ingested over long periods of time, lead deposits in the bone marrow of the long bones.
        (1) Lead lines can be seen on x-rays.
e. Central nervous system: adverse effects may be irreversible.
    i. Lead ingestion results in fluid shifts in the brain and increased intracranial pressure resulting in cortical atrophy and lead encephalopathy.
    ii. Signs and symptoms.
        (1) Lower levels: hyperactivity, learning disabilities, and lowered IQ.
        (2) Higher levels: convulsions, paralysis, blindness, mental retardation, coma, and death.

D. Diagnosis.

1. In many states, it is the law to assess blood lead levels (BLLs) during early childhood.
    a. All children receiving Medicaid are mandated to receive a blood lead assessment at 12 months and 24 months of age.
2. CBCs, urinalyses, and x-rays.
3. BLLs.
    a. BLL of 5 mcg/dL or higher is considered abnormal.
    b. BLL greater than or equal to 45 mcg/dL is dangerously elevated and requires medical intervention (see "Treatment").
4. Lead mobilization tests.

E. Treatment.

1. Prevention.
    a. Healthy diet.
        i. Lead has a strong affinity for combining with the heme portion of the red blood cell. Children who consume diets that are low in iron and vitamin C are, therefore, at higher risk of developing lead toxicity than are children with diets high in iron and vitamin C.
        ii. A diet high in calcium helps to protect the long bones from lead deposition.
    b. Water.
        i. Water in every home, especially those with well water, should be assessed for lead contamination.
        ii. If lead is found in the water.
            (1) Only cold water should be used for drinking and cooking because lead leaches more rapidly into hot than cold water.
            (2) Before using the cold water, it should be allowed to run into the sink for 1 full minute because lead leaches more rapidly into standing water than into flowing water.
            (3) If lead levels are still high after the above interventions, only bottled water should be consumed.
    c. Other exposures.
        i. Dissuade **pica** (i.e., the ingestion of nonfood substances, such as dirt).
        ii. Frequently cleanse such things as hands, floors, windowsills, and toys to remove lead dust.
        iii. Remove children and pregnant and lactating women from environs undergoing renovations.
2. Treatment guidelines, as recommended by the Centers for Disease Control and Prevention (CDC), for BLL at the following levels:
    a. BLL 5 to 9 mcg/dL.
        i. The health-care provider should investigate the possible sources of exposure to lead.
        ii. The parents and others should be educated on ways to reduce lead exposure.
        iii. BLL should be reassessed in 3 to 6 months.
    b. BLL 10 to 14 mcg/dL.
        i. All of the above, except that the BLL should be reassessed in 1 to 3 months
    c. BLL 15 to 44 mcg/dL.
        i. A representative from the department of health may visit the home to:
            (1) Assess the home for possible sources of lead exposure.
            (2) Educate the parents about lead exposure.
            (3) Encourage the parents to provide the child with foods high in iron, vitamin C, and calcium.
    d. BLL greater than or equal to 45 mcg/dL.
        i. All of the above plus chelation therapy.
    e. Chelation therapy.
        i. **Chelation therapy** is performed to remove heavy metals from the body. Because the therapy itself may result in adverse effects,

it should be conducted **only** under medical supervision.

Children who are receiving chelating agents should have their BLLs monitored carefully. In some instances, BLLs actually rise while on chelating agents because lead enters the bloodstream from the bones or gastrointestinal system for excretion through the kidneys. Nephrotoxicity and neurotoxicity may result.

ii. Chelation medications commonly administered are:
(1) Chemet (succimer): may be administered on an outpatient basis.
(a) Dosage.
(i) 10 mg/kg PO every 8 hr × 5 days, then every 12 hr × 14 days or
(ii) 350 mg/m^2 PO every 8 hr × 5 days, then every 12 hr × 14 days.
(b) Adverse effects.
(i) Serious: neutropenia and arrhythmias.
(ii) Common: nausea and vomiting, rash, pruritus, and elevated liver enzymes.
(2) Cuprimine (d-penicillamine) may be administered on an outpatient basis.
(a) Dosage.
(i) 30 to 40 mg/kg/day PO divided tid to qid × 4 to 12 wk or
(ii) 600 to 750 mg/m^2/day PO divided tid to qid × 4 to 12 wk.
(iii) Maximum: 1.5 g/day.
(b) Adverse effects.
(i) Many serious side effects, including thrombocytopenia, leukopenia, aplastic anemia, hypersensitivity reaction, and pancreatitis.
(ii) Common side effects include anorexia, epigastric pain, nausea and vomiting, diarrhea, proteinuria, and pruritic rash.
(3) BAL in oil (dimercaprol): administered while the child is in the hospital.
(a) Dosage.
(i) 75 mg/m^2 IM every 4 hr × 3 to 7 days.
(ii) Maximum: 5 mg/kg/dose.
(iii) BLLs should be assessed after 48 hr to determine whether therapy is still needed.
(b) Adverse effects.
(i) Severe side effect: neutropenia.
(ii) Many common side effects, including pain at the injection site, nausea and vomiting, hypertension, tachycardia, conjunctivitis, and paresthesias.
(4) Calcium disodium versenate (edetate disodium calcium or $CaNa_2EDTA$).
(a) Dosage is individualized for each child.
(b) Adverse effects.
(i) Severe side effects include dangerously low hypoglycemia, hypocalcemia, kidney failure, and seizures.
(ii) Common side effect: malabsorption of vitamins, including vitamin C and the B vitamins.

$CaNa_2EDTA$ should not be confused with Na_2EDTA (disodium ethylenediaminetetraacetic acid), a chemical compound that appears as a white powder.

BAL and $CaNa_2EDTA$ rarely are administered for a BLL less than 70 mcg/dL unless the child is exhibiting signs of encephalopathy.

F. Nursing considerations.
1. Deficient Knowledge/Risk for Altered Growth and Development.
a. Educate the parents and child regarding the importance of handwashing and the avoidance of pica.
b. Educate the parents regarding the importance of house cleaning and cleaning of the child's toys and furniture.
c. Educate the parents regarding the need to let water run and the need to use cold rather than hot water for consumption.
d. Educate the parents regarding the signs and symptoms of lead poisoning.
e. Remind the parents of the importance for BLL testing.
f. Monitor the child's growth and development using growth charts and development assessments (e.g., DDST II, at each well-child visit).

2. Risk for Injury related to chelation therapy.
   a. Monitor laboratory values carefully, including BLLs and renal function tests.
   b. Monitor for central nervous system changes, including Glasgow assessments.
   c. Monitor strict intake and output.
3. Risk for Impaired Coping/Anxiety/Guilt.
   a. Allow the parents and child to express concerns and fears.
   b. Allow the parents to ask important questions regarding prevention and treatment strategies.
   c. Educate the parents regarding the reason for administering chelating agents, if needed.

VIII. Drowning

A. Incidence.
1. Drowning is the number one cause of death by injury for children aged 1 to 4.

B. Etiology.
1. Children can drown in any large body of water, including pools, lakes, and creeks, or in relatively small bodies of water, including bath tubs, toilets, and mop buckets.

C. Pathophysiology.
1. When children are submerged, they try to hold their breath.
2. Eventually, they swallow the water, which results in a choking bronchospasm.
3. The bronchospasm results either in:
   a. Inhalation of water or
   b. Laryngospasm leading to "dry drowning."
4. Signs and symptoms.
   a. Dependent on the age of the child, temperature of the liquid, and the length of time submerged.
   b. Signs and symptoms range from mild hypothermia and slight dyspnea to full cardiopulmonary collapse.

D. Diagnosis.
1. Clinical picture.

E. Treatment.
1. Prevention.
   a. Water safety education is essential! All children, ideally beginning in the preschool period, should complete swim lessons.
   b. Young children should never be left unattended in bath water, near water buckets, near toilets, near any outdoor body of water, or any other potential drowning hazard.
2. Emergency intervention (see earlier).
   a. Airway obstruction protocols should not be performed with drowning victims because they delay the administration of rescue breaths and, if needed, cardiac compressions.

F. Nursing considerations.
1. At the time of the drowning.
   a. Impaired Gas Exchange/Impaired Breathing Pattern.
      i. Rescue breathing and CPR should be performed, as needed.
      ii. When appropriate, parents should be allowed to be present during resuscitation.
2. Following resuscitation.
   a. Risk for Hypothermia.
      i. Core temperature should be monitored carefully.
      ii. Wet clothing should be removed and warm blankets provided.
      iii. Warmed IV fluid should be administered, as needed.
   b. Risk for Deficient Fluid Volume.
      i. Vital signs and fluid and electrolyte balance should be monitored carefully.
      ii. IV fluids should be administered, per order.
      iii. Intake and output should be monitored carefully.
   c. Risk for Injury/Altered Growth and Development.
      i. Cardiac and oxygenation status should be monitored carefully.
      ii. Oxygen should be administered, per order.
      iii. Level of consciousness should be assessed, using the Glasgow scale.
      iv. The child should be carefully monitored for signs of increased intracranial pressure (see Chapter 22, "Nursing Care of the Child With Neurological Problems").
      v. Head of bed should be elevated 20 to 30 degrees.
      vi. The child should be monitored for altered cognitive function.
3. Following resuscitation and/or if the child dies.
   a. Risk for Altered Coping/Anxiety/Guilt.
      i. Parents should be provided opportunities to express fears and guilt.
      ii. Parents should be given clear, accurate explanations of the interventions, including the rationales for treatments.
      iii. Health-care practitioners should provide the parents with honest information regarding the child's status.
   b. Grieving/Risk for Complicated Grieving (Box 10.2).

CASE STUDY: Putting It All Together

Acute poisoning: 4-year-old Caucasian male brought to the ED by his mother

Subjective Data

- Mother states,
  - "My son was playing with his best friend who went home 3 hours ago."
  - "He started vomiting about 1 hour ago, right after I found an empty Children's Tylenol bottle on his bedroom floor. I usually keep it in my purse in case he has a 'boo boo' when we're out."
  - "He must have taken all of it about 4 hours ago."
- Child states,
  - "I hurted my arm so I taked my medicine all by myself!!"

Objective Data

Nursing Assessments

- Vomiting

Vital Signs

Blood pressure:	80/55 mm Hg
Temperature:	98.6°F
Heart rate:	100 bpm
Respiratory rate:	28 rpm

Lab Results

CBC, ALT, AST:	all normal
Serum acetaminophen concentration:	300 mcg/mL

Health-Care Provider's Orders

- Admit to pediatrics
- Begin IV D_5W ½ NS
- IV acetylcysteine 150 mg/kg over 60 min
  - **THEN** 12.5 mg/kg per hour for 4 hr
  - **THEN** 6.25 mg/kg per hour for next 16 hr
- Zofran (ondansetron) 0.1 mg/kg IV STAT
- Repeat CBC, ALT, and AST in a.m.

Case Study Questions

A. Which *subjective* assessments are important in this scenario?

1. ______
2. ______
3. ______
4. ______

B. Which *objective* assessments are important in this scenario?

1. ______
2. ______
3. ______
4. ______

C. After analyzing the data that has been collected, what **primary** nursing diagnosis should the nurse assign to this client?

1. ______

D. What interventions should the nurse plan and/or implement to meet this child's and his family's needs?

1. ______
2. ______
3. ______
4. ______
5. ______
6. ______
7. ______
8. ______
9. ______

Continued

CASE STUDY: Putting It All Together *cont'd*

Case Study Question

E. What client outcomes should the nurse evaluate regarding the effectiveness of the nursing interventions?

1. ____________________
2. ____________________
3. ____________________
4. ____________________
5. ____________________
6. ____________________
7. ____________________
8. ____________________

F. What physiological characteristics should the child exhibit before being discharged home?

1. ____________________
2. ____________________
3. ____________________

REVIEW QUESTIONS

1. A nurse observes a 6-year-old child fall from a 3rd-story window. The area is safe for the nurse to intervene. There is no one else in the area. Which of the following actions should the nurse perform first?
   1. Assess for breathing.
   2. Assess carotid pulse.
   3. Access emergency assistance.
   4. Administer rescue breaths.

2. A nurse is administering cardiopulmonary resuscitation as a 1-person rescuer to an infant who was found not breathing and with no pulse. Which of the following actions should the nurse perform?
   1. Compress the child's chest with the palm of 1 hand.
   2. Obtain an automated external defibrillator (AED) as soon as possible.
   3. Access emergency assistance (call 911) as soon as possible.
   4. Perform resuscitation in a 30 compressions to 2 breaths ratio.

3. Two nurses are providing cardiopulmonary resuscitation on a 6-year-old child who collapsed on the school playground. Which of the following actions should the nurses perform?
   1. Perform resuscitation in a 30 compressions to 2 breaths ratio.
   2. Compress the child's chest to a depth of 2 inches.
   3. Obtain the automated external defibrillator after 2 minutes.
   4. Continue cardiopulmonary resuscitation for at least 2 hours.

4. While supervising lunchtime in an elementary school, a school nurse observes a child abruptly stand up and appear to be gagging. Which of the following actions should the nurse perform at this time?
   1. Inform the child that she should remain seated while eating.
   2. Assess whether the child is able to cough effectively.
   3. Slap the child five times between the shoulder blades.
   4. Stand behind the child and place both fists under the rib cage.

5. A nurse has determined that a 10-month-old child has an obstructed airway. The child is making no vocalizations and is not breathing. Which of the following actions by the nurse is appropriate at this time?
   1. While tipping the child's head down, slap the child five times between the shoulder blades.
   2. Peer inside the child's mouth and look for the obstruction.
   3. Insert the pinky finger into the child's mouth and sweep the mouth.
   4. While standing behind the child, perform upward thrusts with fists placed under the rib cage.

6. A nurse has completed an emergency assessment on a 3-year-old child who has just started to cry. While conducting the secondary assessment, the nurse should ask the parent which of the following questions? **Select all that apply.**
   1. "Where is the child's injury?"
   2. "Does your child have allergies?"
   3. "When is your child due to eat next?"
   4. "Does your child know how to swim?"
   5. "What was the child doing before he was injured?"

7. A child, who is bleeding heavily, is in hypovolemic shock. The nurse determines that the child is currently compensating for the loss of blood when the nurse notes which of the following?
   1. Tachycardia
   2. Hypotension
   3. Bradypnea
   4. Cyanosis

8. A nurse is caring for a 3½-year-old child who consumed a bottle of aspirin 10 minutes earlier. Which of the following findings would the nurse expect to see?
   1. Hyperglycemia
   2. Hyperpnea
   3. Hyperthermia
   4. Hypernatremia

9. A preschool child was administered activated charcoal in the emergency department after a poisoning event. The child is being discharged home. Which of the following adverse reactions to the medication should the parent be advised to report to the child's primary health-care provider?
   1. Rash
   2. Conjunctivitis
   3. Lethargy
   4. Constipation

10. A nurse working in a preschool discovers that a 2½-year-old child has drunk a bottle of red paint. Place the following nursing actions in the correct order of priority.
1. Notify the child's parents.
2. Question the child's teacher regarding the incident.
3. Call the poison control center.
4. Assess the child for adverse effects from the ingestion.

11. A 2-year-old child's blood lead level is 4 micrograms per dL. Based on the data, which of the following actions should the nurse take?
1. Notify the department of health regarding the value.
2. Recommend to the primary health-care provider that the child receive chelation therapy.
3. Educate the child's teacher regarding ways to prevent another incident.
4. Remind the parents of the importance of frequently washing their child's hands, especially prior to eating.

12. A child is receiving oral Chemet (succimer) for a BLL of 48 micrograms/dL. For which of the following side effects should the child be monitored?
1. White blood cell count below 5,000 cells/mm^3
2. Platelet count below 400,000 cells/mm^3
3. Serum potassium above 3.5 mEq/L
4. Serum sodium above 135 mEq/L

13. A child is receiving IV calcium disodium versenate ($CaNa_2EDTA$). For which of the following serious side effects should the child be monitored? **Select all that apply.**
1. Seizures
2. Hypertension
3. Hyperglycemia
4. Hypercalcemia
5. Elevated serum creatinine

14. A 3-year-old child's blood lead level measures 12 micrograms/dL. The nurse would expect the child to exhibit which of the following signs/symptoms?
1. Hyponatremia
2. Polycythemia
3. Aggression
4. Polyphagia

15. A nurse discovers an 8-month-old child face down in a puddle of water. The child is not breathing and has no pulse. Which of the following actions should the nurse perform at this time?
1. 5 back slaps followed by 5 cardiac compressions
2. 30 cardiac compressions followed by 2 rescue breaths
3. A series of rescue breaths every 3 to 5 seconds
4. Call 911 to activate the emergency response team.

REVIEW ANSWERS

1. ANSWER: 1

Rationale:

1. The nurse should assess for breathing.
2. The nurse should assess the carotid pulse after it is determined whether or not the child is breathing.
3. The nurse should access emergency assistance either once it is determined that the child is breathing and that the child's heart is contracting or after the nurse has performed CPR for 2 full minutes.
4. Rescue breaths should be administered only after it is determined that the child is not breathing but that the child's heart is contracting.

TEST-TAKING TIP: The American Heart Association (2010) has developed a protocol for emergency care. Nurses should follow the set protocol. See Figure 10.1.

Content Area: *Pediatrics—School Age*
Integrated Processes: *Nursing Process: Assessment*
Client Need: *Physiological Integrity: Physiological Adaptation: Medical Emergencies*
Cognitive Level: *Application*

2. ANSWER: 4

Rationale:

1. The nurse should compress the child's chest with two fingers.
2. An automated external defibrillator (AED) should be obtained after performing CPR for 2 min.
3. The nurse should call for emergency assistance (call 911) after performing CPR for 2 min.
4. As a single rescuer, CPR should be performed in a 30 compressions to 2 breaths ratio.

TEST-TAKING TIP: The American Heart Association (2010) has developed a protocol for emergency care. Nurses should follow the set protocol. See Figure 10.1.

Content Area: *Pediatrics—Infant*
Integrated Processes: *Nursing Process: Implementation*
Client Need: *Physiological Integrity: Physiological Adaptation: Medical Emergencies*
Cognitive Level: *Application*

3. ANSWER: 2

Rationale:

1. Child CPR by two rescuers should be performed in a 15 compressions to 2 breaths ratio.
2. The child's chest should be compressed to a depth of 2 in.
3. One of the rescuers should obtain the AED as soon as it is determined that the child needs resuscitation.
4. CPR should be continued until emergency personnel are on the scene or until the child is revived.

Content Area: *Pediatrics—School Age*
Integrated Processes: *Nursing Process: Assessment*
Client Need: *Physiological Integrity: Physiological Adaptation: Medical Emergencies*
Cognitive Level: *Application*

4. ANSWER: 2

Rationale:

1. This child is in distress. It would be inappropriate to inform the child that she should remain seated while eating.
2. This action is appropriate. The nurse should first assess whether the child is able to cough effectively.
3. Back blows and cardiac compressions are performed when an infant has an airway obstruction.
4. It would be appropriate to stand behind the child and place both fists under the rib cage only if the child is unable to cough effectively.

TEST-TAKING TIP: When a child over 1 year of age is experiencing an airway obstruction and is able to cough effectively, a rescuer should not intervene physically, but rather should stand by the child and give the child encouragement. Only if the child is unable to cough effectively should the rescuer perform the Heimlich maneuver.

Content Area: *Pediatrics—School Age*
Integrated Processes: *Nursing Process: Assessment*
Client Need: *Physiological Integrity: Physiological Adaptation: Medical Emergencies*
Cognitive Level: *Application*

5. ANSWER: 1

Rationale:

1. This action is appropriate. The rescuer should then follow the back blows with five chest compressions.
2. The rescuer should look for the obstruction after delivering a series of back blows and chest compressions.
3. A rescuer should insert only the pinky finger into the child's mouth and sweep the mouth if the object is visible in the mouth.
4. The Heimlich maneuver should be performed only on children over 1 year of age.

TEST-TAKING TIP: Because infants are relatively small, it is safer and more effective to deliver back blows and chest compressions to dislodge an airway obstruction than to perform the Heimlich maneuver.

Content Area: *Pediatrics—Infant*
Integrated Processes: *Nursing Process: Implementation*
Client Need: *Physiological Integrity: Physiological Adaptation: Medical Emergencies*
Cognitive Level: *Application*

6. ANSWER: 1, 2, and 5

Rationale:

1. The nurse should ask, "Where is the child's injury?"
2. The nurse should ask, "Does your child have allergies?"
3. The nurse should ask, "When and what did your child last eat?" rather than "When is your child due to eat next?"
4. This question is not appropriate. After the emergency is over and if the child's injury occurred near water, then it might be appropriate to ask whether the child is able to swim.
5. The nurse should ask, "What was the child doing before he was injured?"

TEST-TAKING TIP: To determine whether an injured child needs immediate medical attention, it is important for a nurse to ask a number of important questions. The acronym SAMPLE will help the nurse to remember which questions should be asked.
Content Area: *Pediatrics*
Integrated Processes: *Nursing Process: Implementation*
Client Need: *Physiological Integrity: Physiological Adaptation: Medical Emergencies*
Cognitive Level: *Application*

7. ANSWER: 1
Rationale:
1. Tachycardia is a compensatory response.
2. Hypotension is a late sign of shock.
3. Bradypnea is a late sign of shock.
4. Cyanosis is a late sign of shock.
TEST-TAKING TIP: Initially, when a child is losing blood, his or her body will compensate for the blood loss by increasing the heart rate, the respiratory rate, and by constricting the blood vessels. After the child has lost a significant quantity of blood and is in shock, the body no longer is able to compensate. Shock is a life-threatening event.
Content Area: *Pediatrics*
Integrated Processes: *Nursing Process: Analysis*
Client Need: *Physiological Integrity: Physiological Adaptation: Medical Emergencies*
Cognitive Level: *Application*

8. ANSWER: 2
Rationale:
1. The nurse would not expect the child to be hyperglycemic.
2. The nurse would expect the child to be hyperpneic.
3. The nurse would not expect the child to be hyperthermic.
4. The nurse would not expect the child to be hypernatremic.
TEST-TAKING TIP: The chemical term for aspirin is acetylsalicylic acid. In the period immediately after the ingestion, in an attempt to compensate for the acidosis, the child will instinctively increase his or her respiratory rate to exhale large quantities of carbon dioxide, which often results in respiratory alkalosis. When a large quantity of the drug is ingested, however, the child ultimately develops metabolic acidosis.
Content Area: *Poisoning*
Integrated Processes: *Nursing Process: Analysis*
Client Need: *Physiological Integrity: Physiological Adaptation: Medical Emergencies*
Cognitive Level: *Application*

9. ANSWER: 4
Rationale:
1. Rash is not a side effect of activated charcoal ingestion.
2. Conjunctivitis is not a side effect of activated charcoal ingestion.
3. Lethargy is not a side effect of activated charcoal ingestion.
4. Constipation is a common side effect of activated charcoal ingestion.
TEST-TAKING TIP: Activated charcoal is administered to absorb an ingested poison from the gastrointestinal tract. The charcoal also, however, absorbs large quantities of fluid from the tract. As a result, constipation is a common side effect of the therapy.
Content Area: *Poisoning*
Integrated Processes: *Nursing Process: Implementation*
Client Need: *Physiological Integrity: Physiological Adaptation: Medical Emergencies*
Cognitive Level: *Application*

10. ANSWER: The correct order of nursing actions is 4, 3, 1, 2
Rationale:
4. Assess the child for adverse effects from the ingestion.
3. Call the poison control center.
1. Notify the child's parents.
2. Discuss with the teacher ways to prevent another child from ingesting paint.
TEST-TAKING TIP: 4. The nurse must first determine whether the child is in immediate need of resuscitation. The teacher should resuscitate, if needed. 3. Once the child is determined to be breathing and in no immediate distress, the nurse must call the poison control center to determine if an antidote or other intervention should be administered or if the child should be transported to the emergency department. (PCC may also advise the nurse that the substance is not poisonous and, therefore, will not injure the child.) 1. The child's parents should then be notified that their child has ingested a nonfood substance and of the actions that are being taken to care for the child. 2. Finally, in order to prevent the situation from happening again in the future, the nurse should discuss poison prevention strategies with the child's teacher.
Content Area: *Poisoning*
Integrated Processes: *Nursing Process: Implementation*
Client Need: *Physiological Integrity: Physiological Adaptation: Medical Emergencies*
Cognitive Level: *Analysis*

11. ANSWER: 4
Rationale:
1. It is not necessary to notify the department of health regarding the value.
2. Chelation therapy is not needed.
3. It is not necessary to question the parents regarding possible sources of the child's lead ingestion.
4. It would be important to remind the parents regarding the need for frequent handwashing.
TEST-TAKING TIP: Frequent handwashing often is thought to be exclusively an infection control action. However, it also is important as a means of preventing lead ingestion. The soil of much of the United States has been contaminated with lead. Because young children often place their hands in their mouths, especially when eating, it is important for them to wash their hands frequently.
Content Area: *Poisoning*
Integrated Processes: *Nursing Process: Implementation*
Client Need: *Physiological Integrity: Health Promotion/ Disease Prevention*
Cognitive Level: *Application*

12. **ANSWER: 1**
Rationale:
1. The child should be monitored for neutropenia, a serious side effect of Chemet (succimer).
2. The normal platelet count is 150,000 to 400,000 cells/mm^3.
3. The normal serum potassium level is 3.5 to 5 mEq/L.
4. The normal serum sodium level is 135 to 145 mEq/L.
TEST-TAKING TIP: Chemet (succimer) usually is taken on an outpatient basis. The child should be monitored carefully, returning to the health-care provider's office for frequent BLL and CBC assessments.
Content Area: *Poisoning*
Integrated Processes: *Nursing Process: Assessment*
Client Need: *Physiological Integrity: Pharmacological and Parenteral Therapies: Adverse Effects/Contraindications/ Side Effects/Interactions*
Cognitive Level: *Application*

13. **ANSWER: 1, 4, and 5**
Rationale:
1. The child should be monitored for seizures.
2. Hypertension is not a common side effect of $CaNa_2EDTA$.
3. Hyperglycemia is not a common side effect of $CaNa_2EDTA$.
4. Hypercalcemia is a common side effect of $CaNa_2EDTA$.
5. The child should be monitored for an elevated serum creatinine.
TEST-TAKING TIP: Calcium disodium versenate ($CaNa_2EDTA$) is administered to children with very high BLL (usually over 70 mcg/dL) or for children with lower BLL who are exhibiting signs of encephalopathy. When lead is chelated in these children, the BLL may rise prior to being excreted, placing the children at high risk for renal and central nervous system damage.
Content Area: *Poisoning*
Integrated Processes: *Nursing Process: Assessment*
Client Need: *Physiological Integrity: Pharmacological and Parenteral Therapies: Adverse Effects/Contraindications/ Side Effects/Interactions*
Cognitive Level: *Application*

14. **ANSWER: 3**
Rationale:
1. The nurse would not expect the child to be hyponatremic.
2. The nurse would expect the child to be anemic, not polycythemic.
3. The nurse would expect that child to exhibit aggression.
4. The nurse would not expect that child to exhibit polyphagia.
TEST-TAKING TIP: Lead toxicity, even at low levels, can adversely affect the central nervous system and is exhibited as aggression, hyperactivity, and learning difficulties.
Content Area: *Poisoning*
Integrated Processes: *Nursing Process: Assessment*
Client Need: *Physiological Integrity: Physiological Adaptation: Alterations in Body Systems*
Cognitive Level: *Application*

15. **ANSWER: 2**
Rationale:
1. The nurse should begin CPR in a 30 compressions to 2 rescue breaths ratio.
2. The nurse should begin CPR in a 30 compressions to 2 rescue breaths ratio.
3. The acronym for emergency care is CAB—cardiac compressions, airway, breathing. The nurse, therefore, should begin CPR in a 30 compression to 2 rescue breath ratio.
4. The nurse should wait to call 911 to activate the emergency response team until he or she has performed CPR for approximately 2 min.
TEST-TAKING TIP: Even though liquid is the most common cause of airway obstruction in infants, it is recommended that CPR be instituted when a drowning victim is discovered rather than performing actions to dislodge an obstruction.
Content Area: *Pediatrics*
Integrated Processes: *Nursing Process: Implementation*
Client Need: *Physiological Integrity: Physiological Adaptation: Medical Emergencies*
Cognitive Level: *Application*

Nursing Care of the Child With Immunologic Alterations

KEY TERMS

Active immunity—The body's production of memory B cells to prevent illness caused by an antigen.
Anaphylactic response—A severe, potentially life-threatening response to an allergen.
Antibody—A protein produced by B cells that is encoded to seek and destroy one particular type of antigen.
Antigen—A foreign element in the body.
Atopy—A hypersensitivity reaction to an antigen.
B cell—A type of lymphocyte that produces antibodies in an attempt to eradicate antigens from the body.
Passive immunity—Antibodies produced by a source other than the patient and usually received via the intramuscular or intravenous route.
Systemic lupus erythematosus (SLE)—A chronic, autoimmune disease affecting multiple bodily systems in which the immune system mistakenly attacks healthy tissues in the body rather than foreign invaders.
T cell—A type of lymphocyte that protects the body either by attacking body cells that have been infected by antigens or by coordinating B-cell production.
Vertically acquired passive immunity—Antibodies received from the mother across the placenta and through breast milk.

I. Description

The many functions of the immune system—comprised of a number of organs and tissues, including, but not limited to, the skin, bone marrow, spleen, and lymph system—are integral to the health and well-being of the child. Infants and young children are at particular risk of infection because of the immaturity of their immune systems. They are unable to mount either a rapid or an effective response to invading organisms placing them at high risk for serious illnesses. In fact, children are unable to exhibit adult-level responses until they have reached school age.

II. Physiology

A. Immune system basics.
1. During any day, foreign elements (i.e., **antigens**) attempt to invade the body. In response, the body provides both nonspecific and targeted actions to prevent the antigens from causing disease. First, the skin and cell linings of the respiratory and gastrointestinal tracts provide barriers to prevent the many invaders from entering the body.
2. If viruses, bacteria, or other invading organisms do enter the body, an initial, nonspecific response is activated. Substances (e.g., phagocytes,

interferon, and enzymes) are produced by the body and sent to the site of invasion. An inflammatory response—warmth, redness, and swelling—is noted, and the antigens often are stopped at this point. If, however, the nonspecific response is not completely effective, a targeted response is mounted.

3. During the targeted response, T cell and B cell lymphocytes as well as other substances (e.g., cytokines and complement) are produced. **B cells** are programed to produce and secrete antigen-specific antibodies. Each antigen-specific **antibody** is encoded to seek and destroy one particular type of antigen. Antibodies, named IgA, IgG, and IgM, are primarily responsible for fighting bacteria and viruses. IgE is most responsible for allergic responses in the body.
4. Once an antigen has infected a body cell, however, B cells are unable to fight the infection. Rather, **T cells** protect the body either by attacking body cells that have been infected by antigens or by coordinating B-cell production. In addition, some T cells seek and destroy cancerous body cells.

B. Immunity.

1. **Passive immunity.**
   a. While in utero, babies receive passive immunity, also called **vertically acquired passive immunity,** from their mother via the placenta. Antibodies in the maternal bloodstream pass through the placenta into the fetal system and remain in the baby's system during the first few weeks to approximately 6 months after birth.
   b. Breast milk also contains antibodies, protecting the baby for the duration of time that the baby is breastfed.
   c. Passive immunity may also be conveyed via injection or intravenous (IV) administration of immunoglobulins. If exposed to a dangerous disease, individuals often are administered an organism-specific serum containing antibodies against the disease. Similar to the immunity transferred to babies from their mothers, the injections protect the individuals for a short period of time.
2. **Active immunity:** conferred in one of two ways.
   a. Natural active immunity: when an individual becomes ill with a virus or bacterium, the body develops antibodies against that organism. The antibodies work to eradicate the body of the offending antigen. In addition, memory B cells may also be produced. In the future, when the individual is exposed again to the same disease, the body responds by producing antigen-specific antibodies against the disease. These antibodies protect the individual, preventing the person from again becoming ill from the disease. Some natural immunity (e.g., to mumps or rubella) is lifelong, while other natural immunity (e.g., to influenza) lasts for a short period of time.
   b. Acquired active immunity (see also Chapter 12, "Nursing Care of the Child With Infectious Diseases"): when injected with an altered form of a virus or bacterium (i.e., when immunized against a disease) the body develops memory B cells against the original organism. If exposed to the disease (e.g., varicella [chickenpox] or rubeola [measles]) the antibodies produced by the memory B cells prevent the person from contracting the disease. In a similar fashion as in natural active immunity, some vaccines (e.g., inactivated poliovirus [IPV] and human papillomavirus [HPV]), although given as a series, must be administered only once, while other vaccines must be administered repeatedly in order for individuals to maintain immunity (e.g., tetanus).

III. Human Immunodeficiency Virus (HIV)

HIV infection is exhibited in a variety of ways, from mild to severe, with the most severe form referred to as acquired immunodeficiency syndrome, or AIDS.

A. Incidence.

1. "In 2010, an estimated 217 children younger than the age of 13 years were diagnosed with HIV in the 46 states with long-term, confidential name-based HIV infection reporting since at least 2007; 162 (75%) of those children were perinatally infected" (CDC, 2014).
2. In 2010, "26% of all new infections were among young people ages 13–24 [and] 19% [of that number] were among young men who have sex with men" (CDC, 2010).
3. African American and Hispanic children are infected in much higher numbers than are children from other ethnic and racial groups.

B. Etiology.

1. HIV resides in many fluids in the body, most notably blood, semen, vaginal secretions, cerebral spinal fluid, breast milk, and amniotic fluid.
2. The virus is transmitted when an infected bodily fluid penetrates the mucous membranes of a susceptible individual.
3. The most common means of transmission of HIV are:

a. Vertically, from an infected mother to her unborn fetus.
b. Sexually, during vaginal or anal intercourse.
   i. Men who have sex with men are at highest risk of contracting HIV.

DID YOU KNOW?

Anal intercourse is more dangerous than vaginal intercourse. Although possible, transmission of HIV via oral intercourse is rare.

c. Parenterally, by drug abusers through the sharing of contaminated needles, syringes, or drug paraphernalia.

4. Health-care workers may accidentally become infected when stuck by a needle contaminated with a bodily fluid from a patient infected with HIV.

C. Pathophysiology.
1. HIV is classified as a retrovirus (i.e., an RNA virus). If left untreated, HIV is almost 100% fatal.
2. There are a number of phases of HIV infection.
   a. Initial infection.
      i. Within 1 month of becoming infected with HIV, the body exhibits an inflammatory response, during which time the individual usually exhibits malaise and other flu-like symptoms.
      ii. The virus commandeers the CD4 T cells and replicates rapidly within the body.
         (1) As a result, the number of CD4 cells drops precipitously.
         (2) Once the body's immune response is initiated, the numbers of CD4 cells does begin to recover.
   b. Chronic infection can last for up to 10 years.
      i. During the chronic phase, the viral load is fairly low, and the CD4 count is relatively stable.
      ii. Unless tested, many are unaware that they are infected during the chronic phase because they experience few or no symptoms.
   c. When AIDS (i.e., active HIV infection) is left untreated, the individual's life expectancy is usually less than 1 year is characterized by:
      i. CD4 counts that measure less than or equal to 200 cells/mm^3 (normal CD4 count equals 500 to 1600 cells/mm^3) or
      ii. The development of one or more opportunistic infections or cancers because the body is no longer able to fight invading organisms.
         (1) Common infections and cancers contracted by those with AIDS are *Pneumocystic jirovecii* pneumonia, *Cytomegalovirus* retinitis, and Kaposi's sarcoma.
      iii. Children who exhibit failure to thrive and/or developmental delays.
3. Many HIV-positive patients also are infected with a number of other viruses and bacteria, including hepatitis B, hepatitis C, and tuberculosis.

D. Diagnosis.
1. The Centers for Disease Control and Prevention (CDC) recommend that all individuals between 13 and 64 be tested for HIV.
2. Blood immunoassay tests that screen for the virus.
   a. The CDC (2014) recommends that patients be screened for HIV using the "Recommended Laboratory HIV Testing Algorithm for Serum or Plasma Specimens."
      i. In some instances, Western blot or the indirect immunofluorescence assay (IFA) test, the tests previously recommended, have been shown to provide false-negative data.

E. Treatment.
1. Prevention.
   a. The most important aspect of the treatment plan developed by the CDC and other health-care agencies is to prevent individuals from acquiring the virus.
      i. Vertical transmission.
         (1) All pregnant women are counseled to be tested for HIV.
            (a) In some states, women who refuse to be tested during pregnancy are mandated to be tested when they are in labor.
         (2) All pregnant women who are known to be HIV positive are placed on antiretroviral therapy.
         (3) It is recommended that all babies born to women who are known to be HIV positive be delivered by cesarean section and fed with formula rather than the mother's breast milk.
         (4) All neonates are tested for the presence of HIV antibodies.
         (5) Neonates born to mothers who have been diagnosed as HIV positive or are found to be HIV antibody positive at birth usually are placed on zidovudine, ZDV or AZT (Retrovir), for 6 weeks following birth.
      ii. Sexual transmission.
         (1) Circumcision of the penis has been shown to reduce infection rates in

men and, consequently, infection rates in their partners.
(a) No U.S. health-care organization has recommended that all male babies be circumcised.
(2) Individuals are recommended to restrict intercourse to an individual, ideally only one, who has been shown to be HIV negative.
(3) Individuals are recommended to consistently use latex or plastic condoms whenever having sexual intercourse.
(a) Even if HIV-positive individuals take medication on a daily basis, they are still able to transmit the virus to uninfected individuals.
(b) Natural, lambskin condoms do not protect individuals from infection.
(c) Condom users must be taught how to correctly apply and remove condoms.

! Even if the partner is HIV positive, a condom should be worn because an additional strain of HIV can be contracted, which can increase the speed of progression to AIDS and increase the susceptibility to other sexually transmitted infections.

iii. Infection via IV drug use.
(1) Ideally, drug abusers should seek treatment for their addictions.
(2) If drug abusers continue to inject drugs, they should use clean, sterile supplies.
(a) Many communities sponsor clean needle programs to help reduce the incidence of HIV infection.

b. Postexposure prophylaxis.
i. Health-care workers, sexual partners, and rape victims should be offered postexposure prophylaxis as a means of preventing transmission of the virus.
(1) First, an attempt must be made to determine whether the source of the contamination is HIV positive.
(a) Testing is voluntary; patients cannot be forced to be HIV tested.
(b) If the source is HIV negative, no further care is needed.
(2) If the source is HIV positive, or if the source's infection status is unknown, antiretroviral medication should be started within 72 hr of exposure and continued for a minimum of 4 weeks.
(3) Most commonly, two or three nucleotide reverse transcriptase inhibitors (NRTIs) are recommended as postexposure medication prophylaxis.
(a) The individual should be advised of the many medication side effects that he or she may experience.
(4) Baseline testing for the virus should be performed at the time of exposure, and follow-up testing should occur 3 weeks, 6 weeks, and 6 months later.

2. Treatment: there currently is no cure for HIV. Rather, treatment is aimed at controlling the viral load of individuals infected with the virus.
i. The gold standard for current HIV treatment is referred to as HAART (highly active antiretroviral therapy).
ii. There are six classes of antiretroviral medications (Table 11.1).
iii. HAART regimen entails taking three or more of the medications from at least two of the classes.
(1) The combination therapy significantly decreases the likelihood that HIV will mutate, resulting in a virus that is immune to one or more of the medications.
(2) There are medications that combine two or more of the six category drugs into one tablet.
iv. Many of the medications cause severe side effects, including nausea and vomiting, cardiac arrhythmias, osteoporosis, skin rashes, and breathing difficulties.

F. Nursing considerations.
1. Anxiety/Fear/Risk for Altered Coping.
a. Allow the family and child, if appropriate, to voice concerns regarding the need for HIV testing and, if applicable, regarding the HIV diagnosis.
b. Maintain confidentiality of HIV-positive diagnosis, if applicable.
2. If HIV negative.
a. Deficient Knowledge.
i. Educate all pregnant women regarding their own need to be tested for HIV and that their newborns will be tested for HIV.

Table 11.1 Antiretroviral Medications

Drug Class	Drug
Non-nucleotide reverse transcriptase inhibitors (NNRTIs)	delavirdine (DLV) (Rescriptor) and efavirenz (EFV) (Sustiva)
Nucleotide reverse transcriptase inhibitors (NRTIs)	abacavir (ABC) (Ziagen) and zidovudine (ZDV or AZT) (Retrovir)
Protease inhibitors (PIs)	atazanavir (ATV) (Reyataz) and darunavir (DRV) (Prezista)
Fusion inhibitors	enfuvirtide (T-20) (Fuzeon)
CCR5 antagonists	maraviroc (MVC) (Selzentry)
Integrase inhibitors	raltegravir (RAL) (Isentress)

ii. Educate all pregnant women who have tested positive for HIV regarding the importance of taking HAART, as prescribed.
iii. Educate all children by early adolescence regarding the HIV disease and prevention strategies.
iv. At each well-child visit, beginning in early adolescence, query the child regarding his or her sexual practices and other high-risk behaviors.
v. At each well-child visit, beginning in early adolescence, reinforce safe sex and other prevention strategies.
vi. Strongly recommend that each child 13 years old and older be tested for HIV.

3. If HIV positive:
   a. Deficient Knowledge/Risk for Injury/Risk for Delayed Development.
      i. Educate the parents and child, if appropriate, regarding the need strictly to adhere to the treatment plan.
      ii. Educate the parents and child, if appropriate, regarding the side effects of medications and the need to report all side effects to the primary health-care provider.
      iii. Educate the parents and child, if appropriate, regarding signs and symptoms of opportunistic infections that are suggestive of an AIDS diagnosis.
      iv. Educate the parents and child, if appropriate, to maintain standard infection control precautions at all times.
      v. Educate the parents to keep the child's immunizations up to date.
      vi. Educate the child, if sexually active, regarding the need to always use a condom during sexual intercourse.

IV. Systemic Lupus Erythematosus

Systemic lupus erythematosus (SLE) is a chronic autoimmune disease affecting multiple bodily systems.

A. Incidence.
1. SLE is relatively rare in young children.
2. Children who develop the disease are usually 11 years of age or older.
3. Females are about 10 times more likely to develop SLE than are males.
4. Children of color are more likely to develop SLE than are Caucasian children.

B. Etiology.
1. Although the etiology of SLE is unknown, it is known that the immune systems of those with the disease mistakenly attack healthy tissues in the body rather than foreign invaders.

C. Pathophysiology.
1. Antibodies against healthy bodily tissues are produced in large numbers.
   a. Results in inflammatory response in virtually all organ systems, including the cardiovascular, renal, musculoskeletal, respiratory, and central nervous systems.
2. The prognosis of SLE is good in children, but some experience developmental delays, osteoporosis, and a reduced quality of life.
3. Signs and symptoms are dependent on which organ systems are most affected. They include:
   a. Rashes: most notably, a distinctive butterfly rash (Fig. 11.1) that appears over the cheeks and nose.
   b. Arthritis.
   c. Seizures.
   d. Carditis.
   e. Anemia and thrombocytopenia.
   f. Hematuria and proteinuria.

D. Diagnosis.
1. There is no single test that is conducted to diagnose SLE.

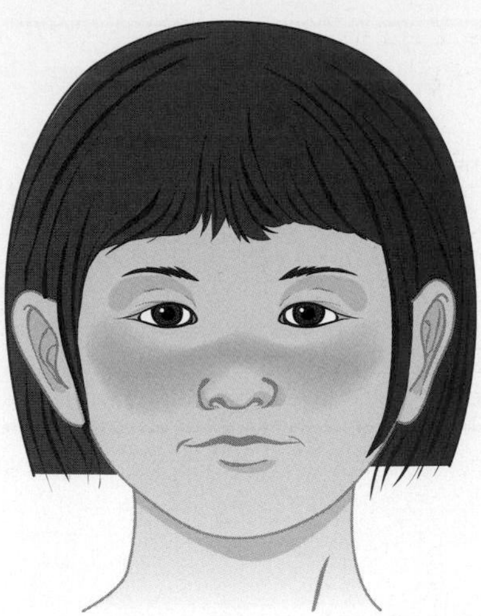

Fig 11.1 Butterfly rash.

2. The disease is highly suggestive if a patient exhibits four or more of the following 11 symptoms: joint pain; chest pain on inspiration; fatigue; elevated temperature without a reason; malaise; alopecia; sores in the mouth; photophobia; butterfly rash, which worsens when exposed to the sun; lymphadenopathy; and arthritis.
3. Blood tests that can be conducted include:
   a. Positive ANA (antinuclear antibody) test.
   b. Positive anti-DNA antibody test.
   c. Positive antiphospholipid antibody test.
4. Tissue biopsies often are conducted as confirmatory assessments.

E. Treatment.
1. There is no cure for the disease.
2. Mild disease is treated with nonsteroidal anti-inflammatory medications and/or corticosteroids.
3. Moderate to severe disease often is treated with high dosages of corticosteroids and/or antineoplastic medications.
4. System-specific medications, when needed, for example:
   a. If CNS involvement, anticonvulsants may be prescribed.
   b. If renal involvement, antihypertensives may be prescribed.
5. Many patients with SLE who experience depression find talk therapy helpful.

F. Nursing considerations.
1. Anxiety/Anger/Risk for Altered Coping/Disturbed Body Image/Deficient Knowledge.
   a. Educate the parents and child regarding physiological changes of SLE and chronicity of the illness.
   b. Allow the child and parents to discuss their fears and concerns regarding bodily changes and living with a chronic illness.
   c. Provide emotional support when needed.
   d. Educate the parents and child regarding the need to adhere to the therapeutic regimen.
      i. Administration of safe dosages of prescribed medications.
      ii. Sunscreen worn at all times to protect the skin.
   e. Recommend membership in a national support organization (e.g., Lupus Foundation of America).
2. Pain/Activity Intolerance.
   a. Use age-appropriate pain tools, and assess management of pain.
   b. Use nonpharmacological pain remedies in conjunction with pharmacological methods, if appropriate.

V. Allergies

Allergy, or **atopy**, is a hypersensitivity reaction to an antigen. Many hypersensitivity reactions are relatively minor, resulting in sneezing, watery eyes, rashes, and other such symptoms. A severe allergic response (i.e., an **anaphylactic response**), however, can be life threatening.

A. Incidence.
1. Approximately 5 out of every 100 children has a documented food allergy.
2. Numbers of other children are allergic to environmental substances (e.g., pets, plants, clothing materials).

B. Etiology.
1. Most children have a genetic predisposition to the allergen.
2. Food allergy is the most common cause of anaphylaxis in children.
   a. Commonly allergenic foods are peanuts, tree nuts, soy, eggs, wheat, fish, and cow's milk.
3. Ingestion of food allergens.

C. Pathophysiology.
1. Circulating IgE combines with the offending antigen resulting in, most importantly, massive quantities of histamine to be released.
2. Histamine production may lead to severe, systemic inflammatory responses of the:
   a. Respiratory tract, resulting in bronchospasm and laryngeal edema.
   b. Skin, resulting in rashes and pruritus.
   c. Gastrointestinal system, resulting in increased peristalsis.

MAKING THE CONNECTION

For a number of years, for families with a strong history of atopy, it has been the practice to restrict the intake of highly allergenic foods by pregnant and lactating women and to introduce highly allergenic foods to children at least 1 year after birth. Because food allergies have increased dramatically since 2000, however, the Adverse Reactions to Foods Committee of the American Academy of Allergy, Asthma & Immunology (Fleischer, Spergel, Assa'ad, & Pongracic, 2013) has developed new recommendations.

- Pregnant and lactating women should no longer maintain diet restrictions, except in the case of the ingestion of peanuts. (There currently is not enough information to determine whether it is safe for pregnant women with a strong history of atopy to ingest peanuts.)
- Breastfeeding for all babies for a minimum of 4 months and, ideally, for at least 6 months.
- Hydrolyzed formula for high-risk babies who are unable to be breastfed.
- Introduction of solid foods, including highly allergenic foods, beginning at 4 to 6 months of life. It is recommended that high-allergy foods be introduced at home, not at a day care or other location.
- Foods should be introduced slowly with low-allergy foods introduced first.
- Except in baked goods and the like, whole milk should not be added to the baby's diet until after 1 year of age.
- If a child should exhibit a severe response to a food, the child should not be reoffered the food, and a health-care professional should be consulted.

 d. Circulatory system, resulting in severe hypotension and, in some cases, death.

D. Diagnosis.
 1. If a child exhibits anaphylaxis, immediate intervention is required, and diagnosis is made ex post facto.
 2. Serum tests for elevated IgE, RAST (radioallergosorbent test), skin patch tests, and skin prick tests are all used to diagnose allergies.

E. Treatment of anaphylaxis.
 1. Prevention.
  a. To prevent anaphylaxis, the child must avoid all contact with a known allergen.
 2. If the child is experiencing an anaphylactic reaction, immediate treatment is essential.
  a. Parenteral epinephrine is the drug of choice.
   i. Children at high risk for anaphylaxis should have a prescription for an EpiPen (i.e., a syringe containing epinephrine that can be used by the child, parent, or other person who witnesses the child in anaphylaxis).
   ii. If epinephrine is unavailable, diphenhydramine (Benadryl) or corticosteroids may be administered.
  b. Oxygen is administered, and the child is intubated, if needed.
  c. Supine positioning is maintained.
  d. IV infusion is maintained.

F. Nursing considerations.
 1. For pregnant and lactating women and parents of infants.
  a. Deficient Knowledge.
   i. Educate individuals regarding the established recommendations (Fleischer et al., 2013, see Making the Connection).
 2. For families whose child has had an anaphylactic reaction.
  a. Anxiety/Fear/Risk for Altered Coping/Risk for Allergic Response/Deficient Knowledge.
   i. Educate the parents, child, school officials, and all other adults in contact with the child regarding the cause of anaphylactic reaction and the need to avoid all contact with the offending antigen.
   ii. Allow the child and parents to discuss their fears and concerns regarding life-threatening illness.
   iii. Provide emotional support, as needed.
   iv. Educate the parents and child, if appropriate, regarding how to use an EpiPen and how to inject the medication (Fig. 11.2).
    (1) Make sure that the medication is safe to administer.
     (a) The medication comes in two strengths; the appropriate strength for the child should be used.
      (i) EpiPen Jr. for children weighing 33 to 66 lb (15 to 30 kg).
      (ii) EpiPen for children weighing more than 66 lb (over 30 kg).
      (iii) No EpiPen is available for children weighing less than 33 lb (15 kg).

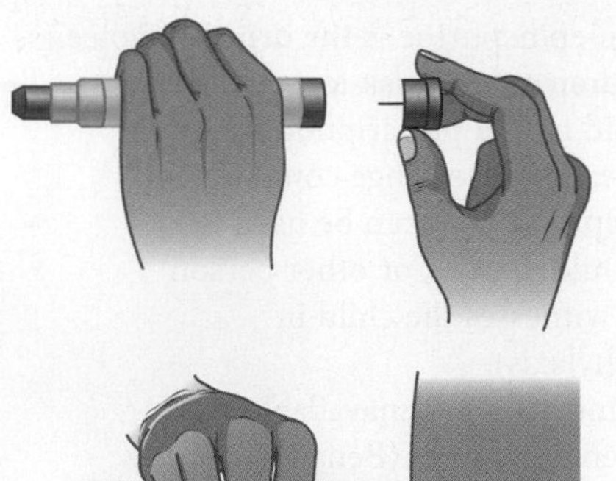

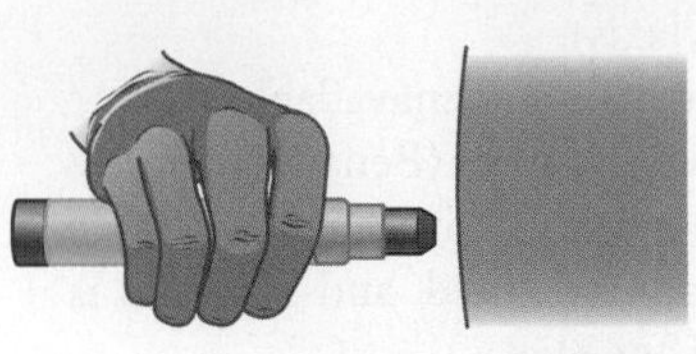

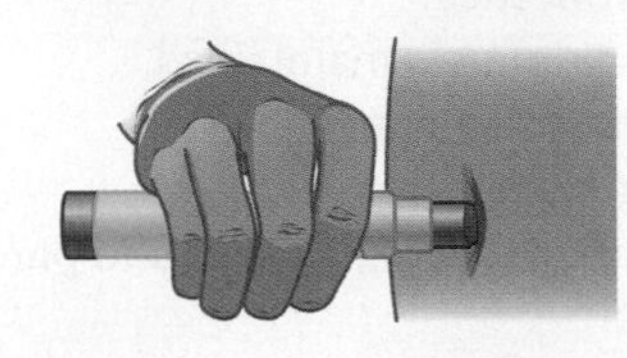

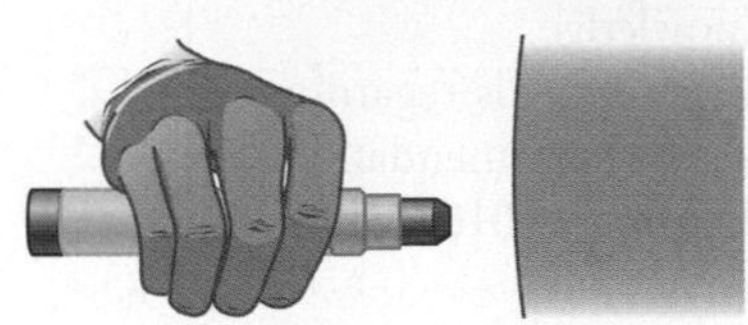

Fig 11.2 Administering an EpiPen injection.

(b) Routinely check the expiration date on the medication, and refill the prescription, if needed.

(c) Routinely check to make sure that the medication is clear, and refill the prescription, if needed.

(2) Injecting procedure.

(a) Remove cap and slide injector out of the case.

(b) Grab the syringe firmly without putting hands or fingers over the tip.

(c) Point the orange tip down, and take off the blue cap on the other end of the syringe.

(i) Firmly and rapidly, inject the orange tip at a right angle to the outer thigh.

(ii) The injection can be given through clothing, if needed.

(iii) A click should be heard indicating that the medication is being released.

(iv) The syringe should be held in place for about 10 sec.

(3) Emergency medical assistance should be obtained immediately after injecting.

When an EpiPen is used, the medication must be injected only into the outer thigh. No other site is safe.

3. Ineffective Airway Clearance/Impaired Gas Exchange/Deficient Fluid Volume.
   a. Perform cardiopulmonary resuscitation (CPR), if needed.
   b. Assist with intubation, if needed.
   c. Administer oxygen, per order.
   d. Obtain and maintain IV fluids.
   e. Administer safe dosages of epinephrine medication via EpiPen or IV, corticosteroids, and/or antihistamines employing the five rights, per order.
   f. Provide needed reassurance to the child and family throughout.

CASE STUDY: Putting It All Together

16-year-old male of Hispanic heritage with HIV

Subjective Data

- Being seen for scheduled checkup; no one accompanies the patient
- During nursing interview,
  - Nurse asks,
    - "How are things going?"
  - Patient replies,
    - "I'm getting fed up with taking all those medications. None of my friends have to take a fistful of pills every day!!"
  - Nurse asks,
    - "During your last appointment, you mentioned that you had a girlfriend. Are you intimate with her?"
  - Patient replies,
    - "Yeah, we're still together. If you mean, do we do it—yeah, we do it."
  - Nurse asks,
    - "Does she know you have HIV? And are you using a condom every time you 'do it'?"
  - Patient replies,
    - "She doesn't know. It would screw everything up. And, I usually wear a rubber."
  - Nurse comments,
    - "You seem a bit tired today."
  - Patient replies,
    - "You'd be tired, too, if you had this damned disease!"

Objective Data

History

- HIV diagnosed at 1 year of age, secondary to vertical transmission
- Mother died of AIDS when child was 10
- Patient currently lives with maternal grandmother
- Patient and grandmother have received extensive education regarding progression of the illness as well as means of preventing transmission to others
- Patient on HAART since diagnosis—current therapy is:
  - Lamivudine (NRTI class medication): 300 mg PO daily
  - Zidovudine (NRTI class medication): 300 mg PO bid
  - Nevirapine (NNRTI class medication): 200 mg PO bid

Vital Signs	
Blood pressure:	98/50 mm Hg
Temperature:	100.4°F
Heart rate:	110 bpm
Respiratory rate:	20 rpm

Lab Results	
CD4 count:	300 cells/mm^3
Hematocrit:	28%
Hemoglobin:	9 G/dL
AST:	200 IU/L (normal 10–34 IU/L)
ALT:	250 IU/L (normal 10–40 IU/L)
Bilirubin:	6 mg/dL (normal 0–0.2 mg/dL)
White blood cell count:	3,500 cells/mm^3

Nursing Assessment

- Physical findings
  - Maculopapular rash

Health-Care Provider's Orders

- Medication revision
- Repeat lab values in 1 week
- Provide needed counseling regarding:
  - The possible worsening of his disease
  - His obligations to his girlfriend
  - The need for a support system

Continued

CASE STUDY: Putting It All Together *cont'd*

Case Study Questions

A. What *subjective* assessments indicate that this client is experiencing a health alteration?

1. ______
2. ______
3. ______
4. ______

B. What *objective* assessments indicate that this client is experiencing a health alteration?

1. ______
2. ______
3. ______
4. ______
5. ______
6. ______
7. ______
8. ______
9. ______
10. ______

C. After analyzing the data that has been collected, what **primary** nursing diagnosis should the nurse assign to this client?

1. ______

D. What interventions should the nurse plan and/or implement to meet this child's and his family's needs?

1. ______
2. ______
3. ______
4. ______
5. ______

E. What client outcomes should the nurse evaluate regarding the effectiveness of the nursing interventions?

1. ______
2. ______

F. What physiological characteristics should the child exhibit before leaving the clinic?

1. ______

G. What subjective characteristics should the child exhibit before leaving the clinic?

1. ______

REVIEW QUESTIONS

1. A child has been exposed to a viral illness. The child's B cells have been activated. The nurse determines that the child's body has undergone which of the following physiological responses?
   1. Red blood cells have increased in number.
   2. Platelets are migrating to the respiratory tract.
   3. Lymphocytes have begun to produce antibodies.
   4. Interferon and enzyme production is inhibited.
2. A 10-month-old infant has been exposed to chickenpox. The nurse would expect the baby's primary health-care provider to order which of the following interventions to prevent the baby from contracting the illness?
   1. Intravenous antibiotics
   2. Varicella zoster immune globulin
   3. Varicella immunization
   4. Nothing because the baby is protected by the mother's antibodies
3. A nurse is coordinating an educational session for middle school students regarding human immunodeficiency virus (HIV). The nurse should advise students that which of the following behaviors place them at high risk of contracting HIV? **Select all that apply.**
   1. Eating food prepared by an individual with HIV.
   2. Engaging in oral intercourse with an individual with HIV.
   3. Sharing marijuana cigarettes with an individual with HIV
   4. Using natural skin condoms while having sex with an individual with HIV.
   5. Drinking alcoholic beverages out of the same container as an individual with HIV.
4. A young woman is being seen in the women's health clinic. She states that she had unprotected intercourse about one month earlier, and she is worried that she may have contracted HIV. Which of the following signs/symptoms would indicate that her worries may be correct?
   1. Macular papular rash covering her thorax
   2. Severe abdominal cramps accompanied by diarrhea
   3. Exhaustion accompanied by muscle aches and pains
   4. Abnormally heavy menstrual period
5. An 18-year-old man reports to a nurse that he had unprotected anal intercourse with a man 3 years earlier. When the nurse suggests that the patient have an HIV test, he states, "Why, I'm fine. I don't have any symptoms at all." Which of the following responses by the nurse would be appropriate to make?
   1. "You are probably correct because unless you had gastrointestinal symptoms after you had intercourse, you are probably not infected."
   2. "You are probably correct because having intercourse with an infected woman is much more dangerous than with a man."
   3. "I understand that there is virtually no chance that you are infected, but it is recommended that all who are 13 and older be tested."
   4. "You should be tested anyway because it can take up to 10 years before any symptoms of the disease are detected."
6. The nurse is providing HIV education to a group of individuals. During the session, the nurse discusses actions that have been shown to reduce the transmission of HIV. Which of the following information did the nurse include in her discussion?
   1. Circumcised men are less likely to contract and transmit HIV than are uncircumcised men.
   2. HIV is eradicated from the body when 2 to 3 different antiretroviral medications are taken for at least one year.
   3. The HIV vaccination has been approved for men and women between the ages of 16 and 26 years of age.
   4. Babies born to HIV positive mothers are less likely to contract HIV if they are exclusively breastfed.
7. A nurse, caring for a client in the emergency department, is stuck by a contaminated needle. Which of the following actions should the nurse perform? The nurse should:
   1. advise the client that a law requires that an HIV test be performed on the client as soon as possible.
   2. wait at least 7 days before having HIV baseline testing performed.
   3. be prepared to receive an intravenous infusion of HIV immune globulin in the emergency department.
   4. begin postexposure prophylactic treatment within 72 hours of the HIV exposure.

8. A nurse is providing a teaching session for adolescents and their parents regarding HIV. Which of the following information should the nurse include in the teaching session? **Select all that apply.**
   1. It is recommended that all individuals aged 18 and older be tested for HIV.
   2. The potential for contracting HIV increases when a person has intercourse with multiple partners.
   3. A person can contract more than one strain of HIV, increasing the likelihood of the disease progressing to AIDS.
   4. Although HAART helps to delay the onset of AIDS, all patients with HIV will die within approximately 20 years of the time of the initial infection.
   5. Anyone who is diagnosed with hepatitis B or hepatitis C is at high risk for also being infected with HIV.

9. A 12-year-old girl has just been diagnosed with systemic lupus erythematosus (SLE). Which of the following information should the nurse include when educating her and her parents regarding the disease?
   1. The cure rate for SLE is between 90% and 95%.
   2. SLE is caused by a virus that permeates 100% of the cells of the kidneys and liver.
   3. The pain of SLE arthritis will likely be controlled with nonsteroidal anti-inflammatories.
   4. SLE antibodies were triggered by pubertal changes.

10. A nurse is providing education to parents of young children regarding the children's potential for developing allergies. The nurse informs the parents that which are the most common allergies of childhood?
    1. Medicines
    2. Foods
    3. Pets
    4. Plants

11. The nurse is providing education to pregnant women who have a family history of severe allergies. Which of the following information should the nurse convey regarding actions the women should take to minimize their children's potential for developing allergies?
    1. Remove high-allergy foods from their diet during their pregnancy and while breastfeeding.
    2. If they decide not to breastfeed their baby, to feed the baby a soy-based rather than a cow's milk–based formula.
    3. Delay feeding their infant any solid foods until the infant is seven to eight months of age.
    4. When they begin to feed their infant solid foods, to begin serving high-allergy foods shortly after low-allergy foods have been introduced.

12. A child, weighing 80 lb, has been prescribed an EpiPen. Which of the following information should the nurse include in the medication teaching for the parents and the child?
    1. To keep the medication in a refrigerator at all times.
    2. Inject the medication at a 45 degree angle to the body surface.
    3. Administer the medication into the dorsogluteal muscle.
    4. Continue to inject the medication for at least 10 seconds duration.

13. A school nurse is called to a third grade classroom because a child, with no previous history, is in anaphylaxis. Which of the following actions should the nurse perform?
    1. Notify the parents to pick up their child as soon as possible.
    2. Take the AED to the classroom, and begin emergency intervention.
    3. Have the child lie quietly in the nurse's office for the next 30 minutes.
    4. Inform the health department that the child has a reportable illness.

REVIEW ANSWERS

1. ANSWER: 3

Rationale:

1. This statement is false.
2. This statement is false.
3. **It is correct that lymphocytes have begun to produce antibodies.**
4. This statement is false.

TEST-TAKING TIP: When the body is exposed to a foreign antigen like a virus, the immune response is activated. B cells, a type of lymphocyte, begin to produce antibodies in an attempt to eradicate the viruses that are proliferating in the body.

Content Area: *Infectious Disease*

Integrated Processes: *Nursing Process: Diagnosis*

Client Need: *Physiological Integrity: Physiological Adaptation: Pathophysiology*

Cognitive Level: *Comprehension*

2. ANSWER: 2

Rationale:

1. The nurse would not expect the primary health-care provider to order IV antibiotics. Antibiotics are not effective against viral illnesses.
2. **The nurse would expect the primary health-care provider to order varicella zoster immune globulin (VZIG), which contains antibodies against the varicella virus.**
3. The nurse would not expect the primary health-care provider to order varicella immunization. The varicella vaccine is recommended to be administered at 12 months or later.
4. The nurse would expect the primary health-care provider to order VZIG be administered to the child. The passive immunity from the mother likely is no longer effective.

TEST-TAKING TIP: The administration of disease-specific immunoglobulins to a patient who has been exposed to a disease provides the patient with passive immunity.

Content Area: *Communicable Disease*

Integrated Processes: *Nursing Process: Implementation*

Client Need: *Physiological Integrity: Pharmacological and Parenteral Therapies: Expected Actions/Outcomes*

Cognitive Level: *Application*

3. ANSWER: 2 and 4

Rationale:

1. HIV is not transmitted via eating food prepared by an individual with HIV.
2. **Although an individual is less likely to acquire HIV when engaging in oral intercourse with an individual with HIV than during vaginal or anal intercourse, it is possible.**
3. HIV is not transmitted when sharing marijuana or nicotine cigarettes with an individual with HIV.
4. **Using natural skin condoms while having sex with an individual with HIV is a high-risk behavior.**
5. HIV is not transmitted when sharing alcohol or any other beverage with an individual with HIV. Alcohol consumption does lower one's inhibitions, however, increasing the probability of engaging in sexual intercourse.

TEST-TAKING TIP: Although latex condom use during intercourse is protective of HIV transmission, wearing natural skin condoms is not. The virus can migrate through small pores in natural skin condoms and enter the mucous membranes of the genital tract.

Content Area: *Communicable Disease*

Integrated Processes: *Nursing Process: Implementation*

Client Need: *Health Promotion and Maintenance: High-Risk Behaviors*

Cognitive Level: *Application*

4. ANSWER: 3

Rationale:

1. Macular papular rash is not characteristic of early HIV infection.
2. Severe abdominal cramps accompanied by diarrhea are not characteristic of early HIV infection.
3. **Exhaustion accompanied by muscle aches and pains may indicate that she is HIV positive.**
4. Abnormally heavy menstrual period is not characteristic of early HIV infection.

TEST-TAKING TIP: Early HIV infection is characterized by flu-like symptoms and malaise approximately 1 month after becoming infected with the virus.

Content Area: *Communicable Disease*

Integrated Processes: *Nursing Process: Assessment*

Client Need: *Physiological Integrity: Physiological Adaptation: Alterations in Body Systems*

Cognitive Level: *Application*

5. ANSWER: 4

Rationale:

1. It can take up to 10 years after becoming infected with HIV to exhibit any symptoms of the disease.
2. This statement is false. Men having sex with men are more likely to become infected during intercourse than are men having sex with women.
3. This statement is false. If the man with whom the patient had intercourse was infected with HIV, the patient may have become infected.
4. **This statement is correct. It can take up to 10 years after becoming infected with HIV to exhibit any symptoms of the disease.**

TEST-TAKING TIP: Early HIV infection is characterized by flu-like symptoms and malaise approximately 1 month after becoming infected with the virus.

Content Area: *Communicable Disease*

Integrated Processes: *Nursing Process: Implementation*

Client Need: *Physiological Integrity: Physiological Adaptation: Alterations in Body Systems*

Cognitive Level: *Application*

6. ANSWER: 1
Rationale:
1. This statement is true. Circumcised men are less likely to contract and transmit HIV than are uncircumcised men.
2. This statement is false. There is no cure for HIV. Antiretroviral medications simply control the viral load of individuals infected with the virus.
3. This statement is false. There is no vaccination to protect individuals against HIV.
4. This statement is false. Breast milk of women infected with HIV can transmit the disease. It is recommended that babies born to women infected with HIV be formula fed.

TEST-TAKING TIP: Although research has shown that circumcised men are less likely to contract and to transmit HIV, no agency or health-care association in the United States has declared that all babies be circumcised at birth.
Content Area: *Communicable Disease*
Integrated Processes: *Nursing Process: Implementation; Teaching/Learning*
Client Need: *Health Promotion and Maintenance: Health Promotion/Disease Prevention*
Cognitive Level: *Application*

7. ANSWER: 4
Rationale:
1. The nurse may ask the client to be HIV tested, but the patient may refuse.
2. The nurse should wait no longer than 72 hours before having HIV baseline testing performed.
3. There is no HIV immune globulin for IV infusion.
4. The nurse should begin postexposure prophylactic treatment within 72 hours of HIV exposure.

TEST-TAKING TIP: Because health-care personnel are at risk of contracting HIV if they are stuck with a contaminated needle, they should engage in safe practices when performing high-risk treatments. For example, only syringes with safety caps should be used.
Content Area: *Communicable Disease*
Integrated Processes: *Nursing Process: Implementation*
Client Need: *Safe and Effective Care Environment: Safety and Infection Control: Handling Hazardous and Infectious Materials*
Cognitive Level: *Application*

8. ANSWER: 2, 3, and 5
Rationale:
1. This statement is false. It is recommended that all individuals aged 13 and older be tested for HIV.
2. It is true that the potential for contracting HIV increases when a person has intercourse with multiple partners.
3. It is true that a person can contract more than one strain of HIV, increasing the likelihood of the disease progressing to AIDS.
4. This statement is false. HAART therapy has changed HIV from a fatal disease to a chronic illness.
5. This statement is true. Anyone who is diagnosed with hepatitis B or hepatitis C is at high risk for also being infected with HIV.

TEST-TAKING TIP: Hepatitis B and hepatitis C both are blood-borne illnesses and are transmitted via the same route as HIV. Those infected with the illnesses are frequently also infected with HIV and vice versa.
Content Area: *Communicable Disease*
Integrated Processes: *Nursing Process: Implementation; Teaching/Learning*
Client Need: *Physiological Integrity: Physiological Adaptation: Alterations in Body Systems*
Cognitive Level: *Application*

9. ANSWER: 3
Rationale:
1. This statement is false. There is no cure for SLE.
2. This statement is false. The cause of SLE is unknown.
3. This statement is true. The pain of SLE arthritis likely will be controlled with nonsteroidal anti-inflammatories.
4. This statement is false. The cause of SLE is unknown.

TEST-TAKING TIP: SLE is an autoimmune illness that affects virtually all organ systems of the body. The disease is usually controlled with the intake of nonsteroidal anti-inflammatory medications and corticosteroids.
Content Area: *Pediatrics—Autoimmune*
Integrated Processes: *Nursing Process: Implementation; Teaching/Learning*
Client Need: *Physiological Integrity: Pharmacological and Parenteral Therapies: Expected Actions/Outcomes*
Cognitive Level: *Application*

10. ANSWER: 2
Rationale:
1. Although many children are allergic to medicines, the most common childhood allergens are foods.
2. Foods are the most common childhood allergens.
3. Although many children are allergic to pets, the most common childhood allergens are foods.
4. Although many children are allergic to plants, the most common childhood allergens are foods.

TEST-TAKING TIP: It is important for parents to be aware that foods are the most common allergens for children. Because of this fact, it is recommended that new foods be introduced at home so that the parents can monitor their children's responses to the new foods.
Content Area: *Pediatrics—Autoimmune*
Integrated Processes: *Nursing Process: Implementation; Teaching/Learning*
Client Need: *Physiological Integrity: Physiological Adaptation: Alternation in Body Systems*
Cognitive Level: *Comprehension*

11. ANSWER: 4

Rationale:

1. It is no longer recommended that women remove high-allergy foods from their diets during their pregnancy and while breastfeeding.
2. It is recommended that babies who are not breastfed be fed hydrolyzed formula, not soy formula, during their infancy.
3. It is recommended that babies start to be fed solid foods between 4 and 6 months of age.
4. **It is recommended that when solid foods are introduced into infants' diets, that high-allergy foods be introduced shortly after low-allergy foods have been introduced.**

TEST-TAKING TIP: For a number of years, it was recommended that pregnant women, lactating women, and infants refrain from consuming high-allergy foods. That is no longer the recommendation. Pregnant and lactating women may consume high-allergy foods with no restrictions, and when solid foods are introduced into infants' diets, high-allergy foods should be introduced shortly after low-allergy foods have been introduced. The only exception to this recommendation is in relation to peanuts. It is still recommended that pregnant and lactating women whose family histories are high risk for allergies and their infants refrain from eating peanuts.
Content Area: *Maternity; Newborn; Pediatric—Infant*
Integrated Processes: *Nursing Process: Implementation; Teaching/Learning*
Client Need: *Health Promotion and Maintenance: Health Promotion/Disease Prevention*
Cognitive Level: *Application*

12. ANSWER: 4

Rationale:

1. It is recommended that the EpiPen be kept with the person with the severe allergy at all times. It need not be refrigerated.
2. The medication should be injected at a 90-degree angle.
3. The medication should be administered into the outer thigh (i.e., vastus lateralis).
4. **The medication should continue to be injected for at least a 10-sec duration.**

TEST-TAKING TIP: EpiPens are prescribed for anyone over 33 lb who experiences anaphylaxis after ingesting or coming in contact with a specific allergen. It is essential that the nurse educate the child and parents regarding the proper use of the EpiPen.
Content Area: *Pediatrics—Medication*
Integrated Processes: *Nursing Process: Implementation; Teaching/Learning*
Client Need: *Physiological Integrity: Pharmacological and Parental Therapies: Medication Administration*
Cognitive Level: *Application*

13. ANSWER: 2

Rationale:

1. Anaphylaxis is an emergent situation. The nurse should begin emergency intervention.
2. **The nurse should take the AED to the classroom and begin emergency intervention.**
3. Anaphylaxis is an emergent situation. The nurse should begin emergency intervention.
4. Anaphylaxis is an emergent situation. The nurse should begin emergency intervention. Anaphylaxis is not a reportable illness.

TEST-TAKING TIP: After ingesting or coming in direct contact with specific allergens, highly allergic individuals go into anaphylactic shock. Massive production of histamine results in a systemic inflammatory response. Emergency intervention is required to resuscitate and maintain physiological function.
Content Area: *Pediatrics*
Integrated Processes: *Nursing Process: Implementation*
Client Need: *Physiological Integrity: Physiological Adaptation: Medical Emergencies*
Cognitive Level: *Application*

Nursing Care of the Child With Infectious Diseases

KEY TERMS

Airborne isolation—Precautions to prevent transmission of communicable disease particles that remain in the air for long periods of time and over wide distances.
Contact isolation—Precautions to prevent transmission of diseases that are communicable by direct contact with the pathogen.
Droplet isolation—Precautions to prevent transmission of diseases that are communicable when contaminated respiratory secretions come in contact with the respiratory tract or mucous membranes.
Koplik spots—White spots on the buccal mucosa.
Parotitis—Swelling of the parotid gland.
Prodrome—The early symptoms or precursors of disease.

I. Description

Historically, many children suffered from and succumbed to communicable diseases. Because of immunizations, the vast majority of the diseases are seen infrequently today. Indeed, smallpox has been eradicated from the world, and the wild form of polio has been eradicated from the United States as well as the rest of the Americas, Europe, and Eastern Pacific regions. Even though the incidence of the rest of the diseases is relatively small as compared to the incidence in the early half of the 20th century and before, it is important for nurses to be familiar with them. Even more essential, however, is the importance for nurses to be aware of the many vaccines available for children and the immunization schedule as recommended by the Advisory Committee on Immunization Practices (ACIP) (CDC, 2014), which was established as a result of an act by the U.S. Public Health Service.

II. Diseases

There are many communicable illnesses that children may acquire. Some (e.g., *Streptococcus pyogenes* pharyngitis [see Chapter 16] and rotavirus [see Chapter 14]) are discussed elsewhere in the text. This chapter primarily focuses on viral illnesses that result either in significant rashes or in bacterial illnesses that cause severe, life-threatening manifestations. Table 12.1 provides an easy format for accessing information about the diseases. It references the pathogen causing the disease, the classic manifestations of the disease, the site of the infection, the incubation period of the illness, the communicability of the illness, major complications that may develop, and the medical management and the nursing management. In some cases, a picture of a patient with the rash is included.

A. Isolation: isolation practices as developed by the Centers for Disease Control and Prevention (CDC) are required when caring for children with many of the diseases.
   1. Standard Precautions: at all times, health-care providers are expected to perform basic infection control measures that prevent the transmission of infectious organisms between patients and themselves. The cornerstone of standard precautions is hand hygiene. Wearing gloves,

gowns, masks, and eye protection and engaging in needle safety are aspects of the precautions. For a full discussion of the guidelines see www.cdc.gov/hicpac/2007ip/2007ip_table4.html.

2. **Contact isolation:** to prevent the transmission of diseases that are communicable by direct contact with the pathogen.
    a. The child must be placed in a single-patient room or, only if a private room is not available, cohorted with other children with the same disease.
    b. Health-care practitioners must wear gown and gloves when providing care to the child.
    c. Special ventilation in the room is not required.
3. **Droplet isolation:** to prevent the transmission of diseases that are communicable when contaminated respiratory secretions come in contact with the respiratory tract or mucous membranes.
    a. The child must be placed in a single-patient room or, only if a private room is not available, cohorted with other children with the same disease.
    b. Health-care practitioners must wear a standard operating room mask when entering the patient's room.
    c. If the child must be transported out of the room, he or she must wear a standard operating room mask.
    d. Special ventilation in the room is not required.
4. **Airborne isolation:** to prevent the transmission of communicable disease particles that remain in the air for long periods of time and over wide distances.
    a. The child must be placed in a single-patient room with the door closed.
    b. Health-care practitioners must wear a special N95 mask or respirator. This type of mask filters at least 95% of the contagious particles of the air breathed in by the practitioner. Special education is required to learn how to don the masks.
    c. If the child must be transported out of the room, he or she must wear a standard operating room mask.
    d. Special ventilation, with multiple air exchanges per hour, is required.
5. For additional information, see CDC Isolation Guidelines at www.cdc.gov/hicpac/pdf/isolation/Isolation2007.pdf.

B. Immunizations (vaccines): a number of vaccines are available to prevent childhood communicable diseases.

1. ACIP: each year, the members of ACIP consult with each other to determine whether the immunization schedule should be altered, including changing the ages when the vaccines should be administered, adding new vaccines to the schedule, and/or other recommendations (e.g., combining vaccines into one injection).
    a. The most up-to-date schedule is available for easy download from the CDC Web site, www.cdc.gov/vaccines/schedules/hcp/child-adolescent.html.
    b. Also available on the CDC Web site is a list of contraindications and precautions for the administration of some of the vaccines (www.cdc.gov/vaccines/recs/vac-admin/contraindications-vacc.htm).
2. Immunizations in the ACIP-recommended schedule for 2014 are:
    a. Hepatitis B (HepB)—administered in a three-dose series.
        i. Minimum age for first injection: birth.
    b. Rotavirus (RV).
        i. Available in two oral forms.
            (1) RV1: trade name Rotarix, which is administered in a two-dose series.
            (2) RV5: trade name RotaTeq, which is administered in a three-dose series.
        ii. Minimum age for first administration: 6 weeks.
    c. Diphtheria, tetanus, and acellular pertussis (DTaP)—administered in a five-dose series.
        i. A combination vaccine containing diphtheria, tetanus, and acellular pertussis vaccines.
        ii. Minimum age for first injection: 6 weeks.
        iii. This form of the vaccine is recommended for children under 7 years of age.
    d. Tetanus, diphtheria, and acellular pertussis (Tdap).
        i. Same vaccines as DTaP, but this form of the immunization is administered to children (and adults) 10 years of age and older.
            (1) Once the Tdap has been administered, adults should receive booster vaccines of tetanus and diphtheria toxoids every 10 years.
        ii. Available in two forms: trade names Boostrix and Adacel.
        iii. Minimum age for first injections: 10 years for Boostrix, 11 years for Adacel.

DID YOU KNOW?

Because infants under 6 months of age are not fully immunized against pertussis (whooping cough), until they receive the third injection, the CDC recommends that all pregnant women, irrespective

MAKING THE CONNECTION

It is important to distinguish between *Hemophilus influenza* type b (*H. flu)* and influenza. They are two distinct organisms that cause different illnesses. *H. flu* is a bacterium that causes many illnesses, including otitis media, pneumonia, and meningitis. Influenza is caused by a virus and is typically referred to as the flu. The vaccines for these illnesses, therefore, are also different (see Table 12.1).

of their previous immunization history, should receive the Tdap vaccine between 27 and 36 weeks' gestation. In addition, it is recommended that all family members—including teenage relatives, fathers, grandparents, and all other caregivers—receive the vaccine at least 2 weeks before coming into direct contact with young infants.

e. *Hemophilus influenzae* type b (Hib).
   i. Available in a number of forms.
      (1) Depending on the form of the vaccine, Hib is administered in either a three- or a four-dose series.
   ii. Minimum age for first injection: 6 weeks.
f. Pneumococcal conjugate vaccine (PCV)—administered in a four-dose series.
   i. Minimum age for first injection: 6 weeks.
g. Inactivated poliovirus vaccine (IPV)—administered in a four-dose series.
   i. Minimum age for first injection: 6 weeks.
h. Influenza vaccines—administered yearly beginning at 6 months of age.
   i. Inactivated influenza vaccine (IIV) may be administered to any aged child once the child reaches 6 months of age.
   ii. Live, attenuated influenza vaccine (LAIV) may be administered only to healthy children 2 years and older (and to healthy adults up to 49 years of age).
i. Measles, mumps, rubella (MMR)—administered in a two-dose series.
   i. A combination vaccine containing measles, mumps, and rubella vaccines.
   ii. Minimum age for first injection: 12 months.
   iii. It is important to note that, because of the rubella vaccine's teratogenicity, women who receive this immunization must use an excellent form of birth control for 4 weeks following the injection.
j. Varicella (VAR)—administered in a two-dose series.
   i. Minimum age for first injection: 12 months.
k. Hepatitis A (HepA)—administered in a two-dose series.
   i. Minimum age for first injection: 12 months.
l. Human papillomavirus (HPV) vaccines—administered in a three-dose series.
   i. There are two forms of the HPV vaccine.
      (1) HPV4: trade name Gardasil, may be administered either to males or females.
      (2) HPV2: trade name Cervarix, may only be administered to females.
   ii. Minimum age for first injection: 9 years for both forms.
m. Meningococcal conjugate vaccines (MCV)—administered in a two-dose series.
   i. There are three forms of the MCV vaccine.
      (1) Minimum ages for first injection
         (a) Six weeks for Hib-MenCY.
         (b) Nine months for MCV4-D: trade name Menactra.
         (c) Two years for MCV4-CRM: trade name Menveo.

3. To reduce the number of injections a child receives, some vaccinations have been combined. Whenever a child must receive more than one vaccination, the nurse should determine the availability of combined forms.

C. Mandated reporting.
1. Every state in the United States has a list of diseases that licensed health-care providers must report to the health department.
   a. Mandatory written reporting: some states require certain diseases to be reported in writing.
   b. Mandatory telephone reporting: some states require certain diseases to be reported via telephone.

It is the responsibility of each licensed health-care provider to know the legal requirements in his or her state and to respond accordingly.

D. Reye syndrome (see Chapter 22, "Nursing Care of the Child With Neurological Problems").
1. It is important to remind parents that aspirin is contraindicated for children suffering from viral illnesses because of the potential for them to develop Reye syndrome.
2. The two viral illnesses that place children at most high risk for Reye syndrome are influenza and chickenpox.

Table 12.1 Children's Communicable Illnesses, Viral and Bacterial

Diseases Listed in the Same Order as They Appear on the ACIP Immunization Schedule

Disease (Common Name)/Pathogen	Classic Signs and Symptoms	Site of Transmission of the Infection
Hepatitis B **Hepatitis B virus (HBV)** *Blood-borne and sexually transmitted infection*	*Signs and symptoms can range from complete absence of symptoms to marked response, including flu-like symptoms, severe jaundice, clay-colored stools, and dark-colored urine.*	*Introduction of the virus into the body via mucous membranes or skin wound, e.g., via contaminated needles, during sexual intercourse, and via vertical transmission.* *Virus is in its highest concentration in the blood of an affected individual, but the virus can be found in all bodily fluids.* *Some individuals who have recovered from the acute illness will continue to carry the antigen (HBsAg+) in their blood and be able to transmit the disease.* *Virus can live on inanimate surfaces for up to 7 days.*
Diphtheria ***Corynebacterium diphtheria* (gram positive bacillus)** 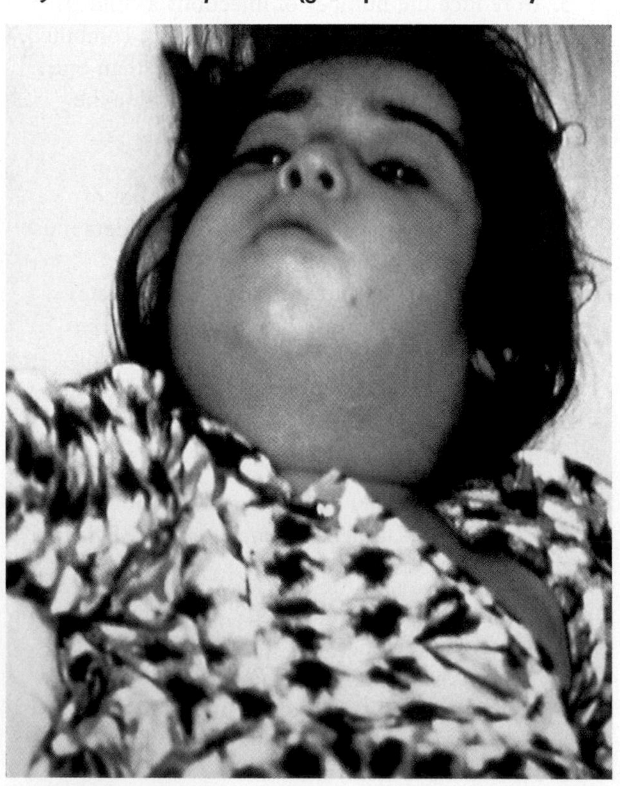	*Initially, sore throat, fever, and chills.* *Eventually, a toxin is produced by the bacteria that results in a grayish-blue membrane at the back of the throat that may cover the trachea, resulting in respiratory compromise, including stridor and bull neck (markedly edematous neck).*	*Discharge from respiratory tract of infected persons.*

Incubation Period	Communicability	Complications	Treatments	Nursing Considerations*
6 weeks to 6 months, with an average of 90 days.	*An individual is communicable once the virus is active in the body.*	*Cirrhosis, liver failure, and hepatocarcinoma.* *Complications occur in up to 90% of affected infants and 50% of children under 5 years of age.*	*Prevention: HepB vaccine.* *To prevent chronic illness in children whose mothers' are HBsAG+, newborns should receive the first dose of the HepB vaccine plus an injection of Hepatitis B immune globulin (HBIG) within 12 hours of delivery. (The injections should be administered in different thighs.)* *The remaining HepB injections should be administered at 1 month and 6 months of age.* *Treatment: postexposure prophylaxis—HBIG.* *Antiviral therapies are available for the acute illness.*	*Educate parents regarding the importance of vaccination.* *Administer antiviral medication, as ordered.* *Maintain bedrest and reduced activity, as needed.* *Monitor liver function tests.* *Educate parents and child, if appropriate, regarding communicability, if chronic antigen carrier, including via vertical transmission.*
2–5 days, with a range of 1–10 days.	*Until bacilli are absent from cultures on three separate occasions (usually over 2–4 weeks).*	*Toxin may also result in cardiac and neurological complications, including heart failure and paralysis.* *Death occurs in 10%–20% of cases.*	*Prevention: D portion of the DTaP and Tdap immunizations.* *Treatment: diphtheria antitoxin (DAT), which can be obtained only from CDC.* *Antibiotics: patients are usually no longer contagious once on antibiotics for 2 full days.*	*Droplet Isolation* *Administer IV DAT and antibiotics, per order.* *Monitor respiratory function.* *Provide humidified oxygen, per order.* *Suction, as needed. Maintain bedrest.* *Have emergency equipment available.*

Continued

Table 12.1 Children's Communicable Illnesses, Viral and Bacterial *cont'd*

Disease (Common Name)/Pathogen	Classic Signs and Symptoms	Site of Transmission of the Infection
Tetanus (Lockjaw) ***Clostridium tetani*** **(anaerobic bacterium found everywhere in the environment)** 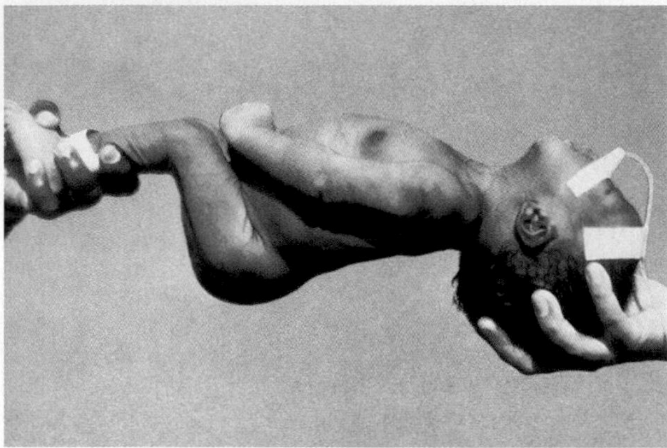	*Early symptoms: lockjaw, neck stiffness, and difficulty swallowing.* *Later symptoms: muscle spasms, seizures, dysrhythmias, and pulmonary emboli.*	*Dirt, animal bites, rusty objects, burns—transmitted when the bacterium is introduced deep into a wound.* *Neonatal tetanus may occur when the bacteria enter via the umbilical cord.*
Pertussis (Whooping Cough) ***Bordetella pertussis*** **(gram negative bacterium)**	*Bacteria attach to the cilia of the respiratory tract and produce a paralyzing toxin, resulting in marked inflammation of the tissues.* *Pertussis is a three-stage illness:* Catarrhal stage *Begins like an upper respiratory infection (e.g., coryza, sneezing, tearing, cough, and slight fever) that usually lasts for 1 to 1½ weeks.* Paroxysmal stage *Cough (usually at night) that starts short and rapid and culminates with inspirations that sound like "whoops."* *During coughs, child becomes flushed or cyanotic, eyes bulge, and tongue protrudes. Coughs often end when the patient vomits. The stage usually lasts for 1–6 weeks, with the shorter length usually seen in those having previously been vaccinated.* Convalescent stage *The patient slowly recovers, with coughing and paroxysms eventually fading. The stage lasts for 1 to 1½ weeks.*	*Discharge from respiratory tract of infected persons.*

Incubation Period	Communicability	Complications	Treatments	Nursing Considerations*
3–21 days (10 days, on average).	*None.*	*Laryngospasms, fractures, dysrhythmias. Death occurs in up to 20% of cases.*	*Prevention: T portion of the DTaP and Tdap immunizations. Treatment: human tetanus immune globulin (TIG) and antibiotics. Clean all wounds well, removing any foreign debris.*	*No special isolation requirements needed because not transmitted person to person. Administer TIG and antibiotics, as ordered. Provide IV fluids and nourishment. Maintain seizure precautions. Monitor for signs of airway obstruction. Have emergency equipment available.*
5–21 days (usually 10 days).	*Greatest during catarrhal stage, but, unless on antibiotics, communicability may last for 4 weeks from the onset of paroxysms.*	*Pneumothorax, pneumonia, otitis media, convulsions, hemorrhages (subarachnoid, subconjunctival, epistaxis), weight loss, dehydration, hernias, encephalopathy, fractured ribs, and prolapsed rectum. Death may occur, especially in children under 1 year of age.*	*Prevention: aP portion of the DTaP and Tdap immunizations. All pregnant women between 27 and 37 weeks' gestation and anyone who is to be in close contact with an infant should be immunized at least 2 weeks prior to the contact. Treatment: aggressive antibiotic therapy. CDC recommends that those, especially infants, who have been exposed to a known case of pertussis should receive prophylactic antibiotic therapy.*	*Maintain droplet isolation during catarrhal stage. Observe for signs of airway obstruction. Maintain bedrest, as needed. Decrease exposure to respiratory irritants (e.g., dust and smoke). Provide fluids, as ordered (e.g., IV and/or frequent, small amounts of oral fluids). Provide humidified oxygen, as ordered. Suction, as needed, to prevent choking. After discharge, visiting nurse service should monitor the child's progress. Monitor for signs of complications. Have emergency equipment available.*

Continued

Table 12.1 Children's Communicable Illnesses, Viral and Bacterial *cont'd*

Disease (Common Name)/Pathogen	Classic Signs and Symptoms	Site of Transmission of the Infection
Poliomyelitis (Polio) **Three types of poliovirus (enteroviruses)** 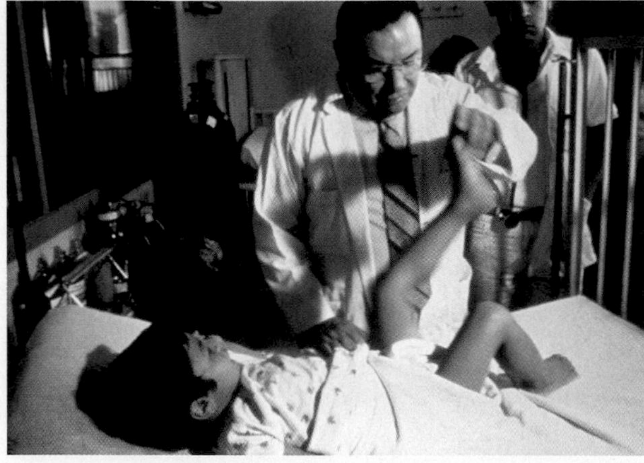	*Three different forms of the disease:* Abortive or Inapparent *Fever, sore throat, headache, anorexia, vomiting, and abdominal pain. May last for a few hours to a few days.* Nonparalytic *Same as abortive form, but the patient experiences more severe symptoms, with pain and stiffness in the neck, back, and legs.* Paralytic *Initially appears to be the same as the nonparalytic form, but ultimately the patient develops paralysis of the nerves, enervating major muscle groups resulting in, e.g., respiratory and/or limb paralysis.*	*Feces and oropharyngeal secretions of infected persons, especially young children.*
Influenza (Flu) **Variety of viruses**	*Influenza is a full-body illness characterized by any or all of the following symptoms: body aches, upper respiratory symptoms, fever, and sore throat. To distinguish the flu from other illnesses, specific testing must be performed (e.g., culturing, serologic assessments, or DNA analysis).*	*Secretions of the upper respiratory system are aerosolized during coughing and sneezing.*

Incubation Period	Communicability	Complications	Treatments	Nursing Considerations*
5–35 days (usually 7–14 days).	*Unknown exact period, but the virus is present in the throat (persists for about 1 week) and feces (persists for 4–6 weeks).*	*Persistent paralysis, respiratory arrest, hypertension, and kidney stones from demineralization of bone during prolonged immobility.* *Death may occur.*	*Prevention: IPV and oral poliovirus vaccine (OPV) (because the wild form of polio has been eradicated from the United States, OPV is no longer administered in the United States).* *Treatment: palliative care only, including assisted ventilation, if respiratory paralysis, and physical therapy following the acute stage.*	*Contact isolation.* *Monitor for signs of respiratory paralysis.* *Have tracheostomy and other emergency equipment at bedside.* *Maintain complete bedrest.* *Position patient to promote body alignment and to prevent contractures and decubiti.* *Administer analgesics and sedatives, as ordered.* *Assist with physiotherapy procedures, including moist hot packs and range of motion exercises.* *Tracheostomy tray at bedside, if needed.*
On average, the incubation period is 2 days long.	*One day before symptoms develop to about 5 days after the onset of symptoms.*	*Ear infections, sinus infections, bronchitis, and pneumonia.* *On average, approximately 35,000 individuals in the United States die from the flu each year.*	*Prevention: yearly, DNA-specific vaccinations.* *Treatment: once an accurate diagnosis is made, antiviral therapy may be administered.* *If a bacterial infection is suspected, the child may initially be prescribed antibiotics.*	*Maintain droplet isolation.* *Administer antiviral agents, antipyretics, and/or analgesics, as ordered and needed.* *Maintain bedrest, as needed.* *Encourage fluid intake, and monitor for signs of dehydration and imbalanced electrolytes.* *Monitor for signs of complications.* *Because of the potential for Reye syndrome, parents should be reminded never to administer aspirin to a child with the flu.*

Continued

Table 12.1 Children's Communicable Illnesses, Viral and Bacterial *cont'd*

Disease (Common Name)/Pathogen	Classic Signs and Symptoms	Site of Transmission of the Infection
Rubeola (Regular Measles) ***Morbillivirus*** 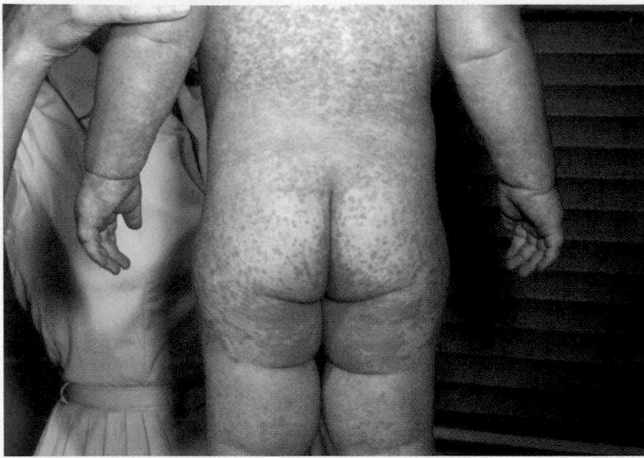	*Highly contagious virus.* ***Prodrome*** (symptoms that precede the disease): *fever, cough, runny nose, malaise, and conjunctivitis with photophobia.* *2–3 days later,* ***Koplik spots*** *appear (white spots on the buccal mucosa).* *Up to 5 days later, red or reddish-brown rash appears, beginning on the face and then progressively descending downward. During the rash phase, the temperature may rise to 104°F or higher.*	*Mucoid discharge of the nose and the mouth that is aerosolized when someone with measles coughs or sneezes.* *The virus can live on inanimate objects for up to 2 hours. Vertical transmission to the fetus may occur.*
Mumps **Type of rubulavirus** 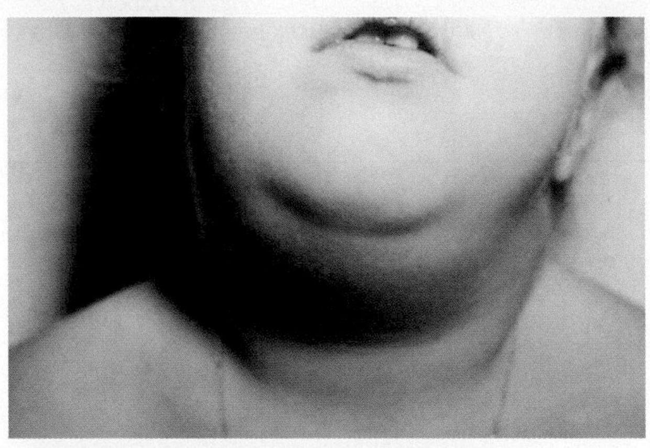	*Prodrome: fever, achiness, and malaise.* *After about a week,* ***parotitis*** *(swelling of the parotid gland)—may be unilateral, bilateral, or absent.*	*Discharge from respiratory tract of infected persons.* *Can be transmitted by contact with contaminated surfaces.*
Rubella (German Measles) ***Rubivirus*** 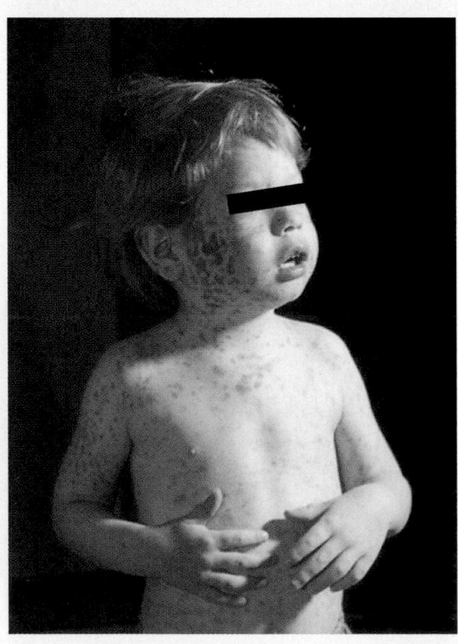	*Prodrome: 1–5 days, subsides 1 day after rash.* *Prodrome is often absent in children but present in adults and teens—fever, headache, malaise anorexia, conjunctivitis, coryza, sore throat, cough, and lymphadenopathy.* *Rash: discrete, pinkish-red maculopapular exanthema. First appears on face. Rapidly spreads downward to neck, arms, trunk, and legs.* *By end of the 1st day, body is covered. Usually lasts for only 3 days.*	*Primarily, nasopharyngeal secretions of infected person.* *Vertical transmission to unborn fetus.*

Incubation Period	Communicability	Complications	Treatments	Nursing Considerations*
7–18 days.	Patients are contagious from about 4 days before to 4 days after the rash appears.	Ear infections, diarrhea. Approximately 5% of patients develop pneumonia and 1/1000 develops encephalitis. Death occurs in about 1/1000 children. (measles kills about 1,000,000 children in developing countries each year). Can lead to miscarriage or preterm labor in pregnant woman.	Prevention: first M portion of the MMR vaccine. Treatment: immune globulin may be given prophylactically if a child is exposed to someone with rubeola. Age-specific doses of vitamin A should be administered to anyone with rubeola.	Practice airborne isolation. Administer antipyretics and vitamin A supplementation, as ordered. Dim lights and warm compresses to the eyes. Maintain bedrest, as needed. Monitor carefully for signs of complications: pneumonia and encephalitis.
16–18 days but may be as long as 25 days.	5 days before to 5 days after the appearance of swelling.	Orchitis in males (most commonly postpuberty—infertility is uncommon), inflammation of the ovaries or breasts, septic meningitis, encephalitis, deafness.	Prevention: second M portion of the MMR vaccine. Treatment: palliative care. If CNS involvement, hospitalization is often required.	Maintain droplet isolation. Provide child with nonirritating fluids (i.e., nonacidic liquids) and soft foods. Place ice or warming collar around the child's neck, whichever is more soothing. Maintain bedrest, especially if orchitis is present. Administer analgesics, as ordered and needed. Monitor carefully for signs of CNS involvement.
14 days with a range of 12–23 days.	7 days before to about 5 days after appearance of rash.	Most benign of all preventable childhood illnesses, with rare complications of arthritis, encephalitis, and purpura. Highly injurious to the unborn fetus, including cardiac defects, deafness, and congenital cataracts.	Prevention: R portion of the MMR vaccine. Treatment: palliative care.	Practice droplet isolation. Reassure parents of benign nature of illness in child. Provide comfort measures, as necessary and ordered, including antipyretics and analgesics. Advise parents to inform any pregnant women with whom the child has had contact.

Continued

Table 12.1 Children's Communicable Illnesses, Viral and Bacterial *cont'd*

Disease (Common Name)/Pathogen	Classic Signs and Symptoms	Site of Transmission of the Infection
Varicella (Chickenpox) ***Varicella zoster*** **(member of the herpes family)** 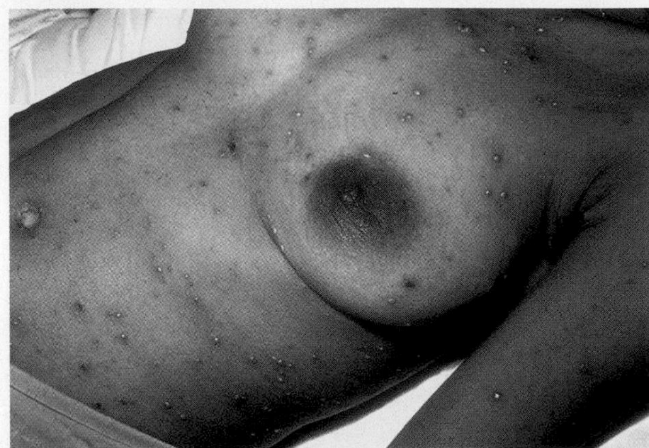 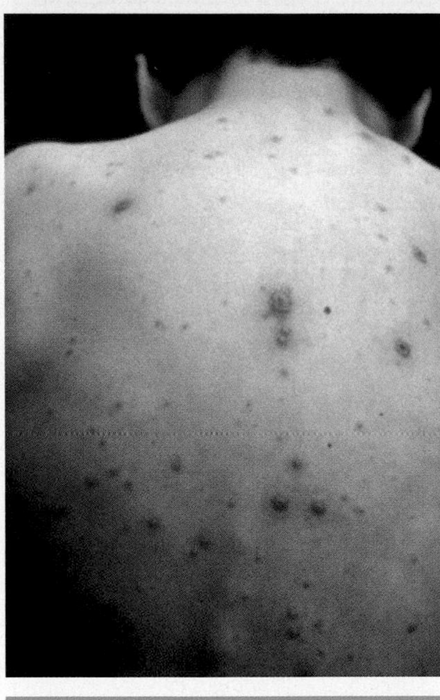	*Prodrome: fever, malaise, and anorexia—may be absent.* *Rash: four stages.* *All stages are eventually present simultaneously—macular, papular, vesicular, and crusted. Rash is highly pruritic and appears cephalopedally and from the chest and back outward to the extremities.*	*Infected respiratory secretions and skin lesions.* *Vertical transmission to the fetus may occur.*

Incubation Period	Communicability	Complications	Treatments	Nursing Considerations*
11–16 days (with a range of 10–21 days).	*Up to 2 days before rash appears until all lesions are fully crusted (about 1 week after outbreak begins).*	*Although rare, secondary bacterial infection, encephalitis, varicella pneumonia, hemorrhagic varicella, and thrombocytopenia.* *Shingles can occur at any time after chickenpox has resolved (herpes virus reactivates in the body).*	*Prevention: varicella vaccine.* *Treatment: VZIG, varicella zoster immune globulin, may be administered after exposure to infected person.* *Specific: usually palliative care. Acyclovir may be administered to immune-compromised or chronically ill children.* *Supportive: oatmeal baths, Benadryl (diphenhydramine).* *Aspirin is contraindicated.*	• *Airborne plus contact isolation.* • *If hospitalized, the nurse caring for the child should not care for any immunosuppressed children.* • *Trim fingernails and cover hands with white mittens to reduce itching and to prevent secondary infection.* • *Provide oatmeal baths/lotions, as needed.* • *Administer antihistamines, analgesics, and antipyretics, as ordered.* • *Because of the potential for Reye syndrome, parents should be reminded never to administer aspirin to a child with chickenpox.*

Continued

Table 12.1 Children's Communicable Illnesses, Viral and Bacterial *cont'd*

Disease (Common Name)/Pathogen	Classic Signs and Symptoms	Site of Transmission of the Infection
Hepatitis A ***Picornavirus* (RNA virus)**	*Flu-like symptoms (i.e., fever, anorexia, nausea, and abdominal pains) followed a few days later by jaundice.*	*Feces of infected individuals.*
Human Papillomavirus (HPV) **Many types of the human papillomavirus. Most common sexually transmitted infection in the United States.**	*Majority of those infected will exhibit no signs or symptoms.* *Depending on the strain of the virus, infected individuals can develop condylomata or warts.* *Other strains can alter the DNA of the cells and cause cancer.* *The changes are most frequently seen in the genital area, but they can also occur in the throat.*	*Sexual contact with infected individual.* *Also can be transmitted vertically from pregnant woman to her newborn during delivery.*
Meningococcal Disease ***Neisseria meningitidis* (bacteria)**	*Many individuals carry the bacteria as normal flora in their throats.* *Symptoms relate to the specific disease caused by the bacteria—pharyngitis, meningitis, and/or meningococcemia.*	*Direct contact with secretions of the respiratory tract of affected individuals.*

Incubation Period	Communicability	Complications	Treatments	Nursing Considerations*
28 days on average.	*Communicable for up to 2 weeks before appearance of symptoms.*	*Death rate in children is less than 1%.*	*Prevention: HepA vaccine.* *Cooking foods and drinks for at least 1 full minute to 185°F.* *Treatment: Postexposure immune globulin.* *Otherwise, palliative care only.*	*Maintain contact isolation for age-specific time frames.* *Educate parents in high-risk areas to heat all potentially contaminated foods and beverages.* *Monitor child carefully for signs of dehydration and/or altered electrolytes. (See Chapter 14, "Nursing Care of the Child With Gastrointestinal Problems.")* *Monitor liver function tests.*
Averages 2–3 months.	*Those with active infection are presumed to be highly communicable, but no specific information is available.*	*Warts in the throat that can lead to respiratory compromise.* *Cancer.*	*Prevention: HPV vaccine (because of the prevalence of HPV in the United States and to maximize the vaccine's effectiveness, it is recommended that boys and girls be immunized at 11 or 12 years of age).* *Treatment: Pap smears and/or HPV tests are performed to monitor for the presence of HPV.* *Medications and surgical procedures are available to treat either the warts or the cellular changes.*	*Educate parents and children regarding the prevalence of the virus and the importance of immunization.* *Educate older school-age children and teens regarding sexual transmitted infections, including the potential for infectivity from HPV during oral and rectal intercourse in addition to genital intercourse.*
Average incubation period is 4 days but may be as long as 10 days.	*About 7 days before symptoms appear to 1 full day following the initiation of antibiotic therapy.*	*Up to 15% of cases are fatal.*	*Prevention: MCV vaccine.* *Treatment: postexposure antibiotic prophylaxis.* *Antibiotic therapy.*	*Practice droplet isolation until the child has been on antibiotic therapy for a full 24 hours.* *If meningococcal disease is suspected, the child should be seen by the primary health-care provider as soon as possible.* *Administer IV antibiotics, as ordered.* *Administer antipyretics and analgesics, as needed and ordered. (See Chapter 16, "Nursing Care of the Child With Respiratory Illnesses" and Chapter 22, "Nursing Care of the Child With Neurological Problems.")*

Continued

Table 12.1 Children's Communicable Illnesses, Viral and Bacterial *cont'd*

Disease (Common Name)/Pathogen	Classic Signs and Symptoms	Site of Transmission of the Infection
Diseases for Which There Are No Immunizations		
Erythema Infectiosum (Fifth Disease) **Parvovirus B19** 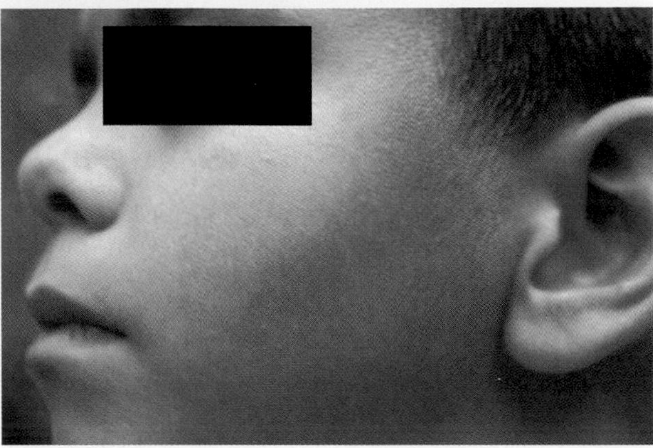	*Prodrome: mild feelings of malaise.* *Rash: bright-red rash on the cheeks that looks like the cheeks were slapped. A few days later, a rash may appear on the trunk that becomes lacy in appearance as it fades. The rash often intensifies in color when the child is warm or has been in the sun.*	*Multiple bodily fluids, including respiratory secretions and blood.*
Hepatitis C **Hepatitis C Virus (HCV)** *Blood-borne organism*	*Vast majority of individuals are asymptomatic until they develop serious liver involvement.*	*Introduction of the virus into the body via a break in the skin, e.g., via contaminated needles. Virus is in its highest concentration in the blood of an affected individual, but the virus can be found in other bodily fluids.* *Although not efficient, it can be transmitted sexually and individuals who are unaware that they are infected may transmit the disease. Vertical transmission is possible.*
Infectious Mononucleosis (Mono) **Epstein-Barr Virus**	*Prodrome: Non-specific flu-like symptoms, including fever, headache, sore throat, body aches, and nausea that may last up to 2 weeks.* *Following the prodrome: splenomegaly, lymphadenopathy, and hepatomegaly develop. Elevated liver enzymes with marked pharyngitis and fatigue are usually present. Some children will develop a maculopapular rash, especially if prescribed antibiotics.*	*Oral secretions. The herpes-like virus lies dormant in the body after resolution of the illness.*

Incubation Period	Communicability	Complications	Treatments	Nursing Considerations*
4–14 days but may be as long as 21 days.	*Unclear but likely during prodrome. Not communicable once the rash appears.*	*Joint pain in older children and adults, and chronic anemia in immune-compromised individuals.* *If a woman is pregnant, a small percentage of fetuses will become severely anemic, and fetal loss may result.*	*Prevention: none.* *Treatment: palliative care.*	*No isolation required.* *Administer analgesics, antipyretics, and antihistamines, as needed and ordered.* *Maintain bedrest, as needed.* *Trim fingernails and cover hands with white mittens to reduce itching and to prevent secondary infection.* *Provide oatmeal baths/ lotions, as needed.* *Educate parents to notify any pregnant women with whom the child has had contact.*
Within 3 weeks the virus is detectable seriologically.	*Up to 85% of HCV positive patients will develop liver infections and after many years up to 70% will develop liver disease, e.g., cirrhosis and hepatocarcinoma. Up to 5% of infected persons will die of their disease.*	*Persons are communicable once the virus is active in the blood.*	*Prevention: refrain from engaging in high-risk behaviors, especially intravenous drug use.* *Treatement: antiviral medications. (For the most recent recommendations see: http://hcvguidelines.org/.)*	*Administer antiviral medication, as ordered.* *Educate parents and child, if appropriate, regarding communicability, including possible vertical transmission.* *Monitor liver function tests.*
Approximately 1 to 2 months.	*Children usually become infected while drinking from the same bottle, while kissing, or engaging in other activities that result in a sharing of oral secretions. Children may shed the virus for many months after resolution of the illness.*	*Severe complications are rare, but include: ruptured spleen and respiratory compromise, if markedly enlarged tonsils.*	*Palliative care with activity restriction, until splenomegaly resolves.*	*Maintain bedrest and frequent rest periods, as needed.* *Provide antipyretics and analgesics for symptom relief.* *Maintain adequate hydration.* *Reinforce importance of activity restrictions for duration of the illness.* *Monitor liver function tests.* *Educate parents and child, if appropriate, regarding possible communicability of the virus.*

Continued

Table 12.1 Children's Communicable Illnesses, Viral and Bacterial *cont'd*

Disease (Common Name)/Pathogen	Classic Signs and Symptoms	Site of Transmission of the Infection
Roseola (Sixth Disease) ***Human herpesvirus 6***	*This illness is almost exclusively seen in older infants and toddlers.* *Prodrome: very sudden, very high fever (103°F and above) sometimes accompanied by minor upper respiratory or gastrointestinal symptoms. Because of the rapid rise, febrile seizures may be triggered.* *Rash: once the fever drops after about 5 days, rash appears. The erythematous, confluent rash usually is most prominent on the thorax. The rash blanches when the skin is compressed.*	*Upper respiratory secretions.*
Scarlet Fever (Scarlatina) ***Streptococcus pyogenes* (group A strep)**	*Prodrome: fever, vomiting, pharyngitis, and chills. Swollen tongue that starts with a white coating but changes to bright red.* *Markedly swollen tonsils also often are present.* *Rash: within 24 hours, a sunburn-like rash first appears on the face—often with a clear area around the mouth—then progresses to the body. The rash is usually much more prominent in the creases of the groin, underarms, and other such areas. After about a week, the rash desquamates.*	*Secretions from the respiratory tract of infected persons.*

Incubation Period	Communicability	Complications	Treatments	Nursing Considerations*
Approximately 9–10 days.	*Unclear but likely from beginning of prodrome to appearance of rash. Once the rash appears, the child is no longer contagious.*	*Febrile seizures. Rarely: encephalitis, hemiplegia, and cognitive changes.*	*Prevention: none. Treatment: palliative care. (See care of children with febrile seizures in Chapter 22, "Nursing Care of Child With Neurological Problems.").*	*Administer analgesics and antipyretics, as ordered and needed. Educate parents regarding care of the child with febrile seizures. Provide fluids and monitor child for dehydration.*
1–7 days.	*Communicable during the acute infection until the child has been on antibiotics for a full 24 hours.*	*Rheumatic fever (see Chapter 16, "Nursing Care of Child with Respiratory Illnesses") or acute glomerulonephritis (see Chapter 22, "Nursing Care of Child with Neurological Problems") may develop if the child is not treated with a full course of antibiotics..*	*Prevention: none. Treatment: once the bacteria have been identified, antibiotics are administered.*	*Maintain droplet isolation until the child has been on antibiotics for a full 24 hours. Administer antibiotics and educate parents to complete the full antibiotic course. Administer antipyretics and analgesics, as ordered and needed. Provide fluids and monitor for signs of dehydration. Maintain bedrest, as needed.*

*Unless otherwise noted, the nurse should follow Standard Precautions when caring for a child with the disease. When specific isolation precautions are cited, the nurse should follow both Standard Precautions and the isolation precautions.

CASE STUDY: Putting It All Together

4-year, 6-month-old Caucasian female

The child's mother accompanies the young girl to the pediatric clinic for a preschool physical assessment. The child is being seen 2 months before entering public kindergarten. The law in the state in which the child lives requires that the following immunization series be complete before entering school:

- *Diphtheria, tetanus, and acellular pertussis series (DTap)*
- *Inactivated poliovirus series (IPV)*
- *Measles, mumps, and rubella series (MMR)*
- *Varicella series (VAR)*
- *Hepatitis A series (HepA)*

Subjective Data

- Parent states that the child is entering kindergarten in 2 months

Objective Data

Nursing Assessment

- All physiological assessments are within normal limits
- All laboratory findings within normal limits
- When the nurse checks the child's immunization record, it is noted that the child must receive the following vaccines to be in compliance with the law:
  - One DTaP vaccine
  - One IPV vaccine
  - One MMR vaccine
  - One VAR vaccine
  - One HepA vaccine

Vital Signs

Temperature:	98.6°F
Heart rate:	98 bpm
Respiratory rate:	24 rpm
Blood pressure:	84/58 mm Hg
Body mass index:	24.1

Health-Care Provider's Orders

- Administer all required vaccines
- Complete immunization form and provide copy to the child's parents

CASE STUDY: Putting It All Together

cont'd

Case Study Questions

A. What *subjective* assessments indicate that this client is experiencing a potential health alteration?

1. ____________________

B. What *objective* assessments indicate that this client is experiencing a potential health alteration?

1. ____________________

C. After analyzing the data that has been collected, what **primary** nursing diagnosis should the nurse assign to this client?

1. ____________________

D. What interventions should the nurse plan and/or implement to meet this child's and his or her family's needs?

1. ____________________
2. ____________________
3. ____________________
4. ____________________
5. ____________________
6. ____________________
7. ____________________
8. ____________________
9. ____________________
10. ____________________
11. ____________________
12. ____________________
13. ____________________
14. ____________________
15. ____________________
16. ____________________

E. What client outcomes should the nurse evaluate regarding the effectiveness of the nursing interventions?

1. ____________________
2. ____________________

F. What physiological characteristics should the child exhibit before leaving for home?

1. ____________________

REVIEW QUESTIONS

1. A 1-year-old child is being seen in the pediatrician's office. The child is up to date on all immunizations. The mother asks, "Will my child need to receive any shots today?" Which of the following responses by the nurse is appropriate?
   1. "The measles, mumps, and rubella (MMR); varicella (VAR); and hepatitis A (HepA) vaccines are all given once children reach one year of age."
   2. "The last hepatitis B (HepB) vaccine is due to be administered."
   3. "Children's first influenza vaccination (IIV) is administered at one year of age, and it will be given again every year at this same time."
   4. "The rotavirus (RV) vaccine will be given today to prevent severe diarrhea."
2. The nurse advises a pregnant woman, 30 weeks' gestation, that she should receive a vaccine to protect the baby from a serious infectious disease. Which of the following explanations should the nurse provide the woman?
   1. "Receiving the *Hemophilus influenzae* type B (Hib) vaccine will help to protect the baby from developing meningitis."
   2. "You should receive the tetanus, diphtheria, and pertussis (Tdap) vaccine because babies are very susceptible to *Bordetella pertussis* bacteria that cause whooping cough."
   3. "You will receive the rotavirus (RV) vaccine because diarrheal illnesses are so life threatening to babies."
   4. "If you receive the meningococcal conjugate vaccine (MCV) today you will be preventing your baby from developing bacterial sepsis after delivery."
3. A 5-year-old child who has received no vaccinations is admitted to the pediatric unit with a diagnosis of diphtheria. Which of the following signs/symptoms would the nurse expect to see?
   1. Macular papular rash
   2. Markedly edematous neck
   3. Strawberry-red tongue
   4. Conjunctival hemorrhages
4. A school-age child, whose parents are accompanying him, has been admitted to the pediatric unit on droplet isolation. Which of the following should the nurse include in the admission information for the child?
   1. "It is important that you wear a face mask whenever you leave your room."
   2. "I know that it will be hard for you, but your parents can only stay in your room for fifteen minutes out of every hour."
   3. "You will hear a funny whooshing sound whenever the door to your room opens because the air is kept from going into the hallway."
   4. "Everyone who comes into your room will be wearing a cap, gown, and mask."
5. An unimmunized child with a serious puncture wound has been diagnosed with tetanus. Which of the following actions is critical for the unit charge nurse to perform?
   1. Check that the child is maintained on contact isolation.
   2. Reinforce the need to pad the side rails and headboard of the child's hospital bed.
   3. Assign only fully immunized nurses to care for the child.
   4. Order a hypothermia mattress and prescribed antiviral medications for the child.
6. The parent of an infant who is to receive an injection of the polio vaccine asks, "Why can't my child have the oral vaccine like I did as a child? I really don't want the baby to receive any more injections than are necessary." Which of the following responses would be appropriate for the nurse to give?
   1. "The oral vaccine has been found to be less effective than the injectable vaccine."
   2. "The baby will be protected from getting polio in a shorter period of time with the injectable vaccine."
   3. "The oral form of the vaccine is no longer being administered to children in our country."
   4. "It was discovered that many babies were being poorly immunized because they often spit out the bad tasting oral vaccine."
7. An 8-year-old, African immigrant is admitted to the pediatric unit with elevated viral titers for the poliovirus. For which of the following signs/symptoms should the nurse carefully monitor the child?
   1. Tinnitus
   2. Petechial rash
   3. Flank pain
   4. Bradypnea

8. A 10-year-old child, who has been positively diagnosed with influenza, is to be cared for at home by the child's parents. Which of the following client-care information should the nurse include in the teaching?
1. The child should be isolated from all susceptible contacts for 2 full weeks.
2. The entire 10-day course of antibiotics must be administered to the child.
3. If the child complains of a sore throat, the child should be seen in an emergency department.
4. Only acetaminophen should be administered to the child for pain or for febrile episodes.

9. A child, who has been diagnosed with rubeola, is being cared for at home. Which of the following actions should the nurse educate the parents to perform?
1. Keep the lights in the child's room dimmed.
2. Give the child oatmeal baths every 3 to 4 hours.
3. Administer calcium supplements every 12 hours.
4. Maintain the child on contact isolation for one week.

10. The parents of a boy who is diagnosed with mumps ask the nurse whether there is any special care that they should provide their child. Which of the following responses would be appropriate for the nurse to provide? **Select all that apply.**
1. Offer soft foods for the child to eat.
2. Encourage the child to drink citrus fruit juices each day.
3. Monitor the child carefully for signs of testicular discomfort.
4. Place an ice collar or warm compresses around the child's neck.
5. Administer ordered antihistamines for the full course of the disease.

11. The nurse reviewing the record of a woman who is planning to become pregnant notes that the woman is not immune to rubella. In addition to recommending that the client have the MMR (measles, mumps, rubella) vaccine, which of the following actions should the nurse take?
1. Educate the client that she will be fully immune to rubella one year after receiving the injection.
2. Advise the client that she should use birth control for 4 weeks after receiving the vaccine.
3. Inform the client that a baby born after she receives the vaccine will be immune to rubella.
4. Remind the client that she will need to receive 2 more injections of the vaccine during the next few months.

12. A nurse is educating a group of parents regarding ways to prevent disease in their home. Which of the following information should the nurse include regarding preventing the transmission of hepatitis A?
1. Cover mouths and noses when coughing or sneezing.
2. Protect family members from blood of affected individuals.
3. Wash all clothing and bedding and dry in a hot dryer.
4. Carefully wash all fresh fruits and vegetables before eating.

13. A parent asks the nurse, "Why should I have my child immunized for human papillomavirus (HPV) when my child is only 11 years old? Isn't it a sexually transmitted infection?" Which of the following responses by the nurse is appropriate?
1. "I agree with you. I will ask your child's pediatrician if the HPV vaccine could be delayed until she becomes sexually active."
2. "It is recommended that children begin the vaccine series when they are preteen so that they have time to develop full immunity."
3. "Although HPV is defined as a sexually transmitted disease, it can also be transmitted if a person with upper respiratory warts coughs or sneezes."
4. "I understand. It is important to realize though that the majority of people in this country are infected with the virus by the time they are in high school."

14. The mother of a child who has been prescribed antibiotics for a diagnosis of scarlet fever telephones the pediatrician's office and states, "My child's temperature is normal, and the rash is disappearing, but my child has enough antibiotics for another 5 days. Do I really have to give my child all of the antibiotics?" Which of the following responses by the nurse is appropriate?
1. "I will ask the doctor if you can stop because we are trying to keep from giving children too many antibiotics."
2. "Scarlet fever is actually caused by a virus, so you can stop administering your child's antibiotics right away."
3. "As long as your child's temperature remains normal for a full day, you can stop administering the antibiotics."
4. "It is important that you finish giving your child the antibiotics in order to prevent your child from developing a serious complication."

REVIEW ANSWERS

1. ANSWER: 1

Rationale:

1. This statement is correct.

2. The last HepB vaccine usually is administered at 6 months of age.

3. The first influenza vaccine is recommended to be administered at 6 months of age. The vaccine is administered yearly thereafter.

4. The RV vaccine is recommended to be administered at 2, 4, and 6 months of age.

TEST-TAKING TIP: Nurses who work in the pediatric area should be familiar with the recommended vaccination schedule. The schedule, which may change from year to year, can be found on the ACIP webpage on the Centers for Disease Control and Prevention (CDC) Web site, www.cdc.gov/vaccines/schedules/hcp/imz/child-adolescent.html.

Content Area: *Child Health, Immunizations*

Integrated Processes: *Nursing Process: Implementation; Teaching/Learning*

Client Need: *Health Promotion and Maintenance: Health Promotion/Disease Prevention*

Cognitive Level: *Application*

2. ANSWER: 2

Rationale:

1. The baby will receive the Hib vaccine at 2, 4, and 6 months of age. It is not administered to adults.

2. This statement is true. It is recommended that all pregnant women, no matter their previous immunization history, receive the Tdap vaccine between 27 and 36 weeks' gestation.

3. The RV vaccine is administered to babies at 2, 4, and 6 months of age. It is not administered to adults.

4. Although the MCV is administered to preteens and teenagers, it is not administered to pregnant women.

TEST-TAKING TIP: The incidence of pertussis outbreaks has increased in recent years, and the potential for complications and even death is relatively high in unimmunized infants. It is recommended, therefore, that pregnant women between 27 and 36 weeks' gestation as well as close family contacts, at least 2 weeks prior to the delivery of a newborn, be administered the Tdap vaccine.

Content Area: *Child Health, Immunizations*

Integrated Processes: *Nursing Process: Implementation; Teaching/Learning*

Client Need: *Health Promotion and Maintenance: Health Promotion/Disease Prevention*

Cognitive Level: *Application*

3. ANSWER: 2

Rationale:

1. There is no rash associated with a diagnosis of diphtheria.

2. Children with diphtheria often do present with a markedly edematous neck.

3. Strawberry-red tongue is not associated with a diagnosis of diphtheria.

4. Conjunctival hemorrhages are not associated with a diagnosis of diphtheria.

TEST-TAKING TIP: A toxin is produced by the bacteria that causes diphtheria, resulting in the development of a grayish-blue membrane at the back of the throat, that may cover the trachea and may result in a bull, or markedly edematous, neck.

Content Area: *Infectious Disease*

Integrated Processes: *Nursing Process: Assessment*

Client Need: *Physiological Integrity: Physiological Adaptation: Alteration in Body Systems*

Cognitive Level: *Application*

4. ANSWER: 1

Rationale:

1. This statement is true.

2. Parents may remain in the room with the child. They must wear a face mask while in the room.

3. Negative pressure rooms are not required for droplet isolation. A negative pressure room with multiple air exchanges per hour is required for a client on airborne isolation.

4. A mask is required for close contact with the patient. A cap and gown are not required.

TEST-TAKING TIP: If a child on droplet isolation must be transported to another part of the hospital, he or she must wear a surgical mask. The mask will prevent the droplet secretions from entering the environment and placing others at risk of infection.

Content Area: *Infectious Disease*

Integrated Processes: *Nursing Process: Implementation*

Client Need: *Physiological Integrity: Physiological Adaptation: Illness Management*

Cognitive Level: *Application*

5. ANSWER: 2

Rationale:

1. Because tetanus is not transmitted from human to human, no isolation is required.

2. The child is at high risk for seizures. The child's side rails and headboard should be padded.

3. Tetanus is not transmitted from human to human.

4. Tetanus is caused by bacteria, and hyperthermia is not a symptom of the disease.

TEST-TAKING TIP: Tetanus is a serious, potentially fatal illness. Symptoms of the disease are muscle spasms, seizures, dysrhythmias, and pulmonary emboli. Because of the potential for seizures, the child should be placed on seizure precautions.

Content Area: *Infectious Disease*

Integrated Processes: *Nursing Process: Implementation*

Client Need: *Physiological Integrity: Physiological Adaptation: Illness Management*

Cognitive Level: *Application*

6. ANSWER: 3

Rationale:

1. This statement is untrue. The oral vaccine actually is more effective than the injectable form.
2. This statement is untrue.
3. **This statement is correct. The oral form is no longer being administered in the United States.**
4. This statement is untrue.

TEST-TAKING TIP: The wild form of polio has been eradicated from the Americas, Europe, and other parts of the world. It is, however, still found in some developing countries. To protect children who could come in contact with an individual from another country who may be traveling in the United States and who may have polio, the CDC has recommended that children still receive the vaccine but no longer receive the live attenuated, or oral, form of the vaccine.

Content Area: *Child Health, Immunizations*
Integrated Processes: *Nursing Process: Implementation*
Client Need: *Health Promotion and Maintenance: Health Promotion/Disease Prevention*
Cognitive Level: *Application*

7. ANSWER: 4

Rationale:

1. Tinnitus is not associated with a diagnosis of polio.
2. Petechial rash is not associated with a diagnosis of polio.
3. Flank pain is not associated with a diagnosis of polio.
4. **Bradypnea may be evident in a child with polio.**

TEST-TAKING TIP: The paralytic form of the poliovirus can lead to paralysis of the respiratory tract and/or paralysis of other muscle systems of the body. A drop in the respiratory rate of a child could indicate that the child is developing respiratory paralysis.

Content Area: *Infectious Disease*
Integrated Processes: *Nursing Process: Implementation*
Client Need: *Physiological Integrity: Physiological Adaptation: Alteration in Body Systems*
Cognitive Level: *Application*

8. ANSWER: 4

Rationale:

1. This statement is not true. Communicability drops after a child has had symptoms for 5 days.
2. The flu is caused by a virus. Antibiotics are not effective against viral illnesses.
3. This statement is incorrect. Sore throat is an expected symptom of the flu.
4. **This statement is correct. Only acetaminophen should be administered as an antipyretic or as an analgesic.**

TEST-TAKING TIP: The two illnesses most associated with the development of Reye syndrome after being administered aspirin are the flu and chickenpox.

Content Area: *Infectious Disease*
Integrated Processes: *Nursing Process: Implementation; Teaching/Learning*
Client Need: *Physiological Integrity: Physiological Adaptation: Illness Management*
Cognitive Level: *Application*

9. ANSWER: 1

Rationale:

1. **This statement is correct. The lights in the child's room should be kept dimmed.**
2. Rubeola is not markedly pruritic. Oatmeal baths are not indicated.
3. This is incorrect. Vitamin A supplements are administered to those with rubeola.
4. This statement is incorrect. Airborne isolation is required for those with rubeola.

TEST-TAKING TIP: Conjunctivitis and photophobia are associated with a diagnosis of rubeola. Children are much more comfortable when they convalesce in a darkened room.

Content Area: *Infectious Disease*
Integrated Processes: *Nursing Process: Implementation; Teaching/Learning*
Client Need: *Physiological Integrity: Physiological Adaptation: Illness Management*
Cognitive Level: *Application*

10. ANSWER: 1, 3, and 4

Rationale:

1. **The child should be offered soft foods to eat.**
2. The child should not be encouraged to drink citrus fruit juices each day.
3. **The child should be monitored carefully for signs of testicular discomfort.**
4. **An ice collar or warm compress should be placed around the child's neck.**
5. Antihistamines are not administered to children diagnosed with the mumps.

TEST-TAKING TIP: Mumps, also called parotitis, is characterized by inflammation of the parotid gland. It can be quite painful for children with mumps to eat coarse foods or to drink acidic juices. Ice or warm compresses to the neck can be comforting. The child should determine which is more comforting.

Content Area: *Infectious Disease*
Integrated Processes: *Nursing Process: Implementation*
Client Need: *Physiological Integrity: Physiological Adaptation: Illness Management*
Cognitive Level: *Application*

11. ANSWER: 2

Rationale:

1. The woman will become immune to the disease in a shorter period of time
2. **This statement is correct. The client must be advised that she should use birth control for 4 full weeks after receiving the vaccine.**
3. This statement is not correct. The baby will receive passive antibodies from the mother via the placenta, but to become fully immunized, the baby will receive the MMR vaccines.
4. This statement is incorrect. The woman will receive up to two doses of the MMR vaccine.

TEST-TAKING TIP: Because the MMR vaccine is a live, attenuated vaccine, it is possible that a fetus can become ill from the virus via vertical transmission. The woman may become pregnant, with no danger to the fetus, once 4 weeks have passed from the date of the immunization.

Content Area: Child Health, Immunizations
Integrated Processes: Nursing Process: Implementation
Client Need: Health Promotion and Maintenance: Health Promotion/Disease Prevention
Cognitive Level: Application

12. ANSWER: 4
Rationale:
1. Although it is important for people to cover their mouths and noses when they cough or sneeze, hepatitis A is not transmitted via coughing or sneezing.
2. Although the blood of hepatitis B is highly infectious, protecting family members from the blood of individuals with hepatitis A will not protect them from the disease.
3. Washing all clothing and bedding and drying the items in a hot dryer will not protect susceptible individuals from contracting hepatitis A.
4. Carefully washing all fresh fruits and vegetables is one important action to protect susceptible individuals from contracting hepatitis A.
TEST-TAKING TIP: Hepatitis A is contracted via the oral-fecal route (i.e., ingesting foods or fluids that have been contaminated with the feces of an infected individual). Carefully washing fresh fruits and vegetables before eating is a means of preventing the virus from being ingested.
Content Area: Infectious Disease
Integrated Processes: Nursing Process: Implementation; Teaching/Learning
Client Need: Health Promotion and Maintenance: Health Promotion/Disease Prevention
Cognitive Level: Application

13. ANSWER: 2
Rationale:
1. It is inappropriate for the nurse to make this statement.
2. This statement is correct. It is recommended that children begin the vaccine series when they are preteens so that they have time to develop full immunity.
3. This statement is not true. HPV is transmitted only via direct contact.
4. This statement is not true. It is true, however, that 80% of women will be exposed to HPV by the time they are 50 years of age.
TEST-TAKING TIP: Three HPV vaccines must be administered over time in order for full immunity to be developed. In order for clients to become fully immunized before engaging in sexual relationships, it is recommended that boys and girls begin to receive the vaccine series at either 11 or 12 years of age.
Content Area: Child Health, Immunizations
Integrated Processes: Nursing Process: Implementation
Client Need: Health Promotion and Maintenance: Health Promotion/Disease Prevention
Cognitive Level: Application

14. ANSWER: 4
Rationale:
1. It would be inappropriate for the nurse to make this statement. The child must complete the full course of antibiotics.
2. This statement is incorrect. Scarlet fever is caused by *S. pyogenes.*
3. This statement is incorrect. The child must complete the full course of antibiotics.
4. This statement is correct. It is important that the child finish the entire course of antibiotics in order to prevent a serious complication.
TEST-TAKING TIP: If untreated or undertreated, patients with infections from *S. pyogenes* can develop one of two serious complications: rheumatic fever or acute glomerulonephritis. Parents should be counseled to make sure that their children complete the full course of prescribed antibiotics.
Content Area: Infectious Disease
Integrated Processes: Nursing Process: Implementation; Teaching/Learning
Client Need: Physiological Integrity: Physiological Adaptation: Illness Management
Cognitive Level: Application

Nursing Care of the Child With Fluid and Electrolyte Alterations

KEY TERMS

Aldosterone—A hormone that helps maintain fluid balance by stimulating the kidneys to retain sodium, decreasing urinary output.
Ascites—Excess fluid in the peritoneal cavity.
Hypercalcemia—Calcium excess greater than 10.2 mg/dL.
Hyperkalemia—Potassium excess greater than 5.0 mEq/L.
Hypernatremia—Sodium excess greater than 145 mEq/L.
Hyperreflexia—Overactive reflexes.
Hypertonic dehydration—Also called *hypernatremic dehydration.* When water loss exceeds sodium loss.
Hypocalcemia—Calcium depletion less than 8.5 mg/dL.
Hypokalemia—Potassium depletion less than 3.5 mEq/L.
Hyponatremia—Sodium depletion less than 135 mEq/L.
Hyporeflexia—Reduced response of the reflexes.
Hypotonic dehydration—Also called *hyponatremic dehydration.* When sodium loss exceeds water loss.
Isotonic dehydration—Also called *isonatremic dehydration.* An equal loss of both fluid and sodium.
Oliguria—Low urinary excretion.
Renin-angiotensin system (RAS)—The production of the hormones aldosterone and angiotensin to regulate blood pressure and fluid balance.
Tetany—Sudden, painful muscle contractions.

I. Description

Fluid, residing both within and outside of the body's cells, makes up the majority of the content of all individuals. Intracellular fluid (ICF), as the name implies, is housed within the confines of the body's cells. Extracellular fluid (ECF) resides in a number of locations, including the vascular tree, interstitial spaces, and spinal column. The body of adults as well as teenagers is comprised of 55% to 60% fluid. Seventy-five percent of the body of infants and young children and 60% to 65% of the body of preschoolers is comprised of fluid. Because the percentage of fluid is so high, especially in infants and young children, they are more at high risk for becoming dehydrated during periods of illness than are older children and adults.

Circulating within both the ICF and ECF are electrolytes, acids, and bases that are essential for the health and well-being of each individual. This chapter highlights the principles surrounding fluid, electrolyte, and acid-base balance, including specific information related to dehydration, edema, and acid-base imbalance. Illnesses that place children at highest risk for imbalance are discussed in other chapters. For example, diarrhea and vomiting that result in dehydration and electrolyte and acid-base imbalances are discussed in Chapter 14, "Nursing Care of the Child With Gastrointestinal Problems," while congestive heart failure that results in fluid volume overload is discussed in Chapter 17, "Nursing Care of the Child With Cardiovascular Illnesses."

II. Essentials of Water and Fluid Compartments in the Body (Table 13.1)

A. Total composition of the body that is water.
   1. 75% of the weight of infants/young children is fluid.
   2. 60% to 65% of the weight of preschool children is fluid.
   3. 55% to 60% of the weight of older children through adulthood is fluid.

B. ICF compartment.
   1. Percentage of fluid.
      a. Approximately the same in infants and young children as it is in older children through to adulthood.
      b. 35% of the weight of children and adults.

C. ECF compartment.
   1. Percentage of fluid.
      a. The percentage of fluid that resides in extracellular spaces is markedly different in young children than it is in older children through adulthood.
      b. 40% of infants' and young children's weight.
      c. 30% of preschool children's weight.
      d. 20% of older children's, adolescents', and adults' weight.

D. Daily fluid exchange.
   1. Each day there is an exchange of fluid in and out of the body.
      a. Fluid is lost via three main routes.
         i. Insensible loss via the lungs and skin.
         ii. Excreted loss via the kidneys.
         iii. Excreted loss via stool.

DID YOU KNOW?

Water is lost in the form of water vapor when it passes through the skin, called transepidermal diffusion, and during respiration. This type of loss is called insensible loss because it cannot be seen, felt, or easily measured. Insensible loss increases whenever the respiratory rate increases and when one perspires.

   2. Each day, the percentage of fluid that is exchanged in the body is markedly different between young children as it is in older children through adulthood.
      a. 50% of infants' and young children's fluid is exchanged per day.
      b. 16% to 17% of older children's through adults' fluid is exchanged per day.
   3. There is fluid movement between and among the ICF and ECF compartments.

E. Mechanisms in the body that help to maintain fluid balance in response to decreased fluid levels in the body.
   1. Thirst.
      a. Triggers an increase in fluid intake.
   2. Antidiuretic hormone (ADH).
      a. Produced by the posterior pituitary.
      b. Kidneys respond by decreasing urinary output.

Table 13.1 Fluid Composition Differences Between Infant/Young Child to Older Child/Adolescent

	Infant/Young Child	Older Child/Adolescent
Total percentage of body weight that is fluid	60%–75%	55%–60%
Percentage of body weight from fluid in intracellular spaces	35%	35%
Percentage of body weight from fluid in extracellular spaces	30%–40%	20%
Percentage of ECF that is exchanged each day	50%	16%–17%
Factors That Affect Fluid Loss	**Infant/Young Child**	**Older Child/Adolescent**
Respiratory rate (insensible loss)	Normal rate: 20–55 rpm	Normal rate: 15–22 rpm
Renal function	Concentrate urine poorly; retain electrolytes poorly	Concentrate urine effectively; retain electrolytes efficiently
Body surface area (including area of intestinal tract)	2 to 3 times the area of the older child or adolescent	Comparatively small

3. **Aldosterone.**
   a. Produced by the adrenal cortex.
   b. Kidneys respond by retaining sodium and, as a result, decreasing urinary output.
4. **Renin-angiotensin system (RAS).**
   a. Produced by the kidneys.
   b. Results in the production of aldosterone as well as angiotensin, a vasoconstrictor.

F. Factors that impact fluid balance.
1. Factors that place infants and young children at higher risk for fluid imbalance as compared to older children and adolescents.
   a. Body surface area (BSA)
      i. The BSA of infants and young children is two to three times the area of older children and adolescents.
      ii. BSA is composed of the surface of the gastrointestinal tract as well as the surface of the skin.
   b. Metabolic rate.
      i. An increased rate in infants and children is needed to support their rapid growth.
      ii. The increased metabolic rate is evidenced by the pulse and respiratory rates of infants and young children that are markedly faster than those of older children and adolescents.
   c. Immature renal system.
      i. Because of their inability to concentrate and dilute urine efficiently, the immature kidneys of infants and young children retain or excrete urine poorly in response to reduced or elevated fluid volumes.
   d. Fluid needs.
      i. Compared to older children and adolescents, infants and young children proportionately must consume larger quantities of fluids each day in order to maintain optimal fluid balance.
2. Important factors that increase fluid requirements and place children at high risk for dehydration.
   a. From insensible loss.
      i. Fever.
      ii. Tachypnea.
      iii. Phototherapy in neonates.
   b. From excretion.
      i. Vomiting.
      ii. Diarrhea.
      iii. Burns.
3. Important factors that may reduce children's daily fluid needs.
   a. Congestive heart failure (CHF) (see Chapter 17, "Nursing Care of the Child with Cardiovascular Illnesses").
   b. Increased intracranial pressure (ICP) (see Chapter 22, "Nursing Care of the Child with Neurological Problems").

Table 13.2 Concentration of Electrolytes in Fluid Compartments in the Body

Electrolyte	Extracellular Fluid (ECF)—Vascular Tree, Interstitial Space, Spinal Column	Intracellular Fluid (ICF)
Na+	High	Low
Cl–	High	Low
K+	Low	High
Ca++	Low	Moderate

III. Essentials of Electrolyte Composition

A. Sodium, chloride, potassium, and calcium.
1. Concentration of the electrolytes varies in the fluid compartments of the body (Table 13.2).
2. Because fluids of the body are comprised of water and electrolytes, any shift in water balance results in a shift in electrolyte balance.
3. Sodium: Na+.
   a. High concentrations in ECF spaces.
   b. Low concentrations in ICF spaces.
   c. Normal serum (extracellular) level is 135 to 145 mEq/L.
4. Chloride: Cl–.
   a. High concentrations in ECF spaces.
   b. Low concentrations in ICF spaces.
   c. Normal serum (extracellular) level: 98 to 106 mEq/L.

DID YOU KNOW?

Sodium (Na) and chloride (Cl) combine to form the salt compound (i.e., NaCl). The concentrations of sodium and chloride, therefore, are similar in the fluid compartments of the body. In addition, whenever a fluid shift occurs, patients usually will experience a shift in both sodium and chloride.

5. Potassium: K+.
   a. Low concentrations in ECF spaces.
   b. High concentrations in ICF spaces.
   c. Normal serum (extracellular) level is 3.5 to 5 mEq/L.
6. Calcium: Ca++
   a. Low concentrations in ECF spaces.
   b. Moderate concentrations in ICF spaces.
   c. Normal serum (extracellular) level is 8.5 to 10.2 mg/dL.

B. When concentrations of electrolytes change—usually in response to a depletion or excess of fluid—complications can result, for example:

1. Sodium excess, called **hypernatremia:** greater than 145 mEq/L.
   a. Intense thirst.
   b. **Oliguria**, i.e., low urinary output.
   c. Nausea and vomiting.
   d. Dry mucous membranes.
   e. If markedly elevated, disorientation and seizures.
2. Sodium depletion, called **hyponatremia**: less than 135 mEq/L.
   a. Muscle cramps.
   b. Rapid pulse.
   c. Hypotension.
   d. Weakness and dizziness.
3. Potassium excess, called **hyperkalemia:** greater than 5.0 mEq/L.
   a. Cardiac dysrhythmias.
   b. Muscle weakness.
   c. **Hyperreflexia**, i.e., overactive reflexes.
   d. Oliguria.
4. Potassium depletion, called **hypokalemia:** less than 3.5 mEq/L.
   a. Cardiac dysrhythmias.
   b. Muscle weakness.
   c. **Hyporeflexia.**
   d. Fatigue.
5. Calcium excess, called **hypercalcemia:** greater than 10.2 mg/dL.
   a. Bradycardia.
   b. Nausea and vomiting.
   c. Anorexia.
   d. Muscle weakness.
6. Calcium depletion, called **hypocalcemia:** less than 8.5 mg/dL.
   a. Muscle spasms and **tetany,** or sudden, painful contractions.
   b. Seizures.
   c. Hypotension.

C. Nursing considerations.

1. Risk for Imbalanced Fluid Volume.
   a. Assess fluid maintenance needs of the child (Box 13.1).
      i. Maintenance needs may change dramatically in times of fluid loss or fluid excess (see earlier).
   b. Administer fluids, oral and/or parenteral, per child's needs and per orders.
   c. Assess for signs of dehydration or fluid excess (see "Dehydration") and report, if present.
   d. Monitor laboratory values for deviations and report, if present.

Box 13.1 Determining a Child's Fluid Needs

Fluid needs of children are based on their respective weights. The nurse must, therefore, calculate the maintenance fluid needs of each child to make sure that the child is receiving his or her minimum required fluids per day. The formula for daily fluid maintenance takes into consideration the fact that infants and young children require more fluids per kilogram than do older children.

To calculate fluid maintenance:

If child weighs between 0 and 10 kg:
The child's fluid needs = 100 mL times the child's weight (in kg)

If child weighs between 10 and 20 kg:
The child's fluid needs = 1,000 mL (i.e., 100 mL times 10 kg) PLUS 50 mL times the child's weight that is OVER 10 kg

If child weighs over 20 kg:
The child's fluid needs = 1,500 mL (i.e., 100 mL times 10 kg plus 50 mL times 10 kg) PLUS 20 mL times the child's weight that is OVER 20 kg

Example 1

Fluid needs of an infant weighing 4.2 kg.
Because the infant weighs less than 10 kg, the entire weight of the infant is multiplied by 100 mL.

4.2 kg × 100 mL = 420 mL

To maintain his or her fluid balance, the infant must take in a minimum of 420 mL of fluid each day.

Example 2

Fluid needs of a young child weighing 12.5 kg.
Because the child weighs over 10 kg:
First, 10 kg is multiplied by 100 mL
Second, the remainder of the child's weight is multiplied by 50 mL
Third, the amounts are added together

10 kg × 100 mL = 1,000 mL

2.5 kg × 50 mL = 125 mL

1,000 + 125 = 1125 mL

To maintain his or her fluid balance, the young child must take in a minimum of 1,125 mL of fluid each day.

Example 3

Fluid needs of a child weighing 42 kg.
Because the child weighs over 20 kg:
First, 10 kg is multiplied by 100 mL
Second, 10 kg is multiplied by 50 mL
Third, the remainder of the child's weight is multiplied by 20 mL
Finally, the amounts are added together

10 kg × 100 mL = 1,000 mL

10 kg × 50 mL = 500 mL

22 kg × 20 mL = 440 mL

1,000 + 500 + 440 = 1,940 mL

To maintain his or her fluid balance, the child must take in a minimum of 1,940 mL of fluid each day.

IV. Dehydration

The large percentage of body weight that is fluid puts infants and young children at very high risk for fluid loss (i.e., for deficient fluid volume or dehydration).

A. Incidence.
1. Dehydration is a common acute problem in pediatrics.

B. Etiology and pathophysiology of types of dehydration.
1. **Isotonic dehydration** (also called isonatremic dehydration).
   a. When fluid loss and sodium loss are proportionate.
      i. No shift seen between contents of the ICF and ECF compartments.
   b. Commonly seen with minor vomiting and diarrheal illnesses.
2. **Hypotonic dehydration** (also called hyponatremic dehydration).
   a. When sodium loss exceeds the water loss.
      i. Shift of fluid seen from the ECF compartments to the ICF spaces, increasing the severity of the dehydration.
   b. Commonly seen with:
      i. Burns.
      ii. Renal disease.
      iii. Excessive vomiting and diarrhea.
      iv. Intravenous (IV) therapy when no electrolytes are added to the solution.
      v. Plain water given to children under 6 months of age.
3. **Hypertonic dehydration** (also called hypernatremic dehydration).
   a. When water loss exceeds sodium loss:
      i. Shift of fluid is seen from the ICF compartments to the ECF compartments.
      ii. Often, symptoms are delayed, but when they appear, they are very serious, with neurological symptoms usually being noted.
   b. Commonly seen with:
      i. IV therapy when concentrations of electrolytes are too high.
      ii. Tube feedings (or formula feedings) when concentrations of electrolytes are too high.

C. Diagnosis of severity of dehydration.
1. Best determined by calculating the percentage of weight loss (Box 13.2).
   a. Mild: 5% weight loss in infants and young children, 3% to 5% weight loss in older children and adolescents.
   b. Moderate: 5% to 9% weight loss in infants and young children, 6% to 8% weight loss in older children and adolescents.

Box 13.2 Calculating the Percentage of Weight Loss

To calculate percentage of weight loss, the nurse must subtract the child's current weight from the last recorded weight of the child. The remainder is then divided by the last recorded weight of the child and multiplied by 100.

$$\text{\% of weight loss} = \frac{\text{last recorded weight} - \text{current weight}}{\text{last recorded weight}} \times 100$$

Example 1

A child is admitted to the hospital with a diagnosis of dehydration. The child's last recorded weight was 37¼ lb. The child's current weight is 34½ lb. What is the child's percentage of weight loss?

$$\text{\% of weight loss} = \frac{37.25\text{ lb} - 34.5\text{ lb}}{37.25\text{ lb}} \times 100$$
$$= (2.75 \div 37.25) \times 100$$
$$= 0.074 \times 100$$
$$= 7.4\%\text{ weight loss}$$

Example 2

A baby is admitted to the hospital with dehydration. The child's last recorded weight was 4,572 g. The child's current weight is 4,112 g. What is the child's percentage of weight loss?

$$\text{\% of weight loss} = \frac{4{,}572\text{ g} - 4{,}112\text{ g}}{4{,}572\text{ g}} \times 100$$
$$= (460\text{ g} \div 4{,}572\text{ g}) \times 100$$
$$= 0.101 \times 100$$
$$= 10.1\%\text{ weight loss}$$

   c. Severe: 10% or more weight loss in infants and young children, 9% or more weight loss in older children and adolescents.
2. Dehydration is also determined by changes in physiological characteristics. The severity of the changes increases in relation to the severity of the dehydration (Table 13.3).
   a. Poor skin color.
   b. Reduced skin turgor.
   c. Drying of mucous membranes.
   d. Change in vital signs.
   e. Decrease in urinary output.
      i. But the volume of urinary output changes little in infants and young children.
   f. Increase in urine specific gravity.
      i. But the specific gravity changes little in infants and young children.
   g. Soft eyeballs.
   h. In infants, depressed anterior fontanels.

D. Treatment.
1. Oral rehydration therapy (ORT) (e.g., Pedialyte, Infalyte, and Rehydralyte).
   a. Contains water, sugar, sodium, potassium, chloride, and lactate.

Table 13.3 Signs and Symptoms of Dehydration

Age	Criterion	Mild	Moderate	Severe
Infant and young child	Percentage of weight loss	5%	5%–9%	10% or more
	Anterior fontanel	Normal	Slightly sunken	Sunken
Older child and teen	Percentage of weight loss	3%–5%	6%–8%	9% or more
All ages	Skin color	Pale	Gray	Mottled
	Skin turgor	Slightly reduced	Poor	Very poor
	Condition of mucous membranes	Dry	Very dry	Parched
	Tears	Present	Some	Absent
	Eyeballs	Normal	Slightly soft	Very soft
	Urinary output	Reduced	Oliguria	Marked oliguria
	Urine specific gravity	Normal or slightly elevated	Elevated	Marked elevation
	Hematocrit	Normal or slightly elevated	Elevated	Marked elevation
	Blood pressure	Normal	Slightly lowered	Lowered
	Heart rate	Normal or slightly elevated	Elevated	Rapid and thready
	Body temperature	Normal	Elevated	Lowered

Table 13.4 Composition of Commonly Used IV Fluids**

IV	Dextrose g/100 mL	Na+ mEq/L	K+ mEq/L	Cl– mEq/L	Bicarb mEq/L	Ca++ mEq/L
D_5W	5	—	—	—	—	—
NS (0.9%)	—	154	—	154	—	—
Ringer's	0–10	147	4	155.5	—	4
Lactated Ringer's	0–10	130	4	109	28	3

**Variations and combinations of IV fluids are also available. For example, ½ NS (0.45%), ⅓ NS (0.33%), ¼ NS (0.225%) often are administered to reduce the possibility of hypernatremia. Combinations D5NS, D5 ½ NS, D5 ⅓ NS, and D5 ¼ NS provide both calories and electrolytes.

b. Replaces fluids and electrolytes and provides some calories.

2. IV therapy.
   a. Specific fluid required is dependent on the type of dehydration, severity of the dehydration, and/or fluid and electrolyte needs (Table 13.4).

The primary health-care provider may order potassium chloride (KCl) to be added to a child's IV fluid. In 1999, the Joint Commission declared that KCl is a high-alert medication because of the serious complications that can arise from an overdose of the electrolyte. All IV solutions with potassium added, therefore, should be administered only if they have been premixed in the pharmacy. In addition, the nurse must always double check to make sure that the solution is labeled with the right percentage of potassium.

E. Nursing considerations.
3. Deficient Fluid Volume.
   a. Weigh child on admission and daily thereafter.
   b. Assess for signs of dehydration, including skin turgor, condition of mucous membranes, and presence of tears.
   c. Administer oral rehydration therapy and/or IV fluids, per orders.
   d. Monitor intake and output.
   e. Carefully monitor vital signs.
   f. Assess laboratory values.

V. Edema

A. Incidence.
1. Is seen as a symptom of some illnesses (e.g., CHF).

B. Etiology.
1. Related to the inability of the body to excrete excess fluids.

C. Pathophysiology.
1. Problems usually are present in the cardiovascular system, such as:
   a. Decrease in circulating protein, resulting in fluid movement from within the vascular tree to the interstitial spaces.
   b. Failure of the heart to pump efficiently, resulting in:
      i. Pulmonary edema from left-sided failure.

ii. **Ascites** (excess fluid in the peritoneal cavity) from right-sided failure.

c. Excess fluid administration, resulting in fluid overload.

d. Local edema resulting from capillary damage.

e. Excess sodium retention, resulting in fluid retention.

2. Obstruction in the lymphatic system.

D. Diagnosis.

1. In infants, bulging fontanel.
2. Increase in weight above normal.
3. To assess for ascites.
   a. Assess for an increase in the circumference of the abdomen.
4. To assess for pulmonary edema:
   a. Auscultate for presence of rales, rhonchi, and/or crackles.
   b. X-ray.
5. To assess for local edema, with the thumb or first two fingers, press tissue against a solid bony surface (e.g., press down on the anterior surface of the lower leg).
   a. The deeper the indent, the worse the edema.
   b. Degree of edema is based on measurement of indented tissue.
      i. +1 edema: when tissue is pressed in a maximum of 2 mm.
      ii. +2 edema: when tissue is pressed in a maximum of 4 mm.
      iii. +3 edema: when tissue is pressed in a maximum of 6 mm.
      iv. +4 edema: when tissue is pressed in 8 mm or more.

E. Treatment: dependent on the pathophysiology.

F. Nursing considerations.

1. Excess Fluid Volume.
   a. Weigh child on admission and daily thereafter.
   b. Monitor intake and output.
   c. Carefully monitor vital signs.
   d. Auscultate lung fields, and report any adventitious sounds.
   e. Assess laboratory values, including serum protein and urinary protein.
   f. If appropriate, measure abdominal circumference on admission and daily thereafter.
   g. If appropriate, assess areas of local edema using the four-point scale.

VI. Factors Related to Acid-Base Balance

A. Incidence.

1. Change in a child's arterial pH occurs relatively frequently, especially in infants and young children.

B. Etiology and pathophysiology.

1. Normal functioning.
   a. Factors (with normal values) that can impact acid-base balance.
      i. Po_2: 80 to 100 mm Hg.
         (1) Less than 80 mm Hg: hypoxemia.
      ii. Pco_2: 35 to 45 mm Hg.
         (1) Less than 35 mm Hg: alkalosis.
         (2) Greater than 45 mm Hg: acidosis.
      iii. HCO_3: 22 to 26 mEq/L.
         (1) Less than 22 mEq/L: acidosis.
         (2) Greater than 26 mEq/L: alkalosis.
      iv. pH: 7.35 to 7.45.
         (1) Less than 7.35: acidosis.
         (2) Greater than 7.45: alkalosis.
      v. Base excess: ±2.
         (1) Less than −2: acidosis.
         (2) Greater than +2: alkalosis.
   b. Compensatory factors that enable the healthy individual to stay in normal acid-base balance.
      i. Based on the numbers of positive (acidic) hydrogen ions in relation to the negative (alkaline) bicarbonate ions that are circulating in the blood.
      ii. When the body becomes either acidotic or alkalotic, compensatory responses occur to try to move the body back into acid-base balance.
      iii. If the body remains either acidotic or alkalotic for a long period of time, compensatory responses are incapable of moving the body back into balance, resulting in severe illness and possible death.
2. Acid-base imbalances develop as a result of four main causes.
   a. Respiratory acidosis.
      i. Develops as a result of poor pulmonary function, resulting in retention of carbon dioxide.
      ii. When carbon dioxide dissolves in liquid (i.e., the serum), carbonic acid results. The higher the concentration of carbonic acid, the lower the pH.
      iii. In an attempt to compensate for the acidosis, the kidneys can retain plasma bicarbonate and excrete hydrogen ions.
   b. Respiratory alkalosis.
      i. Develops when the respiratory rate increases (i.e., the child hyperventilates), resulting in high levels of carbon dioxide being exhaled.
      ii. Because of the reduced levels of carbon dioxide, the concentration of carbonic acid

in the blood drops, and the pH of the blood rises.

iii. In an attempt to compensate for the alkalosis, the body responds by temporarily decreasing bicarbonate concentrations. The action stabilizes the pH.

c. Metabolic acidosis.
   i. Develops as a result of excess loss of bicarbonate from the body, for example via diarrhea stools.
   ii. Because of the loss of the base from the body, an acidic environment results.
   iii. In an attempt to compensate for the acidosis, the volume of exhalation increases, leading to increased carbon dioxide exhalation and a decrease in circulating carbonic acid.
d. Metabolic alkalosis.
   i. Develops as a result of loss of acid, often acid in the stomach from vomiting.
   ii. Because of the loss of acid from the body, an excess of bicarbonate results.
   iii. In an attempt to compensate for the alkalosis, the respiratory rate and volume of each exhalation decreases, leading to retention of carbon dioxide and an increase in circulating carbonic acid.

3. Additional factors that affect acid-base balance.
   a. Oxygen saturation levels.
      i. During periods of acidosis:
         (1) Hemoglobin is less able to combine with oxygen, resulting in a drop in oxygen saturation levels.
         (2) However, oxygen is released to the tissues more readily.
      ii. During periods of alkalosis:
         (1) Hemoglobin combines with oxygen more readily, increasing oxygen saturation levels.
         (2) However, oxygen is released poorly to the tissues.
   b. Pulmonic function.
      i. During periods of acidosis, pulmonary circulation is reduced.
      ii. During periods of alkalosis, pulmonary circulation is promoted.

C. Diagnosis.

1. There are four steps that the practitioner should perform when analyzing a patient's blood gases in relation to his or her clinical picture and history.
   a. Step one.
      i. Check the pH.
         (1) Determine whether normal, acidic, or alkaline.
   b. Step two.
      i. Check the P_{CO_2} level.
      ii. Determine whether it is normal, acidotic, or alkalotic.
         (1) If high, acidotic.
         (2) If low, alkalotic.
   c. Step three.
      i. Check the HCO_3 level.
      ii. Determine whether it is normal, acidotic, or alkalotic.
         (1) If high, alkalotic.
         (2) If low, acidotic.
   d. Step four.
      i. Using the acronym ROME (respiratory opposite/ metabolic equal), compare the P_{CO_2} level with the pH to distinguish which is the cause of the deviation and which is the compensatory effect.
         (1) When the pCO_2 and pH are in opposite directions, i.e., either the pCO_2 is high and the pH is low OR vice versa—the cause of the problem is respiratory.
         (2) When both the pCO_2 and the pH are either high or low, the cause of the problem is metabolic.
      ii. Low pH, acidotic.
         (1) **Respiratory acidosis**—High P_{CO_2} (cause). If the HCO_3 is high, it is a compensatory response.
            (a) A low P_{O_2} (an hypoxic state) helps to confirm respiratory acidosis.
         (2) **Metabolic acidosis**—Low HCO_3 (cause). If the P_{CO_2} is low, it is a compensatory response.
      iii. High pH: alkalotic.
         (1) **Respiratory alkalosis**—Low P_{CO_2} (cause). If the HCO_3 is low, it is a compensatory response.
         (2) **Metabolic alkalosis**—High HCO_3 (cause). If the P_{CO_2} is high, it is a compensatory response.

D. Treatment: dependent on the etiology of the disturbance.

1. Respiratory acidosis.
   a. Treatment of the underlying respiratory illness (e.g., asthma) (see Chapter 16, "Nursing Care of the Child With Respiratory Illnesses").
   b. Treatment examples: bronchodilators and oxygen.
2. Respiratory alkalosis.
   a. Treatment of the underlying respiratory problem (e.g., hyperventilation).

b. A common therapy: rebreathing carbon dioxide by placing a paper bag over the mouth and nose.

3. Metabolic acidosis.
   a. Treatment of the underlying metabolic illness.
      i. Diarrhea: (see Chapter 14, "Nursing Care of the Child With Gastrointestinal Problems").
      ii. Diabetic ketoacidosis: (see Chapter 21, "Nursing Care of the Child With Endocrine Disorders").
   b. Treatment examples.
      i. For diarrhea, ORT and IV fluids.
      ii. For diabetic ketoacidosis, insulin and IV fluids.
4. Metabolic alkalosis.
   a. Treatment of the underlying metabolic illness (e.g., prolonged vomiting) (see Chapter 14, "Nursing Care of the Child With Gastrointestinal Problems").
   b. Treatment examples: ORT and IV fluids.

E. Nursing considerations: dependent on the etiology of the disturbance.
1. Risk for Injury.
   a. Carefully analyze arterial blood gas results, and report abnormal findings.
   b. Administer appropriate therapy, as needed and/or as prescribed.

CASE STUDY: Putting It All Together

6-year, 6-month-old female, Caucasian, in hospital pre-op for a tonsillectomy

Subjective Data

- IV, 1000 mL D_5NS, inserted 30 min ago. At that time, there were no infusion pumps available. Tubing delivering 10 gtt/mL used, and drip rate set at a KVO (keep vein open) rate of 8 gtt/min.
- Mother rings the call bell. When the nurse enters the room, the mother states,
  - "My daughter seems to be having trouble breathing."

Objective Data

Nursing Assessments

- 30 mL of solution remaining in IV bag
- Physical findings
  - Child sitting erect in bed, gasping for air
  - Eyes wide open, appears anxious
  - Pulmonary wheeze heard on auscultation

Vital Signs

Temperature:	98.7°F
Heart rate:	126 bpm (bounding)
Respiratory rate:	36 rpm
Blood pressure:	118/78 mm Hg
Oxygen saturation:	90%

Lab Results

Stat electrolytes

Sodium:	145 mEq/L
Potassium:	3.5 mEq/L

Blood gases:
- PO_2 70 mm Hg
- PCO_2 50 mm Hg
- HCO_3 27 mEq/L
- Base excess: -3
- pH: 7.30

- Weight 18 kg on admission

Health-Care Provider's Orders

- Diagnosis: fluid volume overload/pulmonary edema
- Cancel surgery
- Bedrest with the head of the bed elevated.
- NPO
- Oxygen via cannula at 2 L/min
- Lasix 15 mg IV STAT (recommended dosage: 0.5–2 mg/kg IM/IV every 6–12 hr; start: 1 mg/kg IM/IV x1).
- Infuse IV solution via IV pump at 10 mL/hr
- Monitor vital signs every 15 min
- Monitor oxygen saturation every 15 min
- Repeat blood gases in 1 hr
- Repeat electrolytes in 12 hr

Continued

CASE STUDY: Putting It All Together *cont'd*

Case Study Questions

A. What *subjective* assessments indicate that this client is experiencing a health alteration?

1. __________
2. __________

B. What *objective* assessments indicate that this client is experiencing a health alteration?

1. __________
2. __________
3. __________
4. __________
5. __________
6. __________
7. __________
8. __________

C. After analyzing the data that has been collected, what **primary** nursing diagnosis should the nurse assign to this client?

1. __________

D. What interventions should the nurse plan and/or implement to meet this child's and her family's needs?

1. __________
2. __________
3. __________
4. __________
5. __________
6. __________
7. __________
8. __________
9. __________
10. __________

CASE STUDY: Putting It All Together *cont'd*

Case Study Question

E. What client outcomes should the nurse evaluate regarding the effectiveness of the nursing interventions?

1. ______________________________
2. ______________________________
3. ______________________________
4. ______________________________
5. ______________________________
6. ______________________________
7. ______________________________

F. What physiological characteristics should the child exhibit before being discharged home?

1. ______________________________
2. ______________________________

G. What subjective characteristics should the child exhibit before being discharged home?

1. ______________________________

REVIEW QUESTIONS

1. An 11-month-old child is seen in the primary health-care practitioner's office with a chief complaint of loose stools. The child's temperature, heart rate, and respiratory rate are: 98.9°F, 148 bpm, and 46 rpm, respectively. Which of the following factors places this child at high risk for the nursing diagnosis: Deficient Fluid Volume? The child's: (**Select all that apply.**)
   1. Age.
   2. Heart rate.
   3. Temperature.
   4. Chief complaint.
   5. Respiratory rate.

2. A 6-year-old child is being assessed by a nurse for possible signs of dehydration. Which of the following assessments should the nurse perform?
   1. Patellar reflexes
   2. Anterior fontanel tension
   3. Skin turgor
   4. Pupil reactivity to light

3. A baby who weighs 4.8 kg is in the hospital. The child's hydration status is within normal limits. The nurse is calculating the minimum volume of fluid the child needs per hour to maintain normal hydration status. **Please calculate the baby's needs to the nearest whole number.**

   __________ mL/hr

4. The parents of a child, whose weight is 64 lb, are advised to make sure that the child consumes the minimum fluid needed to maintain a normal hydration status. The nurse calculates the amount for the full day. **Please calculate the child's needs to the nearest whole number.**

   __________ mL/day

5. A child is admitted to the hospital with diarrhea, vomiting, and dehydration. One week earlier, the child weighed 5.6 kg. On admission to the hospital, the child weighs 4.9 kg. What percentage weight loss has the child experienced? **Please calculate to the tenths place.**

   __________ %

6. A 3-year-old child is being seen for a possible diagnosis of dehydration. Two weeks ago, the child weighed 34 lb 8 oz. The child's current weight is 32 lb 4 oz. Please calculate the percentage of weight loss for this child. **Please calculate to the tenths place.**

   __________ %

7. A nurse is caring for an 18-month-old child who is admitted to the pediatric unit with a diagnosis of diarrhea and a weight loss of 4%. The nurse notes that the child's serum sodium and potassium levels are: 140 mEq/L and 4.8 mEq/L, respectively. Which of the following orders by the primary health-care provider would the nurse expect to receive?
   1. Restriction of all dairy products.
   2. Intravenous fluid with potassium added.
   3. Feedings of oral rehydration therapy.
   4. Bouillon soup for lunch and dinner.

8. A 6-month-old child, with a nursing diagnosis of excess fluid volume, is being seen by the nurse. Which of the following signs/symptoms would the nurse expect to see?
   1. Sunken fontanel
   2. Marked weight gain
   3. Soft eyeballs
   4. High urine specific gravity

9. A child is admitted to the pediatric unit with a serum potassium level of 3.0 mEq/L. For which of the following complications should the nurse carefully monitor the child?
   1. Dysrhythmias
   2. Thirst
   3. Seizures
   4. Dry mucous membranes

10. A 3-month-old child is being assessed in the emergency department. The child's laboratory results are: potassium 5.5 mEq/L and sodium 150 mEq/L. Which of the following is most likely the etiology of the child's results?
    1. Baby is consuming concentrated formula that is not diluted with water.
    2. Child has a cardiac defect.
    3. Child has gastroenteritis.
    4. Parent fed the baby large quantities of plain water on a hot summer day.

11. A primary health-care provider has ordered an IV of D_5 ½ NS for a child with a diagnosis of dehydration. The parent asks the nurse to explain why the child must receive the solution. Which of the following responses by the nurse is appropriate?
    1. "The solution contains all of the substances that should be in your child's bloodstream."
    2. "The solution will replace the most important electrolytes that your child is missing."
    3. "The fluid contains some sugar and some salt. Those, in addition to the fluid, will help to make your child better."
    4. "The fluid is the same as the water that you drink. Your child needs the water in order to get better."

12. The nurse assesses the following blood gas results on an infant in the emergency department. Which of the following conclusions is consistent with the data?

Po_2:	90 mm Hg
Pco_2:	34 mm Hg
HCO_3:	16 mEq/L
Base excess:	−4
pH:	7.28

1. Metabolic acidosis
2. Metabolic alkalosis
3. Respiratory acidosis
4. Respiratory alkalosis

13. The nurse assesses the following blood gas results on a child in the emergency department. Which of the following diagnoses is consistent with the data?

Po_2:	60 mm Hg
Pco_2:	50 mm Hg
HCO_3:	30 mEq/L
Base excess:	−4
pH:	7.28

1. Metabolic acidosis
2. Metabolic alkalosis
3. Respiratory acidosis
4. Respiratory alkalosis

14. A child, who is frightened, is hyperventilating. Which of the following blood gas values would the nurse expect to see? **Select all that apply.**

1. Depressed Pco_2
2. Depressed Po_2
3. Elevated pH
4. Elevated HCO_3
5. Base excess of 0

15. The nurse, who is assessing the blood gas results of a young child in the emergency department, notes that the Pco_2 is elevated and that the pH is low. The nurse will check to see if the child's body has attempted to compensate for the disturbance by doing which of the following?

1. Raising the serum bicarbonate levels
2. Raising the serum oxygen levels
3. Raising the serum carbonic acid levels
4. Raising the serum potassium levels

REVIEW ANSWERS

1. **ANSWER: 1, 2, 4, and 5**

Rationale:

1. The child's age places the child at high risk for deficient fluid volume.
2. The child's heart rate places the child at high risk for deficient fluid volume.
3. The child's temperature is within normal limits. A febrile temperature is a temperature that is 100.4°F or higher.
4. The child's chief complaint places the child at high risk for deficient fluid volume.
5. The child's respiratory rate places the child at high risk for deficient fluid volume.

TEST-TAKING TIP: There are a number of factors that place infants and toddlers at high risk for deficient fluid volume, including their BSA, which is proportionately larger than that of an older child or adult, their immature renal function, and their higher metabolic rate, which is evidenced by their higher heart and respiratory rates. In addition, this child is losing fluids because of the chief complaint of loose stools.

Content Area: *Pediatrics—Infant*
Integrated Processes: *Nursing Process: Analysis*
Client Need: *Physiological Adaptation: Fluid and Electrolyte Imbalances*
Cognitive Level: *Application*

2. **ANSWER: 3**

Rationale:

1. Patellar reflexes are not performed when assessing hydration status.
2. Anterior fontanelle tension should be assessed in infants and young toddlers. This child, however, is 6 years of age.
3. The child's skin turgor should be assessed.
4. Pupil reactivity to light is not checked when assessing hydration status.

TEST-TAKING TIP: To assess skin turgor, the nurse should gently pinch the skin between two fingers. A well-hydrated child's skin should return to its original position without noticeable indentations. When a child is dehydrated, however, the skin will stay in the position where it was released in what appears to be a type of tent. This finding is called tenting.

Content Area: *Pediatrics—School Age*
Integrated Processes: *Nursing Process: Assessment*
Client Need: *Physiological Adaptation: Fluid and Electrolyte Imbalances*
Cognitive Level: *Application*

3. **ANSWER: 20 mL/hr**

Rationale:

4.8 kg × 100 mL/kg = 480 mL, daily minimum fluid needs

480 mL/24 hr = x mL/hr

x = 20 mL/hr

TEST-TAKING TIP: Because this child's weight is under 10 kg, the practitioner must simply multiply the child's weight times 10 mL to determine the 24-hr minimum fluid needs for the child. To determine the hourly needs, the total daily need must be divided by 24.

Content Area: *Pediatrics—Infant*
Integrated Processes: *Nursing Process: Implementation*
Client Need: *Health Promotion and Maintenance: Health Promotion/Disease Prevention*
Cognitive Level: *Synthesis*

4. **ANSWER: 1,682 mL per day**

Rationale:

2.2 lb/1 kg = 64 lb/x kg

2.2x = 64

x = 29.09 kg

10 kg × 100 mL/kg = 1,000 mL

10 kg × 50 mL/kg = 500 mL

9.09 kg × 20 mL/kg = 1,81.8 mL

Total daily minimum = 1,681.8 or 1,682 mL per day

TEST-TAKING TIP: This child's weight is in pounds, therefore the first action that the nurse must perform is to convert the child's weight to kilograms. Next, the nurse should note that the child's weight in kilograms is above 20 kg, and the following calculations must be made:

The first 10 kg are multiplied by 100 mL.
The second 10 kg are multiplied by 50 mL.
The remainder of the child's weight is multiplied by 20 mL.
The volumes are then added together to determine the child's minimum daily volume requirements.

Content Area: *Pediatrics—Infant*
Integrated Processes: *Nursing Process: Implementation*
Client Need: *Health Promotion and Maintenance: Health Promotion/Disease Prevention*
Cognitive Level: *Synthesis*

5. **ANSWER: 12.5%**

Rationale:

5.6 kg previous weight
−4.9 kg new weight
0.7 difference

(0.7 ÷ 5.6) × 100 = 0.125 × 100 = 12.5%

TEST-TAKING TIP: To calculate the percentage of weight loss, the nurse must:

1. Subtract the most recent weight from the previous weight.
2. Divide the difference by the previous weight.
3. Multiply the result by 100.

Content Area: Pediatrics
Integrated Processes: *Nursing Process: Implementation*
Client Need: *Physiological Integrity: Physiological Adaptation: Fluid and Electrolyte Imbalances*
Cognitive Level: *Synthesis*

6. **ANSWER: 6.5%**
Rationale:

34.5 lb
−32.25 lb
2.25 lb difference

$(2.25 \div 34.5) \times 100 = 0.065 \times 100 = 6.5\%$

TEST-TAKING TIP: It is possible to calculate the percentage of weight loss using the English system. The test taker simply must remember that there are 16 oz in every pound. Fractions of a pound can then be determined (e.g., 8 oz = ½ or 0.5 lb; 4 oz = ¼ or 0.25 lb).
Content Area: *Pediatrics*
Integrated Processes: *Nursing Process: Implementation*
Client Need: *Physiological Integrity: Physiological Adaptation: Fluid and Electrolyte Imbalances*
Cognitive Level: *Synthesis*

7. **ANSWER: 3**
Rationale:
1. There is no indication in the question that the intake of dairy products would need to be restricted.
2. The child's potassium level is normal. IV potassium is not indicated.
3. The nurse would expect the child to be fed ORT.
4. Bouillon soup contains high levels of sodium. A high-salt intake is not indicated.
TEST-TAKING TIP: As with the child in the question stem, isotonic dehydration is characterized by fluid loss but with normal serum electrolyte levels. ORT is an oral solution that provides both fluids and electrolytes, in physiological proportions, to sick children. It is the appropriate intervention for a child who is in mild isotonic dehydration.
Content Area: *Pediatrics—Toddler*
Integrated Processes: *Nursing Process: Assessment*
Client Need: *Physiological Integrity: Physiological Adaptation: Fluid and Electrolyte Imbalances*
Cognitive Level: *Application*

8. **ANSWER: 2**
Rationale:
1. A sunken fontanel is seen when a child is dehydrated.
2. Marked weight gain is noted when a child is in a state of fluid volume excess.
3. Soft eyeballs are seen when a child is dehydrated.
4. High urine specific gravity (i.e., concentrated urine) is seen when a child is dehydrated.
TEST-TAKING TIP: When a child is in a state of excess fluid volume, he or she is edematous with marked weight gain. Because pulmonary edema may be present, the nurse should assess the child's lung sounds for the presence of rales and crackles.
Content Area: *Pediatrics—Infant*
Integrated Processes: *Nursing Process: Assessment*
Client Need: *Physiological Integrity: Physiological Adaptation: Fluid and Electrolyte Imbalances*
Cognitive Level: *Application*

9. **ANSWER: 1**
Rationale:
1. The nurse should monitor the child for dysrhythmias.
2. Thirst is noted when the sodium levels are very low.
3. Seizures are seen when sodium levels are very high and when calcium levels are low.
4. Dry mucous membranes are indicative of dehydration.
TEST-TAKING TIP: Dysrhythmias often are noted when a child is hypokalemic (i.e., when the child's serum potassium level is below 3.5 mEq/L). Dysrhythmias also are seen when potassium levels are elevated (i.e., above 5 mEq/L).
Content Area: *Pediatrics*
Integrated Processes: *Nursing Process: Implementation*
Client Need: *Physiological Integrity: Physiological Adaptation: Fluid and Electrolyte Imbalances*
Cognitive Level: *Application*

10. **ANSWER: 1**
Rationale:
1. The most likely etiology is that the child is consuming concentrated formula that has not been diluted with water.
2. A diagnosis of cardiac defect does not put a child at high risk for elevated electrolyte levels.
3. Gastroenteritis usually results in the loss of electrolytes.
4. High water intake by babies can result in low serum electrolyte levels.
TEST-TAKING TIP: Both the serum potassium and sodium levels are elevated. When babies are fed concentrated formula, they can become very ill because they are consuming an undiluted fluid that contains a high concentration of electrolytes as well as a high concentration of fats, proteins, and carbohydrates.
Content Area: *Pediatrics—Infant*
Integrated Processes: *Nursing Process: Analysis*
Client Need: *Physiological Integrity: Physiological Adaptation: Fluid and Electrolyte Imbalances*
Cognitive Level: *Application*

11. **ANSWER: 3**
Rationale:
1. The solution only contains dextrose and saline that is one-half the concentration of the blood.
2. Because this response is made using medical terminology, it will be difficult for the parent to understand. In addition, only sodium and chloride are being replaced.
3. This is an appropriate response for the nurse to provide.
4. This statement is not accurate. The fluid is not the same as drinking water. It contains saline one-half the

concentration of the blood and 5 g of dextrose for every 100 mL of water.

TEST-TAKING TIP: The solution, D_5 ½ NS, is comprised of 77 mEq of both sodium and chloride for every 1,000 mL, and 5 g of dextrose for every 100 mL of water. It is providing the child, therefore, with saline that is one-half the concentration of saline of the blood as well as some dextrose for calories.

Content Area: *Pediatrics*
Integrated Processes: *Nursing Process: Implementation*
Client Need: *Physiological Integrity: Physiological Adaptation: Fluid and Electrolyte Imbalances*
Cognitive Level: *Application*

12. ANSWER: 1

Rationale:

1. **The child is in metabolic acidosis.**
2. The child is in metabolic acidosis.
3. The child is in metabolic acidosis.
4. The child is in metabolic acidosis.

TEST-TAKING TIP: Blood gases should be analyzed systematically.

1. Check the pH: 7.28 is an acidic pH.
2. Check Pco_2: low
3. Using ROME, the pH and the Pco_2 are both low, i.e., they are altered in the same direction. The cause of the altered blood gases, therefore, is metabolic.
4. Check HCO_3: low = cause of the problem.
5. Low Pco_2 = compensatory response.
6. The child is in metabolic acidosis.

A possible medical diagnosis for the metabolic acidosis is diarrhea. Please see Chapter 14, "Nursing Care of the Child With Gastrointestinal Problems" for a complete discussion of diarrhea.

Content Area: *Pediatrics—Infant*
Integrated Processes: *Nursing Process: Analysis*
Client Need: *Physiological Integrity: Physiological Adaptation: Fluid and Electrolyte Imbalances*
Cognitive Level: *Analysis*

13. ANSWER: 3

Rationale:

1. The child is in respiratory acidosis.
2. The child is in respiratory acidosis.
3. **The child is in respiratory acidosis.**
4. The child is in respiratory acidosis.

TEST-TAKING TIP: Blood gases should be analyzed systematically.

1. Check the pH: 7.28 is an acidic pH.
2. Check Pco_2: high
3. Using ROME, the pH and the Pco_2 are in opposite directions. The cause of the altered blood gases, therefore, is respiratory.
4. Check Pco_2: high = cause of the problem.
5. High HCO_3 = compensatory response.
6. The child is in respiratory acidosis.

A possible medical diagnosis for the respiratory acidosis is a severe asthma attack. Please see Chapter 16, "Nursing Care of the Child With Respiratory Illnesses," for a complete discussion of asthma.

Content Area: *Pediatrics—Infant*
Integrated Processes: *Nursing Process: Analysis*
Client Need: *Physiological Integrity: Physiological Adaptation: Fluid and Electrolyte Imbalances*
Cognitive Level: *Application*

14. ANSWERS: 1 and 3

Rationale:

1. **The nurse would expect to see a low Pco_2.**
2. The nurse would expect to see a normal Po_2.
3. **The nurse would expect to see an elevated pH.**
4. The nurse would expect to see an depressed HCO_3.
5. The nurse would expect the base excess to be elevated.

TEST-TAKING TIP: Because the child is exhaling large quantities of carbon dioxide, the concentration of carbonic acid in the blood is reduced. The child, therefore, is in respiratory alkalosis.

Content Area: *Pediatrics*
Integrated Processes: *Nursing Process: Assessment*
Client Need: *Physiological Integrity: Physiological Adaptation: Fluid and Electrolyte Imbalances*
Cognitive Level: *Application*

15. ANSWER: 1

Rationale:

1. **The nurse would assess to see if the serum bicarbonate levels are elevated.**
2. The nurse would not expect a rise in serum oxygen levels.
3. The child already has a high serum carbonic acid level.
4. The nurse would not expect the serum potassium levels to rise.

TEST-TAKING TIP: To compensate for respiratory acidosis, the body should try to compensate by raising the bicarbonate levels.

Content Area: *Pediatrics—Toddler*
Integrated Processes: *Nursing Process: Assessment*
Client Need: *Physiological Integrity: Physiological Adaptation: Fluid and Electrolyte Imbalances*
Cognitive Level: *Application*

Nursing Care of the Child With Gastrointestinal Problems

KEY TERMS

Anoplasty—Surgical repair of the anus.
Celiac disease—Damage of the lining of the small intestine caused by a reaction to the consumption of foods that contain gluten.
Enterobiasis—Pinworms.
Esophageal atresia—Congenital defect characterized by an esophagus that ends in a blind pouch.
Gastroenteritis—Diarrhea.
Gastroschisis—Congenital defect in which the abdominal wall fails to develop, resulting in the intestines protruding from the body.
Hirschsprung's disease—Congenital absence of enervation to the rectum and/or lower intestine, resulting in intestinal blockages.
Ileus—Absence of intestinal peristalsis.
Imperforate anus—Absent, narrowed, or misplaced anal opening. In other cases, the rectum connects to another anatomical structure instead of the anus.
Intussusception—When the intestine, usually the small intestine, invaginates.
Omphalocele—Congenital defect resulting from poor abdominal muscle development in which the intestines or abdominal organs protrude into the umbilicus
Oral rehydration therapy (ORT)—Oral fluid replacement that provides sick children with needed fluids and electrolytes as well as some calories.
Polyhydramnios—Excessive amniotic fluid.
Pyloric stenosis—Tissues of the pyloric sphincter hypertrophy, preventing ingested breast milk or formula to pass into the duodenum.
Pyloromyotomy—Incision of pyloric muscle.
REEDA Assessment—An assessment of surgical sites for signs of infection and/or injury, i.e., redness, edema, ecchymosis, discharge, and approximation of the tissue.
Tracheoesophageal fistula—Congenital defect in which an abnormal passage exists between the distal end of the esophagus and the trachea.

I. Description

A. Anatomy: the gastrointestinal system begins at the mouth and ends at the anus. Between those two structures, a long, circuitous path exists, including the teeth, tongue, salivary glands, esophagus, cardiac sphincter, stomach, pyloric sphincter, small intestines, ileocecal valve, large intestines with the cecum and appendix, and rectum. In addition, the liver, gallbladder, and pancreas enable the digestive system to function optimally.

B. Physiology.

1. Ingestion: the mouth and esophagus ingest foods.
2. Digestion.
   a. Mouth: starch digestion, effected by amylase and ptyalin, begins in the mouth.
   b. Stomach: the stomach continues digestion by mixing foods with digestive juices, producing chyme.
   c. Small intestines: fats, proteins, and carbohydrates are digested in the duodenum, jejunum, and ileum via pancreatic enzymes and bile.
3. Absorption: primarily via the small intestine.
   a. Of carbohydrates, fats, proteins, minerals, and vitamins (vitamin B_{12} is only absorbed via the terminal ileum).
   b. Of water: via the large intestines.
4. Synthesis—of vitamins B_{12} and K—in the large intestine.
5. Elimination: via the large intestines, rectum, and anus.
6. Accessory structures.
   a. Liver: produces bile and stores vitamins and glycogen.
   b. Gallbladder: stores bile.
   c. Pancreas: produces enzymes to break down fats, proteins, and carbohydrates.

C. Types of gastrointestinal illnesses: the problems discussed in this chapter develop from a number of factors.

1. Infectious conditions.
   a. Gastroenteritis.
   b. Vomiting.
   c. Enterobiasis (pinworms).
2. Congenital defects.
   a. Cleft lip/palate.
   b. Esophageal atresia and tracheoesophageal fistula.
   c. Imperforate anus.
   d. Hirschsprung's disease.
   e. Gastroschisis.
   f. Omphalocele.
3. Acquired conditions.
   a. Pyloric stenosis (hypertrophic pyloric stenosis).
   b. Intussusception.
4. Malabsorption illness.
   a. Celiac disease, damage to the small intestine lining caused by a reaction to gluten in food.

II. Gastroenteritis

A. Incidence.

1. **Gastroenteritis** (diarrhea) is a common illness in children. Multiple cases of both acute and chronic diarrhea are seen each year by pediatricians.
2. Diarrhea is the leading cause of death in children in developing countries.

B. Etiology.

1. May be caused by any of a number of agents, including viruses (e.g., rotavirus, norovirus), bacteria (e.g., shigella, salmonella, *Escherichia coli*), and parasites (e.g., giardia lamblia).
   a. Rotavirus is the most common pathogen causing diarrhea in infants and toddlers.
   b. Norovirus is the most common pathogen causing diarrhea in the United States.
   b. Giardia lamblia is the most common pathogen seen in day-care centers.
2. Often accompanied by vomiting (see "Vomiting") and abdominal cramping.
3. Primary complication of diarrhea is dehydration.

DID YOU KNOW?

"D & D," i.e., diarrhea and dehydration, is a common diagnosis seen in pediatrics (see Chapter 13, "Nursing Care of the Child With Fluid and Electrolyte Alterations").

C. Pathophysiology.

1. Condition that results in marked peristalsis and frequent emptying of the gastrointestinal tract.
2. Signs and symptoms.
   a. Multiple stools over a short period of time.
   b. Stools may or may not contain blood.
      i. Stools that are streaked with bright-red blood: sign of recent blood loss, indicating that the bleeding is originating in the lower bowel.
      ii. Stools that are black and tarry: sign of the digestion of blood, indicating that the bleeding is originating in the upper bowel or stomach.
   c. Stools may be foul smelling, mucousy, greasy, or watery.
   d. Fever may be present.
   e. Signs and symptoms of dehydration are often present (see Chapter 13, "Nursing Care of the Child With Fluid and Electrolyte Alterations").

D. Diagnosis.

1. Diagnosis is often made on the clinical picture and history alone.
2. If the child is seriously ill, stool cultures as well as blood cultures may be ordered to determine the exact etiology.
3. If needed, the severity of the illness may be determined by assessing serum electrolytes and arterial blood gasses.

E. Treatment.

1. Prevention is the primary goal.
   a Meticulous handwashing.

b. Rotavirus vaccine is recommended to be administered to infants at 2, 4, and 6 months of age.
c. Babies who are exclusively breastfed are much less likely to develop gastroenteritis than are formula fed babies.

DID YOU KNOW?

All mothers should be strongly encouraged to breastfeed. Not only is breast milk comprised of fats, proteins, and carbohydrates that are ideal for human babies, it also contains many protective properties, including white blood cells, antibodies, and lactobacilli, that help to protect babies from infectious diseases, including gastrointestinal illnesses. When breastfed babies do become ill, they should continue to receive breast milk. If breastfeeding difficulties occur at any time, a referral to a lactation consultant should be made to remedy the problem.

2. Treatment.
   a. Fluid and electrolyte replacement.
      i. The child with diarrhea may require as much as two and a half times his or her daily maintenance volume (DMV) (see Chapter 3, "Nursing Care of the Child With Fluid and Electrolyte Alterations," for the formula to calculate DMV).
      ii. **Oral rehydration therapy (ORT)** is usually prescribed if mild to moderate dehydration is diagnosed and the child can tolerate oral fluids.
         (1) If the child is breastfeeding, ORT is offered as a supplement following each feeding.
         (2) If the child is formula feeding, ORT is usually fed to the child as a replacement rather than as a supplement to the formula.
         (3) If the child is interested in eating solid foods, small frequent feedings of low fat meats, complex starches, and well-cooked vegetables may be offered with the ORT.
      iii. IV infusions are needed if the child is severely dehydrated and/or if the child is unable to tolerate oral fluids.
   b. Antibiotics: may be administered for some bacterial infections.
      i. Antibiotics usually are not administered for a diagnosis of diarrhea from *E. coli* or giardia.

(!) Antidiarrhea medications are not recommended for children because they often develop constipation from the medications. Parents should be advised not to administer any over-the-counter antidiarrhea medications to their children.

F. Nursing considerations.
1. Risk for Imbalanced Nutrition: Less than Body Requirements/Risk for Deficient Fluid Volume.
   a. Take an excellent history of the child's activities preceding the diarrhea, including:
      i. Dietary intake, travel, day-care attendance, and play activities.
   b. Assess the frequency, consistency, appearance, and smell of the child's stools.
      i. Stools may need to be weighed in order to estimate the extent of fluid loss via the gastrointestinal tract.
   c. Assess the frequency, amount, and characteristics of any vomiting.
   d. Carefully monitor the child's hydration status (see Chapter 13, "Nursing Care of the Child With Fluid and Electrolyte Imbalances"), including:
      i. Calculating the percentage of weight loss.
      ii. Assessing for additional physiological signs of dehydration, including low urinary output, poor skin turgor, absence of tears, and altered vital signs and,
      iii. If the child is an infant, assessing for a sunken anterior fontanel.
      iv. Monitoring input and output (I & O).
   e. Carefully assess all pertinent laboratory data, including the complete blood count (CBC), electrolytes, blood gases, and, if performed, stool culture reports.
      i. Metabolic acidosis may develop, secondary to the loss of bicarbonate via the stools.
      ii. Hyponatremia and/or hypokalemia may be present.
   f. Provide ORT and/or IV therapy, as needed, per order.
      i. Calculate the child's DMV knowing that the child will be prescribed up to 2½ times the DMV in order to replace needed fluids.
      ii. If the child is to be managed at home, inform the parents and child, if appropriate, regarding the importance of consuming the rehydration therapy.
      iii. Even if vomiting is present, ORT should be administered in small, frequent, quantities.
   g. Weigh the child daily.
   h. If the child has previously not tolerated oral fluids, once he or she is able, the child should return to a normal diet in addition to the ORT.

i. If formula fed, formula should be offered.
(1) Although it does not occur frequently, if the child's diarrhea seems to worsen after ingestion of formula, transient lactose intolerance should be considered.
ii. Best solid foods to serve: low-fat meats; cooked vegetables; starches, such as potatoes and rice; bananas; and yogurt with live cultures.
2. Infection.
a. Maintain contact isolation precautions at all times, if hospitalized.
i. Place the young child in a private room to reduce the potential for transmission.
3. Deficient Knowledge.
a. Educate the family members and child, if appropriate, of handwashing and isolation precautions during hospitalization and after discharge.
b. Educate the family members and child, if appropriate, regarding the etiology of the disease and actions to prevent future episodes.
c. Educate the family members and child, if appropriate, of possible dietary exposure and dietary recommendations, including ORT.
d. Educate the family members and child, if appropriate, regarding the reintroduction of a normal diet.
e. Educate the parents regarding medication administration, if ordered.

III. Vomiting

A. Incidence.
1. Common illness in childhood.

B. Etiology.
1. Acute episodes are usually a symptom of another problem, most often an infectious syndrome.
2. Chronic cases of vomiting may be related to gastroesophageal reflux.

C. Pathophysiology.
1. Condition that results in involuntary regurgitation of the contents of the gastrointestinal tract.
2. Signs and symptoms.
a. Multiple episodes of regurgitation. Possible characteristics of the vomitus with their likely origin are listed in Table 14.1.
b. Fever may be present.
c. Signs and symptoms of dehydration may develop.

D. Diagnosis.
1. Diagnosis is often made on the clinical picture and history alone.

Table 14.1 Vomitus Characteristics and Origination

Vomitus Characteristics	Origination
Visible undigested matter	Stomach
Bile colored	Small intestines
Smells like feces	Lower intestines
Vomitus may or may not contain blood	
Bright-red blood	Bleeding in the upper gastrointestinal tract
Looks like coffee grounds	Blood has been digested, originating from the intestines

2. If needed, the severity of the illness may be determined by assessing serum electrolytes and arterial blood gasses.

E. Treatment.
1. If the child is diagnosed with mild to moderate dehydration and the child is able to tolerate some oral intake, ORT is administered in small, frequent feedings.
2. If the child is severely dehydrated, and/or if the child is unable to tolerate any oral intake, IV fluids should be administered.
3. Antiemetic medications, if needed (e.g., Zofran [ondansetron]), may be prescribed.

F. Nursing considerations.
1. Imbalanced Nutrition: Less than Body Requirements/Risk for Deficient Fluid Volume.
a. Assess the amount, frequency, and appearance of each vomiting episode.
b. Take an excellent history of the child's activities preceding the illness, including:
i. Dietary intake, travel, day-care attendance, and play activities.
c. Assess the frequency, consistency, and appearance of any stooling.
d. Carefully monitor the child's hydration status, including:
i. Calculating the percentage of weight loss.
ii. Assessing for additional physiological signs of dehydration, including low urinary output, poor skin turgor, absence of tears, and altered vital signs and,
iii. If the child is an infant, assessing for a sunken anterior fontanel.
iv. Monitoring I & O.
e. Assess all pertinent laboratory data, including CBC, serum electrolytes, and blood gases.
i. Metabolic alkalosis may develop, secondary to the loss of hydrochloric acid from the stomach.
ii. Hyponatremia and/or hypokalemia may be present.

f. Provide ORT and/or IV therapy, as needed, per order.
   i. Calculate the child's DMV knowing that the child will be prescribed up to 2½ times the DMV in order to replace needed fluids.
   ii. If the child is to be managed at home, inform the parents and child, if appropriate, regarding the importance of consuming the rehydration therapy.
g. Progress diet, as tolerated (see above).
h. Weigh child daily.
i. Administer antiemetics, as ordered.

2. Infection.
   a. Maintain contact isolation precautions at all times, if hospitalized.
      i. Place the young child in a private room to reduce the potential for transmission.
3. Risk for Injury.
   a. Position the child to prevent aspiration of vomitus.
   b. Rinse the child's mouth and/or brush his or her teeth after each vomiting episode to minimize damage to the enamel of the teeth from the acidic vomitus.
4. Deficient Knowledge.
   a. Educate the family members and child, if appropriate, of handwashing and isolation precautions during hospitalization and after discharge.
   b. Educate the family members and child, if appropriate, regarding the etiology of the disease and actions to prevent future episodes.
   c. Educate the family members and child, if appropriate, of possible dietary exposure and dietary recommendations, including ORT.
   d. Educate the family members and child, if appropriate, regarding the reintroduction of a normal diet.
   e. Educate the parents regarding medication administration, if ordered.

IV. Enterobiasis (pinworms)

There are a number of nematodes (worms) that may be consumed, causing gastrointestinal symptoms. Infection from **enterobiasis**, or pinworms, (*Enterobius vermicularis*) is the most common.

A. Incidence.
   1. Occurs in up to 15% of the population of the United States.

B. Etiology.
   1. Ingestion of the offending nematode.

Box 14.1 Usual Pattern of Pinworm Infestation

1. *Child ingests the eggs via such items as contaminated toys, unclean hands, and dirty clothes.*
2. *The eggs usually hatch in the small intestine, and the females and males then mate.*
3. *Eventually, the females exit the body via the rectum and anus and lay eggs. The movement through the rectum and anus is irritating to the child.*
4. *Children may reinfect themselves by scratching the anus and then placing their soiled hands in their mouths.*

C. Pathophysiology.
   1. Fecal-oral contact.
   2. The infestation pattern is shown in Box 14.1.
   3. Signs and symptoms, triggered by the irritation from the presence of worms in the stool and/or from worms exiting the anus.
      a. Anal itching, especially at night.
      b. Enuresis in an otherwise fully toilet-trained child.

D. Diagnosis.
   1. Tape test.

E. Treatment.
   1. For children over 2 years of age: one dose of Mebendazole 100 mg PO at the time of diagnosis and repeated 2 weeks later.
      a. Treatment of children under 2 years of age is controversial. It is recommended that an expert in infectious diseases be consulted regarding an appropriate course of action.
   2. Because the incidence of transfer of the infection is high, it is recommended that all family members be treated at the same time the child is being treated.

MAKING THE CONNECTION

Parents are taught to perform the tape test as the means of diagnosing the presence of pinworms. To obtain a specimen, they are taught to attach a piece of clear, very sticky tape to a tongue blade. Then, before raising the child from his or her bed in the morning, to press the tape to the child's anus (Fig. 14.1). The tape is placed in a plastic bag or container for transport to the health-care practitioner's office. There, the tape is examined under a microscope for the presence of the worms.

Ideally, the test should be performed before the lights are turned on in the room in the morning. It should be performed before the child stools or bathes for the day. The test may need to be performed for a few days in a row before the worms are captured.

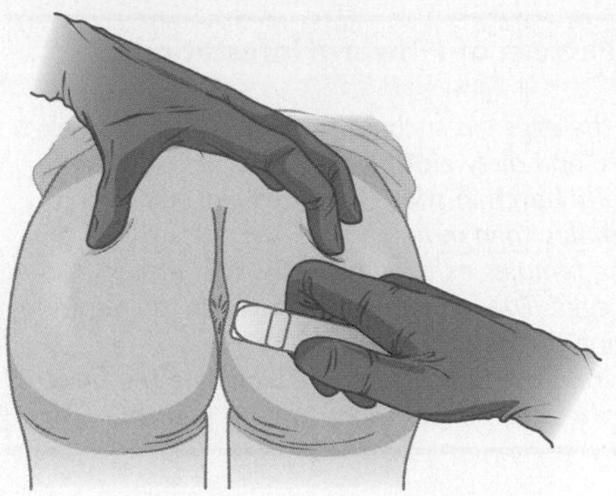

Fig 14.1 Tape test for the presence of pinworms.

F. Nursing considerations.
1. Risk for Infection.
   a. Obtain a thorough history of the child's signs and symptoms as well as his or her activities preceding the illness, e.g., play history and day-care attendance.
   b. Educate the parents regarding how to perform the tape test.
      i. To prevent startling the child, strongly encourage the parents to forewarn their child before going to sleep that the tape test will be performed early the next morning.
   c. Educate the parents regarding medication administration for the child as well as for all members of the family, as prescribed.
2. Deficient Knowledge.
   a. Educate the parents regarding the need to clean clothing and household surfaces well.
      i. Pinworm eggs can live for many weeks on inanimate objects in the child's environment.
   b. Remind the parents and child, if appropriate, regarding the need for frequent handwashing.
   c. Educate the parents to keep their child's fingernails short to prevent eggs from collecting underneath.
   d. Educate the parents to cover sandboxes when not in use.
   e. Educate the parents to keep pets from using sandboxes and other play areas for toileting.
   f. Educate the parents to wash fruits and vegetables well.
   g. Educate the parents to change young children's diapers frequently.
   h. Advise the parents to dress their children in clothing that will reduce the likelihood of the child scratching his or her anal area (e.g., "onesie" pajamas).
      i. If the previously toilet-trained child is wetting the bed, advise the parents and the child that once the child has been treated the child should no longer experience enuresis.
3. Risk for Ineffective Coping.
   a. Allow the parents to express concerns about the diagnosis and about the health of the entire family.
   b. Allow the child, if needed, to express concerns regarding enuresis and anal itching.

V. Cleft Lip/Palate

A. Incidence.
1. Cleft palate alone.
   a. Approximately 2,600 children each year, or 1 in every 1,500 live births.
2. Cleft lip alone.
   a. Over 4,400 children each year, or almost 1 in every 1,000 live births.
3. Children may also exhibit a combination of cleft lip and palate.

B. Etiology.
1. The cause of the majority of cleft birth defects is unknown.
2. There is evidence that:
   a. Women who smoke during pregnancy have a higher likelihood of delivering a baby with a cleft (Little, Cardy & Munger, 2004).
   b. Women who are preexisting diabetics have a higher likelihood of delivering a baby with a cleft (Spilson, Kim & Chung, 2001).
3. There appears to be a multifactorial cause of orofacial clefts (i.e., a combination of genetic predisposition and environmental factors).
   a. Clefts are associated with some chromosomal syndromes (e.g., Pierre Robin syndrome and Down syndrome).
   b. Clefts are seen more frequently in children of Asian, Hispanic, and Native American descent.

C. Pathophysiology (Fig. 14.2).
1. Orofacial clefts occur when the structures of the mouth fail to fuse during the organogenic period of fetal development.
2. Cleft lips develop at approximately 6 to 8 weeks' gestation.
   a. Cleft lips can occur unilaterally or bilaterally.
   b. They may appear as a slight notch in the lip or extend deep into the nasal cavity.
      i. Cleft lips that extend into the nares usually also adversely affect tooth and gum development.
3. Cleft palates occur at approximately 7 to 12 weeks' gestation.

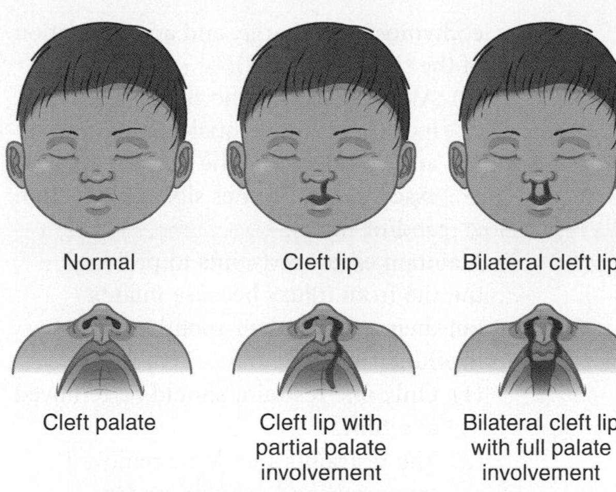

Fig 14.2 Cleft lip and cleft palate.

a. Cleft palates may affect either the hard or the soft palate or may extend through both palates.
b. Because the roof of the mouth is the floor of the nasal passages, when a child has a cleft palate, there is no separation between the child's mouth and the nasal sinuses.
   i. When the child consumes breast milk or formula, the food will frequently drain from the nose.

D. Diagnosis.
1. Cleft lip.
   a. Clinical appearance that may be noted prenatally via ultrasound or at birth.
2. Cleft palate.
   a. May be seen visually when the child's mouth is opened.
   b. Even when the palate appears intact visually, both the hard and soft palates must be assessed carefully with a gloved finger.

E. Treatment.
1. Treatment is multidisciplinary. Frequently, surgeons, nurses, lactation consultants, speech therapists, genetic counselors, emotional therapists, audiologists, otolaryngologists, and orthodontists are all needed to provide the child with comprehensive care.
2. Surgical repairs.
   a. Cleft lip repair.
      i. The initial repair usually is performed by 3 months of age.
      ii. Children often have multiple plastic surgery repairs after the initial closure is completed.
   b. Cleft palate repair.
      i. The initial repair is usually performed by 18 months of age.
      ii. These children, too, often require multiple follow-up surgeries.
3. Speech therapy to assist the children to learn how to pronounce sounds correctly. It is especially difficult for children with cleft lip to pronounce hard consonants like "b," "m," and "p" and for children with cleft palate to pronounce hard consonants like "t," "d," and "n."
4. The family should be referred to a genetic counselor to assess whether there is a possible genetic etiology that could affect any future children.
5. Emotional therapy, including grief counseling for the loss of the perfect child, may be needed for the parents and/or for the child, once he or she ages.
6. Audiology and otolaryngology assessments and therapy, if needed.
   a. Children with cleft palate are especially at high risk for ear infections and hearing loss.
7. Orthodontists to assist with tooth development, dental positioning, and correction of dental malocclusions.

F. Nursing considerations.
1. Preoperative cleft lip and/or palate care.
   a. Risk for Imbalanced Nutrition: Less than Body Requirements/Infection related to structural defect(s).
      i. Breastfeeding.
         (1) Some children with clefts may be able to breastfeed without assistance, but each child must be assessed individually, ideally by an International Board Certified Lactation Consultant.
         (2) If the child is unable to extract milk directly from the breast, the mother should be encouraged to pump her breasts and feed the child the breast milk via an alternate method.
      ii. Alternate feeding methods that may be required.
         (1) Specialized feeding devices may be needed for pumped breast milk or formula feedings (e.g., Haberman feeders, special nipples, obturators, and Breck feeders).
      iii. To enable the child safely to consume sufficient quantities of pumped breast milk or formula, the child must:
         (1) Be fed in an upright position.
         (2) Be fed very slowly with frequent rest periods.
         (3) Be given sufficient time to swallow without choking.
         (4) Be burped frequently.

iv. Milk will exit via the nose when a cleft palate is present.

b. Risk for Altered Family Process/Anxiety/Grieving.
 i. Allow the parents to express grief and loss of the perfect child.
 ii. Assess the parents' responsiveness to the baby.
  (1) Encourage skin-to-skin contact to promote bonding.
  (2) If poor bonding is noted, the nurse should recommend the primary health-care provider to refer the family for counseling.
 iii. Enable the parents to discuss their concerns regarding their feelings of stress and their child's need for surgery.

c. Deficient Knowledge.
 i. Teach the parents regarding feeding techniques, pre- and postsurgery, as needed.
 ii. Provide information regarding corrective surgeries.
 iii. Encourage the primary health-care provider to refer the family for genetic counseling.
 iv. Refer the family to community resources (e.g., Cleft Palate Foundation and Children's Craniofacial Association).
 v. Educate the parents how to provide their child with preoperative teaching prior to surgery, for example:
  (1) Loosely apply elbow restraints on the child for approximately 20 min at a time for a few days prior to surgery. This will accustom the child to the restraints that will be used to prevent the child from injuring the repair.
  (2) Elevate the head of the child's crib for sleep, or place the child in an infant seat for sleep. This will accustom the child to the position that he or she will be placed to reduce inflammation and aspiration and will prevent the child from rubbing his or her face on a hard surface.
  (3) Attach the Logan bow or other protective device that the surgeon may use following surgery to accustom the child to its presence.

2. Postoperative cleft lip repair.

a. Impaired Skin Integrity/Risk for Injury/Risk for Infection
 i. The operative site should be assessed carefully for signs of redness, edema, ecchymosis, discharge, and approximation of the tissue (REEDA).
  (1) Any surgical site, no matter the location, is a potential site of injury and/or infection. The **REEDA assessment** includes signs of infection and/or injury.
 ii. Maintain elbow restraints to protect the site from injury because infants put their hand to their mouths involuntarily.
  (1) Only one restraint should be removed at a time.
  (2) The restraints should be removed frequently and the skin under restraints should be assessed for signs of altered skin integrity.
 iii. Place the infant supine in an infant seat or with the crib head elevated to reduce the potential for injury, edema, and respiratory difficulties.
 iv. Cleanse the lip with sterile water after feedings and apply prescribed antibiotic ointments to the surgical site to prevent infections.
 v. Apply protective devices (e.g., Logan bow), if ordered, to maintain the integrity of the suture line.

b. Pain
 i. Provide both pharmacological and nonpharmacological pain interventions (see Chapter 8, "Nursing Care of the Child in the Health-Care Setting"), as needed and prescribed.
  (1) Very important to reduce crying because stretching of the mouth can lead to suture dehiscence.

c. Risk for Altered Nutrition: Less than Body Requirements.
 i. Infant feedings are usually reintroduced shortly after awaking from surgery.
  (1) Care must be taken to prevent injury to the suture line.
  (2) Cleansing of the suture line following feedings is important to prevent infection (see above).

3. Postoperative cleft palate repair.

a. Impaired Skin Integrity/Risk for Injury/Risk for Infection.
 i. Carefully perform REEDA assessments of the surgical site.
 ii. Keep all objects away from the baby's mouth for 7 to 10 days (e.g., straws, fingers, spoons, forks) to protect the palate repair from injury.

iii. Progress diet as indicated, and protect the site from injury.
(1) Soft solid foods are usually offered from a spoon that is too large to fit into the mouth. The child is taught to slurp the food from the spoon.
(2) Similarly, liquids are usually cup fed, spoon fed from a large spoon, or bottlefed through a short nipple.
iv. Following feedings, rinse mouth with water, per orders, to prevent infection.

b. Pain
i. Provide both pharmacological and nonpharmacological pain interventions, as needed and as prescribed.
(1) Very important to reduce crying because stretching of the mouth can lead to suture dehiscence.

4. Long term: Risk for Altered Health Maintenance.
a. On-going speech, hearing assessments, and dental assessments.
b. Referral to experts in other disciplines (e.g., speech pathologist, orthodontist, otolaryngologist), as needed.

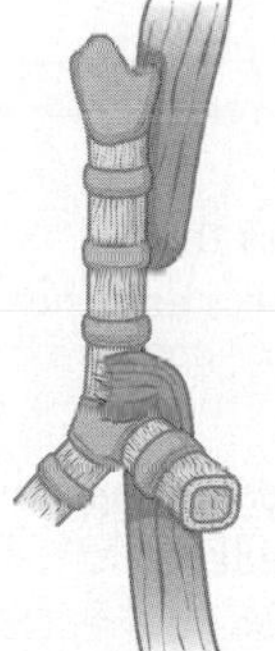
Esophageal atresia with distal TEF

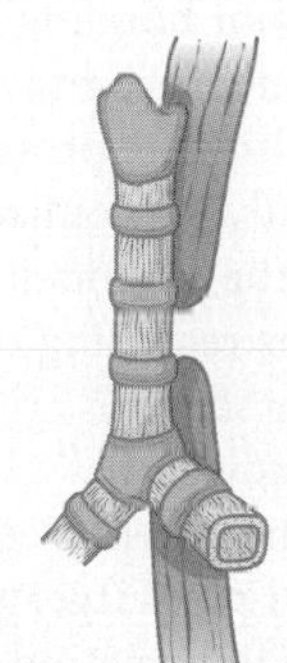
Esophageal atresia without fistula

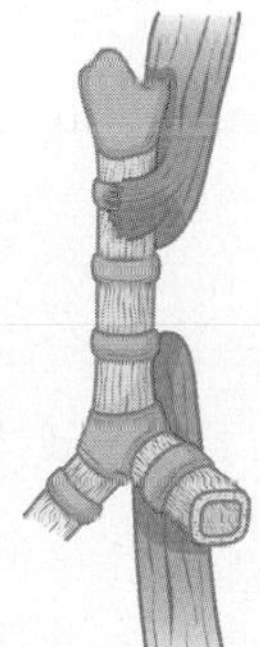
Proximal esophageal fistula with trachea; distal segment has no communication

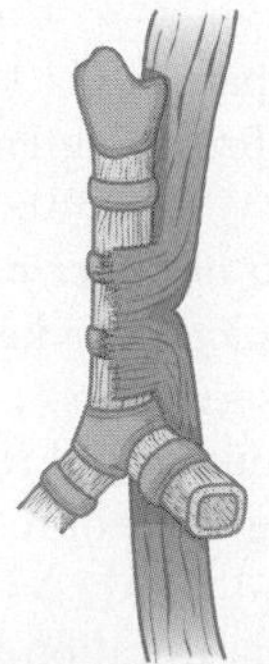
Proximal and distal esophageal fistulas with trachea

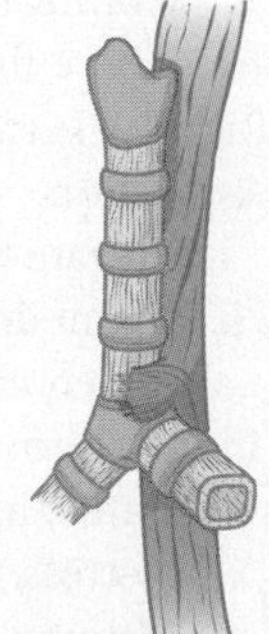
TEF without atresia (also called "H type")

Fig 14.3 Esophageal atresia.

VI. Esophageal Atresia With Tracheoesophageal Fistula (EA/TEF)

A. Incidence.
1. About 1 in 4,000 live births in the United States.

B. Etiology.
1. Exact etiology is unknown.
2. The defect likely has a genetic component because about 50% of babies born with the defect have other anomalies, including babies with chromosomal syndromes and with renal, cardiac, and other gastrointestinal defects.

C. Pathophysiology (see Fig. 14.3).
1. **Esophageal atresia** is characterized by an esophagus that ends in a blind pouch and, most commonly, is accompanied by a defect affecting the trachea.
a. The most common form—EA/TEF—is characterized by an esophagus that ends in a blind pouch and with a fistula between the distal end of the esophagus and the trachea.
i. Because both the esophagus and the trachea are affected, both the

gastrointestinal and the respiratory systems are affected.

b. Other forms of the defect are shown in Figure 14.3.

2. Signs and symptoms.
   a. Maternal **polyhydramnios** (excessive amniotic fluid) noted prenatally is a suspicious finding, especially if the mother is not diabetic.
      i. The fetus with an incomplete gastrointestinal system is unable to swallow amniotic fluid, which results in excess amniotic fluid in the uterine cavity.
   b. Excessive oral mucus production at birth because the baby is unable to swallow his or her saliva.
   c. The three C's of EA/TEF: coughing, choking, and cyanosis at first feeding.
      i. When the gastric secretions enter the trachea, the baby's respiratory system is adversely affected, resulting in the three C's.
   d. Inability to pass a nasogastric (N/G) tube into the stomach.

D. Diagnosis.
1. Clinical picture: suspicious.
2. X-ray and endoscopy: definitive.

E. Treatment.
1. Immediately after birth.
   a. Once the defect is suspected, the child is kept NPO.
   b. An N/G tube is inserted into the esophagus and is attached to low suction in order to remove excess secretions.
   c. Elevate the head of crib to reduce the quantity of secretions entering the trachea.
   d. After calculating the neonate's DMV, administer IV fluids at a safe volume and rate, as prescribed.
2. Within hours or days of birth.
   a. Surgical repair of the fistula to prevent gastric juices from entering the respiratory tree and, if possible, anastomosis of the ends of the esophagus.
   b. If the separation of the ends of the esophagus is too broad, a gastrostomy tube will be inserted for feedings.

F. Nursing considerations
1. Preoperative.
   a. Ineffective Breathing Pattern/Risk for Aspiration (although this is primarily a gastrointestinal defect, the child's respiratory status is **priority**).
      i. Elevate the head of the crib.
      ii. Monitor lung sounds and respiratory status.
         (1) Assessing for signs of respiratory distress including intercostal retractions, grunting, tachycardia, tachypnea, and cyanosis.
      iii. Monitor oxygen saturation levels.
      iv. Monitor blood gases.
      v. Provide oxygen, as ordered.
      vi. Maintain N/G suction to keep the blind pouch clear of secretions.
   b. Imbalanced Nutrition: Less than Body Requirements/Risk for Deficient Fluid Volume.
      i. Keep the child NPO.
      ii. Maintain IV therapy, as prescribed.
      iii. Provide feedings via gastrostomy tube, as ordered.
      iv. Monitor strict I & O.
      v. Monitor the child's weight each day.
   c. Risk for Altered Family Process/Anxiety/Grieving.
      i. Allow parents to express grief and loss of the perfect child.
      ii. Assess the parents' responsiveness to the baby.
         (1) Encourage skin-to-skin contact to promote bonding.
         (2) If poor bonding is noted, the nurse should recommend the primary health-care provider to refer the family for counseling.
      iii. Enable the parents to discuss their concerns regarding their stress and the need for surgery.
   d. Deficient Knowledge.
      i. Teach the parents feeding techniques for pre- and postsurgery, as needed.
      ii. Provide information regarding corrective surgeries.
      iii. Refer to community/parental group resources (e.g., EA/TEF Family Support Connection).
2. Postoperative fistula repair.
   a. Risk for Ineffective Breathing Pattern/Aspiration.
      i. Elevate the head of the crib.
      ii. Maintain N/G suction to keep the blind pouch clear of secretions.
      iii. Monitor lung sounds and respiratory status, including signs of respiratory distress.
      iv. Monitor oxygen saturation levels.
      v. Monitor blood gases.
      vi. Provide oxygen, as ordered.
      vii. Assess patency of the chest tube, if present.

b. Ineffective Thermoregulation.
   i. Monitor temperature because neonatal thermoregulation is often poor.
   ii. Encourage skin-to-skin contact, if possible, or maintain under infant warmer or in Isolette, if needed.
c. Imbalanced Nutrition: Less than Body Requirements/Risk for Deficient Fluid Volume.
   i. Maintain IV, as prescribed.
   ii. Feed breast milk or formula via gastrostomy tube.
   iii. Monitor I & O.
   iv. Monitor weight daily.
   v. Offer pacifiers at each feeding.
      (1) Suckling is a reflex response in neonates providing comfort.
      (2) Oral function must be maintained for future when oral intake will eventually be possible.
      (3) Oral function must be maintained for future speech development.
d. Risk for Impaired Skin Integrity.
   i. Monitor gastrostomy stoma site employing REEDA assessments.
   ii. Monitor surgical site employing REEDA assessments
   iii. Refer the family to a nurse specializing in stoma care or, if no specialist is available, educate the family regarding care of the stoma.
e. Pain:
   i. Provide both pharmacological and nonpharmacological pain interventions, as needed and as prescribed.

3. Long term: Deficient Knowledge.
   a. Educate the parents regarding respiratory assessments, feeding techniques, and skin integrity assessments.
   b. Final repair may be delayed for months.
   c. Educate the parents to offer a pacifier during each feeding.
      i. Associating a pacifier with feeding will help the child in the future when the final repair is completed.
      ii. After the final repair is completed, the child will likely be referred to an occupational therapist to learn how to swallow fluids and to chew and swallow foods.

VII. Imperforate Anus

A. Incidence.
1. **Imperforate anus** affects about 1 in 5,000 live births.

B. Etiology.
1. The etiology is unknown.
2. About one-half of all babies with imperforate anus have other congenital anomalies, including cardiac and urinary tract defects, limb defects, or a chromosomal syndrome (e.g., Down syndrome).

C. Pathophysiology.
1. Absent or markedly narrowed anal opening, a misplaced anal opening, or a rectum that connects to another anatomical structure instead of the anus.

D. Diagnosis.
1. Clinical presentation is suggestive.
   a. No visible anus.
   b. No meconium stool after 24 to 48 hr of life.
   c. Inability to insert rectal thermometer.
2. X-ray, ultrasound, and/or CT scan are diagnostic.

E. Treatment.
1. One-step **anoplasty** (surgical repair of the anus) or
2. Two-stage repair: first step, a temporary colostomy, followed in a second surgery by the anoplasty.
   a. Colostomy will temporarily remain in place after the anoplasty surgery to allow the anoplasty site to heal fully and to prevent infection from gastrointestinal bacteria.

F. Nursing considerations.
1. Risk for Injury.
   a. Monitor for meconium stool after delivery.
      i. If no stool is expelled in 24 hr:
         (1) Report to the primary health-care provider.
         (2) Monitor for abdominal distension.
   b. If diagnosed with imperforate anus, the child is kept NPO until an opening is established (either via anoplasty or colostomy).
2. Imbalanced Nutrition: Less than Body Requirements/Risk for Dysfunctional Gastrointestinal Motility.
   a. Maintain IV as prescribed until oral feeds are allowed.
   b. Advance diet of breast milk, or formula, as indicated postsurgery.
   c. Administer sufficient fluids and provide stool softeners, per orders.
3. Risk for Infection/Risk for Impaired Tissue Integrity.
   a. Monitor surgical site and stoma for evidence of infection using REEDA.
   b. Refer the baby to a stoma therapist and provide stoma care, as ordered.
4. Risk for Altered Family Process/Anxiety/Grieving.
   a. Allow parents to express grief and loss of the perfect child.

b. Assess the parents' responsiveness to the baby.
   (1) Encourage skin-to-skin contact to promote bonding.
   (2) If poor bonding is noted, the nurse should recommend the primary health-care provider to refer the family for counseling.
c. Enable the parents to discuss their concerns regarding their stress and the need for surgery.

5. Deficient Knowledge.
   a. Educate the parents regarding stoma and colostomy care, if needed.
   b. Provide information regarding corrective surgeries.
   c. Educate the parents regarding anal dilatation post anoplasty, if needed.
   d. Refer to community/parental group resources (e.g., Family Resource Center at Cincinnati Children's Medical Center).
      i. Because of the rarity of the defect, local resources specific to imperforate anus are unlikely.
6. Long term: provide guidance to the parents and child regarding toilet training.
   a. Toilet training usually takes much longer than in children with normal anatomy at birth.

VIII. Hirschsprung's Disease (often called megacolon)

A. Incidence.
1. **Hirschsprung's disease** is more common in boys than in girls.

B. Etiology.
1. Cause is usually unknown, although it does occur in relation with some genetic syndromes (e.g. Down syndrome).

C. Pathophysiology.
1. Congenital absence of enervation to the rectum and/or lower intestine.
2. Signs and symptoms.
   a. Delayed expulsion of meconium and/or recurring constipation early in infancy.
   b. Ribbon-like or pellet-like stools.
   c. Failure to thrive.
   d. Distended abdomen.

D. Diagnosis.
1. Highly suspicious if ultrasound shows enlarged upper colon with absence of feces in distal colon and rectum.
2. Definitive diagnosis is made from a biopsy of the affected colon showing absence of nerve fibers.

E. Treatment.
1. One-step surgical repair: removal of the affected colon and the anastomosis of the healthy colon to the anus, or, if needed:
2. Two-stage repair with:
   a. First procedure: removal of the affected colon and the creation of a temporary colostomy, followed by,
   b. Second procedure: removal of the colostomy and the anastomosis of the healthy colon to the anus.

F. Nursing considerations.
1. Preoperative.
   a. Risk for Imbalanced Nutrition/Imbalanced Fluid Volume.
      i. Carefully monitor the child's hydration status, including:
         (1) Calculating the percentage of weight loss.
         (2) Assessing for additional physiological signs of dehydration, including low urinary output, poor skin turgor, absence of tears, and altered vital signs and,
         (3) If the child is an infant, assessing for a sunken anterior fontanel.
      ii. Monitor I & O.
      iii. Monitor biologic growth.
      iv. Monitor laboratory data, including serum electrolytes.
   b. Constipation.
      i. Administer saline edemas to clear.
      ii. After enemas, keep NPO until surgery.
   c. Risk for Infection.
      i. Antibiotic administration (usually per rectum) to decrease bacterial levels in the bowel.
2. Postoperative.
   a. Risk for Infection/Risk for Impaired Skin Integrity.
      i. Monitor vital signs.
      ii. Monitor laboratory data, including CBC and serum electrolytes.
      iii. Provide stoma care, if needed.
      iv. Refer the family to a stoma therapist, if indicated.
   b. Imbalanced Nutrition: Less than Body Requirements/Risk for Imbalanced Fluid Volume.
      i. Keep NPO with N/G tube until peristalsis is present.
      ii. Maintain IV therapy, as prescribed.
      iii. Monitor hydration status and I & O.
   c. Risk for Altered Family Process/Anxiety/Grieving. Deficient Knowledge.
      i. Allow the parents to express grief and loss of perfect child.
      ii. Assess the parents' responsiveness to the child, if colostomy is present.

iii. Educate the parents regarding corrective surgeries.
iv. Enable the parents to discuss concerns regarding their stress and the need for surgery.
v. Refer the family to community/parental group resources (e.g., Intermountain Healthcare System, Salt Lake City, Utah).
(1) Because of the rarity of the defect, local resources specific to Hirschsprung's disease are unlikely.

d. Pain
i. Provide both pharmacological and non-pharmacological pain interventions, as needed and as prescribed.

3. Long-term care:
a. Provide guidance to the parents and child regarding toilet training.
i. Toilet training usually takes much longer than in children with normal anatomy at birth.

IX. Gastroschisis/Omphalocele

A. Incidence.
1. Combined incidence is approximately 1 in every 2,000 live births.

B. Etiology.
1. No specific etiology has been established, however.
a. Higher incidence seen in women who smoke, drink alcohol, and/or take drugs during their pregnancies.
b. There appears to be a lower incidence of abdominal wall defects in women who take folic acid supplements during their pregnancies.

C. Pathophysiology.
1. **Gastroschisis** is a congenital defect in which the abdominal wall fails to develop, resulting in the intestines protruding from the body.
a. The abdominal organs lie outside the body, with no skin or sac covering.
2. **Omphalocele** is a congenital defect resulting from poor abdominal muscle development in which the intestines or abdominal organs herniate into the umbilicus.

D. Diagnosis.
1. Prenatally.
a. Screening test results indicate the possible presence of a defect.
i. Elevated alpha fetoprotein levels.
(1) May be obtained either via serum or amniotic fluid testing.
ii. Ultrasound visualization confirms the diagnosis.
2. Newborn
a. Direct visualization of the defect is possible.
b. X-ray, ultrasound, MRI, and/or CT scan are often performed to determine the severity of the defect.

E. Treatment.
1. Surgical closure, which may be performed either prenatally or after delivery.
a. If done as a newborn, the surgery is usually completed within 48 hr of delivery.
b. Closure may be performed in stages if the defect is large.
i. The defect is covered with sterile gauze and plastic covering.
ii. Once the skin is able to cover the gastric contents, the surgical repair is completed.

F. Nursing considerations.
1. Risk for Injury/Risk for Infection/Risk for Altered Thermoregulation.
a. Maintain N/G tube, as needed.
b. Position the baby supine, taking care to prevent injury to the abdominal contents, including kinking of intestines.
c. Cover the site with moist, sterile gauze and plastic.
d. Monitor for signs of infection.
e. Monitor for hypothermia and hyperthermia because infected neonates may exhibit either temperature shift.
f. Administer safe dosages of antibiotics, per orders.
g. Provide exogenous warmth in Isolette or warming crib to maintain normal temperature.
2. Imbalanced Nutrition: Less than Body Requirements/Risk for Deficient Fluid Volume/ Risk for Dysfunctional Gastrointestinal Motility.
a. Maintain IV, as prescribed.
b. Administer total parenteral nutrition (TPN) through a central line, if prescribed.
c. Monitor strict I & O.
d. Monitor weight daily.
e. Monitor bowel sounds.
i. The baby is at high risk for developing a paralytic **ileus** (i.e., absence of intestinal peristalsis).
3. Risk for Altered Family Process/Anxiety/ Grieving.
a. Allow parents to express grief and loss of the perfect child.
b. Assess the parents' responsiveness to the baby.
i. Encourage frequent visitation to promote bonding.
ii. If poor bonding is noted, the nurse should recommend the primary

health-care provider to refer the family for counseling.
   c. Enable the parents to discuss their concerns regarding their stress and the need for surgery.
4. Deficient Knowledge.
   a. Educate the parents regarding feeding techniques postsurgery, as needed.
   b. Provide information regarding corrective surgeries.
   c. Refer to community/parental group resources.
5. Pain
   a. Provide both pharmacological and nonpharmacological pain interventions, as needed and as prescribed.

X. Pyloric Stenosis (hypertrophic pyloric stenosis)

A. Incidence.
1. Higher incidence of **pyloric stenosis** in males than in females.
2. Age of onset is usually 1 to 2 months of age.

B. Etiology.
1. No specific cause has been identified, but both genetic and environmental causes have been considered.

C. Pathophysiology.
1. The tissues of the pyloric sphincter hypertrophy, preventing ingested breast milk or formula to pass into the duodenum.
2. Signs and symptoms.
   a. Projectile vomiting, which can land 4 to 5 ft from the baby.
      i. Vomiting usually begins 3 to 4 weeks after birth.
      ii. Vomitus is completely undigested and non-bile stained.
      iii. Metabolic alkalosis with below normal serum electrolytes may be present.
   b. Accompanied by:
      i. Visible reverse peristalsis.
      ii. Olive-shaped mass in upper right quadrant.
   c. Baby appears healthy and hungry following vomiting episode.

D. Diagnosis.
1. Clinical signs are highly suggestive.
2. X-ray, which may include a barium swallow, and ultrasound are performed to confirm the diagnosis.

E. Treatment.
1. Prior to surgery, any altered electrolyte, acid/base, and/or fluid states are corrected, if present.
2. Surgery: **pyloromyotomy** (incision of the pyloric muscle) is usually performed via a laparoscope.

F. Nursing considerations.
1. Preoperative.
   a. Risk for Imbalanced Nutrition: Less than Body Requirements/Deficient Fluid Volume.
      i. Maintain NPO.
         (1) Vomiting usually ceases as soon as feedings are stopped.
         (2) If vomiting is still present, document the frequency, amount, and characteristics of the vomitus.
      ii. Maintain IV therapy, as prescribed.
      iii. Monitor serum electrolytes and blood gases and provide electrolyte therapy, if needed and as prescribed.
      iv. Assess the infant's hydration status, including:
         (1) Calculating the percentage of weight loss.
         (2) Assessing for additional physiological signs of dehydration, including low urinary output, poor skin turgor, absence of tears, and altered vital signs and, sunken anterior fontanel.
         (3) Monitoring the infant's I & O.
   b. Risk for Altered Family Process/Anxiety/Deficient Knowledge.
      i. Enable the parents to discuss their concerns regarding their stress and the need for surgery.
      ii. Educate the parents that there was nothing that they did to cause the problem.
      iii. Educate the parents regarding the corrective surgery.
2. Postoperative.
   a. Imbalanced Nutrition: Less than Body Requirements/Deficient Fluid Volume.
      i. Continue preoperative monitoring of blood gases, serum electrolytes, hydration status, and I & O.
      ii. Begin feeds per surgeon's instructions. (Feeds are usually begun soon after the repair is completed.)
         (1) Usual progression of feedings: ORT to half strength formula (if breast milk, no dilution is usually required) to full strength feeds.
      iii. Monitor for vomiting and, if present, document the frequency, amount, and characteristics of the vomitus.
      iv. Monitor for resumption of normal stool pattern.
      v. Assess the incisions for REEDA signs.
   b. Deficient Knowledge.
      i. Advise the parents to advance diet, as prescribed.

ii. Advise the parents to report any vomiting.
iii. Educate the parents regarding postoperative incision assessment and care, and to report any deviations from normal.

XI. Intussusception

A. Incidence.
1. Most commonly seen in children under 2 years of age, with peak age in middle of the first year of life.
2. Most common bowel obstruction problem in children under 5 years of age.
3. Higher incidence in boys than in girls.
4. Babies are high risk for recurrence.

B. Etiology.
1. Majority of cases have an unknown cause.
2. Gastrointestinal pathology of cystic fibrosis (see Chapter 16, "Nursing Care of the Child with Respiratory Illnesses") predisposes affected children to **intussusception**.

C. Pathophysiology.
1. Invagination of bowel, usually at the ileocecal valve (see Fig. 14.4).
2. Signs and symptoms.
   a. Sudden onset of pain, which begins as periodic and rapidly progresses to constant pain, characterized by intense, inconsolable crying.
   b. Abdominal guarding.

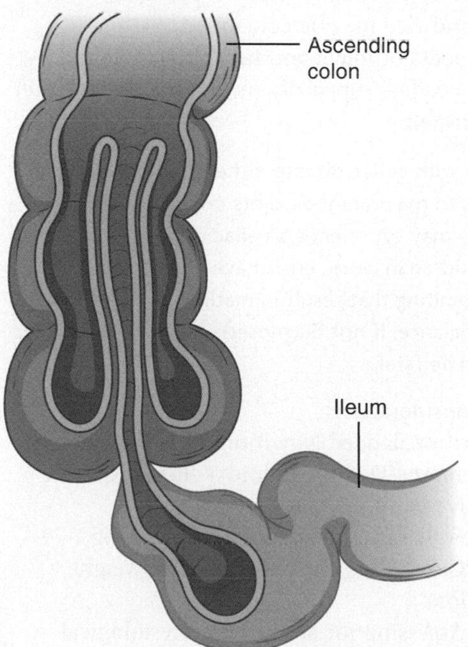

Fig 14.4 Intussusception.

   c. Drawing of knees toward the abdomen.
   d. Vomiting.
   e. Sausage-shaped mass in right upper quadrant.
   f. "Currant jelly" stools, i.e., stools mixed with blood and mucus.

D. Diagnosis.
1. Clinical picture is highly suggestive.
2. X-ray, often with barium contrast, and ultrasound are diagnostic.

E. Treatment.
1. If no signs of shock or sepsis, the bowel is usually restored via air or barium enema.
   a. The force of the enema corrects the intussusception.

DID YOU KNOW?

An intussusception of the bowel is similar to the finger of a rubber glove that invaginates after it is taken off the hand. To correct the invagination, one blows into the glove, and the finger pops back to its original position. Similarly, when the child is given an enema, the bowel is forced open.

   b. Surgical repair, usually via laparoscope, is performed if the clinical picture is poor or if an enema is ineffective.

F. Nursing considerations.
1. Imbalanced Nutrition: Less than Body Requirements/Deficient Fluid Volume.
   a. Assess vital signs for possible shock or sepsis.
   b. Monitor for vomiting and, if present, document the frequency, amount, and characteristics of the vomitus.
   c. Assess hydration status, including.
      i. Calculating the percentage of weight loss.
      ii. Assessing for additional physiological signs of dehydration, including low urinary output, poor skin turgor, absence of tears, and altered vital signs and, sunken anterior fontanel.
      iii. Monitoring the I & O
   d. Maintain the NPO until therapy is instituted, then progress diet, as indicated, following correction of the defect.
   e. Maintain IV therapy, as prescribed.
   f. Monitor serum electrolyte laboratory values.
   g. Administer electrolytes, as prescribed.
   h. Monitor for resumption of normal stooling pattern.
      i. The child should not be discharged until he or she has had a normal stool.
2. Risk for Altered Family Process/Anxiety/Deficient Knowledge.
   a. Enable the parents to discuss their concerns regarding their stress as well as the child's painful episodes and need for surgery.

b. Educate the parents regarding therapeutic procedures.
c. Educate the parents to report any signs of recurrence as soon as possible.
d. Educate the parents to monitor the child's stooling pattern and to report adverse findings as soon as possible.

3. Provide both pharmacological and non-pharmacological pain interventions, as needed and as prescribed.
   a. Assess for signs of abdominal distress, especially inconsolable crying and drawing up of legs.

XII. Celiac Disease

A. Incidence.
1. **Celiac disease** affects approximately one out of every 130 individuals in the United States.

B. Etiology.
1. Many patients with celiac disease carry a genetic mutation on chromosome 6; however, all persons who carry the mutation do not develop celiac disease.
2. Those with type 1 diabetes, Down syndrome, and other preexisting diseases are at high risk of developing celiac.

C. Pathophysiology.
1. Genetic inability to digest the gluten protein (gliadin) found in three grains: barley, wheat, and rye.
2. If gluten is consumed, resultant physiological changes develop.
   a. Atrophy of intestinal villi and ulcerations of the intestinal mucosa.
   b. Dermatitis herpetiformis, which may or may not be accompanied by digestive symptomatology.
      i. Highly pruritic rash that is seen on the knees, elbows, and buttocks. It always is seen bilaterally (i.e., if the rash is present on one knee, it is always also present on the other knee).

DID YOU KNOW?

Many patients are advised not only to avoid consuming foods containing barley, wheat, and rye but also foods containing oats. Oats, however, contain only small quantities of gluten. Instead of advising patients to avoid oats, most health-care practitioners are now advising celiac patients only to consume oats that are milled in plants where the oats are kept completely separate from other grains. The oats must be ground in machines that are never used for grinding any of the three other grains.

3. Signs and symptoms.
   a. Celiac disease may present in a variety of ways.
      i. GI symptoms range from diarrhea to abdominal distention to vomiting.
      ii. Additional symptoms range from irritability to anorexia to muscle wasting to failure to thrive to pruritic rash.
      iii. Adults often present with different symptoms than do children.
      iv. "Children tend to have the more classic signs of celiac disease, including growth problems (failure to thrive, chronic diarrhea/constipation, recurring abdominal bloating and pain, fatigue and irritability)" (University of Chicago Celiac Disease Center [2014]).
4. Patients with celiac disease are at high risk for a number of serious complications, including osteoporosis, gastrointestinal cancers, and seizures.

D. Diagnosis.
1. Signs that are suggestive of the disease:
   a. Positive IgA antibody test (antitissue transglutaminase).
   b. Responsiveness to a diet change.
2. Definitive diagnosis is the finding of atrophy of the intestinal villi seen on histology.

E. Treatment.
1. All wheat, rye, and barley are removed from the diet.
2. Because they contain no gluten proteins, corn, millet, and rice may be consumed.
3. Supplements of folate and fat-soluble vitamins may be needed, especially until a therapeutic diet is established.

(!) If children with celiac disease either are not diagnosed properly or fail to maintain their diets once they are diagnosed, they may experience a celiac crisis. Although uncommon, children in celiac crisis have a rapid onset of diarrhea and vomiting that result in marked dehydration and electrolyte imbalance. If not diagnosed and treated quickly, celiac crisis can be fatal.

F. Nursing considerations.
1. Risk for Imbalanced Nutrition: Less than Body Requirements/Deficient Fluid Volume/Risk for Ineffective Family Coping.
   a. Carefully monitor hydration, including.
      i. Calculating the percentage of weight loss.
      ii. Assessing for additional physiological signs of dehydration, including low urinary output, poor skin turgor, absence

of tears, and altered vital signs and, sunken anterior fontanel.

iii. Monitoring the I & O.

iv. If in celiac crisis, the child may exhibit signs of hypovolemia and shock.

b. Allow the parents to communicate their concerns regarding the child's irritable behavior.

c. Enable the parents to discuss concerns regarding the child's diet and future health.

d. Refer the parents to a dietician for diet counseling.

e. Eliminate all offending foods.

i. Although children's response to gluten varies, as little as one bite of one piece of bread can damage the child's intestines and result in diarrhea and behavioral symptoms.

f. Monitor stooling and growth patterns.

2. Risk for Ineffective Individual Coping.

a. Children, especially teenagers, may resist maintaining the diet.

b. Introduce the child and family to other children with the disease.

DID YOU KNOW?

When children eat and play with friends, it can be embarrassing and/or upsetting to be on a special diet. Older children, especially adolescents, with celiac disease can be encouraged to "negotiate" with their friends about diet choices. For example, one time the teens could decide to go to a pizza parlor where the child with celiac may have to eat a salad or other non-grain item. The next time the teens go out, however, they could go to an Asian restaurant where rice products predominate and, therefore, where the child with celiac can consume the same foods as his or her friends.

3. Deficient Knowledge.

a. The parents and child, if age appropriate, must be carefully educated about the therapeutic diet.

b. Educate the parents to read all food labels carefully for the presence of gluten and gluten-containing grains.

c. Refer the parents to community resource organizations (e.g., American Celiac Society).

CASE STUDY: Putting It All Together

8-year, 2-month-old male Caucasian brought to the pediatrician's office

Subjective Data

- Mother states,
  - "I cannot figure out what is wrong. Our son has always been healthy and easygoing. For the last month or so, he is a completely different child."
  - "Nothing seems to make him happy. He is constantly complaining about something. He won't eat. He yells at his father and me and won't play nice with his brother."
  - "And, he won't let me look, but I think he is having problems going to the bathroom."
  - Child refuses to discuss stool patterns but does state, "My belly hurts sometimes after I eat."

Objective Data

Nursing Assessment

- Physical findings
  - Weight at last doctor visit (6 months earlier): 55th percentile; weight now: 45th percentile
  - Child appears pale; no skin lesions noted and normal skin turgor

Vital Signs	
Temperature:	98.7°F
Heart rate:	100 bpm
Respiratory rate:	20 rpm
Blood pressure:	98/58 mm Hg

Lab Results	
Complete blood count	
Red blood cell count:	3,800,00 cells/mm^3
Hematocrit:	30%
Hemoglobin:	10.0 g/dL
Platelets:	225,000 cells/mm^3
White blood cell count:	8,000 cells/mm^3
Immunoglobulin A-tissue transglutaminase (IgA-tTG): positive	
Small bowel biopsy	
Atrophy of intestinal villi	

Health-Care Provider's Orders

- Diagnosis: celiac disease
- Remove all gluten-containing foods from the diet
- Administer one vitamin supplement daily
- Refer family to a certified dietitian
- Return to pediatrician for follow-up visit in 2 weeks

Continued

Case Study Questions

A. What *subjective* assessments indicate that this client is experiencing a health alteration?

1.
2.
3.

B. What *objective* assessments indicate that this client is experiencing a health alteration?

1.
2.
3.
4.
5.
6.

C. After analyzing the data that has been collected, what **primary** nursing diagnosis should the nurse assign to this client?

1.

D. What interventions should the nurse plan and/or implement to meet this child's and his family's needs?

1.
2.
3.
4.
5.
6.
7.

E. What client outcomes should the nurse evaluate regarding the effectiveness of the nursing interventions?

1.
2.
3.
4.

F. What physiological and psychological characteristics should the child exhibit before being discharged home?

1.
2.
3.
4.
5.
6.

G. What subjective characteristics should the child exhibit before being discharged home?

1.

REVIEW QUESTIONS

1. A 2-month-old infant with a cleft lip is transferred to the pediatric floor immediately following surgical repair of the defect. Which of the following interventions should the nurse perform?
   1. Assess placement of the elbow restraints.
   2. Assess placement of the gastrostomy tube.
   3. Monitor the child for signs of hypokalemia.
   4. Monitor the child for passage of tarry stools.

2. A 7-month-old child who has yet to have a cleft palate repaired is saying a few words. The child's lip is intact. Which of the following words would the nurse expect the child to have the most difficulty saying?
   1. "Ma ma"
   2. "Da da"
   3. "Ba ba"
   4. "Pa pa"

3. The nurse is educating a new mother of a child born with both a cleft lip and a cleft palate regarding formula feeding. Which of the following actions should the nurse include in her teaching session? **Select all that apply.**
   1. Instruct the mother to add rice cereal to the formula.
   2. Encourage the mother to cup feed her baby rather than to bottle feed.
   3. Advise the mother to hold the baby in an upright position during feedings.
   4. Advise the mother to feed the baby slowly to allow the baby time to swallow and to rest.
   5. Notify the mother of the importance of giving the baby pain medicine before each feeding.

4. The nurse in the delivery room suspects that a newly birthed baby may have an esophageal atresia with tracheoesophageal fistula because the baby is exhibiting which of the following signs and symptoms?
   1. Palpable mass in left lower quadrant
   2. Blood-tinged vomitus
   3. Pseudostrabismus
   4. Copious quantities of oral mucus

5. A baby, 12 hours old, in the neonatal intensive care unit, has been diagnosed with esophageal atresia with tracheoesophageal fistula. Which of the following assessments is highest priority for the nurse to make?
   1. Quantity of nasogastric secretions
   2. Oxygen saturation levels
   3. Apical heart rate
   4. Weight of wet diapers

6. A 14-month-old child is in hospital post-op from repair of congenital esophageal atresia (anastomosis of the ends of the esophagus). It is important for the nurse to encourage the surgeon to order a referral for the child to which of the following health-care practitioners?
   1. Speech therapist
   2. Stoma nurse
   3. Otolaryngologist
   4. Occupational therapist

7. A baby was just born with a gastroschisis. Which of the following actions by the nurse is priority?
   1. Inform the parents regarding the etiology of the defect.
   2. Cover the defect with a moist, sterile dressing.
   3. Administer intravenous antibiotics, as ordered.
   4. Educate the parents regarding the surgical repair.

8. A one-month-old baby has been admitted to the pediatric unit with a diagnosis of pyloric stenosis. Which of the following assessments is highest priority for the nurse to report to the baby's primary health-care provider?
   1. Sunken fontanel
   2. Undigested emesis
   3. Apical heart rate of 156 bpm
   4. Serum potassium of 3.6 mEq/dL

9. A one-month-old baby, 8 lb 4 oz, is in the hospital with a diagnosis of pyloric stenosis. The nurse is carefully assessing the child's intake and output. Please calculate the minimum urinary output the baby should excrete per hour. **Please calculate to the nearest tenth.**

   __________ mL/hr

10. A baby, with a history of cystic fibrosis, is admitted to the emergency department. The baby is crying loudly and drawing his legs up toward his abdomen. A diagnosis of intussusception is made. Which of the following orders would the nurse expect to receive at this time?
    1. To administer a corticosteroid medication
    2. To prepare the baby for abdominal surgery
    3. To prepare the baby for an air enema
    4. To administer an antispasmodic medication

11. A baby is admitted with a diagnosis of intussusception. Which of the following signs/symptoms would the nurse expect to see?
    1. Projective vomiting
    2. Acute constipation
    3. Explosive flatus
    4. Currant jelly stools

12. A child has been diagnosed with Hirschsprung's disease. Which of the following findings would the nurse expect the parents to report in the child's history? **Select all that apply.**
1. Ribbon-like stools
2. Chronic constipation
3. Black and tarry stools
4. Distended abdomen
5. Delayed meconium passage

13. A school nurse is monitoring the eating patterns of a child with celiac disease. The nurse counsels the child to choose an alternate lunch when the child picks which of the following foods to put on the lunch tray?
1. Corn taco with refried beans
2. Rice noodles with beef and broccoli
3. Turkey meatloaf with baked potato
4. Roast pork with applesauce

14. A child has just been diagnosed with celiac disease. Which of the following signs and symptoms would the nurse expect the parents to report in the child's history? **Select all that apply.**
1. Irritability
2. Failure to thrive
3. Abdominal pain
4. Excessive hunger
5. Recurring diarrhea

15. A 10-year-old child is diagnosed with enterobiasis (pinworm). Which of the following signs/symptoms would the nurse expect to see?
1. Recurrent vomiting
2. Enuresis
3. Bloody diarrhea
4. Pain

16. The nurse is educating the parents of a 2-month-old infant regarding the immunizations that the child will receive that day. The nurse should educate the parents that which of the following immunizations will protect the child from a serious gastrointestinal infection?
1. Rotavirus vaccine (RV)
2. Diphtheria, tetanus, and acellular pertussis (DTaP)
3. *Haemophilus influenzae* type b (Hib)
4. Pneumococcal conjugate (PCV13)

17. The parent of a 6-month-old calls the child's primary health-care provider and states, "My child has had 5 loose stools since she woke up this morning. What should I do?" The mother is exclusively breastfeeding her baby. Which of the following responses by the nurse is appropriate?
1. "Let's figure out what you may have eaten during the last day that could have caused the diarrhea."
2. "Continue to feed the baby breast milk and give oral rehydration therapy after each feeding."
3. "That's not that unusual for babies who are breastfed but do call again if the stools turn a green color."
4. "Bring the baby in for an appointment with the doctor so that we can weigh and check over the baby."

18. A child is severely dehydrated from a diarrheal illness. The nurse assesses the child's laboratory results. Which of the following results would the nurse expect to find?
1. Hematocrit (Hct) 30%
2. Partial pressure of oxygen (Po_2) 60 mm Hg
3. Potassium (K) 3.0 mEq/L
4. Platelet (Plt) count 100,000 cells/mm^3

19. A 4-year-old child is seen at the primary health-care provider's office with vomiting and diarrhea for the past 24 hours. The primary health-care provider orders a number of interventions. If ordered, the nurse should question the administration of which of the following medications for the child?
1. Lomotil (diphenoxylate/atropine)
2. Zofran (ondansetron)
3. Reglan (metoclopramide)
4. Dramamine (dimenhydrinate)

20. A child is admitted to the pediatric unit. While the nurse was taking the nursing history, the child regurgitated vomitus that looked like coffee grounds and smelled like feces. Which of the following communications would it be appropriate for the nurse to report to the primary health-care provider? "After assessing the vomitus, it appears that the child:
1. has an obstruction proximal to the stomach."
2. has a perforated duodenal ulcer."
3. is vomiting blood from the lower bowel."
4. is exhibiting signs of ruptured esophageal varices."

REVIEW ANSWERS

1. ANSWER: 1
Rationale:
1. **The nurse should assess placement of the elbow restraints.**
2. Gastrostomy tubes are not inserted in children with a diagnosis of cleft lip.
3. The child is not at high risk for hypokalemia.
4. The child is not at high risk for passage of tarry stools.
TEST-TAKING TIP: After surgical repair of a cleft lip, it is important that the sutures not be disturbed. Because babies often put their hands in their mouths, it is important that they be fitted with elbow restraints, but, like all restraints, they must be applied correctly and removed frequently.
Content Area: *Pediatrics*
Integrated Processes: *Nursing Process: Assessment*
Client Need: *Physiological Integrity: Reduction of Risk Potential: Potential for Alterations in Body Systems*
Cognitive Level: *Application*

2. ANSWER: 2
Rationale:
1. The child would be able to say, "Ma ma."
2. **The child would have marked difficulty saying, "Da da."**
3. The child would be able to say, "Ba ba."
4. The child would be able to say, "Pa pa."
TEST-TAKING TIP: When a person makes a number of consonant sounds (e.g., "d," "t," "n") the person must touch the roof of the mouth with his or her tongue. Because a child with a cleft palate has no roof of the mouth, it is virtually impossible for him or her accurately to make those sounds.
Content Area: *Pediatrics*
Integrated Processes: *Nursing Process: Assessment*
Client Need: *Physiological Integrity: Physiological Adaptation: Alteration in Body Systems*
Cognitive Level: *Application*

3. ANSWER: 3 and 4
Rationale:
1. The mother should not be taught to add rice cereal to the formula.
2. This action is not usually included in the teaching sessions.
3. **The mother should be advised to hold the baby in an upright position during feedings.**
4. **The mother should be advised to feed the baby slowly to allow the baby time to swallow and to rest.**
5. The mother should not be notified of the importance of giving the baby pain medicine before each feeding.
TEST-TAKING TIP: Babies with cleft lip and palate must work hard to remove formula from a bottle. Often, alternate feeding methods may be needed, including soft nipples or Breck feeders, but there is rarely a need to cup feed the babies. Because of the difficulty, babies become very tired. They must be given sufficient time to suckle and to swallow. In addition, because of their high risk for ear infections, they should be fed in an upright position.
Content Area: *Pediatrics*
Integrated Processes: *Nursing Process: Implementation*
Client Need: *Physiological Integrity: Reduction of Risk Potential: Potential for Alterations in Body Systems*
Cognitive Level: *Application*

4. ANSWER: 4
Rationale:
1. Palpable mass in left lower quadrant is unrelated to esophageal atresia with tracheoesophageal fistula.
2. Blood-tinged vomitus is unrelated to esophageal atresia with tracheoesophageal fistula.
3. Pseudostrabismus is unrelated to esophageal atresia with tracheoesophageal fistula.
4. **Copious quantities of oral mucus is a classic sign of esophageal atresia with tracheoesophageal fistula.**
TEST-TAKING TIP: Because the baby is unable to swallow the residual amniotic fluid from the lungs as well as his or her saliva, the nurse will note large quantities of mucus continually oozing from the baby's mouth.
Content Area: *Pediatrics*
Integrated Processes: *Nursing Process: Analysis*
Client Need: *Physiological Integrity: Physiological Adaptation: Alterations in Body Systems*
Cognitive Level: *Application*

5. ANSWER: 2
Rationale:
1. Assessing the quantity of nasogastric secretions is important but not of highest priority.
2. **Assessing oxygen saturation levels is highest priority.**
3. Assessing the apical heart rate is important but not of highest priority.
4. Assessing the weight of wet diapers is important but not of highest priority.
TEST-TAKING TIP: When a baby has a tracheoesophageal fistula, there is a direct communication between the baby's gastrointestinal system and his or her pulmonary system. Gastric contents often enter the pulmonary system. Because gas exchange may be compromised, the nurse must carefully monitor the baby's oxygen saturation values.
Content Area: *Pediatrics*
Integrated Processes: *Nursing Process: Assessment*
Client Need: *Safe and Effective Care Environment: Management of Care: Establishing Priorities*
Cognitive Level: *Analysis*

6. ANSWER: 4
Rationale:
1. Speech therapy likely is not required of this child.
2. The child will have had stoma care for his or her gastrostomy tube insertion since birth. A new referral should not be needed.
3. Otolaryngology likely is not required of this child.
4. **The child will need occupational therapy.**
TEST-TAKING TIP: Children who are birthed with esophageal atresia with tracheoesophageal fistula are unable to consume food or drink until the esophageal repair is complete. The 14-month-old child, therefore, has never learned how to swallow food or drink. The child will need to work with an occupational therapist to learn how to perform that behavior.

Content Area: Pediatrics
Integrated Processes: Nursing Process: Implementation
Client Need: Safe and Effective Care Environment: Management of Care: Referrals
Cognitive Level: Analysis

7. ANSWER: 2
Rationale:
1. It is important for the nurse to inform the parents regarding the etiology of the defect, but it is not priority.
2. It is priority for the nurse to cover the defect with a moist, sterile dressing.
3. It is important for the nurse to administer IV antibiotics, as ordered, but it is not priority.
4. It is important for the nurse to educate the parents regarding the surgical repair, but it is not priority.
TEST-TAKING TIP: The abdominal contents of a baby born with gastroschisis are not covered with skin. The abdominal cavity, therefore, is exposed to the air where the contents will dry out and may become infected. It is priority for the nurse to cover the area with a moist, sterile dressing and a plastic covering to reduce the possibility of complications developing.
Content Area: Pediatrics
Integrated Processes: Nursing Process: Implementation
Client Need: Safe and Effective Care Environment: Management of Care: Establishing Priorities
Cognitive Level: Analysis

8. ANSWER: 1
Rationale:
1. It is highest priority for the nurse to report a sunken fontanel.
2. It is not priority for the nurse to report that the child is experiencing undigested emesis.
3. It is not priority for the nurse to report an apical heart rate of 156 bpm.
4. It is not priority for the nurse to report a serum potassium of 3.6 mEq/dL.
TEST-TAKING TIP: A baby with a sunken fontanel is exhibiting signs of dehydration. The physician must be notified. All other findings are within expectations: babies with pyloric stenosis do vomit undigested formula; an apical heart rate of 156 bpm is within normal limits, albeit high normal; and a serum potassium of 3.6 mEq/dL is within normal limits, albeit low normal.
Content Area: Pediatrics
Integrated Processes: Nursing Process: Implementation
Client Need: Safe and Effective Care Environment: Management of Care: Establishing Priorities
Cognitive Level: Analysis

9. ANSWER: 7.5 mL/hr
Rationale:
TEST-TAKING TIP: The minimum output milliliters per hour of an infant is equal to 2 mL times the baby's weight in kilograms (see Table 7.2, Minimum Urinary Outputs, in Chapter 7, "Physical Assessment of Children: From Infancy to Adolescence"). A baby that weighs 8 lb, 4 oz (i.e., 8¼ lb—there are 16 oz in every pound) weighs 3.75 kg (8.25 lb ÷ 2.2 = 3.75 kg). Two times 3.75 kg equals a minimum hourly output of 7.5 mL (3.75 kg × 2 mL/hr = 7.5 mL/hr).

Content Area: Pediatrics
Integrated Processes: Nursing Process: Implementation
Client Need: Physiological Integrity: Reduction of Risk Potential: Potential for Alterations in Body Systems
Cognitive Level: Synthesis

10. ANSWER: 3
Rationale:
1. Corticosteroids are not indicated at this time.
2. The baby likely will not be prepared for abdominal surgery.
3. The nurse would expect to prepare the baby for an air enema.
4. Antispasmodic medication is not indicated at this time.
TEST-TAKING TIP: An air or other type of enema is the usual therapy for a baby with intussusception. Babies with cystic fibrosis are at high risk for the complication.
Content Area: Pediatrics
Integrated Processes: Nursing Process: Analysis
Client Need: Physiological Integrity: Physiological Adaptation: Illness Management
Cognitive Level: Application

11. ANSWER: 4
Rationale:
1. Projective vomiting is not a characteristic symptom of intussusception.
2. Acute constipation is not a characteristic symptom of intussusception.
3. Explosive flatus is not a characteristic symptom of intussusception.
4. Currant jelly stools often are seen in babies with intussusception.
TEST-TAKING TIP: When the bowel invaginates, a narrowing of the lumen results. The fecal material builds up and presses against the intestinal wall. The wall becomes ischemic and begins to break down, resulting in blood mixing with the stool (i.e., currant jelly stools).
Content Area: Pediatrics
Integrated Processes: Nursing Process: Assessment
Client Need: Physiological Integrity: Physiological Adaptation: Alterations in Body Systems
Cognitive Level: Application

12. ANSWER: 1, 2, 4, and 5
Rationale:
1. The nurse would expect the parents to report that the child has ribbon-like stools.
2. The nurse would expect the parents to report that the child has chronic constipation.
3. The nurse would not expect the parents to report that the child has black and tarry stools.
4. The nurse would expect the parents to report that the child has a distended abdomen.
5. The nurse would expect the parents to report that the child has delayed meconium passage.
TEST-TAKING TIP: The lack of enervation to the rectum and/or lower intestine results in the absence of peristalsis in the affected bowel. As a result, in the neonatal period, meconium is passed very late. If the disease remains undiagnosed, the child develops a distended abdomen and chronic constipation with pellet or ribbon-like stools.

Content Area: Pediatrics
Integrated Processes: Nursing Process: Assessment
Client Need: Physiological Integrity: Physiological Adaptation: Alterations in Body Systems
Cognitive Level: Application

13. **ANSWER: 3**
Rationale:
1. A meal of a corn taco with refried beans is compatible with a celiac diet.
2. A meal of rice noodles with beef and broccoli is compatible with a celiac diet.
3. The nurse should counsel a child with celiac disease who chooses meatloaf for lunch.
4. A meal of roast pork with applesauce is compatible with a celiac diet.

TEST-TAKING TIP: Meatloaf is made with breadcrumbs, and breadcrumbs contain gluten protein. Children and parents must be counseled that many foods may look like they are compatible with a celiac diet but are not (e.g., meatloaf that looks like it contains only meat but also contains breadcrumbs).
Content Area: Pediatrics
Integrated Processes: Nursing Process: Implementation
Client Need: Physiological Integrity: Physiological Adaptation: Potential for Alterations in Body Systems
Cognitive Level: Application

14. **ANSWER: 1, 2, 3, and 5**
Rationale:
1. The nurse would expect the parents to report that the child was irritable.
2. The nurse would expect the parents to report that the child experienced failure to thrive.
3. The nurse would expect the parents to report that the child had abdominal pain.
4. The nurse would not expect the parents to report that the child had been excessively hungry. In fact, the child would likely have been anorexic.
5. The nurse would expect the parents to report that the child had recurring diarrhea.

TEST-TAKING TIP: Those with celiac disease can exhibit a variety of signs and symptoms. Children usually exhibit the most common of these: "failure to thrive, chronic diarrhea/constipation, recurring abdominal bloating and pain, fatigue and irritability" (University of Chicago Celiac Disease Center [2014]).
Content Area: Pediatrics
Integrated Processes: Nursing Process: Assessment
Client Need: Physiological Integrity: Physiological Adaptation: Alteration in Body Systems
Cognitive Level: Application

15. **ANSWER: 2**
Rationale:
1. The nurse would not expect to see recurrent vomiting.
2. The nurse would expect the child to be wetting the bed.
3. The nurse would not expect to see bloody diarrhea.
4. The nurse would not expect to see the child in pain.

TEST-TAKING TIP: Pinworm eggs hatch in the small intestines. They then migrate through the remainder of the bowel and exit via the anus during the nighttime hours. The activity of the worms on the perineum and around the anus often results in the child urinating in his or her sleep.
Content Area: Pediatrics
Integrated Processes: Nursing Process: Assessment
Client Need: Physiological Integrity: Physiological Adaptation: Alteration in Body Systems
Cognitive Level: Application

16. **ANSWER: 1**
Rationale:
1. Rotavirus vaccine (RV) is the correct response.
2. Neither diphtheria, tetanus, nor acellular pertussis (DTaP) is a gastrointestinal illness.
3. *Haemophilus influenzae* type b (Hib) protects the baby from an organism that causes pneumonia, meningitis, and sepsis.
4. Pneumococcal conjugate (PCV13) protects the baby from an organism that causes pneumonia, meningitis, and sepsis.

TEST-TAKING TIP: At the 2-month well-baby visit, it is recommended that infants receive a number of vaccinations: rotavirus (RV); diphtheria, tetanus, and acellular pertussis (DTaP); *Haemophilus influenzae* type b (Hib); pneumococcal conjugate (PCV13); and inactivated poliovirus (IPV). Only one of the immunizations protects babies from gastrointestinal illness—the rotavirus vaccine.
Content Area: Pediatrics
Integrated Processes: Nursing Process: Implementation; Teaching/Learning
Client Need: Health Promotion and Maintenance: Health Promotion/Disease Prevention
Cognitive Level: Application

17. **ANSWER: 4**
Rationale:
1. It is unlikely that a change in the mother's diet would result in a child developing acute diarrhea. In addition, the child needs to be evaluated for signs of dehydration.
2. Although the mother may eventually be directed to continue to breastfeed and to supplement the feedings with ORT, the baby first needs to be assessed for signs of dehydration.
3. Breastfeeding stools are relatively loose, but the baby is 6 months old. The mother, by that time, is clearly familiar with the child's bowel habits.
4. The baby does need to be weighed to determine whether the baby is dehydrated.

TEST-TAKING TIP: Percentage of weight loss is the best way to determine the severity of dehydration. The baby should be weighed and the percentage of weight loss calculated. If the baby has mild dehydration, the mother likely will be advised to continue to breastfeed and to give oral rehydration therapy after each feeding. However, if the child is severely dehydrated, the child likely will need IV therapy.

Content Area: *Pediatrics*
Integrated Processes: *Nursing Process: Implementation*
Client Need: *Physiological Integrity: Physiological Adaptation: Alteration in Body Systems*
Cognitive Level: *Application*

18. ANSWER: 3

Rationale:
1. The nurse would not expect to see a hematocrit (Hct) of 30%.
2. The nurse would not expect to see a partial pressure of oxygen (Po_2) 60 mm Hg.
3. The nurse would expect to see a lab report that shows hypokalemia.
4. The nurse would not expect to see a platelet (Plt) count of 100,000 cells/mm^3.

TEST-TAKING TIP: The child has diarrhea, therefore the child is losing fluids. If the child becomes moderately or severely dehydrated, the nurse would expect the Hct to rise. There should be no change in the Po_2 or the Plt count. The nurse would, however, expect that the K level could be low.
Content Area: *Pediatrics*
Integrated Processes: *Nursing Process: Implementation*
Client Need: *Physiological Integrity: Physiological Adaptation: Alteration in Body Systems*
Cognitive Level: *Application*

19. ANSWER: 1

Rationale:
1. Although the child does have diarrhea, Lomotil (diphenoxylate/ atropine) is not recommended to be given to children.
2. Zofran (ondansetron) is an appropriate medication for a child who is vomiting.
3. Reglan (metoclopramide) is an appropriate medication for a child who is vomiting.
4. Dramamine (dimenhydrinate) is an appropriate medication for a child who is vomiting.

TEST-TAKING TIP: If ordered, the nurse should question the administration of an antidiarrhea medication for the child (e.g., Lomotil). Antiemetics often are needed to reduce children's vomiting episodes, but it is recommended that antidiarrhea medications not be administered to young children.
Content Area: *Pediatrics*
Integrated Processes: *Nursing Process: Implementation*
Client Need: *Physiological Integrity: Pharmacological and Parenteral Therapies: Adverse Effects/Contraindications/ Side Effects/Interactions*
Cognitive Level: *Application*

20. ANSWER: 3

Rationale:
1. Vomitus proximal to the stomach would appear as completely undigested food.
2. Vomitus from a perforated duodenal ulcer would appear bile colored and mixed with blood.
3. The vomitus does appear to include blood and feces from the lower bowel.
4. Blood-tinged vomitus from ruptured esophageal varices would appear bright red.

TEST-TAKING TIP: When assessing vomitus, the nurse should consider the location within the gastrointestinal system from where the vomitus likely originated. In addition, the nurse should consider whether the vomitus contained undigested or digested blood.
Content Area: *Pediatrics*
Integrated Processes: *Nursing Process: Implementation*
Client Need: *Physiological Integrity: Physiological Adaptation: Alteration in Body Systems*
Cognitive Level: *Application*

Nursing Care of the Child With Genitourinary Disorders

KEY TERMS

Acute poststreptococcal glomerulonephritis (AGN)—Inflammatory process following a strep infection, affecting the ability of the renal glomerulus to filter the blood.

Anasarca—Generalized swelling of the body.

Bladder exstrophy—A bladder that lies outside of the abdominal cavity.

Chordee—A condition in which the penile shaft curves downward.

Cryptorchidism—Undescended testes.

Enuresis—Urinary incontinence.

Epispadias—A congenital anomaly in which the urethral opening is located on the upper surface of the penile shaft.

Hemoconcentration—Increase in the concentration of the cells and solids in the blood caused by a loss of fluid.

Hyperproteinuria—The presence of large quantities of proteins in the urine.

Hypoproteinemia—A low level of protein circulating in the blood.

Hypospadias—A congenital anomaly in which the urethral opening is located on the underside of the penile shaft.

Nephrotic syndrome (nephrosis)—Inflammation of the glomerulus of the kidneys allowing large molecules, most notably the protein albumin, to be excreted into the urine.

Wilms' tumor (nephroblastoma)—A type of kidney cancer that primarily affects children.

I. Description

The genitourinary (GU) system is comprised of the renal system—kidneys, ureters, bladder, and urethra—and the genitalia. Normal functioning of the system is requisite for the production and excretion of urine as well as for normal reproductive function. Male neonates may be born with congenital defects and/or undescended testes. Boys are also at high risk for enuresis, especially bed-wetting. Acute glomerulonephritis is a disease state that follows infections from *Streptococcus pyogenes,* while the vast majority of time there is no apparent cause of nephrotic syndrome. The primary cancer of the urinary system—nephroblastoma, or Wilm's tumor—also is discussed.

II. Cryptorchidism (undescended testes)

In order to produce healthy sperm, it is essential for the testes to descend into the scrotal sac, an environment that is below the normal temperature of the body.

A. Incidence.
   1. The majority of male infants with **cryptorchidism** are either preterm or lower birth weight babies.

B. Etiology.
   1. Infants' testes descend normally after the 32nd week of gestation.

C. Pathophysiology.
   1. Either one or both testes fail to descend into the scrotal sac.

D. Diagnosis.
   1. The scrotal sacs are gently palpated on admission into the newborn nursery. If the testes are not felt in the sac, ultrasonography is often performed to assess their location.

E. Treatment.
   1. The vast majority of infants' testes will descend on their own by the time they are 6 months of age.
   2. If the testes do not descend naturally, surgery is performed. Undescended testes place the boy at high risk for testicular cancer as well as infertility.

F. Nursing considerations.
   1. Deficient Knowledge/Anxiety.
      a. Educate the parents regarding the condition.
      b. Advise the parents of the strong likelihood that the testes will descend without intervention.
         i. If surgery is required, advise the parents that the procedure usually is performed laparoscopically on an outpatient basis, and enable parents to discuss their concerns regarding their stress and the need for surgery.
   2. Risk for Infection/Risk for Deficient Fluid Volume related to surgery.
      a. Parents must be advised to monitor the laparoscopic incision carefully for bleeding and for redness, edema, ecchymosis, discharge and approximation (REEDA) and to report any deviations from normal.
      b. Educate the parents regarding any prescribed interventions to reduce the possibility of bleeding and infection of the surgical site.

III. Hypospadias/Epispadias: Congenital Anomalies of the Penile Shaft

A. Incidence.
   1. Hypospadias: occurs relatively frequently (in about 1 of every 250 male infants), while epispadias is quite rare.
   2. A small percentage of neonates with hypospadias will also have undescended testes.

B. Etiology.
   1. The incidence runs in families, indicating a hereditary etiology.

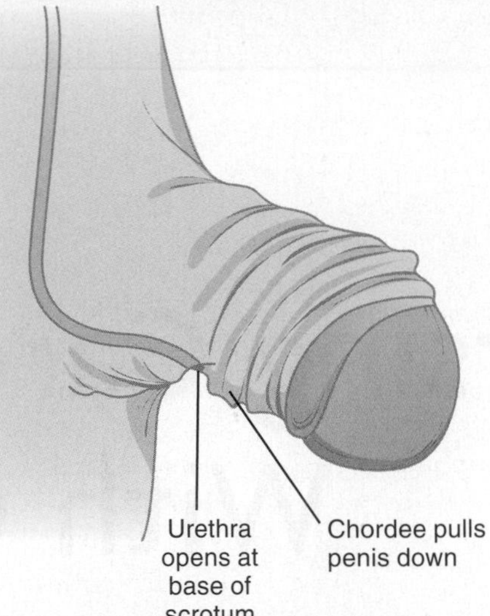

Fig 15.1 Chordee penis with hypospadias.

   2. Also higher incidence in sons of women over 35 years of age.

C. Pathophysiology.
   1. **Hypospadias.**
      a. The urethral opening is located on the underside of the penile shaft.
      b. A **chordee** penis (a penile shaft that curves downward) is frequently seen with hypospadias (Fig. 15.1).
   2. **Epispadias.**
      a. The urethral opening lies on the top side of the penile shaft.
      b. **Bladder exstrophy** (a bladder that lies outside of the abdominal cavity) may also be present.

D. Diagnosis.
   1. Physical examination and visualization of urine flowing from the opening.
      a. Monitoring by nurses of the neonate's urinary stream is important.

E. Treatment.
   1. Surgical intervention: to provide the child with as normal urination and reproductive health as possible.

F. Nursing considerations.
   1. Deficient Knowledge/Anxiety/Grieving/Altered Family Processes.
      a. Allow parents to express grief and loss of the perfect child.
      b. Assess the parents' responsiveness to the baby.
         i. Encourage skin-to-skin contact to promote bonding.
         ii. If poor bonding is noted, the nurse should recommend the primary health-care provider to refer the family for counseling.

c. If requested, advise the parents that the child with hypospadias may not be circumcised at birth.
    i. Foreskin will be used during plastic surgery to construct a urethral opening.
d. Advise the parents that the child with epispadias will likely require extensive reconstructive surgery.

2. Impaired Urinary Elimination/Risk of Infection/Pain.
    a. Provide preoperative education to the parents and child, if appropriate.
    b. Provide the child with adequate hydration.
        i. If oral intake is restricted, the safe administration of IV fluids is required.
    c. Monitor the child carefully for signs of urinary tract infection (UTI) both pre- and postoperatively.
        i. Signs and symptoms of UTI: temperature elevation, urinary frequency, and cloudy or foul-smelling urine.
    d. Employ aseptic technique when caring for the surgical site and for care of any urinary drainage system or stent that is needed.
        i. Monitor the surgical site for REEDA signs and report, if present.
        ii. Provide both pharmacological and nonpharmacological pain interventions (see Chapter 8, "Nursing Care of the Child in the Health-Care Setting"), as needed and prescribed.

IV. Enuresis (urinary incontinence)

A. Incidence.
1. **Enuresis** is a relatively common problem (up to one in five children) up to and through the preschool-age period.
    a. Seen three times more frequently in males than in females.
2. Once children reach 6 years of age, the vast majority of children are completely toilet trained.

B. Etiology.
1. Bed-wetting with daytime dryness is seen predominantly in males.
    a. It usually is related to sleeping soundly and not sensing a full bladder.
2. Daytime wetting with nighttime dryness usually results from becoming too engrossed in activities and waiting too long to go to the toilet.
3. A child who develops enuresis after having been fully toilet trained should be assessed for other pathology (e.g., UTI, enterobiasis, diabetes mellitus).

MAKING THE CONNECTION

It is important to remember the psychosocial milestones of toddlers and preschool-age children: autonomy versus shame and doubt and initiative versus guilt. If children who, for whatever reason, have difficulty becoming fully toilet trained are made fun of or disciplined, they can easily feel ashamed and humiliated. It is important for nurses to communicate empathically with the children and provide appropriate counseling to the parents.

C. Pathophysiology.
1. Toilet training is contingent on mature enervation to the urinary sphincter as well as the attentiveness of the child.
2. The child may either be unable to retain urine or may not be mature enough to retain the urine and to void voluntarily.

D. Treatment.
1. The vast majority of children will become toilet trained without specialized intervention.
2. If appropriate, a full assessment is conducted to determine whether there is a physiological cause for the enuresis.
3. If no physiological cause is noted, behavior modification strategies may be employed to foster toilet training.
4. For the older child who experiences nocturnal enuresis.
    a. Nocturnal alarm system.
        i. A device is attached to pajamas. When the device becomes wet, an alarm sounds awakening the child.
    b. Medication (e.g., desmopressin [DDAVP], a synthetic form of the anti-diuretic hormone [ADH], given either as an oral tablet or as a nasal spray).
        i. Children should be monitored carefully for serious side effects of the medication, including severe hypertension with headaches, blurred vision, and injuries to the nasal mucosa.
        ii. Once the medication is discontinued, many children relapse.

E. Nursing considerations.
2. Deficient Knowledge/Risk for Ineffective Coping/Situational Low Self-Esteem related to delayed toilet training.
    a. Counsel the parents and child that the vast majority of children become completely toilet trained by 6 years of age.
    b. Counsel the parent that punishment is inappropriate.

c. Educate the parents and child, using age-appropriate language, regarding appropriate interventions, for example:
   i. Remind the child to void at regular intervals throughout the day.
   ii. Advise the parent and child to restrict the child's fluid intake in the evening hours.
   iii. Advise the parent and child to refrain from consuming products containing caffeine that can cause bladder irritation.
   iv. Advise the parents to praise the child for periods of dryness.

d. If prescribed, educate the parents and child, using age appropriate language, regarding the safe administration of the nocturnal alarm system and/or medications.

V. Acute Poststreptococcal Glomerulonephritis (Acute Poststreptococcal Glomerular Nephritis)

A. Incidence.
1. Seen most frequently in children at high risk for strep throat (i.e., preschool- and school-age children).
2. **Acute poststreptococcal glomerulonephritis** (AGN) is may also occur following a case of impetigo, scarlet fever, or any other illness caused by *S. pyogenes*. (See Chapter 11, "Nursing Care of the Child With Infectious Diseases," and Chapter 19, "Nursing Care of Children With Integumentary System Disorders.")

B. Etiology.
1. Sequela to a group A beta hemolytic strep infection (see Chapter 16, "Nursing Care of the Child With Respiratory Illnesses").
2. Usually occurs about 1 to 2 weeks post strep infection.

C. Pathophysiology.
1. Inflammatory process that results from a toxin (antigen/antibody complex) produced by the strep bacteria. The complex affects the ability of the glomerulus to filter the blood.
2. Sodium and water are retained by the body, resulting in oliguria and edema. (This rarely results in encephalopathy.)
3. Large molecules are able to be excreted through the injured capillary walls, most notably red blood cells.
4. Signs and symptoms (see Table 15.1).
   a. Gross hematuria.
      i. Urine often turns dark brown (tea or coke colored).
   b. Mild to moderate proteinuria.
   c. Edema.
      i. Especially of the face.
      ii. Most notably in the morning, and edema subsides as the day progresses.
   d. Slight weight gain.
   e. Hypertension: resulting from sodium and water retention.
   f. Elevated ASO antibodies.

DID YOU KNOW?

Streptolysin-O is a toxin released by beta hemolytic streptococcal bacteria that causes hemolysis (i.e., the destruction of red blood cells). In response, the body produces the antibody antistreptolysin-O (ASO), the presence of which indicates that an individual is infected with beta hemolytic streptococci (*S. pyogenes*) or had been infected with the bacteria in the recent past.

Table 15.1 Comparison of Acute Glomerulonephritis With Nephrotic Syndrome

	Acute Glomerulonephritis	Nephrotic Syndrome
Proteinuria	*Mild to moderate*	*Moderate to gross (urine becomes thick and frothy)*
Proteinemia	*Slightly decreased*	*Markedly decreased*
Edema (from fluid retention)	*Abrupt* *Mild to moderate (facial edema that dissipates during the day)*	*Insidious* *Moderate to severe (anasarca)*
Hematuria	*Gross (urine becomes tea or coke colored)*	*Minimal*
Other	*Elevated BUN and other kidney function tests* *Elevated antistreptolysin (ASO) antibodies*	*Elevated BUN and other kidney function tests* *Elevated cholesterol* *Elevated triglycerides*
Blood pressure	*Elevated*	*Normal or slightly reduced*
Etiology	*Post-group A streptococcal infection*	*Idiopathic*
Common age range	*Preschool to school age*	*Toddler to preschool*

D. Diagnosis: clinical history and picture.
1. Gross hematuria with mild to moderate proteinuria.
2. Elevated ASO antibodies. (If the infection presented as impetigo or other skin infection, the child may not have produced ASO antibodies.)
3. Rarely, a culture that is positive for *S. pyogenes.*
   a. The child will culture positive only if the infection is still present.

E. Treatment.
1. Antibiotics, only if the bacteria are still present.
2. Palliative care (there is no cure for AGN).
   a. Control of hypertension.
      i. Antihypertensive medications and/or
      ii. No salt-added diet and
      iii. Fluid restriction.
   b. To protect the kidneys from further injury, the child is restricted from engaging in any contact sports or activities (e.g., rough housing).

F. Nursing considerations.
1. Imbalanced Fluid Volume (interstitial excess and intravascular deficit)/Risk for Impaired Gas Exchange/Risk for Altered Breathing Pattern/Risk for Injury/Imbalanced Nutrition: Less than Body Requirements.
   a. Strict intake and output (I & O).
      i. Report output that is less than minimum for the child.
         (1) Infants and toddlers (although AGN rarely seen at this age): 2 to 4 mL/kg/hr.
         (2) Preschoolers and young school-age children: 1 to 2 mL/kg/hr.
         (3) Older children: 0.5 to 1 mL/kg/hr.
   b. Monitor weight daily.
   c. Monitor blood pressure every 4 hr, using an accurately sized cuff.
   d. Auscultate lung fields and report adventitious sounds.
      i. Pulmonary edema may develop as a result of marked fluid retention.
   e. Restrict fluids, as prescribed.
   f. Restrict salt intake, as prescribed.
      i. Consult with the family and a registered dietitian to develop a menu of low-salt foods that are palatable to the child.
   g. Administer safe dosages of antihypertensive medications employing the five rights of medication administration.
2. Fatigue/Activity Intolerance.
   a. Organize nursing care, allowing for periods of rest and sleep.
   b. Provide interesting, quiet activities (e.g., television, video games, puzzles) to entertain the child.
   c. Place the child with a roommate who also must comply with activity restrictions.
   d. Educate the child, using age-appropriate language, and the parents regarding the need to avoid injury to the kidney until the inflammation is resolved.
3. Risk for Impaired Skin Integrity.
   a. Encourage the child to change positions frequently.
   b. Provide excellent, atraumatic skin care.
   c. Place the child on a lamb skin mattress, if needed.
   d. Monitor skin for signs of dehydration, including poor skin turgor and dry mucous membranes.
4. Anxiety/Fear/Risk for Altered Coping/Deficient Knowledge.
   a. Allow the parents and child to express anxiety and fears.
   b. Reassure everyone that the vast majority of children recover completely and that recurrence is rare.
   c. Provide the parents and child with age-appropriate explanations of the disease process and of the interventions.
   d. Educate the parents that whenever their child has a prolonged sore throat or other possible source of *S. pyogenes* in the future, that he or she should be seen by a health-care provider in order to have the site cultured.
   e. On discharge, educate the parents and child, using age-appropriate language, regarding:
      i. Fluid restrictions,
      ii. Diet modification,
      iii. The need for blood pressure management, including important information regarding antihypertensive medications,
      iv. The need for activity restriction, and
      v. The need to return to the primary health-care provider for frequent blood pressure, urine, and serum assessments.

VI. Nephrotic Syndrome (nephrosis)

A. Incidence.
1. Illness predominately of toddlers and preschool-age children.
2. May recur in the same child.

B. Etiology.
1. The specific cause of nephrosis is usually unknown (i.e., it is usually an idiopathic disease).
2. In rare instances, the disease occurs following another illness.

C. Pathophysiology.
1. **Nephrotic syndrome** is an inflammatory disease. For unknown reasons, the glomerulus of the kidneys becomes enflamed and allows large molecules, most notably the protein albumin, to be excreted into the urine, characterized by marked **hyperproteinuria.**
2. As a result, albumin is lost from the vascular system, resulting in a significant drop in circulating albumin (i.e., **hypoproteinemia,** a low level of protein circulating in the blood).
   a. The marked protein loss also results in a marked drop in the number of circulating antibodies.
3. The hypoproteinemia results in a drop in the colloidal pressure in the vascular tree, resulting in a fluid shift into the child's interstitial spaces, resulting in: **anasarca** (generalized swelling), pulmonary edema, and **hemoconcentration,** an increase in the concentration of the cells and solids in the blood caused by the loss of intravascular fluid.
   a. The hemoconcentration results in the child becoming high risk for thrombus formation.
4. The kidney responds by increasing renin production, which increases renin levels.
5. The high level of renin leads to renal fluid retention, thus exacerbating the edema.
6. In addition, although not completely understood, there is a marked increase in the production of cholesterol and triglycerides, resulting in hypercholesterolemia and a high concentration of circulating triglycerides.

D. Diagnosis.
1. Usually based on the clinical picture, but it is important to note that the edema develops insidiously.
   a. The parents often state that they had recently noticed that the child's clothes were becoming tight.
2. Classic signs and symptoms (see Table 15.1).
   a. Massive hyperproteinuria: 3+ to 4+.
   b. Thick, frothy urine because of a high concentration of protein.
   c. Mild hematuria.
   d. Elevated cholesterol, triglycerides, and hematocrit levels.
   e. No evidence of previous strep infection and a normal blood pressure.

E. Treatment.
1. High-dose steroids (usually prednisone) to control the inflammation.
   a. Usually continued for a few weeks after the proteinuria subsides, then slowly tapered off.
2. If the child responds poorly to steroid administration, antineoplastic medication may be ordered (e.g., cyclophosphamide [Cytoxan]).
3. IV albumin is often administered to restore fluid balances.
   a. Lasix may be given with the albumin to decrease the risk of fluid volume overload.
4. Salt restriction, if needed.
5. Fluid restriction, if needed.
6. Prophylactic antibiotics are often administered to protect the child from infection because of the loss of circulating antibodies.
7. Monitoring for adverse effects resulting from hypercholesterolemia and hemoconcentration (e.g., thrombi).

F. Nursing considerations.
1. Imbalanced Fluid Volume: Interstitial Excess and Intravascular Deficit.
   a. Weigh child daily.
   b. Maintain strict I & O.
   c. Report if the child's output is below minimum per hour (see earlier).
   d. Measure and record abdominal girth measurements daily.
   e. Carefully auscultate lungs for adventitious sounds and report to the primary health-care provider, as needed.
   f. Monitor for signs of dehydration.
   g. Monitor vital signs every 4 hr, especially blood pressure and pulse rate.
   h. Administer safe dosages of IV fluids and/or medications, as ordered (i.e., IV albumin, steroids, and/or diuretics).
   i. Provide palatable foods in a no-added-salt diet, if prescribed.
      i. Nutrition counseling is appropriate.
2. Risk for Infection.
   a. Meticulous handwashing.
   b. To protect the child from complications, screen visitors for signs of infection.
   c. Place in a room with an infection-free roommate.
   d. Administer safe dosages of antibiotics, if prescribed.
   e. Monitor the child for signs of infection (e.g., temperature elevation, elevated white blood cell count).
3. Risk for Impaired Skin Integrity/Activity Intolerance.
   a. Change child's position every 2 hr.
   b. Provide excellent, therapeutic hygiene and skin care.
   c. Provide safe, age-appropriate activities that will not injure or excessively fatigue the child.

d. Place the child on a lamb skin blanket or alternating pressure mattress, if appropriate, to prevent decubiti.

4. Anxiety/Fear/Risk for Altered Coping/Deficient Knowledge.
   a. Allow the parents and child, if applicable, to express anxiety and fears.
   b. Provide the parents and child with age-appropriate explanations of the disease process and of all interventions.
   c. On discharge, educate the parents and child, if applicable, regarding:
      i. Fluid restrictions
      ii. Diet modification
      iii. Skin care and
      iv. The need for activity restriction.
      v. Medication orders.

VII. Wilms' Tumor (nephroblastoma)

A. Incidence.
1. Most common tumor of the renal system.
2. Very rare. **Wilms' tumor** is diagnosed in about 8 out of every 1 million children.
3. Most frequently diagnosed in children aged 3 to 4.
4. Incidence is slightly higher in African American children.

B. Etiology.
1. Most frequently, the etiology is unknown.
2. About 10% of patients who develop Wilms' were born with a birth defect.
3. About 2% of children with Wilms' have a family member who also was diagnosed with the tumor.

C. Pathophysiology.
1. Solid, cancerous tumor.
2. May be present in one kidney—usually the left—or there may be tumors in both kidneys.
3. Tumor arises from slow-growing embryonic tissue.
4. Tumor usually is self-contained (encapsulated), but, if ruptured, will metastasize, usually to the lung.
   a. Prognosis is excellent, if the capsule remains intact.
5. Tumor staging.
   a. Stage I: one kidney involved; tumor removed intact.
   b. Stage II: one kidney involved; cancer spread locally, but no lymph nodes affected; all cancer removed during surgery.
   c. Stage III: one kidney involved; cancer spread to abdomen; surgeon unable to remove all cancer.
   d. Stage IV: one kidney involved; cancer spread throughout the body.
   e. Stage V: tumors in both kidneys.
6. Signs and symptoms.
   a. Abdominal mass noted on palpation that is then viewed via x-ray, MRI, or CT.
      i. Once noted, the tumor should never again be palpated.

(!) As long as the tumor remains fully encapsulated, the kidney and tumor are usually removed intact during surgery, resulting in a very good prognosis for recovery. If the capsule is punctured, however, the possibility of metastasis increases. To reduce the potential for injuring the capsule, a sign should be placed at the child's bedside to remind nurses and other health-care practitioners never to palpate the child's abdomen.

   b. Hematuria, which, if present, may be mild.
   c. Hypertension is noted in about one of four patients.
   d. Definitive diagnosis is determined from a biopsy of the tumor tissue.

D. Treatment.
1. Surgery.
   a. Usually the entire kidney is removed to prevent rupture of the capsule.
2. Chemotherapy usually follows. The type and timing of the chemotherapy is dependent on tumor staging.
   a. See the discussion of acute lymphoblastic leukemia (ALL) in Chapter 18 for information regarding chemotherapy.
3. Radiation may also be added with the type and timing dependent on tumor staging.
4. Dialysis is required if both kidneys are affected and removed.
   a. If both kidneys are removed the child is a candidate for renal transplant.

E. Nursing considerations.
1. Preoperative.
   a. Risk for Injury.
      i. Discourage activities that could result in direct contact with the abdomen.
      ii. Place a sign at the child's bed: "Do not palpate abdomen."
   b. Anxiety/Deficient Knowledge.
      i. Provide age-appropriate information to the parents and child, if appropriate, regarding the tumor and the surgery.
      ii. Allow the parents and child, if appropriate, to express fears and anxiety related to a diagnosis of cancer.
      iii. Advise the parents to refrain from palpating the child's abdomen.
      iv. Answer questions regarding the impact of losing one (or both, if indicated) kidney.

2. Postoperative.
   a. Routine postoperative nursing care, including pain management, REEDA assessment, vital signs assessment, monitoring of gastrointestinal functioning, and bleeding potential.
   b. Risk for Infection/Impaired Skin Integrity.
      i. Perform meticulous handwashing.
      ii. Use aseptic technique when performing dressing changes.
      iii. Monitor the child for signs of infection, at the surgical site as well as urinary and pulmonary infections.
   c. Risk for Imbalanced Fluid Volume.
      i. Strict I & O.
      ii. Report if the child is excreting below the minimum output for his or her weight (see earlier).
      iii. Monitor the child's weight daily.
         (1) Marked increase in weight is a strong indicator of fluid retention.

CASE STUDY: Putting It All Together

Mother brings 3-year, 3-month-old female to be assessed by the primary health-care practitioner

Subjective Data

- Child is seen playing with dolls in the waiting room while pretending to give the baby a bottle and wrapping the baby in a blanket
- Mother states,
  - "Everything seems fine, but I noticed that my daughter's urine is pink. I first saw it yesterday evening."
  - "She has had a couple of colds this year, but nothing out of the ordinary. What do you think is going on?"

Objective Data

Nursing Assessment

- Since birth, the child's well-child checks have been within normal limits, including weight, height, and head circumferences all at the 50th percentile
  - Child is up to date on all immunizations
  - Mass palpated in left upper quadrant—child exhibits minimal guarding
- Ultrasound results
  - Presumed Wilms' tumor noted in left kidney

Vital Signs

Temperature:	98.8°F
Heart rate:	100 bpm
Respiratory rate:	26 rpm
Blood pressure:	106/66 mm Hg

Lab Results

Complete blood count	
Red blood cell count:	3.6 million/mm^3
Hemoglobin:	11 g/dL
Hematocrit:	33%
White blood cell count:	10,000/mm^3
Platelet count:	225,000/mm^3
Urine: within normal limits except	
Red blood cells:	10 (normal less than or equal to 2)

Health-Care Provider's Orders

- Admit to pediatric unit
- Prepare for surgery in a.m.
- NPO after midnight
- Modified bedrest
- Absolutely no one is to palpate the abdomen.

CASE STUDY: Putting It All Together *cont'd*

Case Study Questions

A. What *subjective* assessments indicate that this client is experiencing a health alteration?

1. ______
2. ______

B. What *objective* assessments indicate that this client is experiencing a health alteration?

1. ______
2. ______
3. ______
4. ______
5. ______
6. ______
7. ______

C. After analyzing the data that has been collected, what **primary** nursing diagnosis should the nurse assign to this client?

1. ______

D. What interventions should the nurse plan and/or implement to meet this child's and her family's needs?

1. ______
2. ______
3. ______
4. ______
5. ______
6. ______
7. ______
8. ______
9. ______

E. What client outcomes should the nurse evaluate regarding the effectiveness of the nursing interventions?

1. ______
2. ______
3. ______
4. ______

Continued

CASE STUDY: Putting It All Together *cont'd*

Case Study Question

F. What physiological characteristics should the child exhibit before being discharged home (from the hospital)?

1. ______________________________
2. ______________________________
3. ______________________________
4. ______________________________
5. ______________________________
6. ______________________________
7. ______________________________

G. What subjective characteristics should the child exhibit before being discharged home (from the hospital)?

1. ______________________________

REVIEW QUESTIONS

1. Four babies were delivered in the maternity unit during a 24-hour period. Which of the babies would the nurse most predict would exhibit cryptorchidism?
   1. 34 weeks' gestation, 2,200 grams, Apgar 9/9
   2. 37 weeks' gestation, 4,000 grams, Apgar 8/9
   3. 39 weeks' gestation, 3,500 grams, Apgar 7/8
   4. 42 weeks' gestation, 2,400 grams, Apgar 8/8

2. An Orthodox Jewish couple deliver a baby boy with hypospadias. The parents state, "We are so excited. We are planning the baby's *bris* (ritual circumcision) for next week. Which of the following responses by the nurse is appropriate?
   1. "I know how happy you must be. I know that you will have a wonderful party."
   2. "If you are comfortable sharing the information, what Hebrew name do you plan to give your baby next week?"
   3. "I understand how important it is to have a *bris*, but the baby will not be able to be circumcised next week."
   4. "Do you have a mohel to perform the *bris*? I know how hard it is to locate one who you feel you can trust."

3. A baby is admitted to the newborn nursery with a chordee penis. The nurse carefully assesses the baby for which of the following signs/symptoms?
   1. Blood-tinged urine
   2. Constant dripping of urine from the urethra
   3. Absence of urinary output
   4. Urine flowing from the under surface of the penis

4. A 7-year-old child has been prescribed desmopressin (DDAVP) 20 mcg intranasal (10 mcg in each nostril) for nocturnal enuresis. Which of the following information regarding the medication should the nurse include in the parent/child teaching session?
   1. Child must consume at least five cups of fluid each day.
   2. Medication should be stored in the freezer between administrations.
   3. Severe headaches with blurred vision should be reported to the prescribing practitioner.
   4. Spray should be administered into the nostrils while the child is lying supine with head extended.

5. An 8-year-old child is seen in the pediatrician's office for primary nocturnal enuresis. Which of the following nursing diagnoses should the nurse include in the child's nursing care plan?
   1. Overflow Urinary Incontinence
   2. Risk for Impaired Skin Integrity
   3. Risk for Imbalanced Fluid Volume
   4. Situational Low Self-Esteem

6. The nurse is educating the parents and their 10-year-old child regarding home care for the child's diagnosis of acute glomerular nephritis. Which of the following statements by the child indicate that the child understood the teaching? **Select all that apply.**
   1. "I can't eat any potato chips or other salty foods."
   2. "I can't go to school for a week because I am contagious."
   3. "I won't be able to go back to soccer practice for a long time."
   4. "I'm going to have to go to the doctor's office a lot during the next few months."
   5. "When I get home, I will have to stay in bed, except when I need to go to the bathroom."

7. A child has been diagnosed with acute glomerular nephritis. Which of the following changes would the nurse expect to see in the child's laboratory reports?
   1. Urine white blood cell count: elevated
   2. Urine specific gravity: decreased
   3. Urine creatinine clearance: decreased
   4. Urine red blood cell count: elevated

8. A 6-year-old child with antistreptolysin antibodies and negative cultures is admitted to the pediatric unit with a diagnosis of acute poststreptococcal glomerular nephritis. It would be most appropriate for the nurse to admit the child into which of the following rooms?
   1. Isolation room on droplet isolation with no roommate
   2. Isolation room on droplet and contact isolation with a child with bronchiolitis
   3. Regular patient room with 8-year-old child in traction for a broken femur
   4. Regular patient room with 6-year-old child with diabetes for insulin control

9. A 6-year-old child is admitted to the pediatric unit with a diagnosis of acute poststreptococcal glomerular nephritis. Which of the following toys/activities would be most appropriate for the nurse to provide to the child?
   1. Push and pull toy
   2. Bean bags and target
   3. Crayons and paper
   4. Set of blocks

10. A child is admitted to the pediatric unit with nephrotic syndrome. Which of the following laboratory results would the nurse expect to see?
    1. Thrombocytopenia
    2. Hypoalbuminemia
    3. Neutropenia
    4. Hypermagnesemia

11. A child with nephrotic syndrome has been prescribed prednisone. The nurse should monitor the child for which of the following medication side effects?
    1. Gastric distress
    2. Bradycardia
    3. Hypoglycemia
    4. Weight loss

12. A 2-year-old child with nephrotic syndrome is admitted to the pediatric unit. The following orders have been written in the child's medical record. Which of the actions is highest priority for the nurse to perform?
    1. Place child on alternating pressure mattress.
    2. Administer intravenous albumin.
    3. Weigh all wet diapers.
    4. Administer oral antibiotics.

13. A 3-year-old child is admitted to the pediatric unit for surgery. The child has a tumor in his left kidney. The child is to undergo surgery the next day. Which of the following primary health-care practitioner prescriptions is most important for the nurse to follow?
    1. Maintain the child NPO after midnight.
    2. Place a sign at the head of the bed stating, "Do not touch abdomen."
    3. Send a urine specimen for a urinalysis.
    4. Send a blood specimen for electrolyte analysis.

14. A young girl is being discharged from the pediatric unit after a left nephrectomy for Stage 1 Wilms' tumor of the left kidney and the first round of chemotherapy. The nurse is providing the parents with discharge planning. Which of the following statements should the nurse include?
    1. Child will need to restrict fluids for the rest of his or her life.
    2. Child will require dialysis until a kidney for transplant is found.
    3. Child will be able to live a normal life after the surgical site heals.
    4. Child will have to take antirejection medications after surgery.

15. The parents of a Hispanic American child who has been diagnosed with Wilms' tumor ask the nurse about the origin of the tumor. Which of the following information should the nurse provide the parents?
    1. "Nephroblastoma is a cancer that originated in another part of your child's body."
    2. "The tumor often starts growing in the kidney while the baby is still in the uterus."
    3. "Wilms' tumor is especially prevalent in the Hispanic population."
    4. "The cancer is often seen in children who live in areas near nuclear reactors."

16. The oncologist caring for a child immediately postsurgery for Wilms' tumor reports: the child is in Stage III. The child will go through a series of chemotherapy. Based on the proposed therapy, which of the following patient-care goals should be included in the child's nursing care plan? **Select all that apply.**
    1. The child will be free of infection.
    2. The child will experience no tissue damage.
    3. The child will have regular bowel movements.
    4. The child will not complain of nausea and will not vomit.
    5. The child will regress to the previous level of growth and development.

REVIEW ANSWERS

1. ANSWER: 1

Rationale:

1. Most babies who are born with cryptorchidism are preterm.
2. By 36 weeks' gestation, the testes should be descended.
3. By 36 weeks' gestation, the testes should be descended.
4. By 36 weeks' gestation, the testes should be descended.

TEST-TAKING TIP: The testes develop in the abdomen and slowly descend through the inguinal canal into the scrotal sac. Babies who are born preterm are, therefore, most likely to exhibit cryptorchidism. Apgar and weight do not affect whether or not the testes descend.

Content Area: *Child Health, Infant*
Integrated Processes: *Nursing Process: Analysis*
Client Need: *Health Promotion and Maintenance: Developmental Stages and Transition*
Cognitive Level: *Application*

2. ANSWER: 3

Rationale:

1. It would be appropriate for the nurse to congratulate the couple, but this is not the most appropriate statement for the nurse to make.
2. It is true that the baby's Hebrew name would be bestowed at the *bris,* but this is not the most appropriate statement for the nurse to make.
3. This is the most appropriate statement for the nurse to make. The baby will not be able to be circumcised at the *bris*.
4. It is true that a mohel is the individual who does the circumcision at a *bris,* but this is not the most appropriate statement for the nurse to make.

TEST-TAKING TIP: When a baby is born with hypospadias, circumcisions are postponed until surgical correction of the urethra is performed. The surgeon will use the foreskin from the circumcision as grafting material for the reconstruction.

Content Area: *Pediatrics—Infant*
Integrated Processes: *Nursing Process: Implementation*
Client Need: *Physiological Integrity: Physiological Adaptation: Alterations in Body Systems*
Cognitive Level: *Application*

3. ANSWER: 4

Rationale:

1. Babies with a chordee penis are not at high risk for blood-tinged urine.
2. Babies with a chordee penis are not at high risk for constant urine dripping from the urethra.
3. Babies with a chordee penis are not at high risk for absence of urinary output.
4. Babies with a chordee penis are at high risk for hypospadias.

TEST-TAKING TIP: Nurses should be prepared to assess for birth defects that commonly accompany assessment findings. Babies who are born with a chordee penis (a penis that curves downward) should carefully be assessed for hypospadias, that is, for urine that exits from the underside of the penis.

Content Area: *Pediatrics—Infant*
Integrated Processes: *Nursing Process: Assessment*
Client Need: *Physiological Integrity: Physiological Adaptation: Alterations in Body Systems*
Cognitive Level: *Application*

4. ANSWER: 3

Rationale:

1. This statement is incorrect. The child's fluid intake should be restricted, especially before bedtime.
2. This statement is incorrect. The medication should be kept in the refrigerator but should not be frozen.
3. This statement is correct. If the dosage is too high, the child may develop adverse signs, including severe high blood pressure with headaches and blurred vision.
4. This statement is incorrect. The child should be sitting upright, and the nasal spray bottle should be vertical during medication administration.

TEST-TAKING TIP: Desmopressin is one of the few medications administered to children with nocturnal enuresis. It is important to monitor the child for possible side effects, including severe hypertension with headaches and blurred vision and injuries to the nasal mucosa.

Content Area: *Pediatrics*
Integrated Processes: *Nursing Process: Implementation; Teaching/Learning*
Client Need: *Physiological Integrity: Pharmacological and Parenteral Therapies: Adverse Effects/Contraindications/ Side Effects/Interactions*
Cognitive Level: *Application*

5. ANSWER: 4

Rationale:

1. The child is not experiencing overflow incontinence, which results from an overly distended bladder.
2. The child's skin integrity is intact.
3. The child is not experiencing imbalanced fluid volume.
4. Situational Low Self-Esteem is an appropriate nursing diagnosis for the nurse to include in the care plan.

TEST-TAKING TIP: When older children are still wetting the bed, they often feel guilty and ashamed. Situational Low Self-Esteem is an appropriate nursing diagnosis for the nurse to include in the child's care plan.

Content Area: *Pediatrics*
Integrated Processes: *Nursing Process: Analysis*
Client Need: *Psychosocial Integrity: Therapeutic Environment*
Cognitive Level: *Application*

6. ANSWER: 1, 3, and 4

Rationale:

1. This statement is true. Children with AGN are usually on salt restricted diets.
2. This is not correct. It is rare for children with AGN still to be contagious. If they are still *S. pyogenes* positive, they will be prescribed penicillin. Once they have been on the medication for one full day, they are no longer contagious.
3. This statement is correct. Until the urinalyses are normal, children are restricted from participating in contact sports.

4. This statement is correct. The child will require frequent urinalyses and blood pressure assessments to monitor the progression of the disease.
5. Children with AGN rarely are placed on strict bedrest. In the early days of the disease, they usually modify their own activity level. Once they feel well enough, they are allowed to ambulate.
TEST-TAKING TIP: The nurse should educate both the parents and the child and should evaluate the child's as well as the parents' understanding. The large part of a child's day is spent at school away from parents. It is critically important that sick children be included in age-appropriate discussions about their illnesses as well as their plans of care.
Content Area: *Pediatrics*
Integrated Processes: *Nursing Process: Implementation: Teaching/Learning*
Client Need: *Physiological Integrity: Reduction of Risk Potential: Therapeutic Procedures*
Cognitive Level: *Application*

7. ANSWER: 4
Rationale:
1. The nurse would expect to see white blood cells in the urine if the child had a UTI.
2. Because of the hematuria and proteinuria, the nurse would expect to see an increase in the child's urinary specific gravity.
3. Because the child's kidney function is compromised, the nurse would expect to see reduced creatinine clearance in the urine, but a concurrent rise in the serum creatinine.
4. The number of red blood cells in the urine increases dramatically.
TEST-TAKING TIP: Laboratory data often can provide the nurse with important information regarding a patient's clinical course. It is essential that the nurse become familiar with normal laboratory results and expected changes in relation to disease states.
Content Area: *Pediatrics*
Integrated Processes: *Nursing Process: Assessment*
Client Need: *Physiological Integrity: Physiological Adaptation: Alterations in Body Systems*
Cognitive Level: *Application*

8. ANSWER: 3
Rationale:
1. Isolation is not needed. The child has negative cultures.
2. Isolation is not needed. The child has negative cultures.
3. This would be the most appropriate room to place the child. Children in the early stages of AGN often remain in their beds because of marked fatigue. A child in traction would also be confined to his or her bed.
4. A child in the hospital for insulin control is likely up and about with no medically imposed or self-imposed activity restrictions. Although the children are the same age, their activity levels will be much different.
TEST-TAKING TIP: One of the important actions of the pediatric nurse is the assignment of children to patient rooms. The nurse should take into consideration all aspects of each child's characteristics, including growth and development, activity levels, and potential for transmission of infection.
Content Area: *Pediatrics*
Integrated Processes: *Nursing Process: Implementation*
Client Need: *Psychosocial Integrity: Therapeutic Environment*
Cognitive Level: *Application*

9. ANSWER: 3
Rationale:
1. Push and pull toys are appropriate for active toddlers.
2. Bean bags would be appropriate for an active child who is angry at being confined to a bed.
3. It would be most appropriate to provide the child with crayons and paper. The activity would not be too strenuous, and the child could express his or her feelings about being hospitalized in a drawing.
4. A set of blocks would be appropriate for an active child who could get down onto the floor and build a tower.
TEST-TAKING TIP: Toys and activities provided to sick children should be appropriate to the age without being overly challenging. Materials for drawing and painting are especially appropriate for school-age children because the art supplies enable the child to express him or herself through the art. In addition, puppets and dolls enable children to act out their frustrations through play.
Content Area: *Pediatrics*
Integrated Processes: *Nursing Process: Implementation*
Client Need: *Psychosocial Integrity: Therapeutic Environment*
Cognitive Level: *Application*

10. ANSWER: 2
Rationale:
1. The nurse would expect the platelet count to be within normal limits.
2. The child's serum albumin levels would be markedly decreased.
3. The nurse would expect the serum white blood cell count to be within normal limits.
4. The nurse would expect the serum magnesium levels to be within normal limits.
TEST-TAKING TIP: Children with nephrotic syndrome lose large quantities of albumin into the urine. As a result, the child's serum albumin levels are markedly decreased. Because antibodies are protein, children with hypoalbuminemia are at high risk for infections.
Content Area: *Pediatrics*
Integrated Processes: *Nursing Process: Assessment*
Client Need: *Physiological Integrity: Physiological Adaptation: Alterations in Body Systems*
Cognitive Level: *Application*

11. ANSWER: 1
Rationale:
1. Gastric distress is a common side effect of prednisone.
2. Bradycardia is not a documented side effect of prednisone.
3. Hyperglycemia is seen in patients taking high doses of prednisone.

4. Weight loss is not a documented side effect of prednisone.

TEST-TAKING TIP: It is important for the test taker to read questions carefully. Hyperglycemia is a side effect of prednisone, while hypoglycemia is not.

Content Area: *Pediatrics*

Integrated Processes: *Nursing Process: Implementation*

Client Need: *Physiological Integrity: Pharmacological and Parenteral Therapies: Adverse Effects/Contraindications/ Side Effects/Interactions*

Cognitive Level: *Application*

12. ANSWER: 2

Rationale:

1. It is important to place the child on an alternating pressure mattress, but it is not the priority action.
2. **Administering IV albumin is the priority action.**
3. Weighing all wet diapers is important, but it is not the priority action.
4. Administering oral antibiotics is important, but it is not the priority action.

TEST-TAKING TIP: To determine the priority action, the nurse should determine which action will reverse the problem. The only response that is a treatment that will help to reverse the pathology of nephrotic syndrome is the administration of albumin.

Content Area: *Pediatrics*

Integrated Processes: *Nursing Process: Implementation*

Client Need: *Safe and Effective Care Environment: Management of Care: Establishing Priorities*

Cognitive Level: *Analysis*

13. ANSWER: 2

Rationale:

1. Even if it were within the 12-hr window before surgery, this is not the first order that the nurse should complete.
2. **The nurse should first place a sign at the head of the child's bed stating, "Do not touch abdomen."**
3. The nurse can wait to send the urine specimen for urinalysis.
4. The nurse can wait to send the blood specimen for protein and electrolytes.

TEST-TAKING TIP: The prognosis of Wilms' tumor is dependent on the tumor remaining encapsulated in the kidney. If it were to rupture, the likelihood of metastasis markedly increases. The nurse must place the sign at the head of the child's bed to make sure that no one entering the room palpates the child's abdomen.

Content Area: *Pediatrics*

Integrated Processes: *Nursing Process: Implementation*

Client Need: *Safe and Effective Care Environment: Management of Care: Establishing Priorities*

Cognitive Level: *Analysis*

14. ANSWER: 3

Rationale:

1. The child will not need to restrict fluids for the rest of his or her life.
2. The child still has one kidney. There will be no need for dialysis.
3. **Child will be able to live a normal life after the surgical site heals. This statement is correct.**
4. The child did not receive a transplant. The child will not need to take antirejection medications after surgery.

TEST-TAKING TIP: Stage 1 tumors are tumors that are completely encapsulated, are contained within one kidney, and completely removed during surgery. The prognosis is excellent following successful surgery.

Content Area: *Pediatrics*

Integrated Processes: *Nursing Process: Implementation*

Client Need: *Physiological Integrity: Reduction of Risk Potential: Potential for Complications of Diagnostic Tests/ Treatments/Procedures*

Cognitive Level: *Application*

15. ANSWER: 2

Rationale:

1. Nephroblastomas arise from embryonic tissue and develop over time.
2. **This statement is correct.**
3. Wilms' tumor is slightly more prevalent in the African American population.
4. This statement is untrue.

TEST-TAKING TIP: Usually, the etiology of Wilms' is unknown. About 10% of patients who develop Wilms' were also born with a birth defect, about 2% of children with Wilms' have a family member who also was diagnosed with the tumor, and Wilms' is seen slightly more often in the African American population than in other ethnic groups.

Content Area: *Pediatrics*

Integrated Processes: *Nursing Process: Implementation; Teaching/Learning*

Cognitive Level: *Application*

Client Need: *Physiological Integrity: Physiological Adaptation: Pathophysiology*

16. ANSWER: 1, 2, 3, and 4

Rationale:

1. **This is an appropriate patient-care goal.**
2. **This is an appropriate patient-care goal.**
3. **This is an appropriate patient-care goal.**
4. **This is an appropriate patient-care goal.**
5. Although the child may regress, the goal should be that the child will regain or maintain his or her level of growth and development.

TEST-TAKING TIP: Chemotherapy places children at high risk for a number of complications. The goals of patient care should state that the child will not develop any of the complications, including infection, stomatitis, nausea, vomiting, and constipation.

Content Area: *Pediatrics*

Integrated Processes: *Nursing Process: Planning*

Client Need: *Physiological Integrity: Pharmacological and Parenteral Therapies: Adverse Effects/Contraindications/ Side Effects/Interactions*

Cognitive Level: *Application*

Nursing Care of the Child With Respiratory Illnesses

KEY TERMS

Acute otitis media (AOM)—Acute inflammation of the middle ear.

Asthma—Reversible airway disease characterized by inflammation of the bronchi and lower airway obstruction as a result of edema and mucus production.

Bronchiolitis—Inflammation of the bronchioles seen almost exclusively in infants, primarily caused by respiratory syncytial virus (RSV).

Croup—A group of middle airway illnesses primarily seen in infants and toddlers characterized by a barking cough.

Cystic fibrosis (CF)—An autosomal recessive illness in which sodium and chloride are unable to cross cell membranes, resulting in the development of thick mucus in the organ systems of the body.

Epiglottitis—Life-threatening bacterial croup characterized by inflammation of the epiglottis and potential tracheal occlusion. High fever with a barky cough and inspiratory stridor (i.e., high-pitched squeal on inhalation) are signs of the illness.

Intercostal retractions—The pulling inward of the intercostal muscles (attached to the ribs) during labored breathing.

Laryngotracheal bronchitis (LTB)—A viral croup illness affecting tissue both above and below the vocal cords.

Mucolytic—A class of drugs used to loosen and liquefy mucus.

Myringotomy—Surgical insertion of tympanostomy tubes to drain fluid from the middle ear related to otitis media with effusion (OME).

Otitis media with effusion (OME)—Condition of the middle ear in which fluid is trapped behind the eardrum.

Pharyngitis—Tonsillitis; marked enlargement of the palatine tonsils.

Stridor—A high-pitched wheezing sound resulting from a blockage in the upper airway.

I. Description

The respiratory system can be divided into three distinct areas: upper airway, composed of the ears, nose, sinuses, mouth, and tongue (Fig. 16.1); the middle airway, composed of the throat, epiglottis, and trachea; and the lower airway, composed of the bronchi and lungs (both middle and lower airways are illustrated in Fig. 16.2). The disease states discussed in this chapter are organized by the three different airways.

A number of diagnostic tests are employed to determine the health and well-being of clients with respiratory illnesses. For example, blood gas analyses assess the concentration of oxygen and carbon dioxide as well as the acidity/alkalinity of the blood (see Chapter 13, "Nursing Care of the Child With Fluid and Electrolyte Alterations" for a discussion of blood gas analysis), while pulse oximetry is a noninvasive method of monitoring oxygenation. Pulmonary function tests measure the efficiency of a person's respiratory efforts, while x-rays

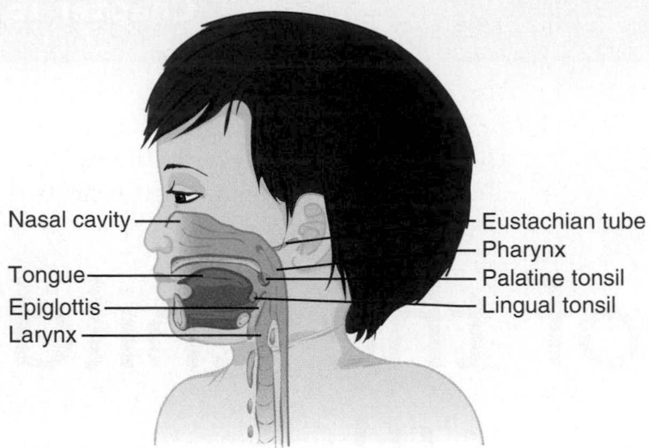

Fig 16.1 Upper airway.

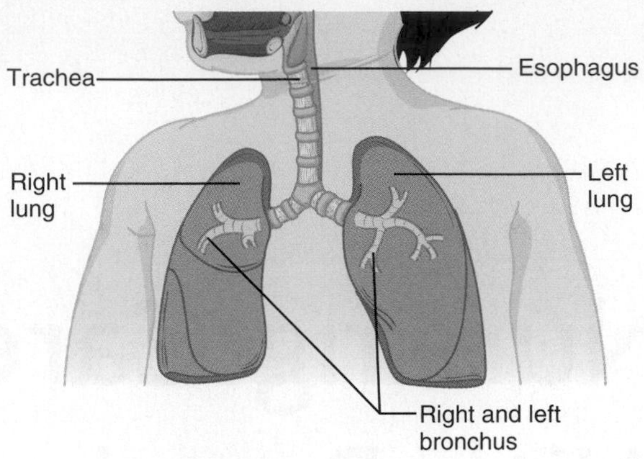

Fig 16.2 Middle and lower airways.

provide practitioners with pictures of the lungs. Practitioners are also able to view the airway directly via bronchoscopies and laryngoscopies.

II. Upper Airway: Otitis Media

Ear infections are some of the most common illnesses seen in young children. The term otitis media primarily refers to two conditions of the middle ear: **acute otitis media (AOM)** and **otitis media with effusion (OME)**. Although the ear may become infected outside of the eardrum, otitis externa, it is not discussed in this chapter.

A. Incidence.
   1. Most common illness of infants and young children, but rarely seen after 6 years of age.

B. Etiology.
   1. Variety of viral illnesses, including the common cold.
   2. Bacteria, especially *Haemophilus influenzae* and *Streptococcus pneumoniae.*
   3. Other risk factors.
      a. Formula feeding.
      b. Attending day care.
      c. Exposure to cigarette smoke.
      d. Anatomy and physiology of the young child's upper airway.
         i. Young children's eustachian tubes are short, wide, and straight, while older children's and adults' are longer, narrower, and slanted (Fig. 16.3).
         ii. Underdeveloped cartilage allows the tube to expand.
         iii. Lymphoid tissue obstructs the opening at the oropharynx.
         iv. Poor immune systems with frequent allergic responses, especially to formula and tobacco smoke.

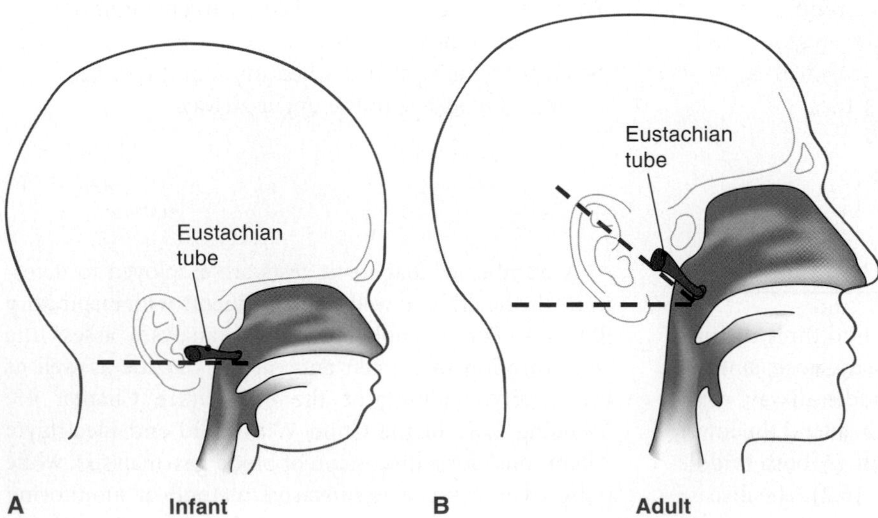

Fig 16.3 Differences in (A) infant and (B) adult ear canal angles.

v. Horizontal positioning of infants during sleep and during feeds that creates pooling of fluids, especially formula, in the pharyngeal cavity.

C. Pathophysiology.

1. Acute otitis media (AOM).
   a. Acute inflammation of the middle ear.
   b. Signs and symptoms.
      i. Acute onset of pain, crankiness, pulling on the ear, and fever.
      ii. Bulging, red tympanic membrane.
      iii. Pus-like drainage.
2. Otitis media with effusion (OME).
   a. Subacute problem with fluid trapped behind the eardrum.
   b. Signs and symptoms.
      i. Hearing loss with tinnitus.
      ii. Dull, retracted tympanic membrane.

D. Diagnosis.

1. Usually by clinical signs alone.
2. Visualization of the tympanic membrane via an otoscope, making sure to employ the correct technique (Fig. 7.2).
   a. Infants.
      i. Because the canal curves upward and the membrane lies horizontal along the upper wall of the canal, the pinnae of the ear must be pulled downward and backward.
   b. Three-year-olds and older.
      i. Because the canal curves downward and forward and the drum slopes inward and forward, the pinnae of the ear must be pulled upward and backward.
3. Culture and sensitivity—If drainage is present.
4. To distinguish OME from AOM.
   a. Pneumatic otoscopy—A test that measures the movement of the tympanic membrane.
   b. Tympanometry—A test that measures the pressures in the middle ear as well as movement of the tympanic membrane.

E. Treatment.

1. Treatment of otitis is controversial.
   a. Because antibiotics have often been administered indiscriminately, resistant organisms have developed.
2. Prevention: like much of pediatric care, prevention is important.
   a. Vaccinations that prevent proliferation of offending organisms should be administered.
      i. *H. influenzae* type b (Hib): administered at 2, 4, and 6 months, with a booster dose administered at 12 to 15 months of age.
      ii. Pneumococcal conjugate (PCV13): administered at the same times as the Hib.
   b. Reducing the child's exposure to factors that place the child at risk of otitis.
      i. Breastfeeding instead of formula feeding (see Chapter 11, "Nursing Care of the Child With Immunologic Alterations," for a discussion of the immunologic benefits of breastfeeding).
         (1) If the child is formula feeding, not propping the bottle or putting the baby to bed with a bottle.
      ii. Not smoking in the baby's vicinity.
      iii. Isolating the baby from sick individuals, especially children.
3. AOM—The current treatment plan recommended by Lieberthal and colleagues (2013) for the American Academy of Pediatrics (American Academy of Family Physicians) is dependent on the age and overall health status of the child.
   a. If the child is younger than or equal to 6 months of age.
      i. Antibiotics (Amoxicillin is recommended as the first-line antibiotic) should be administered at the time of diagnosis.
   b. If the child is between 6 months and 2 years of age.
      i. Administration of antibiotics is determined by the severity of the illness or when a specific bacterial organism has been identified.
   c. If the child is equal to or over 2 years of age.
      i. Palliative care alone provided for up to 3 days, often called watchful waiting, unless the child is severely ill or a specific bacterial organism has been identified.
         (1) Watchful waiting is recommended because many cases of AOM are caused by viruses rather than bacteria.
            (a) If after watchful waiting the AOM is still present, antibiotics are usually prescribed.
         (2) Palliative care.
            (a) Safe dosages of acetaminophen or ibuprofen are administered to control the child's pain. Warm compresses or cold packs (whichever the child prefers) are applied to the outer ear.
         (3) Per the American Academy of Pediatrics (AAP), over-the-counter medications (OTC meds), especially cough and cold medicines, other than acetaminophen, should **not** be administered to children under 2 years of age.

4. OME (AAP, 2004).
   a. Watchful waiting with reexamination approximately every 3 months.
   b. If effusion persists for an extended period of time or if the child is at high risk or exhibiting hearing loss, learning difficulties, and/or speech delay:
      i. **Myringotomy** (i.e., surgical insertion of tympanostomy tubes).

F. Nursing considerations.
1. Acute Pain.
   a. Educate the parents regarding safe dosages of acetaminophen and ibuprofen.
   b. Recommend nonpharmacological pain relief measures (e.g., warm compress to the affected ear).
2. Infection.
   a. If ordered, educate the parents regarding safe dosage of antibiotics **and** the need to complete the entire course of the medication.
   b. If ordered, advise the parents regarding the importance of returning for a follow-up assessment.
3. Risk for Deficient Fluid Volume.
   a. Monitor the child for signs of dehydration.
   b. Encourage the parents to provide the child with increased oral fluids.
   c. Advise the parents to administer oral rehydration therapy (ORT) as needed.
4. Deficient Knowledge.
   a. Educate the parents and child, if appropriate, regarding the rationale for the applicable diagnostic procedures.
   b. If the child is bottlefed, educate the parents to feed the child in a semi-sitting position.
   c. Advise the parents to avoid cigarette smoke and sick individuals in the vicinity of the baby.
   d. Educate the parents regarding precautions if the child has tympanostomy tubes inserted.
      i. Use ear plugs for bathing and swimming.
      ii. Do not allow the child to immerse his or her head underwater.
      iii. Observe for spontaneous loss of the tubes, usually found on the child's pillow.
         (1) Loss should be reported to the physician.

III. Middle Airway: Pharyngitis (tonsillitis)

A. Incidence.
1. **Pharyngitis** (tonsillitis) is most commonly seen in preschool and school-age children.
2. Rarely seen in infants and toddlers.

B. Etiology.
1. Sore throat can be caused by many viruses and bacteria.
2. Group A beta hemolytic strep (*Streptococcus pyogenes*), the exemplar of the chapter, is commonly the only pathogen that is treated.

C. Pathophysiology.
1. Marked enlargement of the palatine tonsils (often called "kissing" tonsils).
   a. The adenoid tonsils may also become infected.
2. Other signs and symptoms.
   a. Very sore throat with painful swallowing.
   b. Enlarged and red tonsils often covered in pus.
   c. Elevated temperature.
   d. Leukocytosis.
   e. May complain of nausea and anorexia.
3. If group A strep is left untreated, the child may develop one of two serious sequelae.
   a. Rheumatic fever (see Chapter 17, "Nursing Care of the Child With Cardiovascular Illnesses") or acute glomerulonephritis (AGN) (see Chapter 15, "Nursing Care of the Child With Genitourinary Disorders").

D. Diagnosis.
1. Clinical picture: suggestive.
2. Throat culture: diagnostic.
   a. Rapid test should be performed, if available, but, because it may result in a false negative, a classic throat culture should also always be performed.

E. Treatment.
1. Antibiotics: if the throat culture is positive for group A strep.
   a. Penicillin is often the antibiotic of choice.
      i. Parents and the child, if appropriate, must be advised to complete the full antibiotic course.
         (1) The child should be kept isolated from other children until he or she has completed a full 24 hr of antibiotic therapy.
2. Tonsillectomy
   a. If the child experiences recurrent group A strep tonsillitis, a tonsillectomy may be performed.
   b. They are often not curative of sore throats.
   c. Tonsillectomies are rarely performed before a child turns 3 years of age because young children often:
      i. Bleed more heavily during the surgery.
      ii. Experience tonsil regrowth.

F. Nursing considerations.
1. Pharyngitis.
   a. Infection/Deficient Knowledge.

i. Educate parents regarding the need to take their child to a health-care provider for a throat culture whenever he or she exhibits symptoms.
ii. Educate the parents regarding the need to complete the full course of antibiotics, if prescribed.
iii. Educate the parents regarding sequelae that may occur if the child does not complete the antibiotics.

2. Tonsillectomy.
   a. Preoperative.
      i. Anxiety/Deficient Knowledge.
         (1) Allow the parents and child, if appropriate, to express their concerns about surgery.
         (2) Educate the parents and child, using age-appropriate language, regarding the surgical experience (Box 16.1).
         (3) Educate the parents regarding postoperative care (see "Postoperative") because the child will be discharged home shortly after the procedure.
   b. Postoperative.
      i. Risk for Bleeding/Risk for Injury.
         (1) Assess the throat for fresh blood being especially vigilant for 1 full day after surgery and 1 week following surgery.
            (a) The back of the throat should be visualized frequently using a flashlight.
            (b) Recurrent swallowing is often an indicator of fresh bleeding
            (c) Any vomitus should be assessed carefully for bright-red blood.
            (d) Any fresh bleeding should be immediately reported to the surgeon.
         (2) Apply ice collar to the child's throat and neck to promote vasoconstriction, to reduce inflammation, and to reduce pain.
         (3) Prevent the child from inserting straws, forks, and any other potentially harmful objects in his or her mouth.
         (4) Advise child not to cough, gargle, or otherwise strain the throat area.
      ii. Pain.
         (1) Regularly assess pain level, using age-appropriate tool.
         (2) Administer safe dosage of pain medications employing the five rights of medication administration, as needed, per orders.
      iii. Risk of Impaired Airway Clearance/Risk for Altered Breathing Patterns.
         (1) Position child in semi-Fowler's position on his or her side to promote drainage of oral secretions and to minimize inflammation.
         (2) Carefully monitor respiratory rate and breathing patterns.
            (a) Any alteration in the child's breathing pattern and/or any color change should be immediately reported.
      iv. Risk for Imbalanced Nutrition: Less than Body Requirements/Risk for Deficient Fluid Volume.
         (1) Begin clear fluids, including ice pops, when the child is awake and alert.
            (a) Because of the color of blood, red-colored liquids should not be served.
            (b) Because they can be painful to swallow, citrus juices should not be served.
         (2) Because dairy products may increase mucus production, coughing, and throat clearing, they usually are not added to the diet until the child is postoperative day 2 or 3.
         (3) The child's diet should be advanced slowly to a soft diet during the week after surgery.

Box 16.1 Preoperative Education of a Child for a Tonsillectomy

- *Using puppets and dolls to convey the information may help to reduce the child's fears.*
- *Have the child try on surgical attire and look at him or herself in the mirror to see how the surgical staff will appear.*
- *Advise the child that pain medicine will be available.*
- *Advise the child that he or she may hold a favorite toy or blanket before and after surgery.*
- *Inform the child about:*
  - *The possible sight of dried blood around his or her mouth.*
  - *The postoperative sore throat.*
  - *IV therapy*
  - *The need for an ice collar.*
  - *The possibility of his or her speech sounding strange.*
  - *The postoperative diet.*
  - *The nursing assessments, including visualizing the back of the throat with a flashlight.*

v. Risk for Infection.
   (1) Monitor the child's temperature for elevations.
   (2) Report signs of infection to the surgeon.

IV. Middle Airway: Croup

Croup is not simply one condition, but rather a group of illnesses, including:

A. Relatively minor, usually viral, illnesses.

1. Spasmodic croup.
   a. Characterized by a barking cough to **stridor** (high-pitched wheezing).
   b. Usually worst during periods of sleep.
   c. Affecting tissues below the vocal cords.
2. **Laryngotracheal bronchitis (LTB).**
   a. Similar symptoms to spasmodic croup.
   b. Affecting tissues both above and below the vocal cords.
3. Treatment: viral croups usually are treated on an outpatient basis by:
   a. Exposing the child to humidified air.
      i. Cool mist vaporizer in the child's bedroom during sleep.
      ii. Sitting with the child in the bathroom with a hot shower running during coughing episodes or
      iii. Sitting outdoors in cool, moist air during coughing episodes.
   b. Calming the child using distractions and other techniques.
      i. Crying increases the possibility of airway obstruction.
   c. Offering warm oral fluids (because cold often exacerbates the problem).
   d. However, if breathing becomes labored or if stridor develops, the child should be transported to the emergency department for immediate evaluation.

B. Serious, bacterial illnesses, most importantly:

1. Acute **epiglottitis.**
   a. Incidence.
      i. Infant and toddler years.
      ii. Rarely seen after age 7.
      iii. Incidence is dropping in the United States because most children are receiving preventive vaccinations.
   b. Etiology.
      i. Bacteria.
         (1) Most commonly: *H. influenzae* and *S. pneumoniae*.
         (2) Also may be caused by *Staphylococcus aureus* and *Haemophilus parainfluenzae*.
      ii. A physiologically narrow airway places young children at high risk for the illness.
   c. Pathophysiology: Epiglottitis is a medical emergency characterized by:.
      i. Infected and markedly inflamed epiglottis.
      ii. Signs and symptoms.
         (1) Abrupt onset.
         (2) Fever.
         (3) Tripod posturing: the child having difficulty respiring sits forward supported by his or her hands in an attempt to breathe as efficiently as possible (Fig. 16.4).
         (4) Four D's (Box 16.2).
   d. Diagnosis.
      i. Suspected.
         (1) Clinical picture.
         (2) Elevated temperature.
         (3) Elevated white blood cell count.
      ii. Definitive diagnosis.
         (1) Visual inspection of a cherry-red, swollen epiglottis.

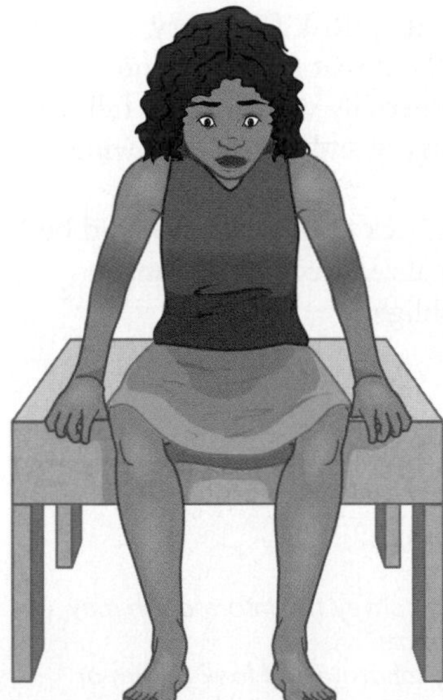

Fig 16.4 A child with epiglottitis in tripod posturing.

Box 16.2 The Four D's for the Diagnosis of Epiglottitis

Dyspnea—*including inspiratory stridor plus other signs of respiratory distress: nasal flaring, intercostal retractions, tachypnea, tachycardia, and cyanosis*
Drooling
Dysphonia—*difficulty in speaking*
Dysphagia—*difficulty in swallowing*

A definitive diagnosis of epiglottitis is made when a cherry-red, swollen epiglottis is visualized. It is, however, dangerous to do so. There is a strong likelihood that when a child with epiglottitis opens his or her mouth wide that the action will result in marked inflammation and total tracheal occlusion. Nurses who suspect that a child has epiglottitis should NEVER assess the child's throat and should seek immediate medical assistance. If a physician performs a visual examination, the nurse should make certain that intubation and tracheostomy trays are immediately available in case they are needed.

(2) The epiglottis should be assessed by a primary health-care provider only.
(3) An intubation and tracheostomy tray should be immediately available.

e. Treatment.
i. Prevention.
(1) Immunizations against *Haemophilus influenzae* type b (Hib) and pneumococcal bacteria (PCV) (see Chapter 11: "Nursing Care of the Child With Immunologic Alterations") have markedly reduced the number of children contracting epiglottitis.

ii. Treatment.
(1) Intubation.
(2) IV epinephrine.
(3) IV antibiotics.
(4) Humidified oxygen administration.

f. Nursing considerations.
i. Infection/Risk of Ineffective Breathing Pattern/Impaired Gas Exchange/Ineffective Airway Clearance.
(1) Assist with intubation.
(2) Safe dosages of the medications, employing the five rights of medication administration, should be administered, per orders.

MAKING THE CONNECTION

The priority nursing actions for a child with epiglottitis who is still breathing effectively is the administration of IV medications (i.e., epinephrine and antibiotics), because the only action that will reverse the illness is the administration of the medications. Primary health-care providers, however, often intubate children before inserting the IV catheter in preparation for the administration of the medications. IV insertion is a painful procedure, leading children to cry and to open their mouths wide, which would likely result in an obstructed airway. Intubating the child before the IV insertion reduces the likelihood of a compromised airway.

(a) Epinephrine rapidly reverses the inflammation, but epinephrine has a very short half-life, so the child must be watched carefully for a return of respiratory distress.
(b) IV antibiotics.

(3) Administer humidified oxygen, as needed and as prescribed.
(4) If intubated, the child's airway should be suctioned, as needed.
(5) The child should be allowed to assume the most comfortable posture.
(6) The child's respiratory effort should be assessed frequently for altered lung sounds and for signs of respiratory distress, including stridor, rales, and wheezing.
(7) Assess the child's oxygenation status via continuous pulse oximetry and blood gas assessments, as ordered.
(8) Administer safe dosage of antipyretics, as ordered.

ii. Anxiety/Fear/Risk for Altered Coping.
(1) Maintain as calm a demeanor as possible while caring for the child.
(2) Allow the parents to remain with the child to provide reassurance and distraction.
(3) Allow the parents to express their concerns/fears.
(4) Calm the child with nonpharmacological means, including, for example, distracting the child, allowing the child to keep a favorite toy/object, and singing to the child.

iii. Risk of Deficient Fluid Volume.
(1) Monitor the child for signs of dehydration (See Chapter 13, "Nursing Care of the Child With Fluid and Electrolyte Alterations").
(2) Administer warm fluids (if safe) and IV fluids, as prescribed.
(3) Monitor the child's temperature at least every 4 hr.

iv. Deficient Knowledge.
(1) Remind the parents regarding the importance of vaccinations.
(2) Advise the parents that viral croup may recur, but bacterial croup rarely does.
(3) Inform the parents regarding actions that should be taken if signs of croup appear and when to proceed to the emergency department.

V. Lower Airway: Bronchiolitis

A. Incidence.
1. Seen almost exclusively in infants.
2. Most frequently seen in babies who were born preterm and chronically ill infants.
3. Most commonly seen in the winter.

B. Etiology.
1. Although other pathogens can cause **bronchiolitis**, respiratory syncytial virus (RSV) is by far the most common pathogen.

C. Pathophysiology.
1. Inflammation of the bronchioles.
2. Signs and symptoms.
   a. Begins like a cold (i.e., rhinitis and loose cough).
   b. Rather than the illness resolving, the child progressively becomes more and more ill and exhibits worsening signs and symptoms:
      i. Wheezing.
      ii. Rales to crackles to rhonchi.
      iii. Tachypnea.
      iv. Signs of respiratory distress: nasal flaring, grunting, and **intercostal retractions**.
      v. Cyanosis.
      vi. Variable temperature.

D. Diagnosis.
1. Clinical picture with a history of prematurity: suggestive.
2. Definitive.
   a. Positive ELISA test for RSV (assesses antigen/antibody response).
   b. X-ray showing hyperinflation of the lung that develops because the child is unable to exhale trapped air.

E. Treatment.
1. Prevention.
   a. Synagis (palivizumab) IM every month for 6 months—usually from November to March, i.e., during the height of RSV season.
      i. The medication is only administered to preterm babies under 6 months of age who were born at less than 36 weeks' gestation.
      ii. Or to acutely and chronically ill infants.
2. There is no specific treatment for an RSV infection; treatment includes:
   a. Cool, humidified oxygen.
   b. IV fluids.
   c. Bronchodilators and steroids.
   d. Virazole (ribavirin), in rare cases.
3. Children with RSV should be maintained both on contact and droplet isolation throughout their hospitalizations.
   a. RSV remains pathogenic on inanimate objects, e.g., tissues, table tops, and bed railings.

F. Nursing considerations.
1. Risk of Ineffective Breathing Pattern/Impaired Gas Exchange/Ineffective Airway Clearance.
   a. Monitor respiratory effort, pulse oximetry, blood gases, and color carefully.
   b. Administer medications, as ordered.
      i. Bronchodilators.
      ii. Steroids.
      iii. Virazole (ribavirin), if prescribed.
         (1) Administered via SPAG (small particle aerosol generator) mist.
         (2) Must be reconstituted with sterile water.
         (3) Pregnancy X category medication: pregnant women must not be in the room when the medication is being administered.
   c. Administer humidified oxygen, per order.
   d. Suction the child's nasal secretions, as needed.
   e. Elevate the head of the bed or crib.
   f. Allow for periods of uninterrupted rest and sleep.
2. Infection/Ineffective Thermoregulation.
   a. To prevent infection:
      i. Administer Synagis (palivizumab) every month to high-risk infants at home or in a clinic, if prescribed.
      ii. Educate the parents to avoid contact with sick children (RSV in older children and adults resembles the common cold).
   b. Meticulous handwashing is essential.
   c. On admission, place the child on contact and droplet isolation.
      i. The child may be placed in a single room or cohorted with other RSV children.
      ii. Educate the parents and other visitors regarding isolation precautions and the rationale for the precautions.
   d. Monitor the child's temperature for alterations.
      i. Young infants and preterm babies may become either hypothermic or hyperthermic.
   c. Administer antipyretics, as needed and as ordered.
3. Risk for Deficient Fluid Volume.
   a. Monitor the child's hydration status.
   b. Administer IV and oral fluids, per orders.
   c. Instill saline nasal drops and bulb suction, as needed, to facilitate oral feedings.
4. Anxiety/Fear/Deficient Knowledge.
   a. Allow the parents to express their concerns/fear regarding the child's illness.

b. Maintain as calm an environment as possible.
c. Provide the parents with information regarding the illness, therapies, and the need for isolation.

VI. Lower Airway: Cystic Fibrosis

A. Incidence.
1. **Cystic fibrosis** (CF) is one of the most common autosomal recessive illnesses.
2. Seen most commonly in those of northern European descent, but mutations are seen in all ethnicities.
3. 1/3,500 live Caucasian births.

B. Etiology.
1. Autosomal recessive illness:
a. Punnett square: example of probability of inheritance if both parents are carriers (Aa) for the illness.

	A	a
A	AA	Aa
a	Aa	aa

Key: A—normal allele; a—CF allele; Aa—carrier genotype; aa—disease genotype
25% probability of disease (aa)

b. CF patients exhibit variable expressivity of the disease, with some children having a very serious form, while others exhibit few symptoms.

C. Pathophysiology.
1. CFTR gene mutation leading to the production of a malfunctioning protein and resulting in the inability of the chloride molecule to cross cell membranes.
a. Because sodium and chloride are markedly attracted to each other, CF basically is an abnormality in salt and water transport across epithelial surfaces.
2. Results in thick mucus developing in the organ systems of the body.
3. Predominately affects the pulmonary, gastrointestinal, and reproductive systems.
4. Signs and symptoms.
a. Respiratory system.
i. Copious amounts of thick mucus that are virtually impossible to cough up without the assistance of chest physical therapy (CPT) and medication.
ii. Frequent bouts of bronchitis and bacterial pneumonia.
iii. Chronic lower airway symptoms, including crackles, wheezing, intercostal retractions, diminished breath sounds, and chronic hypoxia.
iv. Either heart failure or pneumonia are usual causes of death.
b. Gastrointestinal system.
i. Meconium ileus: early sign of the disease.
(1) Meconium stool expelled after 24 hr of age.
ii. Pancreatic involvement.
(1) Absence of pancreatic enzymes resulting in:
(a) Altered fat digestion.
(b) Inadequate absorption of fat-soluble vitamins.
(c) Reduced caloric intake and failure to thrive.
(d) Steatorrhea: fatty, bulky, smelly stools.
(i) Often leads to rectal prolapse and high risk for intussusception (see Chapter 14, "Nursing Care of the Child With Gastrointestinal Problems").
(2) Acquired diabetes mellitus.
(a) From chronic pancreatic involvement.
(3) Liver disease resulting from obstructed bile duct.
c. Reproductive system.
i. Most men are sterile.
(1) From aspermia related to thick mucus production or from congenital absence of the vas deferens.
ii. Females are often infertile.
(1) Secondary to fallopian tube obstruction resulting from mucus production.

D. Diagnosis.
1. Prenatal DNA analysis if family history.
a. Via amniocentesis or chorionic villus sampling (CVS).
2. Newborn screening of the most common CF mutations is performed in all 50 states.
a. Neonates are not always screened for less common mutations.
3. DNA analysis of the child's CFTR genes.
4. Sweat test: reliable assessment.
a. The two-part noninvasive test, which must be performed using a precise technique, measures the quantity of chloride in the child's perspiration.
b. Diagnostic chloride levels vary according to the child's age (Cystic Fibrosis Foundation, 2011).
i. For infants 6 months of age or younger, chloride levels:

(1) Over 60 mEq/L are diagnostic.
(2) Between 30 and 59 mEq/L are suggestive, and the test must be repeated.
(3) Below 30 mEq/L are negative.

ii. For children older than 6 months, chloride levels:
(1) Over 60 mEq/L are diagnostic.
(2) Between 40 and 59 mEq/L are suggestive, and the test must be repeated.
(3) Below 40 mEq/L are negative.

E. Treatment.

1. CF is considered to be an incurable disease, although lung transplantation and gene therapies are being used in some children.
2. Respiratory: maintenance therapies as well as acute illnesses.
   a. Chest physiotherapy.
      i. Percussion and vibration with postural drainage, oscillating therapy devices, and other methods used to mobilize the thick mucus.
      ii. Daily exercise.
         (1) Swimming is often recommended as a daily exercise because while swimming, the child:
            (a) Breathes in humidified air and
            (b) Breathes out into the water.
   b. Medications
      i. Inhaled bronchodilators (e.g., albuterol).
      ii. **Mucolytics** to loosen and liquefy the mucus.
         (1) Pulmozyme (dornase alfa) inhaled via nebulizer, which works by fragmenting the DNA of the extracellular mucus.
         (2) Inhaled hypertonic, sterile saline solution, if over 6 years of age, via nebulizer that helps clear the thick mucus in the lungs.
      iii. Inhaled Tobi (tobramycin) via nebulizer.
         (1) Administered daily to prevent *Pseudomonas aeruginosa* pneumonia infection because most CF patients are chronically colonized with the bacteria.
      iv. Kalydeco (ivacaltor), an oral medication approved by the FDA in 2012, is the first drug to treat the etiology of CF.
         (1) The drug has been approved for children aged 6 and older with specific CF gene mutations.
         (2) The medication enables the affected protein to function, therefore resulting in the salt molecules and water to cross cell membranes.
   c. Anti-inflammatories, to help to maintain lung function (e.g., ibuprofen).
   d. Inhaled corticosteroids (e.g., Flovent or Pulmicort).
3. Gastrointestinal.
   a. High-calorie, high-protein diet.
   b. Pancreatic enzymes with every meal and snack to facilitate fat digestion.
   c. Water-miscible forms of fat-soluble vitamins.
   d. Extra salt intake during times of increased perspiration (e.g., heat and exercise) to enable the child to maintain normal electrolyte balance.

F. Nursing considerations.

1. Ineffective Airway Clearance/Impaired Gas Exchange.
   a. Assess respiratory function.
      i. During routine examinations or during periods of respiratory compromise multiple assessments may be performed (e.g., lung sounds, respiratory rate, oxygen saturations, blood gases, and skin color).
      ii. Assess for signs of chronic hypoxemia (e.g., check for clubbing and polycythemia).
   b. Perform chest physiotherapy two to three times per day or as needed.
      i. At least 1 hr before meals or 2 hr after meals to reduce episodes of nausea and vomiting.
   c. Teach "huffing" technique to increase mucus mobilization.
   d. Administer safe dosages of medications, including bronchodilators, mucolytics, Tobi, and others, per orders.
   e. Administer oxygen, carefully, per order.
      i. Because the child likely is chronically hypercapnic, the child may become apneic if oxygen is administered in high doses.
   f. Allow the child to assume posture of comfort.
   g. When physically able, promote exercise (e.g., swimming).
2. Risk for Infection/Infection.
   a. Perform meticulous handwashing.
   b. Encourage parents and child, if appropriate, to avoid contact with children and adults with active infection.
   c. Administer all childhood vaccinations, per recommended schedule.
   d. Administer safe dosage of Tobi, per order.

e. Monitor for signs of infection: fever, chills, dyspnea, and elevated white blood cell count.
f. If pneumonia has been diagnosed, administer safe dosages of IV antibiotics, as prescribed.

3. Imbalanced Nutrition: Less than Body Requirements/Delayed Growth and Development.
   a. Provide a well balanced diet that is high in calories and protein.
   b. Administer pancreatic enzymes with every food intake.
      i. Infants frequently are fed predigested formula.
      ii. Younger child: open capsules and spread the enzymes on a cracker or other non-protein food.
      iii. Older child: have the child swallow the enzyme capsules.
   c. Administer water-miscible forms of fat-soluble vitamins.
   d. Monitor consistency and frequency of stools.
   e. Chart height and weight progression at each medical checkup.
4. Deficient Knowledge.
   a. Educate the parents and child, when appropriate and using age-appropriate language, regarding the genetic and chronic nature of the illness.
   b. Educate the family, child, and others regarding the importance of maintenance therapies.
   c. Refer the parents to a genetic counselor.
   d. Advise the parents to notify the child's school regarding his or her illness, medications, and the need for chest physiotherapy during the school day.
5. Anxiety/Risk for Altered Coping/Anticipatory Grieving.
   a. Allow the family and child to express their anger, frustration, and guilt regarding the genetic and chronic nature of the disease.
   b. Allow the family and child to discuss the ultimate progression of the disease, including anticipatory grief.
      i. In severely affected patients, death often occurs by the mid-20s.
   c. Encourage the parents and child, when appropriate, to join a support group (e.g., Cystic Fibrosis Foundation).
   d. Encourage the child to wear a MedicAlert bracelet.
   e. Introduce the child and family to others with the disease.
   f. Encourage the parents to allow the child to engage in age-appropriate activities, as tolerated.

VII. Lower Airway: Asthma

Asthma, a reversible obstructive airway disease, is the most common admitting diagnosis in children's hospitals.

A. Incidence.
1. Higher incidence in African American children and children living in crowded, urban locations.
   a. Severity often lessens as the child grows and his or her airway matures.

B. Etiology.
1. A trigger (may be an infection, smoke, change in temperature, food allergy, pet allergy, allergy to pollen, exercise, or another irritant) stimulates an inflammatory response within the bronchi.
2. Each person's trigger is individual and must be identified in order to control the disease.

C. Pathophysiology.
1. Inflammation of the bronchi with concurrent airway obstruction as a result of edema and mucus production.
2. Signs and symptoms.
   a. Minor attack.
      i. Prolonged exhalation: resulting from difficulty in exhaling air from the lungs through the inflamed bronchi.
      ii. Coughing.
      iii. Wheezing.
      iv. Mild shortness of breath.
      v. "Yellow" zone on expiratory flow meter (see below).
   b. Severe attack.
      i. Marked respiratory distress, including intercostal retractions, tachycardia, tachypnea, and cyanosis.
         (1) Initially, tachypnea leads to respiratory alkalosis.
         (2) If respiratory function does not return to normal, respiratory acidosis and hypoxia develop.
         (3) Eventually, when no air exchange is occurring, patients may develop a "silent chest."
      ii. Restlessness, apprehension, and diaphoresis.
         (1) From marked anxiety and hypoxia.
      iii. Tripod positioning.
      iv. Chest tightening: "I can't breathe."
      v. "Red" zone on expiratory flow meter (see below).
      vi. Death is possible if the attack goes untreated or if treatment is delayed.

D. Diagnosis.
1. Clinical signs and clinical history.
2. Peak expiratory flow assessments, that is, measurements of how effectively the child can exhale the air in his or her lungs.

a. Following the assessment, the child's primary health-care provider will determine the child's optimal peak flow.
b. Base on the child's optimal peak flow, the practitioner will determine the child's "yellow" zone, which will indicate when the child is experiencing an early attack, and the child's "red" zone, when the child is experiencing a severe attack.

3. Assessments of vital lung capacity, i.e., measurement of the greatest amount of air that the child is able to exhale after breathing in his or her maximum.
4. Blood gases.
5. Pulse oximetry.
6. RAST testing (radioallergosorbent test) to assess for allergens.

E. Treatment.

1. Treatment regimen to prevent an acute asthma attack.
 a. Identification of the trigger(s) is essential.
 b. Regular exercise (swimming is an excellent respiratory therapy) as an aid in improving pulmonary function.
 c. Immunotherapy (allergy shots) to develop immunity to the trigger.
 d. Monitoring of expiratory peak flow and vital lung capacity.
 e. Medications: individualized in relation to the child's trigger and pattern of attacks.
  i. Inhaled corticosteroids: by nebulizer (if young) or metered dose inhaler (MDI) (for older children, if able).
   (1) Such as Pulmicort (budesonide) and Flovent (fluricasone).
  ii. Leukotriene inhibitor.
   (1) Such as Singulair (montelukast) PO.
  iii. Long-acting beta-2 adrenergic agonists (LABA).
   (1) Such as Serevent (salmeterol) via MDI.
  iv. Short-acting beta-2 agonist (SABA): prior to exercise or exposure to known allergen.
   (1) Such as albuterol or Xopenex (levalbuterol): nebulizer or MDI.
2. Treatments performed during an acute attack.
 a. Assess the child's peak flow using a portable peak flow meter.
  i. If child's peak flow is in the "yellow" zone, the child will likely be able to be treated at home.
   (1) SABA (e.g., albuterol or Xopenex [levalbuterol]) will need to be administered via nebulizer or MDI, as prescribed, as soon as possible.
  ii. If the child's peak flow is in the "red" zone, the child should be transported to the emergency department for emergent care (see below).
 b. Emergent care.
  i. Inhaled bronchodilators every 20 minutes.
  ii. IV steroids, if needed.
  iii. Intubation and ventilator support, if needed.

F. Nursing considerations.

1. Deficient Knowledge/Risk for Injury.
 a. Educate the parents and child, if appropriate, regarding the need to identify trigger(s) of attacks.
  i. Educate the parents and child, if appropriate, to avoid contact with the known trigger(s).
 b. Educate the parents and child, if appropriate, regarding the differences between maintenance and rescue medications.
  i. Educate the parents and child, if appropriate, regarding the importance of taking prevention, i.e., maintenance, medications.
  ii. Educate the parents and child, if appropriate, regarding nebulizer and/or MDI usage (see Chapter 9, "Pediatric Medication Administration").
   (1) Spacers should be used for young children who are to be medicated with an MDI.
 c. Educate the parents and child, if appropriate, regarding pulmonary function tests and the use of a peak flow meter.
  i. Zones are determined and set by the primary health-care practitioner.
 d. Advise the parents to notify the child's school nurse and teacher regarding the illness and medications.
 e. Encourage the child to wear a MedicAlert bracelet.
2. During an attack: Ineffective Airway Clearance/Impaired Gas Exchange/Fatigue/Activity Intolerance.
 a. Assess respiratory effort, including peak flow assessment, auscultation of lung fields, respiratory rate, blood gases, and oxygen saturation.
 b. Administer safe dosage of bronchodilators and other medications, as ordered, and monitor for effectiveness.
 c. Administer humidified oxygen, as ordered.
 d. Assist the child to assume his or her position of choice.
 e. Place intubation and tracheostomy trays at the child's bedside.

f. Administer no food or drink unless breathing improves.
   i. Once the child may drink, provide warm fluids.
g. Provide the child with needed periods of rest.

3. Risk for Deficient Fluid Volume.
   a. Administer IV fluids, as ordered.
   b. Monitor for signs of dehydration.
   c. If safe, administer warmed, clear fluids.
      i. Cold fluids increase bronchospasm, and milk often increases mucus production.
4. Fear/Anxiety/Risk for Altered Coping.
   a. Allow the child and parents to express their fears/concerns.
   b. Maintain a calm environment.
   c. Explain all procedures to the parents and child, using age-appropriate language.
   d. Encourage the parents to remain at the child's bedside for support and comfort.
   e. Provide age-appropriate distractions, and allow the child to retain a favorite toy/object.
   f. Refer the family to a support group/organization.
      i. Such as the American Lung Association and the Asthma and Allergy Foundation of America.

CASE STUDY: Putting It All Together

6-month-old, Caucasian girl in the pediatrician's office with acute otitis media

Subjective Data

- Crying and shaking her head back and forth while in her mother's arms
- Repeatedly tugging at her right ear
- Mother states,
  - "She has had a cold for the past couple of days. Her nose has been all snotty, she's had a hard time breathing through her nose, and she's had a bit of diarrhea, too."
  - "About 3 a.m. this morning she woke up crying. I took her temperature with an armpit thermometer, and it was 101.8°F. She has been miserable all day."
  - "I think she needs antibiotics."
- When asked about factors that place this child at high risk for ear infections, the mother states,
  - "She drinks formula from a bottle."
  - "I try to keep my husband from smoking in the house, but it's hard. He hates to have to go out onto the porch to smoke when it's so cold outside."

Objective Data

Nursing Assessments

- Color pink
- Lungs clear
- Rhinorrhea
- Red, bulging tympanic membrane on right
- Slight bulging of tympanic membrane on left
- Current weight: 15½ lb (consistent growth since last well-child visit)

Vital Signs	
Rectal temperature:	102.0°F
Apical pulse:	165 bpm
Respiratory rate:	48 rpm

Health-Care Provider's Orders

- Acetaminophen 80 mg PO every 6 hr—administer first dose in office
- Ampicillin 150 mg PO every 6 hr for 10 days
- Warm or cold packs to ears, as needed
- Instill saline nasal drops prior to feedings
- Diet change: ORT instead of formula for 2 days
- Return for reassessment after completion of the antibiotic course or earlier, if child shows no improvement.

Continued

CASE STUDY: Putting It All Together *cont'd*

Case Study Questions

A. What *subjective* assessments indicate that this client is experiencing a health alteration?

1. ____________
2. ____________
3. ____________
4. ____________
5. ____________
6. ____________

B. What *objective* assessments indicate that this client is experiencing a health alteration?

1. ____________
2. ____________
3. ____________
4. ____________
5. ____________
6. ____________

C. After analyzing the data that has been collected, what **primary** nursing diagnoses should the nurse assign to this client?

1. ____________
2. ____________

D. What interventions should the nurse plan and/or implement to meet this child's and her family's needs?

1. ____________
2. ____________
3. ____________
4. ____________
5. ____________
6. ____________
7. ____________

E. What client outcomes should the nurse evaluate regarding the effectiveness of the nursing interventions?

1. ____________
2. ____________

F. What physiological characteristics should the child exhibit before being discharged home?

1. ____________

G. What subjective characteristics should the child exhibit before being discharged home?

1. ____________

REVIEW QUESTIONS

1. The mother of an 11-month-old remarks to a nurse at the pediatric clinic, "We are so lucky. Our daughter has never had an ear infection!" Which of the following factors can the nurse tell the mother have protected her daughter from the disease? **Select all that apply.**
   1. The family owns no pets.
   2. No one in the family smokes.
   3. The mother breastfeeds her daughter.
   4. Child attends day care only two mornings a week.
   5. The family lives in the southern part of the country.

2. The mother of a 3-year-old child who has been diagnosed with an ear infection states, "I can't understand why you won't give my child antibiotics. Can't you see that she is sick?" Which of the following responses by the nurse is appropriate at this time?
   1. "I know how you feel, but the best medicine for your daughter right now is acetaminophen."
   2. "Your child will get better on her own in a few days."
   3. "I am also very surprised that the pediatrician didn't order antibiotics."
   4. "It is likely that the ear infection is caused by a virus, and antibiotics do not kill viruses."

3. A child has had tympanostomy tubes inserted. Before discharging the child from the hospital, which of the following should be included in the nurse's discharge teaching?
   1. Elevate the head of the child's bed 30 degrees for the next week.
   2. Bright-red bleeding may drain from the ears for remainder of the day.
   3. Administer narcotic analgesic every 4 hours for the next two days.
   4. Not to allow the child's head to be submerged in bath or pool water.

4. A 7-year-old child has been prescribed penicillin V for streptococcal pharyngitis. Which of the following information should the nurse teach the parents regarding the medication?
   1. Once the child starts the medication, he will no longer be contagious.
   2. The child must take all of the medication.
   3. The child's fever may persist until all of the medicine has been taken.
   4. If given with food, the medicine will be ineffective.

5. The throat culture of an 8-year-old child grew out 4 bacteria. The nurse should request the primary health-care provider to prescribe an antibiotic for the child to treat which of the following bacteria?
   1. *Hemophilus influenzae*
   2. *Streptococcus pyogenes*
   3. *Streptococcus pneumoniae*
   4. *Mycoplasma pneumoniae*

6. A child is being sent home after a tonsillectomy. Which of the following actions should the nurse educate the parents to perform?
   1. Monitor the child for excessive swallowing.
   2. Place warm compresses around the child's neck.
   3. Encourage the child to drink cold citrus juices.
   4. Position the child supine for the next six hours.

7. A 10-year-old child who is receiving pre-op teaching from the surgical nurse states, "My friend told me that I will be given lots of ice cream right after the surgery. I can't wait!" Which of the following responses by the nurse is appropriate?
   1. "You are right. You are going to have to come to the hospital for surgery, but at least we give you a big treat afterwards."
   2. "Your friend is correct that you will be able to eat shortly after the surgery. We will let you eat ice pops, but no ice cream for a day or two."
   3. "I'm afraid that your friend wasn't correct. We don't want you to eat or drink anything cold for at least a week."
   4. "I bet your friend watched an old movie about children having their tonsils out. I'm afraid these days we won't let you eat or drink for two whole days."

8. The parent of an 18-month-old-child calls the child's primary health-care provider and states, "My child coughed all night long. She doesn't seem to be too sick, and she has no temperature. What can I do to help her and the rest of us to sleep tonight?" Which of the following responses is appropriate for the nurse to make?
   1. "It often helps to promote sleep by putting a steam vaporizer right next to the head of the baby's crib."
   2. "There are a number of very good non-prescription cough and cold medications at the pharmacy."
   3. "You could try raising the head of the baby's crib by putting books under the crib's front feet."
   4. "The baby probably needs antibiotics so let's make an appointment for her for this afternoon."

9. A child is seen in the emergency department. The nurse hears a high-pitched squeal every time the child inhales. The parent states that the child's fever is very high and, in addition, the child is gasping for breath and sitting in the tripod position. Which of the following actions would be appropriate for the nurse to perform at this time?
1. Provide the child with warm liquids to drink.
2. Inspect the throat with a flashlight and tongue blade.
3. Check the child's vital signs and lung fields.
4. Get immediate medical attention for the child.

10. A nurse is educating a group of parents regarding the rationales for the administration of vaccinations. The nurse should advise the parents that the vaccine that prevents infections from which of the following diseases has helped to reduce the numbers of children diagnosed with bacterial croup?
1. Hepatitis A
2. *Hemophilus influenzae* type b
3. Rotavirus
4. *Neisseria meningitidis*

11. A newborn baby has been diagnosed with cystic fibrosis (CF). Regarding which of the following characteristics of the disease should the nurse forewarn the parents?
1. Chronic conjunctivitis
2. Rapid weight gain
3. Recurrent vomiting
4. Thick respiratory mucus

12. The parents of a child, who has had multiple respiratory infections since birth, tell the nurse, "When we kiss our child, all we can taste is salt." It would be appropriate for the nurse to suggest to the primary health-care provider that the child be assessed for which of the following illnesses?
1. Cystic fibrosis
2. Asthma
3. Bronchiolitis
4. Pharyngitis

13. A neonate has been diagnosed with cystic fibrosis. The nurse should educate the parents regarding which of the following dietary needs of their baby?
1. The baby must receive a dose of folic acid three times each day.
2. The baby must never consume any milk or milk products.
3. The baby must receive pancreatic enzymes before bedtime every night.
4. The baby must consume a predigested formula that is high in calories.

14. A 10-year-old child has cystic fibrosis. It would be appropriate for the nurse to advise the parents that the child should be monitored yearly for which of the following illnesses?
1. Lupus
2. Arthritis
3. Hyperthyroidism
4. Diabetes mellitus

15. A 4-month-old child is admitted to the pediatric unit with a diagnosis of RSV bronchiolitis. The child is to receive ribavirin (Virazole) every 12 hr × 3 days. Which of the following actions by the nurse are appropriate? **Select all that apply.**
1. Reconstitute the medication with sterile water.
2. Place the child on contact and droplet isolation.
3. Place an oxygen saturation monitor on the child's foot.
4. Administer the medication deep in the vastus lateralis muscle.
5. Advise no pregnant staff or family members to be in contact with the medication.

16. A baby is born 12 weeks preterm. The nurse should determine that which of the following monthly medication injections would be appropriate for this child to receive?
1. Hepatitis B immune globulin
2. Synagis (palivizumab)
3. Pulmozyme (dornase alfa)
4. Varicella-zoster immune globulin

17. A nurse monitoring a preterm baby with RSV bronchiolitis notes that the baby is exhibiting signs of respiratory distress. Which of the following signs did the nurse observe? **Select all that apply.**
1. Huffing
2. Tachypnea
3. Nasal flaring
4. Expiratory grunting
5. Intercostal retractions

18. An 8-year-old child, who has a history of asthma, is seen in the office of the school nurse with coughing and wheezing. Which of the following actions should the nurse perform first?
1. Assess the child's peak expiratory flow.
2. Educate the child to avoid triggers.
3. Transport the child to the emergency department.
4. Notify the child's parents of his condition.

19. A 10-year-old child has been prescribed an MDI administered bronchodilator. Which of the following actions should the nurse teach the child to perform when taking the medication?

1. Take care not to shake the medication container before administering.
2. Wait no more than 10 seconds between administrations of the medication.
3. Exhale completely before placing the medication mouthpiece in the mouth.
4. Compress the container for 30 seconds before inhaling the medication.

20. A 3-year-old child, who has been diagnosed with asthma, is being prescribed albuterol (Ventolin) via nebulizer as a rescue medication for acute episodes. The parents should be advised that the child may exhibit which of the following common side effects of the medication?

1. Insomnia
2. Lethargy
3. Constipation
4. Weight gain

REVIEW ANSWERS

1. **ANSWER: 2, 3, and 4**

Rationale:

1. Pet ownership has not been shown to have any effect on the incidence of ear infections.
2. **Cigarette smoke places children at high risk for ear infections.**
3. **Breastfeeding has been shown to have a protective effect on the incidence of ear infections.**
4. **Day-care attendance places children at high risk for ear infections.**
5. Geographic location has not been shown to have an effect on the incidence of ear infections.

TEST-TAKING TIP: Nurses working with pregnant women and with young children should encourage parents to promote healthful behaviors in the home. Babies who consume breast milk are less likely to develop ear infections as well as a number of other conditions.

Content Area: *Pediatrics—Respiratory*
Integrated Processes: *Nursing Process: Implementation*
Client Need: *Health Promotion and Maintenance: Health Promotion/Disease Prevention*
Cognitive Level: *Application*

2. **ANSWER: 4**

Rationale:

1. This statement is correct, but it does not provide the mother with an explanation of why antibiotics have not been prescribed.
2. This statement is likely correct, but it does not provide the mother with an explanation of why antibiotics have not been prescribed.
3. This statement is not correct. Antibiotics are not prescribed for illnesses that are likely viral in origin.
4. **This is an appropriate statement for the nurse to make.**

TEST-TAKING TIP: The nurse should provide the patient with a clear rationale for the health-care provider's treatment plan.

Content Area: *Pediatrics—Respiratory*
Integrated Processes: *Nursing Process: Implementation; Teaching/Learning*
Client Need: *Physiological Integrity: Physiological Adaptation: Illness Management*
Cognitive Level: *Application*

3. **ANSWER: 4**

Rationale:

1. The child may sleep flat in bed.
2. Little to no blood loss is expected after a myringotomy procedure.
3. Pain medication may be administered, but it is unlikely that the baby will need narcotics for 48 hr.
4. **The child's head should not be allowed to submerge in bath or pool water.**

TEST-TAKING TIP: Tympanostomy tubes are inserted through the eardrum to enable fluid to drain from the middle ear. Unfortunately, fluid can also travel into the middle ear. To prevent fluid from entering the middle ear, children should refrain from submerging their heads in water.

Content Area: *Pediatrics—Respiratory*
Integrated Processes: *Nursing Process: Implementation; Teaching/Learning*
Client Need: *Physiological Integrity: Reduction of Risk Potential: Potential for Complications of Diagnostic Tests/ Treatments/Procedures*
Cognitive Level: *Application*

4. **ANSWER: 2**

Rationale:

1. This statement is incorrect. The child will no longer be contagious once he or she has been on the medication for a full 24 hr.
2. **This statement is correct. In order to prevent the child from developing rheumatic fever or acute glomerular nephritis, he or she must complete the full course of antibiotics.**
3. The child's temperature will likely be normal within 24 hr of medication administration.
4. Penicillin V may be administered with food.

TEST-TAKING TIP: The only sore throat bacteria that is usually treated is *S. pyogenes* or group A beta hemolytic strep because, if left untreated, children may develop serious sequelae from the infection, either rheumatic fever or acute glomerular nephritis.

Content Area: *Pediatrics—Respiratory*
Integrated Processes: *Nursing Process: Implementation; Teaching/Learning*
Client Need: *Physiological Integrity: Pharmacological and Parenteral Therapies: Medication Administration*
Cognitive Level: *Application*

5. **ANSWER: 2**

Rationale:

1. It is unlikely that a child would be treated for a throat culture that grew out *H. influenzae.*
2. **A child would be treated if his or her throat culture grew out *S. pyogenes.***
3. It is unlikely that a child would be treated for a throat culture that grew out *S. pneumoniae.*
4. It is unlikely that a child would be treated for a throat culture that grew out *M. pneumoniae.*

TEST-TAKING TIP: The nurse should be familiar with pathogenic bacteria that are especially dangerous. Although *H. influenzae* and others do cause disease under some circumstances, antibiotics are not routinely administered to children who have the bacteria in their throats. Because of the serious sequelae that can develop after a *S. pyogenes* infection, however, children will always be treated when sick from that organism.

Content Area: *Pediatrics—Respiratory*
Integrated Processes: *Nursing Process: Implementation*
Client Need: *Safe and Effective Care Environment: Management of Care: Collaboration With Interdisciplinary Team*
Cognitive Level: *Application*

6. ANSWER: 1
Rationale:
1. The parents should be taught to monitor the child for excessive swallowing.
2. It is contraindicated to place warm compresses around the neck of a child who has just undergone a tonsillectomy.
3. It is contraindicated to offer citrus juices to a child immediately following a tonsillectomy.
4. It is contraindicated to position a child supine who has just undergone a tonsillectomy.

TEST-TAKING TIP: It could be very painful for children post-tonsillectomy to drink citrus juices. Ice collars are applied to children post-tonsillectomy to reduce inflammation and the risk of excessive bleeding. Children post-tonsillectomy should be elevated and placed in the side-lying position to reduce inflammation and the potential for aspiration. If the child is bleeding from the surgical site, he or she may be swallowing excessively.
Content Area: *Pediatrics—Respiratory*
Integrated Processes: *Nursing Process: Implementation; Teaching/Learning*
Client Need: *Physiological Integrity: Reduction of Risk Potential: Potential for Complications From Surgical Procedures and Health Alterations*
Cognitive Level: *Application*

7. ANSWER: 2
Rationale:
1. This statement is not correct. Clear liquids are given on the day of surgery.
2. This statement is correct, the child will be given ice pops on the day of surgery, but no ice cream for a day or two.
3. This statement is not correct. Children are usually not kept NPO after tonsillectomies.
4. This statement is not appropriate. It provides the child with no positive feedback, and children are not kept NPO after tonsillectomies.

TEST-TAKING TIP: Unless they are experiencing nausea or are vomiting, children are allowed to have clear liquids shortly after a tonsillectomy. It is recommended that the fluids not be red (because blood is red) and should be cold to reduce the bleeding potential. When milk products are consumed, children often need to clear their throats because of increased mucus production. Any aggressive action, such as gargling, crying, coughing, or throat clearing, is contraindicated post-tonsillectomy because of the potential for injuring the surgical site.
Content Area: *Pediatrics—Respiratory*
Integrated Processes: *Nursing Process: Implementation; Teaching/Learning*
Client Need: *Physiological Integrity: Reduction of Risk Potential: Potential for Alterations in Body Systems*
Cognitive Level: *Application*

8. ANSWER: 3
Rationale:
1. Steam vaporizers should not be placed in children's rooms.
2. Over-the-counter cough and cold therapies are contraindicated for young children.
3. Raising the head of the bed can be helpful for children who are likely suffering from spasmodic croup.
4. This child has no fever and appears well. It is unlikely that the child has a bacterial infection.

TEST-TAKING TIP: Positioning cool mist vaporizers near a child's bed is an excellent way to provide humidified air that can often relieve the symptoms of spasmodic croup. On the other hand, children can be seriously burned when steam vaporizers are used.
Content Area: *Pediatrics—Respiratory*
Integrated Processes: *Nursing Process: Implementation*
Client Need: *Physiological Integrity: Physiological Adaptation: Illness Management*
Cognitive Level: *Application*

9. ANSWER: 4
Rationale:
1. With the signs and symptoms listed, it would be inappropriate to provide the child with something to drink.
2. Inspecting the throat of a child with the noted signs and symptoms could result in total occlusion of the trachea.
3. Vital signs and lung sounds are appropriate, but not at this time.
4. The nurse should obtain immediate medical attention for the child.

TEST-TAKING TIP: This child is exhibiting three signs/symptoms of epiglottitis. Inspiratory stridor is especially concerning. The child should be examined immediately by a primary health-care provider.
Content Area: *Pediatrics—Respiratory*
Integrated Processes: *Nursing Process: Implementation*
Client Need: *Physiological Integrity: Physiological Adaptation: Illness Management*
Cognitive Level: *Application*

10. ANSWER: 2
Rationale:
1. Hepatitis A vaccine prevents a fecal-oral viral illness that affects the liver.
2. *H. influenzae* type b vaccine prevents upper respiratory infections, including bacterial croup.
3. Rotavirus vaccine prevents a serious gastrointestinal infection.
4. Meningococcal vaccine prevents bacterial meningitis and meningococcemia.

TEST-TAKING TIP: The vast majority of cases of epiglottitis are caused by *H. influenzae.* Administration of the vaccine to infants has markedly reduced the numbers of childhood cases of the disease.
Content Area: *Pediatrics—Respiratory*
Integrated Processes: *Nursing Process: Implementation; Teaching/Learning*

Client Need: *Health Promotion and Maintenance: Health Promotion/Disease Prevention*
Cognitive Level: *Application*

11. **ANSWER: 4**
Rationale:
1. Chronic conjunctivitis is not a sign/symptom of CF.
2. Children with CF often exhibit poor weight gain.
3. Recurrent vomiting is not a sign/symptom of CF.
4. Thick respiratory mucus is seen in children with CF.
TEST-TAKING TIP: Because of a genetic defect, the chloride molecule of children with CF is incapable of diffusing across the cell membrane. As a result, thick mucus production is noted in the organ systems of the body, especially the pulmonary, gastrointestinal, and reproductive systems.
Content Area: *Pediatrics—Respiratory*
Integrated Processes: *Nursing Process: Implementation; Teaching/Learning*
Client Need: *Physiological Integrity: Physiological Adaptation: Alteration in Body Systems*
Cognitive Level: *Application*

12. **ANSWER: 1**
Rationale:
1. There is a high concentration of salt in the sweat of children with CF.
2. There is not a high concentration of salt in the sweat of children with asthma.
3. There is not a high concentration of salt in the sweat of children with bronchiolitis.
4. There is not a high concentration of salt in the sweat of children with pharyngitis.
TEST-TAKING TIP: The sodium molecule has a high affinity for the chloride molecule. In CF, the chloride molecule of children with CF is incapable of diffusing across the cell membrane. As a result, sodium chloride, or salt, is in high concentrations in the sweat of children with CF.
Content Area: *Pediatrics—Respiratory*
Integrated Processes: *Nursing Process: Implementation*
Client Need: *Safe and Effective Care Environment: Management of Care: Collaboration With Interdisciplinary Team*
Cognitive Level: *Application*

13. **ANSWER: 4**
Rationale:
1. Children with CF are not routinely supplemented with folic acid.
2. Children with CF may consume milk or milk products.
3. Children with CF must receive pancreatic enzymes each time they consume food.
4. Babies with CF usually are fed a predigested formula that is high in calories.
TEST-TAKING TIP: Children with CF digest fats and proteins poorly. They also gain weight slowly. To ensure optimal nutrition, infants frequently are fed a predigested formula.
Content Area: *Pediatrics—Respiratory*
Integrated Processes: *Nursing Process: Implementation; Teaching/Learning*
Client Need: *Physiological Integrity: Physiological Adaptation: Illness Management*
Cognitive Level: *Application*

14. **ANSWER: 4**
Rationale:
1. Children with CF are not especially at high risk for lupus.
2. Children with CF are not especially at high risk for arthritis.
3. Children with CF are not especially at high risk for hyperthyroidism.
4. Children with CF often become type 1 diabetics.
TEST-TAKING TIP: The thick mucus caused by CF results in the inability of the pancreas to produce insulin. Children with CF, therefore, frequently develop type 1 diabetes.
Content Area: *Pediatrics—Respiratory*
Integrated Processes: *Nursing Process: Implementation; Teaching/Learning*
Client Need: *Physiological Integrity: Reduction of Risk Potential: Potential for Alterations in Body Systems*
Cognitive Level: *Application*

15. **ANSWER: 1, 2, 3, and 5**
Rationale:
1. Ribavirin should be reconstituted with sterile water.
2. Children with RSV should be placed on contact and droplet isolation.
3. A pulse oximeter should be placed on the child's foot.
4. The medication is administered via a SPAG nebulizer.
5. Pregnant women should not be in the room when the medication is administered.
TEST-TAKING TIP: Ribavirin is teratogenic, and, because it is administered via a SPAG nebulizer, the medicine becomes aerosolized. Pregnant women, therefore, should not be in the same room when the medication is administered.
Content Area: *Pediatrics—Respiratory*
Integrated Processes: *Nursing Process: Implementation*
Client Need: *Physiological Integrity: Pharmacological and Parenteral Therapies: Adverse Effects/Contraindications/Side Effects/Interactions*
Cognitive Level: *Application*

16. **ANSWER: 2**
Rationale:
1. Hepatitis B immune globulin is administered only to babies whose mothers are hepatitis B surface antigen positive.
2. It would be appropriate for the baby to receive Synagis (palivizumab).
3. Pulmozyme (dornase alfa) is administered to children with CF.
4. Varicella-zoster immune globulin is only administered to babies born to mothers who have chicken pox.

TEST-TAKING TIP: Synagis is a medication that helps to protect preterm and/or chronically ill infants from developing a serious infection from RSV.
Content Area: *Pediatrics—Respiratory*
Integrated Processes: *Nursing Process: Analysis*
Client Need: *Physiological Integrity: Pharmacological and Parenteral Therapies: Expected Actions/Outcomes*
Cognitive Level: *Application*

17. ANSWER: 2, 3, 4, and 5
Rationale:
1. Huffing is a technique taught to children with CF to enable them to expectorate thick mucus.
2. Tachypnea is a sign of respiratory distress in infants.
3. Nasal flaring is a sign of respiratory distress in infants.
4. Expiratory grunting is a sign of respiratory distress infants.
5. Intercostal retractions are seen in infants who are in respiratory distress.
TEST-TAKING TIP: In the beginning, infants infected with RSV often appear to be sick with a common cold. Over time, the infection may enter the bronchioles, causing bronchiolitis. If so, they may exhibit signs of respiratory distress, including tachypnea, nasal flaring, expiratory grunting, intercostal retractions, and cyanosis.
Content Area: *Pediatrics—Respiratory*
Integrated Processes: *Nursing Process: Assessment*
Client Need: *Physiological Integrity: Physiological Adaptation: Alterations in Body Systems*
Cognitive Level: *Application*

18. ANSWER: 1
Rationale:
1. The nurse should assess the child's peak expiratory flow.
2. The child does need to be educated to avoid triggers, but this should not be the nurse's first action.
3. The child may need to be transported to the emergency department, but this should not be the nurse's first action.
4. The child's parents should be notified of the child's condition, but this should not be the nurse's first action.
TEST-TAKING TIP: This child's condition must be thoroughly assessed, including assessment of lung sounds, respiratory rate, and peak expiratory flow. Depending on the assessment, the child's condition may be reversed with prescribed medication, or the child may need to be transported to the emergency department. Educating the child regarding triggers should be performed when the child is well, not during an attack. The child's parents must be notified as soon as the assessment is complete and, if needed, any immediate intervention has been provided.
Content Area: *Pediatrics—Respiratory*
Integrated Processes: *Nursing Process: Implementation*
Client Need: *Safe and Effective Care Environment. Management of Care: Establishing Priorities*
Cognitive Level: *Analysis*

19. ANSWER: 3
Rationale:
1. The container should be shaken well prior to the medication administration.
2. It is appropriate to wait approximately two minutes between MDI administrations.
3. This statement is correct. The child should place the medication mouthpiece in the mouth after exhaling.
4. The container should be compressed at the same time that the child inhales.
TEST-TAKING TIP: The order of the actions during MDI medication administration are: shake the MDI; exhale as completely as possible; secure lips around mouthpiece in the mouth; inhale at the same time as the container is compressed; and, if a second dose is ordered, wait 2 minutes before the second inhalation. If young children are unable to inhale on command, a spacer or a nebulizer should be used to administer their medication.
Content Area: *Pediatrics—Respiratory*
Integrated Processes: *Nursing Process: Implementation; Teaching/Learning*
Client Need: *Physiological Integrity: Pharmacological and Parenteral Therapies: Medication Administrations*
Cognitive Level: *Application*

20. ANSWER: 1
Rationale:
1. Albuterol is a short-acting beta-2 agonist. Insomnia is a common side effect of the medication.
2. Lethargy is not a common side effect.
3. Constipation is not a common side effect.
4. Weight gain is not a common side effect.
TEST-TAKING TIP: If the medication is prescribed to be taken repeatedly during the day, it may be difficult for the parents to get the child to go down for sleep. They should be made aware of this as well as all other common side effects.
Content Area: *Pediatrics—Respiratory*
Integrated Processes: *Nursing Process: Evaluation*
Client Need: *Physiological Integrity: Pharmacological and Parenteral Therapies: Adverse Effects/Contraindications/Side Effects/Interactions*
Cognitive Level: *Application*

Chapter 17

Nursing Care of the Child With Cardiovascular Illnesses

KEY TERMS

Acyanotic defects—Cardiac defects that allow the blood to traverse freely through the pulmonary system and, therefore, enable the blood to become oxygenated.

Atresia—A passageway that should be open that is closed or completely undeveloped.

Congestive heart failure (CHF)—A disease process characterized by the inability of the heart to pump blood effectively.

Cyanotic defects—Cardiac defects that result in blood bypassing the pulmonary system and, therefore, preventing the blood from being oxygenated.

Obstructive defects—Cardiac defects that are characterized by an intact vascular system but with an obstruction preventing the free flow of blood through the heart.

Stenosis—Abnormal narrowing.

I. Description

The cardiovascular system is comprised of the heart as well as the arteries, veins, and capillaries. The majority of cardiac illnesses seen in children are related either to congenital cardiac defects or to inflammatory processes affecting the heart or the blood vessels. Some of the congenital defects actually are residual ducts that were present during fetal circulation (see Fig. 17.1). The fetal circulatory system is distinguished by the presence of three ducts—ductus venosus, foramen ovale, and ductus arteriosus—and mixed blood. The ducts enable the majority of the blood to bypass the lungs because fetal blood is oxygenated via the placenta. Once the baby is born and takes a breath, the ducts should close spontaneously. In some instances, however, the foramen ovale or the ductus arterious remain open. The inflammatory illnesses that are discussed in this chapter usually are seen in children after the infancy period.

II. Cardiac Defects

The heart develops very early in the fetal period. Initially, it is a single tube through which single cells pass. Rapidly, two sets of chambers form—atria and ventricles. By the end of the 8th week of fetal development, the atrial and ventricular septa have formed and the pulmonary artery, aorta, and vena cava are all in place. Unfortunately, many different cardiac defects can develop within the first 8 weeks of pregnancy because many women remain unaware that they are pregnant through this period and may take medications, drink alcohol, or even develop an

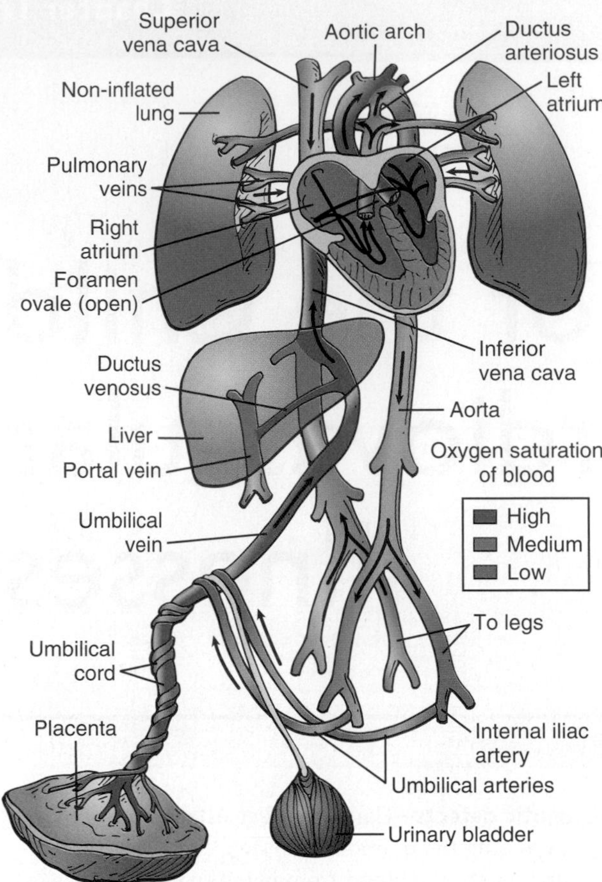

Fig 17.1 The fetal circulatory system.

infectious disease, all of which can cause defects. The most common heart defect seen in neonates is the ventricular septal defect.

A. Incidence.

1. Cardiac defects are seen in 4 to 10 out of every 1,000 live births.

B. Etiology.

1. Although the cause of the vast majority of defects is unknown, they can be caused by a number of factors, including:
    a. Prenatal rubella infection.
    b. Maternal alcohol consumption.
    c. Advanced maternal age.
    d. Maternal diabetes.
    e. Genetic diseases, such as Down syndrome, Klinefelter's syndrome, and Turner syndrome.

C. Pathophysiology.

1. There are three types of congenital cardiac defects (see Table 17.1).

DID YOU KNOW?

The best way to remember the pathophysiology of each cardiac defect is carefully to break down the name of the defect. For example, a ventricular septal defect is a defect (or hole) in the septum (or wall) between the ventricles. Similarly, aortic **stenosis** is a narrowing of the aortic valve.

Table 17.1 Types of Congenital Cardiac Defects

Acyanotic Defects

Characterized by defects that result in blood being shunted from the left to the right side of the heart. As a result, the blood enters and reenters the pulmonary system.

Name	Signs and Symptoms	Treatment
Atrial septal defect (ASD) Hole between the atria. May be a foramen ovale that has not closed or a defect unrelated to the fetal duct.	Most have no symptoms, but the child may develop CHF, if the ASD is large. A murmur may be present.	Many ASDs close spontaneously. If not, surgery or interventional cardiology may be performed. 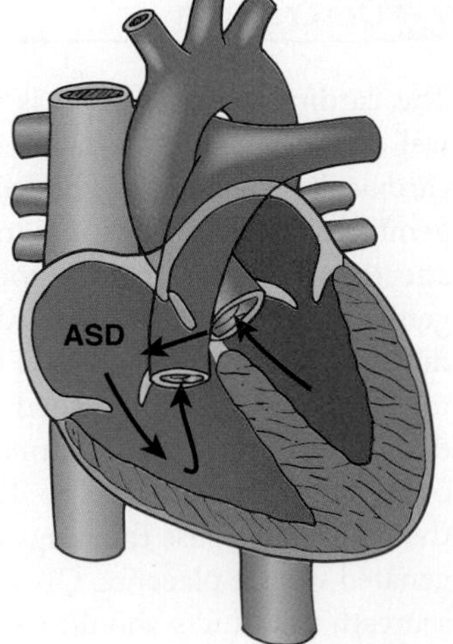

Table 17.1 Types of Congenital Cardiac Defects *cont'd*

Name	Signs and Symptoms	Treatment	
Ventricular septal defect (VSD) A hole between the ventricles; the most common cardiac defect.	Most have no symptoms, but the child may develop CHF if the VSD is large. A murmur may be present.	Small VSDs close spontaneously. If not, surgical repair will be needed.	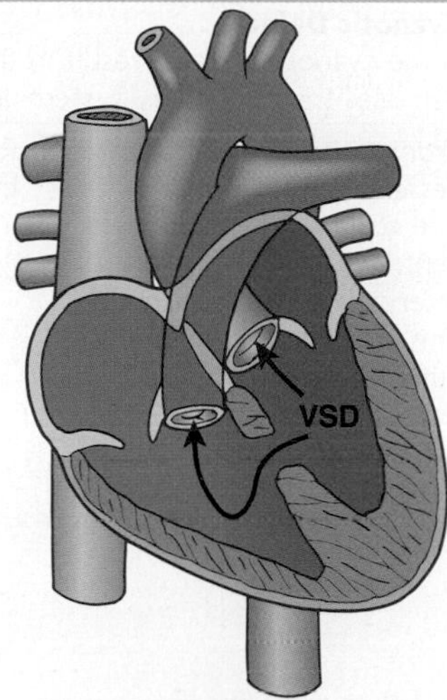
Patent ductus arteriosus (PDA) Most commonly seen in premature infants, especially when they weigh less than or equal to 1,500 g at birth. The fetal duct between the pulmonary artery and the aorta fails to close.	May have no symptoms, but a murmur may be heard, and the child may develop CHF.	The defect may close spontaneously. If not, it may be closed medically with the administration of indomethacin (Indocin), a prostaglandin inhibitor. If the medication is unsuccessful, surgery may be needed.	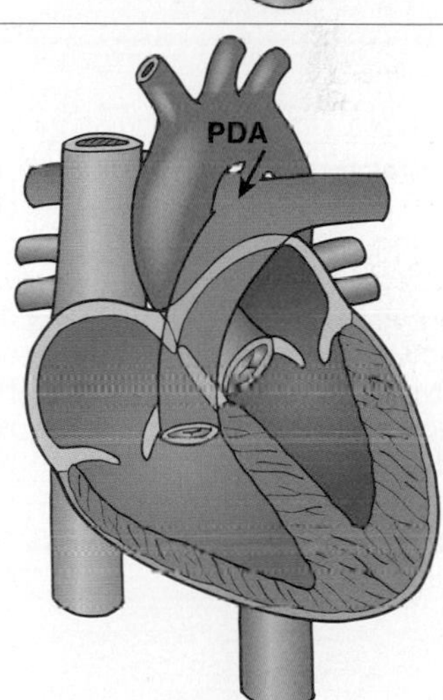
Atrioventricular canal (AVC) A large hole in the middle of the heart.	Signs and symptoms: progressively worsening CHF.	Surgical repair is required.	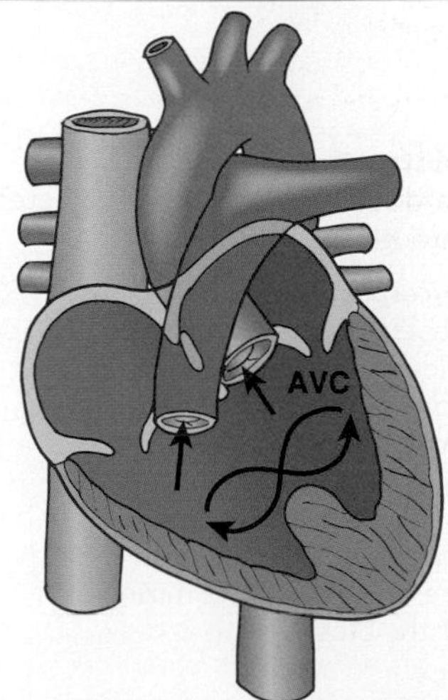

Continued

Table 17.1 Types of Congenital Cardiac Defects *cont'd*

Name	Signs and Symptoms	Treatment	
Cyanotic Defects Some cyanotic defects result in the blood being shunted from the right to the left side of the heart. As a result, the blood bypasses the pulmonary system. In other cyanotic defects, deoxygenated blood never reaches the pulmonary system.			
Transposition of the great vessels (TGV) The aorta exits off the right ventricle and the pulmonary artery off the left ventricle. This defect is incompatible with life unless another defect is present that allows the mixing of blood.	Rapid and sustained cyanosis.	Surgery to create an intact vascular system.	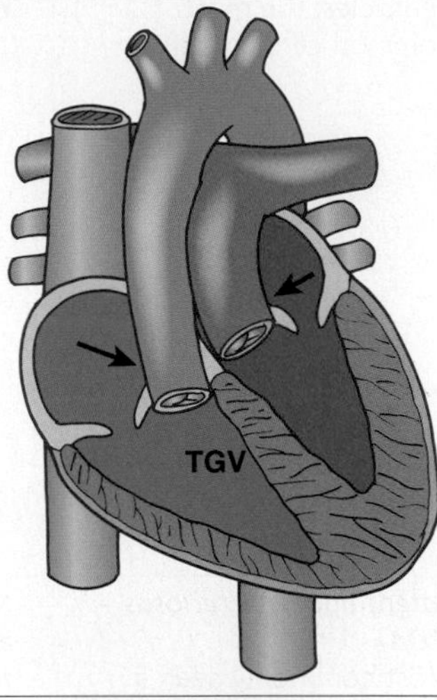
Tetralogy of Fallot (ToF) The most common cyanotic defect, consisting of four defects: VSD, overriding aorta, pulmonary stenosis, and right ventricular hypertrophy. The right ventricular hypertrophy develops over time because the ventricle is working extra hard to circulate the blood.	TET spells, in which the child becomes cyanotic, especially when crying and while eating (infancy) and during play (in older children); additional changes that develop if the defect is not repaired include polycythemia, a greater than normal number of circulating red blood cells, and clubbing of the fingers. These signs develop as a result of chronic hypoxic.	Surgical repair. The cyanosis that develops during a TET spell can be relieved when the legs and knees are bent, resulting in reduced blood flow to the lower body and improved blood flow to the vital organs. Infants should be placed in a knee-chest position. If the defect has not been repaired, older children usually squat instinctively.	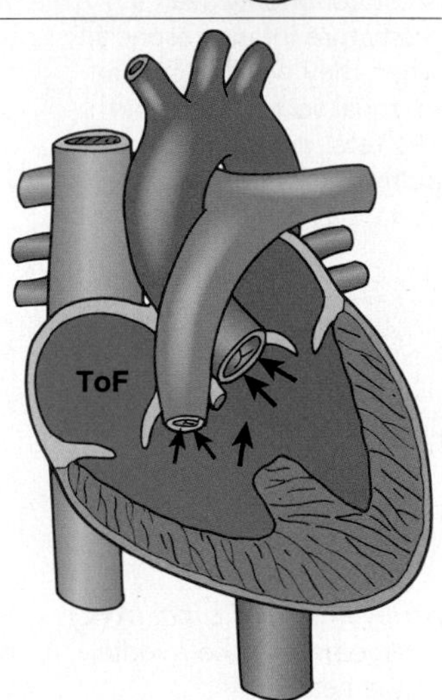
Obstructive Defects Cardiac defects that are characterized by an intact vascular system but with an obstruction preventing the free flow of blood through the heart.			
Tricuspid atresia (TA) Characterized by a closed tricuspid valve, resulting in no movement of blood from the right atrium to the right ventricle. This defect is incompatible with life unless another defect is present that allows mixing of the blood.	Rapid and sustained cyanosis.	Surgical repair.	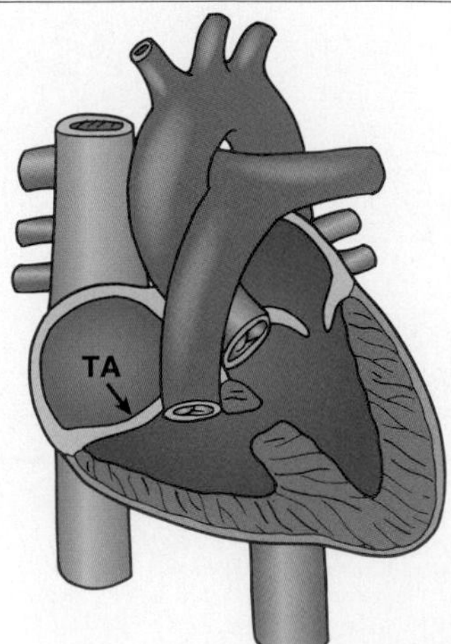

Table 17.1 Types of Congenital Cardiac Defects *cont'd*

Name	Signs and Symptoms	Treatment
Pulmonic stenosis (PVS) A narrowing of the pulmonary artery or valve.	Cyanosis during times of activity to severe CHF.	Balloon angioplasty or surgical repair. 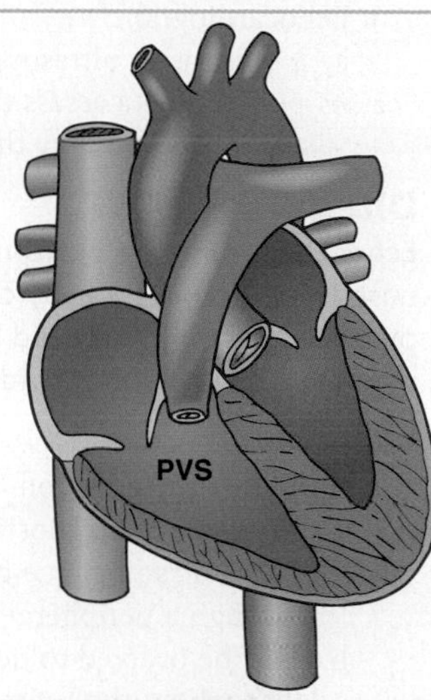
Aortic stenosis (AS) A narrowing of the aorta or aortic valve.	Murmur to CHF.	Balloon angioplasty or surgical repair. 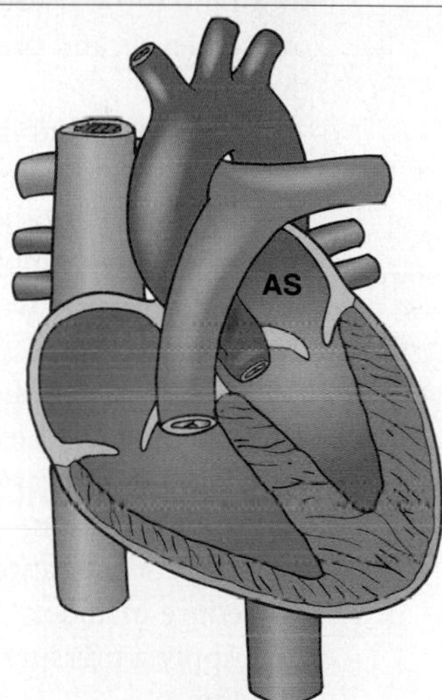
Coarctation of the aorta (CoA) A narrowing of the aorta, usually distal to the ascending vessels.	Markedly higher blood pressures and pulses in the upper extremities as compared to those in the lower extremities. If left uncorrected, older children suffer from recurrent episodes of epistaxis and complaints of leg cramps or leg pain, especially during periods of activity.	Surgical repair. 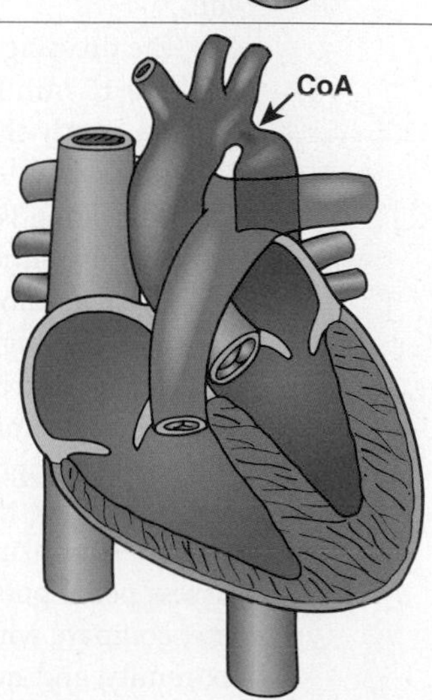

D. Diagnosis—A number of specialized tests are performed in order to accurately diagnose a cardiac defect:

1. Echocardiogram.
   a. Noninvasive ultrasound of the heart that is performed to assess the structures of the heart and the blood flow through the heart.

DID YOU KNOW?

Echocardiograms are performed on babies who are unsedated. To keep a baby content during the procedure the nurse should keep the baby as warm as possible and provide the baby with a pacifier.

2. Cardiac catheterization.
   a. An invasive diagnostic procedure during which a radiopaque catheter is threaded through a peripheral vessel to the heart.
   b. May be ordered to determine blood flow throughout the heart as well as to assess oxygen levels and pressures in the chambers of the heart.
      i. Dye is injected into the heart, and x-rays are taken to determine circulation patterns. Periodically during the procedure, samples of blood for analysis and pressures within the chambers of the heart are taken.
   c. Babies are sedated during the procedure.
   d. The parents must be educated regarding the procedure and regarding care of the baby postcatheterization.
   e. Nursing considerations following the procedure include:
      i. Apply a pressure dressing to the puncture site.
         (1) The dressing must be assessed every 5 to 15 min for the first hour and frequently throughout the remainder of the day.
         (2) If bleeding is noted on the dressing, pressure should be applied and the physician notified.
         (3) The dressing must be protected from fecal and urine contamination.
      ii. Keep the extremity where the puncture was made straight for 4 to 6 hr. It often is helpful to have the child rest on his or her parent's lap during this time.
      iii. Assess pedal pulses distal to the puncture site, compare with those on the opposite extremity, and notify the physician of any disparity.
      iv. Assess the temperature and color of the affected extremity distal to the puncture site, compare with those on the opposite extremity, and notify the physician of any disparity.
      v. Assess the child for signs of pain using an age-appropriate pain rating scale.

E. Nursing considerations.

1. Cardiac defects often are not evident until after birth. During the assessment performed on the neonate on admission to the newborn nursery, the nurse must, therefore, assess for signs and symptoms associated with cardiac defects including signs and symptoms of congestive heart failure (see below):
   a. Assess the baby's skin color, especially when the baby is crying and feeding, for duskiness, circumoral cyanosis, i.e., a bluish discoloration around the mouth, and peripheral cyanosis.
   b. Listen to the apical heart rate for a full minute, noting whether the heart rate deviates from normal (110 to 160 bpm) and/or whether any heart murmurs are present.
   c. Listen to the lung fields for a full minute for adventitious sounds, noting whether the respiratory rate deviates from normal (30 to 60 rpm).
   d. Palpate the brachial and femoral pulses to note any variations in intensity between them.
   e. Perform pulse oximetry on the baby, preferably at least 24 hr after birth. (The number of false-positive results drop when the test is performed after 24 hr of life.)
      i. The probes should be placed on the right hand and on one foot.
      ii. An algorithm to determine actions following the screening test is available in Kemper and associates (2011), "Strategies for implementing screening for critical congenital heart disease."
   f. If indicated, assess the blood pressures (normal 60 to 80 mm Hg/40 to 50 mm Hg) in all four quadrants, and note any disparity between the pressures in the arms versus the pressures in the thighs. (Blood pressures often are not assessed unless other signs/symptoms are present.)
   g. Notify the neonatologist if any of the signs or symptoms are present. If present, an echocardiogram likely will be ordered.

III. Congestive Heart Failure

Congestive heart failure (CHF) is the failure of the heart effectively to circulate the blood. It can develop as a result of either right-sided or left-sided failure.

MAKING THE CONNECTION

The quantity of blood ejected from one of the cardiac ventricles each minute is called the cardiac output (CO). It is equal to the product of the stroke volume (SV), which is the quantity of blood ejected from the left ventricle each time the heart beats, and the heart rate (HR), or CO = SV × HR.

The SV of children changes little during pathologic events; therefore one must monitor HR carefully. A fluctuation of HR that cannot be explained often is an indication of disease.

A. Incidence.
1. The most common complication of patients with congenital heart disease.
2. Dependent on the severity of the cardiac defect.

B. Etiology.
1. In children, CHF most commonly results from altered blood flow secondary to a cardiac defect.

C. Pathophysiology.
1. Signs and symptoms (see Box 17.1 for a complete list).

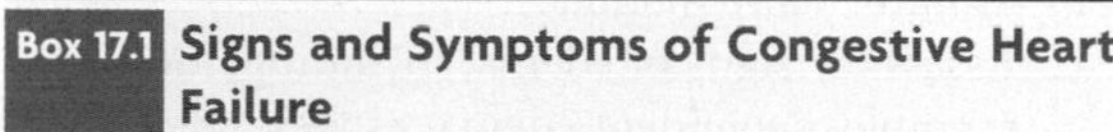

Box 17.1 Signs and Symptoms of Congestive Heart Failure

Cardiovascular
- *Tachycardia: rapid heart rate.*
- *Altered pulses: variation in intensity between the brachial and femoral pulses.*
- *Cardiomegaly: enlarged heart.*
- *Polycythemia: excessive number of circulating red blood cells.*
- *Clubbing: fingertips and nails that are abnormally broad and rounded (Fig. 17.2).*
- *Hypertension: high blood pressure.*

Respiratory
- *Dyspnea: difficulty breathing.*
- *Tachypnea: rapid respiratory rate.*
- *Retractions: drawing in of the skin between the ribs during each inspiration.*
- *Recurrent upper respiratory infections.*
- *Posturing: taking on a body position that helps to improve respiratory function. For example, when a child assumes a tripod posture, he or she sits upright and slightly forward with his or her arms straight and places his or her hands on a surface to support the body (Fig. 16.4).*

Renal
- *Fluid retention: secondary to poor renal perfusion that leads to edema—dependent, pulmonary, and/or central—and weight gain.*

Other Symptoms (related to poor oxygenation)
- *Infants: refusal to eat.*
- *Toddlers and older children: sitting or squatting rather than standing; walking or crawling rather than running; taking frequent rest periods.*

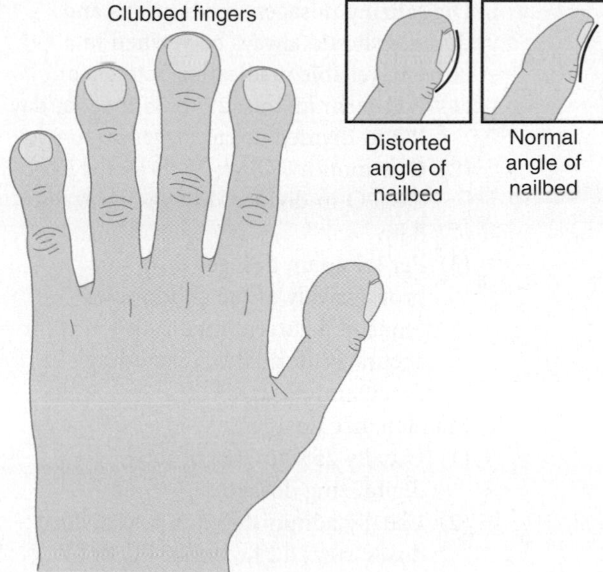

Fig 17.2 Clubbed fingers.

a. The classic signs and symptoms of CHF are:
   i. Tachycardia.
   ii. Tachypnea.
   iii. Weight gain.
b. When right-sided failure is present.
   i. The right ventricle is unable effectively to pump blood into the pulmonary artery, which leads to decreased oxygenation of the blood and increased pressure in the right atrium and systemic system.
   ii. In addition to the classic signs and symptoms, the child will exhibit systemic signs and symptoms, e.g., dependent edema, ascites, and hypertension.
c. When left-sided failure is present.
   i. The left ventricle is unable to pump blood through the aorta, which leads to pulmonary congestion.
   ii. In addition to the classic signs and symptoms, the child will exhibit signs and symptoms of pulmonary edema, e.g., rales, rhonchi, wheezes, and orthopnea.

D. Diagnosis.
1. Based on the severity of the clinical picture (see "Signs and symptoms").

E. Treatment.
1. Treatment of the underlying defect.
2. Oxygen, as needed.
3. Medications.
   a. Digoxin (Lanoxin): to improve the cardiac output by increasing the contractility of the cardiac muscle and slowing the heart rate.

i. Digitalizing dosages (medications and dosages should always be verified in a current, reliable medication reference).
   (1) Full-term infants: 25 to 35 mcg/kg/day PO in divided dosages every 6 to 8 hr.
   (2) One month to 2 yr: 35 to 60 mcg/kg/day PO in divided dosages every 6 to 8 hr.
   (3) Per kilogram dosages drop progressively as the child grows (consult a current medication text for accurate information, including parenteral dosages).

ii. Maintenance dosages.
   (1) Usually 25% to 35% of total digitalizing dosages.
   (2) Usually administered in two divided doses every 12 hr, either PO or IV.

Digoxin may be ordered either as a mg dosage or as a mcg dosage. Nurses must, therefore, carefully read a digoxin order and carefully calculate the amount to be administered (see Chapter 9, "Pediatric Medication Administration," for guidelines on safe dosage calculations). To avoid errors, two nurses must ALWAYS check the recommended dosage for the child's weight, the ordered dosage, and the requisite safe dosage calculations. Only after both nurses agree that the calculations are accurate, should the nurse administer the medication.

b. Furosemide (Lasix): diuretic that promotes fluid excretion by inhibiting the reabsorption of sodium and chloride.

c. ACE inhibitors, such as captopril (Capoten): may be added to relax smooth muscles by blocking the conversion of angiotensin I to angiotensin II, thereby reducing vasoconstriction and sodium retention.

F. Nursing considerations.

1. Decreased Cardiac Output.
   a. Monitor vital signs, EKG, and oxygen saturation levels.

MAKING THE CONNECTION

Before administering digoxin, the apical pulse must always be taken for 1 full minute. If the heart rate is below the cut-off heart rate, the medication is held and the rate reported to the physician. For children, the cut-off heart rate will usually be included in the medication order. If not, the nurse should check to make sure that a correct cutoff is being used. Common apical heart rate cutoffs before administering digoxin are:

- Infants and toddlers: 100 bpm.
- Preschoolers and school-age children: 70 bpm.
- Adolescents: 60 bpm.

   b. Monitor peripheral perfusion by assessing peripheral pulses, skin color, and capillary refill.
   c. Cluster nursing interventions together to allow the child undisturbed rest periods.
   d. If possible, feed the patient small amounts frequently to decrease the workload of the heart.
   e. When administering digoxin (Lanoxin), note:
      i. Digoxin has a narrow therapeutic range: 0.8 to 2 ng/mL; it is important that dig blood levels be checked regularly and when any signs of dig toxicity are noted. For example, dig levels should be drawn if a child exhibits vomiting, arrhythmias, bradycardia, or hypokalemia.

A common sign of digoxin toxicity is vomiting. Digoxin should NEVER be administered to a child who is vomiting until it is confirmed that the digoxin level is within therapeutic range.

2. Excess Fluid Volume.
   a. Monitor strict intake and output.
   b. Monitor daily weights.
   c. Assess for signs of edema, including, for example, dependent edema, ascites, rales, and rhonchi.
   d. Administer safe dosages of Lasix or other diuretic, as prescribed.

Serum potassium levels must be monitored carefully in children with CHF. Not only must potassium levels be monitored carefully whenever Lasix, a potassium-loser, is administered, but because the child is also receiving digoxin. Hypokalemia places the child at increased risk for cardiac arrhythmias. Normal serum potassium levels in children older than 1 year of age are 3.5 to 5.0 mEq/L. In newborns and infants, values are slightly higher; hospital lab data should be consulted for accurate values.

   e. If the child is old enough to consume food, encourage the intake of potassium-rich foods, such as bananas and orange juice.
   f. If an older child is on fluid restriction, provide fluids in small cups (e.g., medicine cups) to reduce feelings of frustration.

3. Ineffective Breathing Pattern/Altered Tissue Perfusion.
   a. Monitor breathing pattern, lung sounds, and respiratory rate.
   b. Administer oxygen as prescribed, but this intervention may not be as effective as one would expect because the pathophysiology is in the circulatory system, **not** the respiratory system.

c. Assist the child with position changes, such as elevating the head of the bed and assisting an older child to the tripod position.
d. Cluster nursing interventions to allow for rest periods.
e. Prevent exposure of the child to others with infectious diseases.

4. Risk for Infection.
   a. Monitor the child carefully for signs of infection because infection increases the workload on the heart.
   b. Report temperature elevations, and request treatment for all infections.
   c. If inpatient, place the child in a room with a noncontagious roommate.
   d. Maintain meticulous hand washing.
5. Activity Intolerance/Fatigue
   a. If an older child, limit physical activity by encouraging quiet activities (e.g., video games, board games, puzzles).
   b. Organize nursing actions to allow for rest periods.
   c. Intervene immediately to decrease the child's frustrations, such as anticipating demands and needs.
   d. Cuddle and give the older child explanations to reduce anxiety.
6. Imbalanced Nutrition: Less than Body Requirements.
   a. Provide small, frequent feeds to reduce exertion time (babies may breastfeed or formula feed).
   b. Alter the feeding method as needed, such as gavage feed or increase the hole in a bottle's nipple.
   c. Feed in the upright posture to facilitate breathing.
   d. For the older child, provide highly nutritious, easily digested but palatable foods, such as milk shakes and frozen yogurt.
   e. Use incentives to encourage the child to eat, including the use of picnic-style lunches and book readings during the meal.
7. Deficient Knowledge/Anxiety/Altered Family Processes.
   a. Allow the parents and child, if appropriate, to express their concerns and feelings.
      i. Parents become frightened when a newborn is diagnosed with a heart defect.
   b. Educate the parents, using understandable language or pictures, regarding the child's condition.
   c. Educate the parents regarding all medications, including how to take the apical pulse; how to administer the medications; side effects of the medications; and times to notify the pediatrician of adverse effects.
   d. Include the child's siblings and other family members in the discussions.
   e. Always use language that is appropriate to the child's developmental level.

IV. Rheumatic Fever (RF)

RF, an illness that develops subsequent to a bacterial illness, is included in this chapter because the most serious complication that can result from the illness is scarring and permanent damage to the mitral valve.

A. Incidence.
1. Highest incidence is in school-aged children in lower socioeconomic groups, especially those living in crowded housing.

B. Etiology.
1. The consequence of an autoimmune response resulting from antibody development following an infection from group A beta-hemolytic streptococci.
   a. Although there are many different strains of streptococci, including *Streptococcus pneumoniae* that causes ear infections and pneumonia and *Streptococcus mutans* that is one of the leading causes of tooth decay, *Streptococcus pyogenes* (i.e., group A beta-hemolytic strep) is the only one that causes RF.
   b. RF may occur following a case of strep throat (see Chapter 16, "Nursing Care of the Child With Respiratory Illnesses"), impetigo (See Chapter 19: "Nursing Care of the Child With Integumentary System Disorders), scarlet fever (See Chapter 11: "Nursing Care of the Child With Immunologic Alterations), or any other illness caused by *S. pyogenes.*
2. RF is usually seen about 2 weeks following the infection.

C. Pathophysiology.
1. A serious inflammatory disease affecting the heart, joints, central nervous system, and subcutaneous tissues.
2. The inflammation may lead to chronic valvular stenosis and/or regurgitation.

D. Diagnosis.
1. Diagnosed using the Jones criteria (see Table 17.2).

E. Treatment.
1. Antibiotics.
   a. If group A beta-hemolytic strep is still present, the strep infection is treated with oral penicillin V (drug of choice) for 10 full days or one dose of penicillin G benzathine IM.

Table 17.2 Jones Criteria

Rheumatic fever is diagnosed if:
- **Two or more major manifestations are present,** OR
- **One major manifestation and two or more minor manifestations are present WITH evidence of recent group A strep infection,** such as recent scarlet fever, positive throat culture, elevated antistreptolysin antibodies, or other strep antibodies.

Major Manifestations	
Carditis Inflammation of the heart muscle	*Most serious manifestation of RF.* *Characterized by tachycardia, cardiomegaly, new murmurs, muffled heart sounds, precordial friction rub, precordial pain, and/or EKG changes.* *Can also present as CHF.*
Migratory polyarthritis Inflammation of the joints	*Most common symptom of RF.* *Characterized by swollen, red, hot, painful joints; usually affects the large joints, such as the elbows, knees, and hips.* *Swelling migrates around the body, with different joints being affected every couple of days.*
Erythema marginatum Demarcated rash	*Characterized by transient, macular rash with a wavy, well-demarcated border and a clear center.* *Rash is seen on the trunk and inner surfaces of the extremities.*
Chorea Involuntary movements	*Also called St. Vitus' Dance, Sydenham's chorea.* *Characterized by aimless, involuntary movements; speech disorders; and profound muscle weakness.* *Very frightening to children because they are unable to control their own bodies.*
Subcutaneous nodules	*Characterized by painless, subcutaneous bumps that appear over bony surfaces and tendons, most commonly on the back of the wrist, over the elbows, and on the knees.*

Minor Manifestations

Fever.
Arthralgias: Joint pains.
Elevated erythrocyte sedimentation rate (ESR): blood test that measures the speed at which erythrocytes (red blood cells) sink in a tube of blood. An elevated rate is a nonspecific indicator of the presence of an inflammatory process in the body.
Positive C-reactive protein: blood test that measures the amount of protein in the blood. The protein is a nonspecific indicator of the presence of an inflammatory process in the body.
Prolonged P-R interval on EKG.

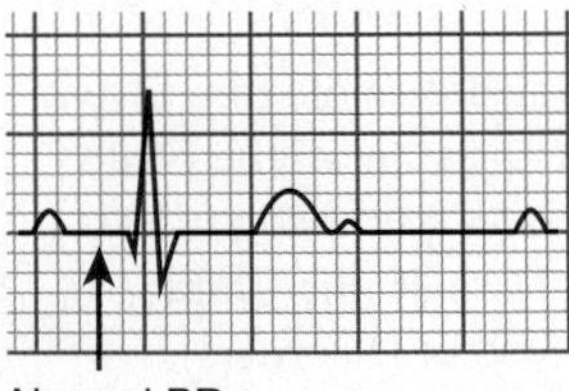
Normal PR

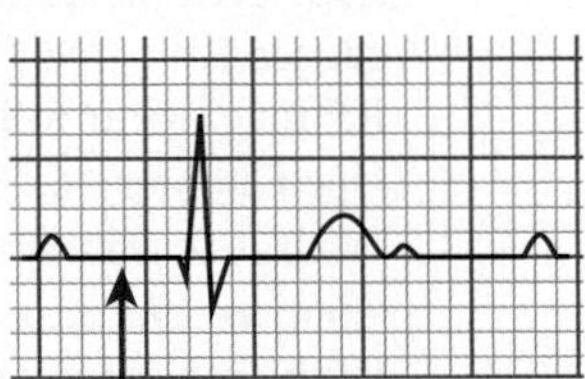
Prolonged PR

b. Children who are allergic to penicillin usually receive erythromycin.
c. Antibiotics must be taken until all the medication is gone.
d. Prophylactic penicillin (either monthly IM or daily PO) usually is prescribed to prevent a recurrence of the disease in children who have had RF.

2. Anti-inflammatories.
   a. Aspirin and corticosteroids: administered to prevent cardiac damage and to treat arthritis and other inflammatory symptoms.

DID YOU KNOW?

To prevent the development of Reye syndrome, aspirin is contraindicated in children who have viral infections, especially flu and chickenpox. It is, however, an excellent therapy for children who have been diagnosed with inflammatory illnesses such as RF. The nurse must carefully educate the parents regarding the rationale for the administration of the aspirin.

3. Bedrest.
   a. To reduce the workload on the heart.

F. Nursing considerations.
1. Infection.
   a. Culture the possible source of infection (e.g., throat, skin) per accepted technique. (The culture may come back negative because the child's strep infection already may have been eradicated from the body.)

MAKING THE CONNECTION

RF is a preventable disease. Because of the lack of good medical care, the vast majority of children who develop RF today live in developing countries. It does still exist in the United States, however, when children are not diagnosed with a group A strep infection in a timely fashion. It is important, therefore, for nurses to advise parents that if their child complains of a sore throat for more than 2 days, the child should be seen by a health-care provider so that a culture can be taken.

b. If the culture is positive for group A strep, place the child on droplet isolation for the first 24 hr of antibiotic therapy—either in a private room in the hospital or quarantined at home if outpatient.
c. If the culture is positive for group A strep, administer a safe dose regimen of antibiotics per the health-care provider's prescription.
   i. Educate the parents regarding safe medication administration practices if the child is to be cared for at home.
2. Deficient Knowledge/Anxiety/Fear.
   a. Educate the parents, child, and others regarding the disease process, especially in relation to cardiac involvement.
   b. Educate the parents, child, and others regarding the potential dangers associated with sore throats and the need for culturing.
   c. If oral medication is ordered, educate the parents regarding the need to complete the entire antibiotic course to make sure that the disease has been completely eradicated from the body.
   d. Allow the parents, child, and others to express their concerns regarding the health and well-being of the child.
3. Risk for Injury.
   a. Maintain bedrest.
   b. Educate the parents regarding the need for on-going prophylaxis, when prescribed.
   c. Maintain seizure precautions, if chorea is present.
4. Acute Pain/Activity Intolerance.
   a. Assess pain using an age-appropriate pain tool.
   b. Provide pharmacological and non-pharmacological pain management, as needed and as prescribed.
   c. Encourage quiet activities (e.g., video games, board games, puzzles, books).
   d. Apply heat or cold to affected joints, as needed.

V. Kawasaki Disease

Kawasaki disease is a potentially fatal three-phase disease. If left untreated, it can progressively weaken the walls of the child's blood vessels.

A. Incidence.
1. Primarily seen in children during the toddler period.

B. Etiology.
1. Unknown etiology, but it is likely caused by an infectious agent.

C. Pathophysiology.
1. Stage 1.
   a. Lasts between 10 and 14 days.
   b. Characterized by high fever; conjunctivitis (Fig. 17.3); strawberry tongue; cracks and fissures in the lips; pervasive erythematous rash, including on the palms and soles; and edema of hands and feet.
2. Stage 2.
   a. Lasts about 10 days.
   b. Characterized by fever and resolution of the rash (hands and feet desquamate); irritability and anorexia; arthritis and arthralgias; and, most seriously, cardiovascular changes, including CHF, arrhythmias, and development of coronary aneurysms.
3. Stage 3.
   a. Lasts until the elevated sedimentation rate returns to normal.
   b. Grooves on the fingernails are often noted.

D. Diagnosis.
1. Diagnosis usually is made using the following criteria:

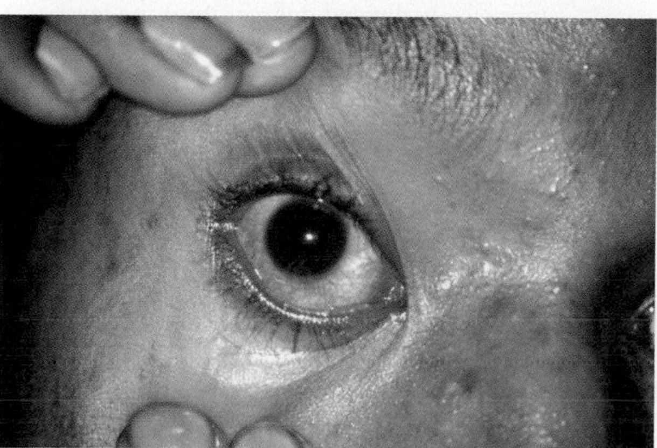

Fig 17.3 Conjunctivitis.

a. No other disease can explain the findings.
b. Fever that lasts for at least 5 days **plus** the presence of four of the following five signs/symptoms:
   i. Nonpurulent conjunctivitis.
   ii. Changes in the oral mucosa (see above).
   iii. Erythematous palms and soles, followed by desquamation.
   iv. Characteristic rash on trunk.
   v. Cervical lymphadenopathy.
c. Other tests that are performed.
   i. Laboratory findings, including elevated white blood cell (WBC) count, elevated erythrocyte sedimentation rate (ESR), and elevated C-reactive protein.
   ii. Electrocardiogram (EKG): heart block may be seen during phase 1.
   iii. Echocardiogram—to assess for coronary aneurysms

E. Treatment.

1. The goal of therapy is to minimize the cardiovascular pathology. Results are much better when the intervention is administered within 10 days of the onset of the fever.
   a. High-dose IV immune globulin (IVIG): 2 g/kg once over 10 to 12 hr. (See Chapter 9, "Pediatric Medication Administration," regarding the administration of IV infusions and blood products.)
      i. A nonspecific immune globulin is administered because the exact organism, and therefore the exact antibody, has not yet been identified.
      ii. The IVIG should be clear with no sediment or cloudiness.
      iii. The nurse should check and document the expiration date and lot number of the IVIG.
   b. High-dose aspirin: 80 to 100 mg/kg/day in four evenly divided dosages until the fever resolves, then 3 to 5 mg/kg once per day for approximately 8 more weeks.

F. Nursing considerations.

1. Deficient Knowledge/Anxiety/Altered Family Processes.
   a. Educate the parents regarding the pathophysiology of the disease and reason for IV intervention.
   b. Allow the parents to express their fears, concerns, and feelings.
   c. Educate the parents regarding all medications that are administered to the child.
   d. Include the child's siblings and other family members in the discussions. Always use language that is appropriate to the children's developmental levels.
2. Risk for Injury.
   a. Monitor temperature and dress the child in lightweight, cotton clothing.
   b. Monitor vital signs, EKG, skin color, and oxygen saturation levels for deviations from normal.
   c. Administer IVIG as prescribed and as per hospital protocol.
      i. Monitor the child closely for signs of transfusion reaction.
      ii. Have diphenhydramine (Benadryl), acetaminophen (Tylenol), and epinephrine available in case of a transfusion emergency.
3. Altered Skin Integrity.
   a. Monitor rash.
   b. Cleanse affected areas with water only—no soap or other irritants.
   c. Use salve on cracked lips, as needed.
   d. Report excessive pruritus, and request an order for antipruritic medication, if needed.
4. Imbalanced Nutrition: Less than Body Requirements.
   a. Provide favorite foods in attractive ways.
   b. Provide bland foods, and avoid citrus or other irritating foods/drinks.
5. Risk for Deficient Fluid Volume.
   a. Monitor temperature elevation.
   b. Carefully monitor the child's hydration status (see Chapter 13, "Nursing Care of the Child With Fluid and Electrolyte Alterations"), including:
      i. Calculating the percentage of weight loss.
      ii. Assessing for additional physiological signs of dehydration, including low urinary output, poor skin turgor, absence of tears, and altered vital signs.
   c. Maintain adequate fluid intake, including IV and oral fluids.
   d. Monitor laboratory data, especially electrolyte values.
6. Acute Pain.
   a. Assess pain level using an age-appropriate pain rating tool.
   b. Monitor for arthritic changes.
   c. Administer aspirin, as prescribed, using safe medication administration protocol.
   d. Maintain bedrest, as needed.
7. Fear/Anxiety.
   a. Allow for regression of developmental behavior during the hospital stay.

b. Provide transition object and activities appropriate to the age level of the child (e.g., favorite doll, blanket, videos).
c. Encourage the parents to provide support and comfort.
d. Provide nap and nighttime rituals to maintain consistency of care and to promote needed rest periods.

CASE STUDY: Putting It All Together

8-year-old Native American boy is brought to the emergency department by his father

Subjective Data

- The child says that he feels sick and:
  - "Yesterday, my elbow and now my knees hurt. And I'm really scared because my face keeps moving, and I don't want it to."
- The father says,
  - "He's been having a fever for the past 2 days now."
  - "He had a sore throat 3 weeks ago and was prescribed to take antibiotics here in the emergency department. He didn't finish the whole bottle, though, because he was fine after a couple of days."
  - "I became really scared when he started to complain of pain in his chest."
- Father also states that the child's mother is currently at work as a waitress and that his son:
  - takes a children's multivitamin every morning,
  - has no known drug allergies, and
  - had his last checkup 3 years ago when he received his pre-public school immunizations.

Objective Data

Nursing Assessments

- Febrile, temperature 101.9°F
- Pain in the elbow and knees when moving
- Red, demarcated skin lesion noted on trunk
- Facial twitching
- Murmur heard primarily at the apex of the heart

Vital Signs	
Temperature:	101.9°F
Heart rate:	110 bpm
Respiratory rate:	27 rpm
Blood pressure:	88/60 mm Hg
Weight:	80 lb
O_2 saturation:	98%

Lab Results	
Throat culture:	positive for group A streptococcus
ESR:	15 mm/hr (normal 3–13 mm/hr)
EKG:	prolonged P-R interval
WBC:	12,500 cells/mm^3

Health-Care Provider's Orders

- Transfer child to pediatrics
- Maintain child on complete bedrest
- Institute continuous cardiac monitoring
- Provide normal diet
- Administer penicillin V 500 mg PO tid for 10 days
- Administer aspirin 325 mg PO every 4 hr while in hospital
- Institute seizure precautions

Continued

CASE STUDY: Putting It All Together *cont'd*

Case Study Questions

A. What *subjective* assessments indicate that this client is experiencing a health alteration?

1. ______
2. ______
3. ______
4. ______
5. ______
6. ______

B. What *objective* assessments indicate that this client is experiencing a health alteration?

1. ______
2. ______
3. ______
4. ______
5. ______
6. ______
7. ______
8. ______
9. ______
10. ______

C. After analyzing the data that has been collected, what **primary** nursing diagnosis should the nurse assign to this client?

1. ______

D. What interventions should the nurse plan and/or implement to meet this child's and his family's needs?

1. ______
2. ______
3. ______
4. ______
5. ______
6. ______
7. ______
8. ______
9. ______
10. ______
11. ______
12. ______

CASE STUDY: Putting It All Together

cont'd

Case Study Question

E. What client outcomes should the nurse evaluate regarding the effectiveness of the nursing interventions?

1. ______________________________

2. ______________________________

3. ______________________________

F. What physiological characteristics should the child exhibit before being discharged home?

1. ______________________________

2. ______________________________

3. ______________________________

REVIEW QUESTIONS

1. A nurse is assessing a 1-day-old sleeping baby in the well-baby nursery. Which of the following assessments should the nurse report to the neonatologist?
   1. Temperature 97.9°F
   2. Blood pressure 77/46
   3. Respiratory rate 52
   4. Apical heart rate 179

2. A baby, exhibiting no obvious signs of congestive heart failure, has been diagnosed with a small ventricular septal defect. Which of the following information should the nurse explain to the baby's parents?
   1. The baby will likely need open-heart surgery within a week.
   2. The defect will likely close without therapy.
   3. The defect likely developed early in the second trimester.
   4. The baby will likely be placed on high-calorie formula.

3. A nurse is educating the parents of a child with an atrial septal defect regarding the child's condition. Which of the following information would be appropriate for the nurse to provide?
   1. The baby becomes cyanotic because the blood is flowing through a hole from the right side of the heart to the left side of the heart.
   2. The baby has a murmur because there is a hole between the aorta and the pulmonary artery.
   3. The baby's heart is working harder than a normal heart because some of its blood is reentering the pulmonary system.
   4. The baby's heart rate is slowed because of the high number of red blood cells in the blood.

4. A newborn baby is receiving digoxin (Lanoxin) and furosemide (Lasix) for congestive heart failure. Which of the following actions would be appropriate for the nurse to perform?
   1. Hold digoxin if the apical heart rate is 170 bpm.
   2. Hold digoxin for a digoxin level of 1 ng/mL.
   3. Hold both the digoxin and furosemide for a weight increase of 5% in one day.
   4. Hold both the digoxin and the furosemide for a potassium 3.2 mEq/L.

5. A baby that was born 5 minutes earlier is tachypneic, tachycardic, and markedly cyanotic. A STAT echocardiogram confirms the presence of a cyanotic congenital cardiac defect. Which of the following defects would be consistent with the assessment findings?
   1. Patent ductus arteriosus
   2. Transposition of the great vessels
   3. Atrial septal defect
   4. Ventricular septal defect

6. The neonatal cardiologist orders digoxin (Lanoxin) for a newborn in congestive heart failure. The baby weighs 7 lb 8 oz and is 21 inches long. The drug reference states: for full-term newborns, 8 to 10 mcg/kg/day in divided doses every 12 hr. Which of the following orders would be safe for the nurse to administer?
   1. 10 mcg PO every 12 hr
   2. 15 mcg PO every 12 hr
   3. 20 mcg PO every 12 hr
   4. 25 mcg PO every 12 hr

7. A 7-year-old child has been diagnosed with rheumatic fever. Which of the following physical findings would the nurse expect to assess?
   1. Vesicular rash over the face and chest
   2. Warm and swollen knees and elbows
   3. Palpable mass in the upper right quadrant of the abdomen
   4. Yellow pigmentation of the sclerae of the eyes

8. A 12-year-old child has been diagnosed with group A strep pharyngitis. The primary health-care provider has ordered penicillin V 500 mg PO tid for 10 days. Which of the following questions is important for the nurse to ask the parents and the child before giving them the prescription?
   1. "Is there any reason why you will not be able to take medicine 3 times a day for 10 days?"
   2. "Would you rather get 1 shot or take 40 pills?"
   3. "Have you ever had strep throat before?"
   4. "Do you know of any other children in your school who have recently had sore throats?"

9. A child who has been diagnosed with chorea has been admitted to the pediatric unit with a diagnosis of rheumatic fever. Immediately prior to admission, the child's throat culture was positive for group A strep. Which of the following actions should the nurse perform when admitting the child? **Select all that apply.**
   1. Cover the headboard with a soft material.
   2. Put the child on droplet precautions.
   3. Place a tracheostomy tray in the child's room.
   4. Have the child perform active range of motion exercises.
   5. Assess the child's apical heart rate for one full minute.

10. The EKG of a child diagnosed with rheumatic fever is shown:

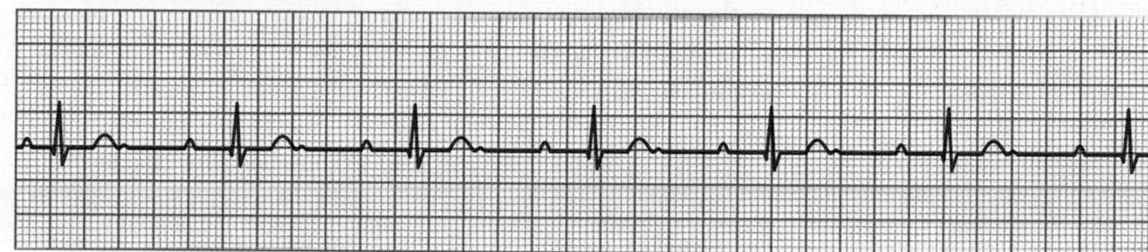

After examining the strip, which of the following conclusions would the nurse make? The strip shows evidence of:
1. Atrial fibrillation.
2. Premature ventricular contraction.
3. Prolonged P-R interval.
4. Flattened T wave.

11. A 10-year-old child is in the hospital on bedrest with a diagnosis of rheumatic fever complicated by carditis. When the nurse responds to the child's call bell, the child states, "I hate this! I want to get up and play!" Which of the following responses is appropriate for the nurse to make at this time?
1. "I know that you are unhappy, but you must stay in bed so that you can get better and go home."
2. "What if we make a deal and I promise to let you get up for 10 minutes every 2 hours if you are very good the rest of the day?"
3. "I am sure that I can get the doctor to let you go to the playroom for 1 to 2 hours this afternoon."
4. "I am so sorry that you are unhappy, but what if I contact the play lady and have her bring you a selection of video games to play with?"

12. An 8-year-old girl, who is complaining of a "really bad" sore throat and whose temperature is 102.2°F, is seen in the school nurse's office. The nurse has the child lie down in a room away from other children. Which of the following statements is most important for the nurse to convey when calling the child's parents?
1. "Your child should be seen by her primary care provider."
2. "Your child is very uncomfortable with a sore throat."
3. "Your child is crying and asking for mommy and daddy."
4. "Your child may be contagious to the other children."

13. A child has been diagnosed with Kawasaki disease. Which of the following signs and symptoms would the nurse expect to see? **Select all that apply.**
1. Diarrhea
2. Vertigo
3. Purpural rash over torso
4. Reddened and crusty eyes
5. Skin peeling from hands and feet

14. A 2½-year-old child is in the hospital with Kawasaki disease. Which of the following actions by the nurse is important for the child's psychosocial care?
1. Place the child in a single-bedded room.
2. Make sure the child always has his transitional object with him.
3. Supply the child with board games for play.
4. Let the child see what he looks like in a surgical mask and cap.

15. A toddler with Kawasaki disease is to receive IV immune globulin. Which of the following actions must the nurse perform? **Select all that apply.**
1. Discard the immune globulin if it appears cloudy.
2. Check the expiration date of the immune globulin.
3. Secure the arm to the arm board with a clear shield.
4. Document the lot number of the infusion in the child's medical record.
5. Allow the refrigerated immune globulin to warm in the microwave for 1 full minute.

16. A child with Kawasaki disease is to receive IV immune globulin on day 7 of the illness. A parent asks the nurse, "I am so scared. Will my child be cured after getting the medicine?" Which of the following responses by the nurse is appropriate?
1. "I cannot promise, but children have been shown to have the best results from the medicine when it is given before the 10th day of the illness."
2. "I am sure that your child will be fine. This medicine has been shown to work well for children with Kawasaki disease."
3. "I really do not know. We will find out more when your child has follow up testing in 1 or 2 days."
4. "I know that you are scared, but it is important for you to have faith in your doctors because they are doing all that they can do."

REVIEW ANSWERS

1. ANSWER: 3

Rationale:

1. The temperature of 97.9°F is normal in a neonate.
2. The blood pressure of 77/46 mm Hg is normal in a neonate.
3. **The respiratory rate of 52 is normal in a neonate.**
4. The normal heart rate in a newborn is 110 to 160 bpm. A rate of 179 is well above normal.

TEST-TAKING TIP: Tachycardia in a neonate may indicate the presence of cardiac disease.

Content Area: *Newborn*
Integrated Processes: *Nursing Process: Assessment*
Client Need: *Health Promotion and Maintenance: Ante/Intra/Postpartum and Newborn Care*
Cognitive Level: *Application*

2. ANSWER: 2

Rationale:

1. The majority of small VSDs close spontaneously. Surgery is performed only when babies' defects fail to close and/or if signs and symptoms of CHF develop.
2. **The majority of small VSDs close spontaneously.**
3. The heart is formed early in fetal development—by the 8th week of gestation.
4. Babies usually are maintained on a normal diet—either breast milk, if the mother is breastfeeding, or over-the-counter formula.

TEST-TAKING TIP: The vast majority of babies with VSDs are discharged from the well-baby nursery and are seen periodically by a cardiologist on an outpatient basis. This can be frightening to the parents who are told that their baby has a hole in his or her heart. It is important, therefore, for the nurse to reassure the parents that most VSDs do close spontaneously. However, the nurse must educate the parents regarding signs of CHF in case the baby does begin to go into cardiac failure.

Content Area: *Pediatrics—Cardiac*
Integrated Processes: *Nursing Process: Implementation*
Client Need: *Physiological Integrity: Physiological Adaptation: Alterations in Body Systems*
Cognitive Level: *Application*

3. ANSWER: 3

Rationale:

1. An ASD is an acyanotic defect. If the child should develop cyanosis, which is rare unless the defect is very large, the symptom is not due to a right-to-left shunt. In the case of an ASD, the blood flows through the defect from left to right.
2. The murmur heard when a baby has an ASD is due to blood moving through the septal defect. A hole between the pulmonary artery and the aorta is a patent ductus arteriosus (PDA).
3. **This response is correct. In the case of an ASD and other acyanotic defects, the blood is reentering the pulmonary system as a result of left to right shunting.**
4. Babies with ASDs usually have normal heart rates. If they do go into CHF, however, they would exhibit tachycardia rather than bradycardia. Elevated RBC counts are seen in babies with cyanotic defects as a result of chronic hypoxia.

TEST-TAKING TIP: Left-to-right shunt refers to the path the blood takes through the heart. When there is a hole in the heart—ASD, VSD, or PDA—the blood travels from the left side to the right side simply because the left ventricle is stronger than the right ventricle. Because the blood travels repeatedly into the right ventricle, it enters the pulmonary system repeatedly via the pulmonary artery. In some cyanotic diseases, most notably Tetralogy of Fallot, the blood travels from the right side of the heart to the left side. This occurs in Tetralogy of Fallot because the stenotic pulmonic valve prevents the blood from entering the pulmonary artery. Rather the blood is "shunted" through the overriding aorta, thereby bypassing the lungs.

Content Area: *Pediatrics—Cardiac*
Integrated Processes: *Nursing Process: Implementation; Teaching/Learning*
Client Need: *Physiological Integrity: Physiological Adaptation: Pathophysiology*
Cognitive Level: *Application*

4. ANSWER: 4

Rationale:

1. Tachycardia is one sign of CHF and is an indication for the administration of digoxin.
2. A dig level of 1 ng/mL is within the therapeutic range of the medication (0.8 to 2 ng/mL).
3. Fluid retention is a sign of CHF and is an indication for the administration of both digoxin and furosemide.
4. **A serum potassium level of 3.2 mEq/L is well below the normal for a newborn of 3.7 to 5.9 mEq/L. The nurse should hold both medications and notify the health-care provider who ordered them.**

TEST-TAKING TIP: Hypokalemia, or a serum potassium level that is lower than normal, places the body at high risk for cardiac arrhythmias. In addition, when digoxin is taken, the potential for the cardiac arrhythmias increases. Furosemide increases the excretion of potassium. It is essential, therefore, that the nurse not administer the medications until the hypokalemia has been reported and action has been taken to return the electrolyte level to normal.

Content Area: *Pediatrics—Cardiac*
Integrated Processes: *Nursing Process: Implementation*
Client Need: *Physiological Integrity: Pharmacological and Parenteral Therapies: Medication Administration*
Cognitive Level: *Application*

5. ANSWER: 2

Rationale:

1. PDA is an acyanotic defect that results in a left-to-right shunt.
2. **Transposition of the great vessels (TGV) is a cyanotic defect. Unless another defect is also present, the defect is incompatible with life.**
3. ASD is an acyanotic defect that results in a left-to-right shunt.

4. VSD is an acyanotic defect that results in a left-to-right shunt.

TEST-TAKING TIP: The only cyanotic defect listed is TGV. If the test-taker were not to know that fact, however, he or she could deduce the correct response. Septal defects and PDAs result in left-to-right shunts, resulting in the blood reentering the pulmonary system in which it is oxygenated.

Content Area: Pediatrics—Cardiac
Integrated Processes: Nursing Process: Assessment
Client Need: Physiological Integrity: Physiological Adaptation: Pathophysiology
Cognitive Level: Application

6. ANSWER: 2

Rationale:

1. Ten mcg PO every 12 hr is below the recommended dosage range for digoxin.
2. **Fifteen mcg PO every 12 hr is between the minimum and the maximum recommended dosages for digoxin and is the correct response.**
3. Twenty mcg PO every 12 hr is above the recommended dosage range for digoxin.
4. Twenty-five mcg PO every 12 hr is above the recommended dosage range for digoxin.

TEST-TAKING TIP:

Ratio and proportion method:

The baby in the scenario weighs 7 lb 8 oz, or 7½ lb (there are 16 oz per pound).

$$1 \text{ kg}: 2.2 \text{ lb} = x \text{ kg}: 7.5 \text{ lb}$$

$$x = 3.409, \text{ or } 3.41 \text{ kg}$$

Minimum safe dosage:

$$8 \text{ mcg}: 1 \text{ kg} = x \text{ mcg}: 3.41 \text{ kg}$$

$$x = 27.28 \text{ mcg, per day dosage}$$

$$27.28 \div 2 = 13.64 \text{ mcg, every 12 hr dosage (two doses per day)}$$

Maximum safe dosage:

$$10 \text{ mcg}: 1 \text{ kg} = x \text{ mcg}: 3.41 \text{ kg}$$

$$x = 34.1 \text{ mcg, per day dosage}$$

$$34.1 \div 2 = 17.05 \text{ mcg, every 12 hr dosage (two doses per day)}$$

Dimensional analysis method:

Minimum safe dosage:

$$\frac{8 \text{ mcg}}{1 \text{ kg/day}} \times \frac{1 \text{ kg}}{2.2 \text{ lb}} \times \frac{7.5 \text{ lb}}{} \times \frac{1 \text{ day}}{2 \text{ doses (every 12 hr)}} = \frac{13.64 \text{ mcg}}{\text{every 12 hr}}$$

Maximum safe dosage:

$$\frac{10 \text{ mcg}}{1 \text{ kg/day}} \times \frac{1 \text{ kg}}{2.2 \text{ lb}} \times \frac{7.5 \text{ lb}}{} \times \frac{1 \text{ day}}{2 \text{ doses (every 12 hr)}} = \frac{17.05 \text{ mcg}}{\text{every 12 hr}}$$

The only dosage that falls between the minimum and the maximum safe dosages is 15 mcg every 12 hr.

Content Area: Pediatrics—Cardiac
Integrated Processes: Nursing Process: Implementation
Client Need: Physiological Integrity: Pharmacological and Parental Therapies: Dosage Calculation
Cognitive Level: Synthesis

7. ANSWER: 2

Rationale:

1. Erythema marginatum is one of the major manifestations of RF; however, it is not a vesicular rash. It is a well-demarcated macular rash that is seen on the torso and inner surfaces of the extremities.
2. **Polyarthritis, one of the major manifestations of RF, is manifested by warm, swollen, and painful joints.**
3. Abdominal masses are not associated with RF.
4. Yellow pigmentation of the sclerae is not associated with RF.

TEST-TAKING TIP: When a child presents with a specific diagnosis, the nurse, unless it is contraindicated, should assess for the common signs and symptoms of the disease. In the case of RF, for example, the nurse should assess for the manifestations as listed in the Jones criteria.

Content Area: Pediatrics—Cardiac
Integrated Processes: Nursing Process: Assessment
Client Need: Physiological Integrity: Physiological Adaptation: Alterations in Body Systems
Cognitive Level: Application

8. ANSWER: 1

Rationale:

1. **It is important to be sure that the child will receive the entire 10 days of medication. If the parents or child state that they will be unable to complete the prescribed medication, the nurse should notify the ordering practitioner and suggest that an injection of penicillin G benzathine be administered instead.**
2. This question is a poor way for the nurse to determine whether it would be best to administer the penicillin orally or parenterally.
3. The nurse should ask the parents and child whether this is the first bout of strep A or whether the child has had the infection previously. That information, however, is unrelated to providing them with the prescription.
4. Noting whether other children have had sore throats is unrelated to providing the child and parents with the medication prescription.

TEST-TAKING TIP: If either the parents or the child indicates an unwillingness or inability to complete the full course of oral antibiotics, the nurse should suggest to the ordering practitioner that it would be best to administer an injection. Because only one injection of penicillin G is needed, the nurse and ordering health-care practitioner can then be assured that the child's infection will be treated adequately.

Content Area: Pediatrics—Cardiac
Integrated Processes: Nursing Process: Implementation
Client Need: Physiological Integrity: Pharmacological and Parenteral Therapies: Medication Administration
Cognitive Level: Application

9. ANSWER: 1, 2, and 5

Rationale:

1. A child with chorea from RF should be placed on seizure precautions. The headboard should be covered.

2. The child's throat culture is positive for group A strep. The child should be placed on droplet isolation until he or she has received a full 24 hr of medication.

3. There is no need to place a trach tray in the child's room. Tracheal occlusion is a rare complication of strep pharyngitis.

4. It is inappropriate to have the child perform active ROM exercises. The child may have carditis and/or polyarthritis. ROM exercises could aggravate either of the manifestations of the disease.

5. The nurse should assess the child's apical pulse for 1 full minute to assess whether or not a murmur is present. A murmur would indicate that the child likely has carditis.

TEST-TAKING TIP: This is a multiple response item. Each of the items should be reviewed independently to determine which of them is related to the stem of the question. Because the child in the scenario has been diagnosed with RF and has been found to have a positive culture for group A strep, responses 1, 2, and 5 are correct.

Content Area: *Pediatrics—Cardiac*
Integrated Processes: *Nursing Process: Implementation*
Client Need: *Physiological Integrity: Physiological Adaptation: Illness Management*
Cognitive Level: *Application*

10. ANSWER: 3

Rationale:

1. The strip shows a prolonged P-R interval.
2. The strip shows a prolonged P-R interval.
3. The strip shows a prolonged P-R interval.
4. The strip shows a prolonged P-R interval.

TEST-TAKING TIP: Although pediatric nurses are not expected to be expert EKG readers, they should be able to identify some characteristic changes. A prolonged P-R interval (i.e., a P-R interval that lasts longer than 0.2 sec) is one of those changes.

Content Area: *Pediatrics—Cardiac*
Integrated Processes: *Nursing Process: Analysis*
Client Need: *Physiological Integrity: Physiological Adaptation: Pathophysiology*
Cognitive Level: *Application*

11. ANSWER: 4

Rationale:

1. Although accurate, the statement is not supportive of the young child's frustration with having to remain on bedrest. There is a much better response.

2. This response is not appropriate. The activity may be damaging to the child's heart.

3. This response is not appropriate. The doctor may not allow the child to go to the playroom, even if transported in the hospital bed. The child, then, may not trust the nurse after the promise has been broken.

4. This is an appropriate statement. The nurse is empathetic and is offering a realistic solution to the child's unhappiness.

TEST-TAKING TIP: It is important for nurses to be honest with children. When a promise is made to a child and not kept, the child often will not trust any future statements the caregiver makes.

Content Area: *Pediatrics—Cardiac*
Integrated Processes: *Nursing Process: Implementation*
Client Need: *Psychosocial Integrity: Therapeutic Environment*
Cognitive Level: *Application*

12. ANSWER: 1

Rationale:

1. This is the most important statement. The child may have a group A strep infection that will need to be treated.

2. This is an important statement but not the most important.

3. This is an important statement but not the most important.

4. This is an important statement but not the most important.

TEST-TAKING TIP: Anytime a test question includes the word "most," all of the actions in the responses are correct. The examiner, however, is asking the test-taker to pick the one best response to the question. Because any infection caused by group A strep that is untreated may result in the child developing rheumatic fever, the nurse must advise the parents to have their child assessed by the child's primary health-care provider.

Content Area: *Pediatrics—Cardiac*
Integrated Processes: *Nursing Process: Implementation*
Client Need: *Physiological Integrity: Reduction of Risk Potential: Potential for Alterations in Body Systems*
Cognitive Level: *Application*

13. ANSWER: 4 and 5

Rationale:

1. Diarrhea is not a classic symptom of Kawasaki disease.
2. Vertigo is not a classic symptom of Kawasaki disease.
3. Purpural rash is not a classic sign of Kawasaki disease.
4. Children with Kawasaki disease do have conjunctivitis.
5. The palms and soles of children with Kawasaki do desquamate.

TEST-TAKING TIP: Kawasaki disease is diagnosed from a series of signs and symptoms, including prolonged fever, conjunctivitis, strawberry tongue, rash on the palms and soles that desquamates, and cardiac changes.

Content Area: *Pediatrics—Cardiac*
Integrated Processes: *Nursing Process: Assessment*
Client Need: *Physiological Integrity: Physiological Adaptation: Alteration of Body Systems*
Cognitive Level: *Application*

14. ANSWER: 2

Rationale:

1. A single-bedded room is not indicated in this situation and will not help to promote the psychosocial well-being of the toddler.

2. Transition objects (e.g., blankets, dolls, pacifiers) help toddlers to deal with stressful situations. Unless medically contraindicated, nurses should make sure that young children are in possession of their transition objects at all times while in the hospital.

3. Toddlers usually engage in parallel play. They rarely play with board games.

4. There is no reason to have the child wear a surgical mask. Kawasaki disease is not contagious and children with Kawasaki rarely need surgery.

TEST-TAKING TIP: When caring for children, nurses must consider not only their physiological illness, but also the child's growth and development needs. Toddlers engage in parallel play and often are strongly attached to transition objects.

Content Area: *Pediatrics—Cardiac*

Integrated Processes: *Nursing Process: Implementation*

Client Need: *Psychosocial Integrity: Therapeutic Environment*

Cognitive Level: *Application*

15. ANSWER: 1, 2, 3, and 4

Rationale:

1. Immune globulin should be clear with no cloudiness or sediment. If either is present, the solution should be discarded.

2. It is essential for nurses to check the expiration date of any medication administered to patients.

3. Toddlers may unintentionally injure an IV site. To maintain its patency, therefore, the arm should be taped to an arm board, and a clear shield should be placed above the site for easy inspection.

4. The lot number of the immune globulin should be documented in case serious side effects occur. All other bags of that lot number can then be examined and/or destroyed.

5. If the immune globulin has been refrigerated, it should be warmed. The only safe way to warm the solution, however, is to leave it at room temperature for 30 min. The solution should never be placed in the microwave.

TEST-TAKING TIP: Administering immune globulin requires similar safety practices as those performed when administering blood products. Although no matching of blood type is involved as it is when blood is infused, there is a potential for allergic responses and other signs/symptoms seen in transfusion reactions (e.g., flank pain and elevated temperature).

Content Area: *Pediatrics—Cardiac*

Integrated Processes: *Nursing Process: Implementation*

Client Need: *Physiological Integrity: Pharmacological and Parenteral Therapies: Medication Administration*

Cognitive Level: *Application*

16. ANSWER: 1

Rationale:

1. This is an appropriate response for the nurse to give. The nurse is providing correct information without making false promises.

2. Even when immune globulin is administered, some children still develop aneurysms. The nurse should not give the mother promises that may not be correct.

3. This statement dismisses the mother's question. If the nurse is uncertain regarding what the answer should be, he or she should have someone with knowledge speak with the mother.

4. This statement does not answer the mother's question. Having trust in the health care providers is not the issue. The child's health is the issue.

TEST-TAKING TIP: Nurses must communicate to parents honestly but with compassion. It is inappropriate to give parents false promises, but to provide them with realistic hope for a successful outcome is appropriate.

Content Area: *Pediatrics—Cardiac*

Integrated Processes: *Nursing Process: Implementation*

Client Need: *Psychosocial Integrity: Therapeutic Communication*

Cognitive Level: *Application*

Nursing Care of the Child With Hematologic Illnesses

KEY TERMS

Acute lymphoblastic leukemia (ALL)—Also called acute lymphocytic leukemia, ALL is the most common form of childhood cancer and is characterized by a proliferation of lymphoblasts, or immature white blood cells.

Acute sequestration crisis (ASC)—A complication of sickle cell anemia characterized by markedly reduced blood volume and shock that may lead to cardiovascular collapse due to pooling of large quantities of blood in the spleen.

Aplastic crisis—A marked reduction in circulating red blood cells, resulting in profound anemia, which is seen in some patients with sickle cell anemia when fighting an infection.

Extravasation—Damage to the tissue surrounding a vessel when a vesicant infiltrates during an IV infusion.

Hemarthrosis—Bleeding into the joint.

Hemophilia—A group of hereditary illnesses characterized by slowed to markedly altered blood clotting resulting from a deficiency of one of the factors necessary for blood coagulation.

Iron-deficiency anemia—A blood disorder caused by insufficient iron intake in which the body produces inadequate quantities of hemoglobin.

Ischemia—Poor tissue perfusion.

Sickle cell disease (SCD)—An autosomal recessive hereditary disease in which red blood cells become malformed, causing them to clump, leading to thromboses, decreased tissue perfusion, and organ damage.

Vaso-occlusive crisis—The sickling of hemoglobin S (HgbS) when a child with sickle cell anemia (SCA) becomes dehydrated, hypoxic, and/or acidotic.

Vesicant—An IV medication that, when exposed to healthy tissue, causes it to blister.

I. Description

Hematology is the study of the blood and blood products. Relatively few hematologic illnesses are predominately seen in children. Iron-deficiency anemia, although seen throughout the life span, often is seen in infants and toddlers who consume large quantities of milk instead of foods that contain iron. Teenagers, too, are at high risk for anemia. They often have poor eating habits at the same time that young women start to menstruate, and all teens are experiencing rapid growth. SCA and hemophilia are genetic illnesses that are diagnosed in childhood. Thankfully, although not true in the past, because of improved therapies, many children affected with these illnesses are living well into adulthood. Acute lymphoblastic leukemia is the most common cancer in children. (Because cancer is so rare in children, this cancer and other solid tumor cancers are discussed in the chapters relating to the origin of the cancer rather than in a separate chapter.)

Although it is important to note that laboratories may report slight variations of hematologic values, nurses must have a working knowledge of the normal values for each of the most important items reported in a complete blood count (CBC) (see Table 18.1, and note age differences).

II. Iron-Deficiency Anemia

Iron deficiency anemia is a preventable illness resulting from a diet containing an insufficient supply of iron.

A. Incidence.
   1. The highest incidence of iron-deficiency anemia (anemia) is seen in preterm infants, infants of multiple pregnancies, toddlers, and teenagers.

B. Etiology.
   1. In infants.
      a. Breast milk (the ideal food for the developing infant) and iron-fortified formula contain iron supplies needed by the developing infant. Once full-term infants reach 4 to 6 months of age, however, they need additional foods for their nourishment.
         i. Iron-fortified cereals are usually the first foods recommended by children's health-care providers because they provide babies with needed supplementation. If infants do not consume these foods, they are at high risk of becoming anemic.

DID YOU KNOW?

Preterm babies are at very high risk for iron-deficiency anemia because iron is not stored by the fetus until well into the third trimester. Preterm babies, therefore, are born with insufficient iron supplies.

      b. Babies who are born preterm as well as twins and triplets can develop anemia at earlier ages.
   2. In toddlers.
      a. Once formula-fed babies reach one year of age, they are shifted from formula, which often is fortified with iron, to milk that contains no iron, placing them at high risk of anemia.
      b. Some toddlers, whether breast- or formula fed, drink excessive quantities of milk, eat poorly, and are therefore at high risk for anemia.
      c. Other toddlers, known as finicky eaters, eat "white" foods (e.g., cheese, yogurt, mashed potatoes), most of which is iron-poor. These children are at high risk for anemia.
   3. In adolescents.
      a. Teens, especially those who prescribe to vegetarian diets and girls who are beginning to menstruate, are at high risk for anemia.

C. Pathophysiology.
   1. Hemoglobin is the oxygen-carrying portion of the red blood cell (RBC). Iron intake is essential for the production of hemoglobin. Iron-deficiency anemia results when an insufficient quantity of iron is consumed, resulting in hemoglobin that is iron poor (i.e., hemoglobin values that are below the normal values [see Table 18.1]).

D. Diagnosis.
   1. RBC count, reticulocyte count, hemoglobin, and hematocrit are assessed and compared with the normal values. Below normal values are consistent with iron-deficiency anemia.
   2. Blood for analysis may be obtained by a number of methods (i.e., via heelstick, fingerstick, or venipuncture).

DID YOU KNOW?

Children are at more high risk for iron-deficiency anemia than are adults because adults' bodies reuse iron that is available from the normal destruction of RBCs. Children, especially during periods of rapid growth, such as during adolescence, because they are producing RBCs for maintenance as well as to accommodate growth, need supplies of iron over and above what they obtain from normal RBC destruction.

E. Treatment.
   1. Because iron-deficiency anemia is preventable, the American Academy of Pediatrics (AAP) recommends the following:
      a. Birth to 6 months: exclusively breastfeed babies. If not breastfed, feed the child iron-fortified formula.
      b. Six months to 1 year: continue to breastfeed or formula feed—refrain from feeding infants cow's milk—while adding iron-fortified foods, such as cereals and meats, to the diet.
      c. Toddlerhood: after 1 year of age, cow's milk may be fed to children, but the quantity should be limited. Children should obtain the majority of their nutrition from solid foods, including iron-rich foods, such as meat, eggs, and dark green leafy vegetables.
      d. Remainder of life: consume a varied diet that includes needed nutrients.
   2. For those with documented deficiency.
      a. Diet counseling: educating the parents of young children and teenagers as well as the teens themselves regarding:

Table 18.1 Normal Lab Values in Childhood for CBC Blood Cell Types

Cell Type	Important Statistics Related to the Cell Type	Definition of Each Statistic	Normal Values of Important Statistics With Important Age Differences
Erythrocytes (Red Blood Cells [RBCs])	*RBC count.*	*Number of RBCs in 1 cubic millimeter (mm^3) of venous blood.*	*3.0 to 4.5 million/mm^3: 1 to 6 months* *3.7 to 5.3 million/ mm^3: 6 months to 6 years* *4.0 to 5.2 million/ mm^3: 6 to 12 years* *4.5 to 5.3 million/ mm^3: male adolescents* *4.1 to 5.1 million/ mm^3: female adolescents*
	Hematocrit (Hct).	*Percent of RBCs in total blood volume.*	*28% to 42%: by 2 months* *35% to 45%: until 12 years* *37% to 49%: male adolescents* *36% to 46%: female adolescents*
	Hemoglobin (Hgb).	*Total amount of hemoglobin, the oxygen-carrying protein, in the RBCs.*	*9.0 to 14.0 g/ dL: by 2 months* *11.5 to 15.5 g/ dL: until 12 years* *13.0 to 16.0 g/ dL: male adolescents* *12.0 to 16.0 g/ dL: female adolescents*
Reticulocytes (Immature RBCs)	*Reticulocyte count.*	*Percent of RBCs that are reticulocytes.*	*0.5% to 1.5%: after 12 weeks of age*
Leukocytes (White Blood Cells [WBCs])	*Total WBC count.*	*Cells whose chief action is to protect the body from microorganisms (divided into two categories—granulocytes and agranulocytes).*	*By 1 mo: 5,000 to 19,500 cells/mm^3* *1 to 3 yr: 6,000 to 17,500 cells/mm^3* *4 to 7 yr: 5,500 to 15,500 cells/mm^3* *8 to 13 yr: 4,500 to 13,500 cells/mm^3* *Adolescents: 4,500 to 11,000 cells/mm^3*
	Differential report:	*Includes the percentage of each type of WBC in the blood.*	
	Granulocytes.	*WBCs that contain granules in the cytoplasm. They are produced in the bone marrow.*	
	Neutrophils: primary function is to kill and digest bacteria.		*Neutrophils: 57% to 67% of total WBC count*
	Eosinophils: primarily assist the body during allergic episodes.		*Eosinophils: 1% to 3% of total WBC count*
	Basophils: contain histamine and heparin; improve circulation to injured tissues while also preventing coagulation.		*Basophils: up to 0.75% of total WBC count*
	Agranulocytes.	*WBCs that contain no granules in the cytoplasm.*	
	Monocytes: phagocytic cells that act like neutrophils.		*Monocytes: 3% to 7% of total WBC count*
	Lymphocytes: *T Lymphocytes (also called T-cells): involved with cellular immunity.* *B Lymphocytes: involved with humoral or antibody immunity.*	*(See the discussion on HIV in Chapter 11, "Nursing Care of Children With Immunologic Alterations.")*	*Lymphocytes: 25% to 33% of total WBC count*
Thrombocytes (Platelets)	*Platelet count.*	*Cells that are essential in the blood clotting process. They collect together en masse to prevent blood from leaking from small breaks in blood vessels.*	*150,000 to 400,000 cells/mm^3: throughout life*

i. Foods high in iron.
ii. The need to restrict the intake of large quantities of cow's milk and other substances that are iron-poor.

b. Iron supplementation: 3 to 6 mg/kg/day in three divided doses.

c. RBC transfusion: only in severe cases when cardiovascular compromise is present or is likely to develop.

F. Nursing considerations.

1. Ineffective Peripheral Tissue Perfusion.
   a. Monitor for signs of ineffective perfusion (e.g., fatigue, decreased activity, tachycardia, pallor).
   b. Assess and monitor blood counts.
      i. Once therapy is begun, reticulocyte count should increase quickly, indicating a rise in RBC production.
   c. Provide needed rest periods.
2. Deficient Knowledge/Imbalanced Nutrition: Less than Body Requirements.
   a. Educate the parents and/or child, if appropriate, regarding the function and composition of RBCs.
   b. Obtain a diet history from the parents and/or child, if appropriate.
   c. Provide the parents and/or child, if appropriate, with education regarding foods that are high in iron.
   d. If prescribed, educate the parents regarding the safe dosage and administration of iron supplements.
      i. Only administer dosage as ordered.
      ii. If liquid supplements, give through a straw to prevent discoloration of the child's teeth.
      iii. If pills, have the child swallow the pill whole; iron supplements should not be crushed, broken, or chewed.
      iv. Eggs, milk, and calcium supplements, substances that interfere with iron absorption, should not be consumed at the same time as the supplement.
      v. Administer iron supplements with a vitamin C (ascorbic acid) source (e.g., orange juice) because vitamin C fosters iron absorption.
      vi. Administer supplements at least 1 hr before bedtime to reduce gastric irritation.
      vii. Forewarn the parents that the child's stools will turn black and tarry.
      viii. Keep supplements locked and out of the reach of young children because excessive intake can result in heavy metal poisoning.
   f. If indicated, refer the family to a registered dietician and/or to a federal and/or state nutrition program, e.g., U.S. Department of Agriculture Special Supplemental Nutrition Program for Women, Infants, and Children.

III. Sickle Cell Disease

Sickle cell disease (SCD) is a hereditary illness that can lead to multisystem compromise and death.

A. Incidence: the vast majority of children with SCD are of African descent, although those of Mediterranean descent are also at high risk for the disease.

1. About 1 of every 500 African Americans has SCA.
2. Approximately 8% of African Americans have sickle cell trait.

B. Etiology.

1. SCD is an autosomal recessive genetic disease (i.e., the child must carry two recessive genes—one from each parent—in his or her genome to exhibit the disease, SCA).
2. The carrier or trait state is characterized by the presence of one recessive gene in the genome.
   a. Punnett square: examples of the probability of inheritance.
      i. If one parent is a carrier (Aa) for the illness and one parent is disease free (AA). (Key: A—normal gene; a—sickle gene)

	A	A
A	AA	Aa
A	AA	Aa

(1) 50% probability of an offspring being disease free (AA).
(2) 50% probability of an offspring being a carrier for the disease (Aa).

ii. If both parents are carriers (Aa). (Key: A—normal gene; a—sickle gene)

	A	A
A	AA	Aa
a	Aa	aa

(1) 25% probability of an offspring being disease free (AA).
(2) 50% probability of an offspring being a carrier (Aa).
(3) 25% probability of an offspring having SCA (aa).

DID YOU KNOW?

It is believed that SCD developed as a result of evolutionary changes. Although those who have SCA are afflicted with a serious, debilitating disease, those who carry one sickle cell gene are afforded some protection against malaria, a devastating illness that is endemic in the same geographic locations as those who are at high risk for SCD.

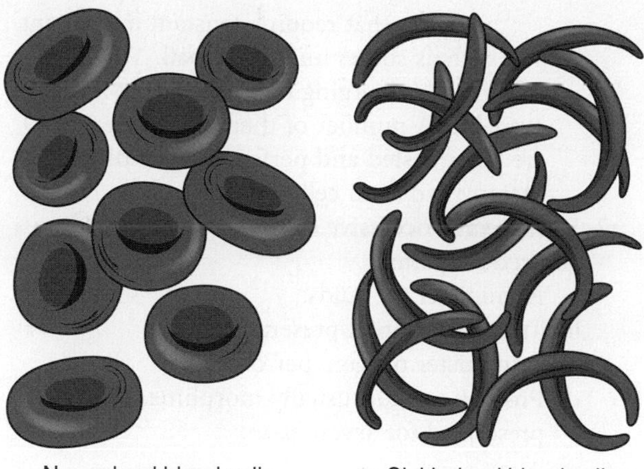

Fig 18.1 Normal red blood cells versus sickle cells.

C. Pathophysiology.
1. One amino acid in the normal beta chain of the hemoglobin molecule is altered, resulting in the body producing hemoglobin S (HgbS). (Valine sits in the sixth position of the chain instead of glutamic acid.)
2. When a child is well hydrated, well oxygenated, and has a normal pH, RBCs take on their normal, smooth shape and appearance (Fig. 18.1).
3. **Vaso-occlusive crisis:** a change in the molecular structure of HgbS in a child with SCA who is dehydrated, hypoxic, and/or acidotic. The change in structure causes the child's RBCs to sickle and results in a cascade of physiological changes (Fig. 18.1).
   a. The clumping of sickled RBCs results in thromboses that obstruct blood vessels and leads to ischemia distal to the clumping.
      i. Concurrently, because of clumping in the vessels, RBCs are destroyed, resulting in the characteristic anemia.
      ii. Severe pain develops as a result of altered peripheral perfusion and tissue hypoxia.
   b. The **ischemia** (i.e., poor tissue perfusion) resulting from the clumping of RBCs is noted throughout the body.
      i. Spleen: in the early stages of the disease, the spleen maintains its function, but after multiple vaso-occlusive crises, splenic infarcts and scarring develop, resulting in a nonfunctioning organ.
         (1) In addition, the spleen may need to be removed if the congestion of blood in the organ becomes life threatening (see "Acute sequestration crisis").
         (2) Because the spleen is important in fighting infection, patients with nonfunctioning spleens are susceptible to infection.
      ii. Liver: ischemia of the liver can lead to altered liver function and, eventually, liver necrosis.
      iii. Kidneys: signs of kidney ischemia are hematuria, enuresis, and the inability to concentrate urine.
      iv. Skeletal system: poor perfusion to the bones results in osteoporosis, kyphosis, lordosis, and osteomyelitis.
      v. Central nervous system: cognitive deficits and stroke, which may be fatal, are seen.
      vi. Cardiac: the cardiac muscle must work harder than normal to maximize tissue perfusion with an anemic blood supply. As a result, cardiomegaly and, eventually, heart failure are noted.
      vii. Genitals: males often complain of priapism from the congestion of sickle cells in the vessels of the penis.
      viii. Other complications of vaso-occlusive crises and SCD are altered skin integrity from poor circulation and growth retardation from chronic hypoxia.
4. **Acute sequestration crisis (ASC):** usually seen in children under 4 years of age, an ASC is characterized by pooling of large quantities of blood in the spleen, resulting in markedly reduced blood volume and shock. ASCs can result in total cardiovascular collapse.
5. **Aplastic crisis:** when fighting an infectious event, SCD children can develop a marked reduction in circulating RBCs, resulting in profound anemia.

D. Diagnosis.
1. Most children are diagnosed at birth: all 50 of the United States assess for SCD in the newborn screen.
2. If the newborn screen is positive, hemoglobin electrophoresis is performed to confirm the diagnosis and determine whether the child is a carrier or has SCA.
3. SCD can be diagnosed prenatally via chorionic villus sampling or amniocentesis.

E. Treatment.
1. Prevention of crises is the primary goal.
   a. Prevent infection.
      i. Avoid others with viral or bacterial illnesses.
      ii. Administer prophylactic penicillin (either monthly IM or daily PO).

(1) Because of splenic dysfunction, resulting in high risk for infection, penicillin is frequently prescribed to prevent bacterial infections and subsequent crises.

iii. Administer vaccinations per recommended schedule, especially *Haemophilus influenzae* type b (Hib), hepatitis B, pneumococcal, and yearly flu vaccinations.

b. Promote normal RBC production.

i. Administer folic acid supplementation (dosage is dependent on age): folic acid is essential for RBC production.

ii. Infuse transfusions, if needed to maintain adequate RBC levels.

(1) Because iron is a heavy metal, SCD patients who receive multiple blood transfusions must be monitored for excessive iron deposition. If excess heavy metal is noted, the child may need chelation (see Chapter 10, "Pediatric Emergencies").

iii. Administer safe dosages of Droxia (hydroxyurea), as prescribed:

(1) Hydroxyurea promotes the production of fetal hemoglobin in the bone marrow.

(a) Fetal hemoglobin binds with oxygen much more readily than adult hemoglobin and fetal hemoglobin does not sickle.

(2) The medication is administered with caution in children because of its potential carcinogenicity and because the medication inhibits DNA synthesis and, therefore, can interfere with normal growth.

c. Maintain adequate hydration.

i. Provide sufficient fluids, which must be calculated precisely (see Chapter 13, "Nursing Care of the Child With Fluid and Electrolyte Alterations").

ii. To prevent dehydration, fluid intake must be increased above daily maintenance levels during periods of increased need (e.g., during hot weather, febrile illnesses, and marked activity).

d. Maintain adequate oxygenation to prevent both hypoxia and respiratory acidosis.

i. Provide needed rest periods, especially during periods of marked activity.

ii. Encourage the child to engage in activities that include periods of rest, such as baseball and sprint swimming, rather than activities that require constant movement, such as soccer and basketball.

e. Administer emerging therapies, when available: A number of therapies to treat SCD are being tested and perfected, including gene therapy and stem cell transplantation.

2. During vaso-occlusive crises, to reverse sickling and reduce pain:

a. Administer IV fluids.

b. Treat infection, if present.

c. Administer oxygen, per order.

d. Provide opioids, usually morphine, as prescribed for severe pain.

DID YOU KNOW?

Although the pain felt by some patients in sickle cell crisis is minimal, many patients state that their pain is excessive, measured at 9/10 or 10/10 on a numeric pain rating scale. Narcotics, preferably morphine, should be prescribed and administered, as needed. As the patient's pain level lessons, the medication should be titrated downward slowly to prevent the return of the severe pain.

i. Opioids may be prescribed to be administered via a number of routes, e.g., as an IV bolus, as patient-controlled analgesia (PCA), IM, intrathecally, or transdermally.

e. Transfuse to reverse anemia, if needed and prescribed.

(!) Although oxygen is administered during vaso-occlusive crises, it rarely alters the child's pain. The oxygen does help to reduce the sickling of the RBCs that enter the pulmonary system, but it cannot relieve the sickling of the cells already in the periphery. The priority nursing actions are to provide hydration and to administer pain medications. Increasing the blood volume helps to relieve the clumping and promote blood flow, and narcotics provide the child with needed comfort.

F. Nursing considerations.

1. Deficient Knowledge/Risk for Infection/Risk for Injury.

a. Educate the parents and/or child, if appropriate, regarding fluid needs, including exactly how many glasses of fluid must be consumed each day, and the need to increase fluids during high-risk periods.

b. Educate the parents and/or child, if appropriate, regarding infection control measures (e.g., meticulous handwashing; penicillin, as ordered; timely vaccinations; avoidance of others with contagious illnesses).

c. Educate the parents and/or child, if appropriate, regarding activities that increase the potential for hypoxia, acidosis, and/or dehydration (e.g., prolonged periods in the sun, hyperthermia, intensive aerobic activities).

d. Educate the parents and/or child, if appropriate, regarding the need to wear a MedicAlert bracelet.
e. Refer the family to genetic counseling.

2. Ineffective Peripheral Tissue Perfusion/Risk for Decreased Cardiac Tissue Perfusion during crises.
   a. Monitor vital signs and oxygen saturation.
   b. Administer IV fluids, as prescribed.
   c. Administer oxygen, per order.
   d. Monitor strict intake and output (I&O).
   e. Administer blood transfusion, as prescribed.
   f. Assess laboratory values: RBC count, hemoglobin, hematocrit, and reticulocyte count.
3. Pain during crises.
   a. Monitor pain level using an age-appropriate pain rating scale.
   b. Administer narcotic analgesics, as prescribed and as needed.
   c. Utilize nonpharmacological pain-relieving measures (e.g., warmth, guided imagery, distraction).
   d. Encourage quiet activities (e.g., video games, board games, puzzles).
   e. Perform passive range-of-motion exercises.
4. Ineffective Coping/Anxiety/Fear.
   b. Educate the parents, child, and others regarding the disease process.
   c. Allow the parents, child, and others to express concerns regarding the health and well-being of the child.
      i. Include the child's siblings and other family members in the discussions.
      ii. Always use language that is appropriate to the children's developmental levels.
   b. Inform the parents, child, and others regarding the importance of following the prevention regimen.
   c. Refer the family to a local chapter of the Sickle Cell Foundation, and introduce the family to other families whose children have SCD.

IV. Hemophilia

Hemophilia is a group of hereditary illnesses characterized by slowed to markedly altered blood clotting resulting from a deficiency of one of the factors necessary for blood coagulation.

A. Incidence.

1. Von Willebrand disease: one in 100 to 1 in 10,000 individuals; most common bleeding disorder.
2. Hemophilia A: one in 4,000 to 1 in 5,000 males.
3. Hemophilia B: approximately 1 in 20,000 males.

B. Etiology.

1. Von Willebrand disease.
   a. Three types: type 1, autosomal dominant inheritance; type 3, autosomal recessive inheritance; type 2 may be either autosomal dominant or recessive inheritance.
   b. The mutated gene results in a deficiency or altered functioning of the Von Willebrand factor.
2. Hemophilia A: also called classic hemophilia.
   a. X-linked recessive inheritance.
   b. The mutated gene results in factor VIII deficiency or an altered form of factor VIII.
3. Hemophilia B: also called Christmas disease.
   a. X-linked recessive inheritance.
   b. The mutated gene results in either factor IX deficiency or an altered form of factor IX.

DID YOU KNOW?

Many genetic illnesses exhibit a range of expressivity. Expressivity refers to the severity of the disease. Some children with hemophilia will exhibit mild expressivity (i.e., will bleed only when seriously injured). Others will exhibit moderate or severe expressivity (i.e., will bleed with mild to moderate injury or spontaneously with no injury at all).

C. Pathophysiology.

1. Altered clotting mechanism: specific to the type of hemophilia, resulting in inability to form a blood clot, especially during periods of trauma.
2. Signs and symptoms include:
   a. **Hemarthrosis,** or bleeding into the joint: most common problem.
      i. Can lead to crippling deformities.
      ii. Early signs: stiffness, tingling, and achiness in the joint.
      iii. Later signs: decreased range of motion, signs of inflammation (warmth, redness, swelling, severe pain).
   b. Subcutaneous (subcu) and intramuscular hemorrhages.
   c. Spontaneous hematuria.
   d. Even more serious manifestations.
      i. Bleeding into the neck, mouth, and/or thorax, any of which may lead to respiratory compromise.
      ii. Intracranial hemorrhage that may lead to stroke.
      iii. Bleeding into the GI tract that may lead to severe hypovolemia or obstruction.
      iv. Hematomas in the spinal column that may lead to paralysis.

D. Diagnosis.
1. Clinical picture and family history.
2. Prolonged partial thromboplastin time (PTT).
3. Genetic testing: prenatal testing is available.
4. Factor assay assessment.

E. Treatment: dependent on the severity of the disease.
1. Regular administration of IV factor replacement: currently recombinant factors are available.
   a. Frequency and timing of the administration is dependent on the severity of the disease.
2. DDAVP (desmopressin acetate), administered either subcu or IV, provides a short-term rise in factor VIII and von Willebrand factor.
3. Antifibrinolytic medications that are administered at times of trauma (e.g., prior to dental visits and surgery).
   a. Amicar (aminocaproic acid) PO.
   b. Cyklokapron (tranexamic acid) PO.

DID YOU KNOW?

To prevent bleeding on a daily basis, the majority of hemophiliacs must receive replacement of their missing factor on a regular basis (i.e., 2 to 3 times per week). Both factor VIII and IX are available as fresh frozen plasma or as a concentrate. During periods of bleeding, the children require an additional emergency infusion of their missing factor.

F. Nursing considerations.
1. Deficient Knowledge/Anxiety/Altered Family Processes.
   a. Allow the parents, child, and others to express their concerns and feelings.
   b. Educate the parents and child, when appropriate, regarding the pathophysiology of the disease and the signs and symptoms of bleeding episodes.
   c. Educate the parents and child, when appropriate, never to ingest aspirin or any products containing aspirin.
   d. Educate the parents regarding alterations to the home environment to maximize safety (e.g., padding corners of tables, adding joint padding to clothes, providing the child with a soft-bristled toothbrush).
   e. Educate the parents regarding the procedures for the safe administration of the factor replacement and of DDAVP (See Chapter 9: "Pediatric Medication Administration").
      i. Educate the child, when he or she is developmentally ready, to perform replacement him- or herself.
   f. Include the child's siblings and other family members in the discussion, and always use language that is appropriate to the children's developmental levels.
   g. Refer the family to a local chapter of the Hemophilia Foundation, and introduce the family to other families with a child with hemophilia.
   h. Educate the parents and/or child, if appropriate, regarding the need to wear a MedicAlert bracelet.
   i. Refer the family to genetic counseling.
2. Risk for Deficient Fluid Volume during bleeding episodes.
   a. Administer blood transfusions, as prescribed, employing safe technique.
   b. Maintain adequate fluid intake, including IV and oral fluids.
   c. Monitor laboratory data, including CBC and PTT.
3. Risk for Injury during bleeding episodes.
   a. Educate the parents and/or child, if appropriate, to report signs of spontaneous bleeding (e.g., black and tarry stools, hematuria, altered level of consciousness).
   b. Apply pressure to small injuries for a minimum of 15 min, and monitor for prolonged bleeding.
   c. If hemarthrosis or bleeding into the joint develops, institute RICE (rest, ice, compression, elevation) protocol, as prescribed.
   d. Encourage the child to engage in a joint-strengthening program to help to prevent joint injuries.

V. Acute Lymphoblastic Leukemia

Acute lymphoblastic leukemia (ALL) is characterized by a proliferation in the production of lymphoblasts, or immature white blood cells, in the bone marrow.

A. Incidence.
1. Leukemia is the most common form of cancer in children, and ALL is the most common leukemia seen in children.
2. Cancer is very rare in children: only 1% of new cancers each year are in children. However, cancer is the leading cause of death from disease in children.
3. ALL is more common in males than in females.
4. Peak age of onset of ALL is between 2 and 6 years of age.
5. Currently, there is a 90% cure rate in children under 15 years of age.

B. Etiology.
1. Unknown, but chromosomal anomalies predispose some children to leukemia.
   a. Trisomy 21 (Down syndrome): 15 times the risk of general population.
   b. Translocation of chromosomes 7 and 14: frequently seen in children with ALL.

DID YOU KNOW?

All cancers are genetic in origin. That does not mean that all cancers are inherited; very few cancers are inherited. Rather, it means that all cancers develop as a result of a mutation in the DNA of the respective cells. In the case of ALL, for example, a mutation in the bone marrow, the etiology of which is unknown, results in the proliferation in the production of lymphoblasts. Concurrently, the bone marrow fails to produce mature WBCs, RBCs, and platelets.

C. Pathophysiology.
1. Hyperproduction of immature white blood cells (WBCs), called blast cells, in the bone marrow.
2. Poor production of other blood cells and inadequate maturation of WBCs in the bone marrow, resulting in:
   a. Reduced erythrocyte production resulting in anemia characterized by fatigue and lack of energy.
   b. Reduced platelet production resulting in thrombocytopenia characterized by petechiae and bruising.
   c. Reduced number of mature WBCs resulting in neutropenia characterized by low-grade fevers, recurring infections, and lymphadenopathy.

D. Diagnosis.
1. Initial suspicions from:
   a. Clinical picture.
   b. Altered findings on CBC (see Table 18.1):
      i. RBC count less than normal.
      ii. Platelet count less than normal.
      iii. Altered WBC count.
2. Bone marrow biopsy with DNA analysis is performed to confirm the diagnosis.
   a. Staging of the disease is based on the results of the bone marrow biopsy as well as the results of a lumbar puncture. When blast cells are found in the cerebral spinal fluid, the prognosis is less favorable.

E. Treatment.
1. Chemotherapy (chemo) is the conventional therapy.
   a. Exact combination of drugs is dependent on the specific protocol for the specific genetic type of leukemic cells.

MAKING THE CONNECTION

Because of the following considerations, only nurses who have been especially trained in the administration of chemo may administer these drugs:

Vesicants: many chemotherapeutic agents cause serious blistering when exposed to healthy tissue.

Extravasation: if an IV infiltrates while the chemo is infusing, the tissue surrounding the vessel can become seriously damaged, resulting in minor symptoms of discomfort, pain, and rash to severe complications related to tissue necrosis, including permanent damage.

In addition, chemotherapeutic medications can result in severe, life-threatening allergic reactions, called anaphylactic reactions, that are characterized by hyperthermia, tracheal swelling, and respiratory compromise.

   b. The chemotherapy regimen for children with ALL is divided into three phases: induction, consolidation, and maintenance.
      i. Goal of the induction phase: remission (i.e., to reduce the percentage of blast cells in the blood to 5% or less).
         (1) Response to the medications is monitored by serial bone marrow aspirations.
         (2) If the child does not go into remission, the protocol is changed to a different set of chemotherapeutic agents.

DID YOU KNOW?

When ALL patients receive chemo, the therapeutic goal is to inhibit the production of lymphoblast cells by the bone marrow. Concurrently, however, the chemo inhibits the bone marrow from producing all blood cells, including RBCs and platelets. As a result, the medication causes the patients to become even more severely anemic, thrombocytopenic, and neutropenic than they had been from the disease. The neutropenia, or immunosuppression, is especially concerning because the patients are at very high risk of contracting severe, potentially life-threatening infections. All health-care professionals must engage, therefore, in excellent infection control and caregiving practices when caring for patients who are receiving chemo.

      ii. Goal of the consolidation phase: maintain remission and prevent the progression of the disease to the central nervous system and/or the testes, in males.

(1) During this phase, the chemo is usually administered intrathecally (i.e., into the spinal column) to prevent migration of the cells into the CNS.

(2) The testes are radiated if blast cells are found in that organ.

iii. Goal of the maintenance phase: continued remission.

(1) Chemo is administered periodically—PO and/or IV—over the next few years.

(2) Periodic blood counts and bone marrow biopsies are performed to monitor for possible relapse.

2. Bone marrow and/or cord blood transplants may be performed
   a. A transplant may be either autologous (patient's own cells) or allogeneic (donor cells).
   b. If the transplant is allogeneic, to prevent rejection, antirejection medications are administered, (e.g., prednisone, cyclosporine, tacrolimus).
3. Additional medications/interventions that may be administered while the child is undergoing chemo and/or transplant include antibiotics, antifungals, antivirals, RBC production stimulators (e.g., Epogen), white blood cell production stimulators (e.g., Leukine), and blood transfusions.

F. Nursing considerations.

1. Anxiety/Fear/Pain.
   a. Allow the parents and child, if appropriate, to discuss their fears and concerns regarding the diagnosis, including the fear of dying (See Chapter 8, "Nursing Care of the Child in the Health-Care Setting")
   b. Provide adequate pain and emotional support when needed, especially during painful and scary procedures.
      i. Lumbar punctures and bone marrow aspirations, both of which are painful, also are especially frightening to children because they are performed out of one's field of vision.
      ii. Use age-appropriate pain rating tools, and assess pain on a regular basis.
      iii. Use nonpharmacological pain remedies in conjunction with pharmacological methods, if appropriate and as prescribed.
   c. Query the parents/family regarding whether they are using complementary and/or alternative therapies.
      i. These therapies may be beneficial or harmful to the child's recovery.
2. Infection or Risk for Infection resulting from periods of neutropenia.
   a. Monitor vital signs frequently, especially temperature.
   b. Practice meticulous handwashing and aseptic technique when performing procedures.
   c. Monitor the child for signs of infection, such as:
      i. Thrush with stomatitis (inflammation of the mucous membranes in the mouth).
      ii. Diarrhea.
      iii. Urinary tract infections.
   d. Obtain cultures to identify the pathogen, when appropriate.
   e. Practice safe but meticulous oral hygiene.
      i. Soft toothbrushes should be provided.
   f. Administer antibiotics, antivirals, and/or antifungals, as prescribed.
   g. Avoid contact with other children/adults with active infections or objects that may carry pathogens.
   h. If febrile, administer anti-pyretic medications, as prescribed.
      i. Because of the potential for bleeding, aspirin should be avoided.
   i. Administer dead, attenuated vaccines as recommended by ACIP.
      i. Live, attenuated vaccines should not be administered.

(!) As long as a child is immunosuppressed, all live vaccines (i.e., varicella, MMR, and nasal flu) are contraindicated. Immunosuppressed children who receive live vaccines could die from the unchecked production of the virus in their bodies. Even though the viruses had been attenuated, or made much less potent, immunosuppressed children's bodies are unable to control the infection.

3. Risk for Altered Tissue Perfusion/Activity Intolerance/Fatigue resulting from the anemia.
   a. Monitor vital signs carefully.
   b. Monitor for signs of ineffective perfusion (e.g., fatigue, decreased activity, tachycardia, pallor).
   c. Assess and monitor blood counts.
   d. Provide the child with needed rest periods.
   e. Encourage quiet, age-appropriate activities (e.g., video games, puzzles, reading books).
4. Bleeding or Risk for Bleeding resulting from the thrombocytopenia.
   a. Assess skin for petechiae, purpura, and bruising.
   b. Assess stools and urine for the presence of blood.
   c. Apply gentle pressure to injuries, including puncture sites.

d. Avoid contact injuries, especially potential head injuries.
e. Provide stool softeners to prevent straining at stool.
f. Pinch and ice nose bleeds, if they occur.

5. Risk for Imbalanced Nutrition: Less than Body Requirements/Risk for Deficient Fluid Volume resulting from complications of illness and medical therapies (e.g., poor appetite, stomatitis, nausea and vomiting).
   a. Administer antiemetics with chemo, as needed and as prescribed.
   b. Administer chemo at night, if possible.
   c. Monitor for signs of dehydration.
   d. Maintain strict I&O.
   e. Assess weight regularly.
   f. Obtain a referral to a nutritionist.
   g. Offer favorite foods and fluids in as appealing a manner as possible.
   h. Refrain from serving foods or fluids that irritate the oral mucosa, e.g., citrus juices, highly salted foods.
   i. Provide the child with high-calorie, high-protein supplements.
      i. Milk shakes are often excellent foods because they are nutritious and appealing. In addition, because they are cold they are less irritating to the mucous membranes.
6. Risk for Impaired Skin Integrity/Altered Body Image resulting from side effects of the illness and of the medications.
   a. Assess oral mucosal for ulceration.
   b. Provide the child with saline or sodium bicarbonate mouthwashes to maintain oral health.
   c. Monitor tooth eruption (delayed tooth eruption is common).
   d. Use nonirritating lotions and soaps, wash cloths, and towels.
   e. Change the child's position frequently, if bedbound.
   f. Warn the child and monitor for loss of hair.
      i. Educate the child that his or her hair will regrow, although it may look and feel different.
      ii. Encourage the child to wear colorful headgear and/or wigs.
7. Risk for Injury related to side effects of medications.
   a. Monitor for signs of injury—short term as well as long term—related to chemotherapeutic agents, including:
      i. Constipation.
      ii. Foot drop.
      iii. Cognitive dysfunction.
      iv. Reproductive dysfunction.
      v. Skeletal changes.
      vi. Altered growth and development.
8. Deficient Knowledge.
   a. Use pictures, microscopes, and all other available visual tools to provide the child and parents with as complete an understanding of how the blood works as possible.
   b. Keep the parents and child, if appropriate, informed of the progress of the disease and treatments, including side effects of the treatments.
   c. Allow time for repeated discussions related to topics such as the disease process, treatment needs, and pain management.

CASE STUDY: Putting It All Together

A 6-year-old, African American boy is brought to the emergency department by his father

Subjective Data

- The child is in his father's arms and is crying in pain.
- The father states,
  - "Our son has sickle cell anemia. He had his first crisis when he was 2 years old. He has had six or seven since then. He woke up with a fever this morning and now this!"
- When queried about his fluid intake, the father states,
  - "He has drunk a little, but I can't get him to drink as much as he should. I gave him acetaminophen, but you can see that that didn't help at all."
- Father states that the child was to receive his flu shot next week. Otherwise, father states that the child is up to date on his vaccinations and takes penicillin and folic acid daily.

Objective Data

Nursing Assessment

- Febrile, temperature 102.4°F
- Profuse pain of the elbows, knees, and abdomen
  - Child chooses "Hurts Worst" face on the Wong-Baker Pain Scale.
- Elbows and knees: swollen, warm, red
- Enlarged spleen

Vital Signs

Temperature:	102.4°F
Heart rate:	130 bpm
Respiratory rate:	25 rpm
Blood pressure:	94/56 mm Hg
Weight:	18 kg (10th percentile)
Height:	109 cm (10th percentile)
O_2 saturation:	89%

Lab Results

RBC:	3.0 million/mm^3
Reticulocytes:	0.2%
Hematocrit:	28%
Hemoglobin:	9.1 g/dL
Platelets:	200,000 cells/mm^3
WBC:	15,500 cells/mm^3

Health-Care Provider's Orders

- Place client on bedrest
- IV D5 ¼ NS at 90 mL/hr
- Clear fluids, as tolerated
- Perform throat culture STAT
- Administer penicillin G 600,000 units IV every 6 hr
- Administer morphine 3 mg IV STAT, may repeat every 2 hr, as needed
- Oxygen 2 L/min
- Monitor oxygen saturations

Case Study Questions

A. What *subjective* assessments indicate that this client is experiencing a health alteration?

1. ______
2. ______
3. ______
4. ______

B. What *objective* assessments indicate that this client is experiencing a health alteration?

1. ______
2. ______
3. ______
4. ______
5. ______
6. ______
7. ______

CASE STUDY: Putting It All Together *cont'd*

Case Study Question

C. After analyzing the data that has been collected, what **primary** nursing diagnosis should the nurse assign to this client?

1. ______________________________

D. What interventions should the nurse plan and/or implement to meet this child's and his family's needs?

1. ______________________________
2. ______________________________
3. ______________________________
4. ______________________________
5. ______________________________
6. ______________________________
7. ______________________________
8. ______________________________
9. ______________________________
10. ______________________________
11. ______________________________
12. ______________________________
13. ______________________________

E. What client outcomes should the nurse evaluate regarding the effectiveness of the nursing interventions?

1. ______________________________
2. ______________________________
3. ______________________________
4. ______________________________
5. ______________________________

F. What physiological characteristics should the child exhibit before being discharged home?

1. ______________________________
2. ______________________________
3. ______________________________
4. ______________________________

G. What subjective characteristics should the child exhibit before being discharged home?

1. ______________________________

REVIEW QUESTIONS

1. A toddler has been diagnosed with iron-deficiency anemia. Which of the following information should the nurse educate the parents regarding medication administration?
   1. Add the iron elixir to his morning bottle.
   2. Have the child drink orange juice right after he takes his medicine.
   3. Administer the medicine right before his meals.
   4. Crush the tablets and mix the medicine with his applesauce.

2. The maximum safe dosage of elemental iron for a child 6 months to 2 years of age is 6 mg/kg/day in divided doses tid or qid. Which of the following prescriptions is safe for an 18-month-old child weighing 22 pounds?
   1. 15 mg qid
   2. 20 mg qid
   3. 25 mg tid
   4. 30 mg tid

3. A child has been prescribed 20 mg of elemental iron tid. The nurse has determined that the dosage is safe for the child. Ferrous sulfate elixir is available as: 44 mg/5 mL. How many mL of medication will the child consume each day? **(If rounding is needed, please calculate to the nearest tenth.)**

   __________ mL

4. A 12-week-gestation African American woman asks her obstetrician's nurse whether her baby could be born with sickle cell disease. Which of the following replies is appropriate for the nurse to give?
   1. It is possible because one out of every 500 African Americans is diagnosed with sickle cell anemia.
   2. If either you or the baby's father has sickle cell anemia, your child may be born with the disease.
   3. The baby could only have sickle cell anemia if both you and the baby's father carry a sickle cell gene.
   4. If the child is a boy, he could have sickle cell anemia, but if the child is a girl, she will definitely be healthy.

5. A young child is admitted to the emergency department in vaso-occlusive crisis. Which of the following orders is the highest priority for the nurse to perform?
   1. Morphine 1 mg subcu STAT
   2. IV D_5W ¼ NS at 90 mL/hr
   3. Oxygen 2 L/min
   4. Arterial blood gases STAT

6. A school-age child has sickle cell anemia. The child's parents ask the school nurse regarding the high-risk nature of 4 activities the child is requesting to participate in. Which of the following activities should the nurse advise the parents is most high risk for the child to perform?
   1. Perform the lead role in the school play.
   2. Play the violin in the school orchestra.
   3. Create an oil painting in art class.
   4. Join the after-school wrestling team.

7. A child with sickle cell anemia weighs 68 lb. How many mL of fluid should this child consume per day (i.e., what are this child's daily maintenance fluid needs)? **(If rounding is needed, please calculate to the nearest tenth.)**

   __________ mL

8. A 12-year-old boy with a history of sickle cell anemia and a diagnosis of vaso-occlusive crisis is being assessed by the admitting nurse in the emergency department. Which of the following signs/symptoms would the nurse expect to see? **Select all that apply.**
   1. Priapism
   2. Pain level of 2/10
   3. Hematuria
   4. Elevated liver enzymes
   5. Hematocrit 39%

9. A 10-year-old child, diagnosed with hemophilia A, is in the emergency department after experiencing a fall on the school playground. Which of the following laboratory data would the nurse expect to see?
   1. Leukocyte count 15,000 cells/mm^3
   2. Platelet count 75,000 cells/mm^3
   3. Partial prothrombin time (PTT) 90 sec (normal 60–70 sec)
   4. Prothrombin time (PT) 9 sec (normal 11–12.5 sec)

10. A pregnant woman with a family history of hemophilia B and who has been seen by a genetic counselor makes the following statements. The nurse must clarify the information in which of the statements?
    1. "Because the disease is X-linked, only my daughters can be born with hemophilia B."
    2. "Prenatal testing can be performed to determine whether my fetus has hemophilia B."
    3. "Some children with hemophilia B have worse bleeding problems than other children with the same genetics."
    4. "Children with hemophilia B are lacking one of the important factors needed to clot blood."

11. A 16-year-old male has hemophilia A. The nurse is assessing the actions performed by the family when administering the teen's medications. Which of the following actions would the nurse expect to see?
   1. His mother draws up the factor replacement into a syringe.
   2. The young man washes his hands carefully and puts on sterile gloves.
   3. The missing factor is infused every night while the teen sleeps.
   4. Antifibrinolytic medication is taken before each factor infusion.

12. The nurse is taking a health history from a young adult with hemophilia. The nurse should ask the client whether he is experiencing any signs and symptoms of which of the following chronic illnesses?
   1. Osteoarthritis
   2. Diabetes mellitus
   3. Asthma
   4. Hypothyroidism

13. A child has been diagnosed with acute lymphoblastic leukemia (ALL). With which of the following signs/symptoms did the child likely present to the primary health-care provider? **Select all that apply.**
   1. Bruising
   2. Lethargy
   3. Jaundice
   4. Leukopenia
   5. Erythema

14. A child is receiving chemotherapy for a diagnosis of acute lymphoblastic leukemia (ALL). The nurse monitors the child for which of the following common side effects? **Select all that apply.**
   1. Malaise
   2. Alopecia
   3. Priapism
   4. Anorexia
   5. Epistaxis

15. The nurse is caring for a child with stomatitis after receiving chemotherapy. Which of the following food items would be appropriate for the nurse to provide the child?
   1. Orange juice
   2. Whole-grain crackers
   3. Dried apple chips
   4. Milkshake

16. An 11-month-old child is receiving chemotherapy for a diagnosis of acute lymphoblastic leukemia (ALL). Which of the following vaccinations is safe for the nurse to administer to the child?
   1. Var (varicella)
   2. MMR (measles, mumps, rubella)
   3. LAIV (live attenuated influenza vaccine)
   4. PCV (pneumococcal)

17. The mother of a child with acute lymphoblastic leukemia (ALL) states that their family is employing complementary therapies to improve the child's chances of survival. The child is also receiving chemotherapy. The nurse should discuss with the mother that which of the following therapies may actually be in conflict with the child's medical care?
   1. Therapeutic touch
   2. Healing meals
   3. Pet therapy
   4. Folic acid supplements

REVIEW ANSWERS

1. **ANSWER: 2**

Rationale:

1. Iron elixir can stain a child's teeth. It should not be added to the child's bottle.
2. **Ascorbic acid (vitamin C) promotes the absorption of iron. Orange juice is high in vitamin C.**
3. Iron is absorbed best when administered between meals.
4. Iron supplements should be taken whole. They should not be broken, crushed, or chewed.

TEST-TAKING TIP: Toddlers who need iron supplements should be administered the elixir. It should be consumed via a straw to minimize the potential for tooth discoloration.

Content Area: *Pediatrics—Hematological*
Integrated Processes: *Nursing Process: Implementation; Teaching/Learning*
Client Need: *Physiological Integrity: Pharmacological and Parenteral Therapies: Medication Administration*
Cognitive Level: *Application*

2. **ANSWER: 1**

Rationale:

1. **15 mg qid.**
2. 20 mg qid.
3. 25 mg tid.
4. 30 mg tid.

TEST-TAKING TIP: *Ratio and proportion method:* The recommended pediatric dosage is stated as per kilogram. The weight calculation formula must be used:

convert 22 lb to kg: 22/2.2 = 10 kg

Calculate the maximum safe daily dose per day:

6 mg/1 kg = x mg/10 kg

x = 60 mg

Calculate the maximum safe dosage for each administration, dividing the daily dosage by 3 (tid) and by 4 (qid):

tid: 60 mg/3 = 20 mg is the maximum tid dosage

qid: 60 mg/4 = 15 mg is the maximum qid dosage

Dimensional analysis method:

Calculate both the tid and the qid dosage levels:

tid:

6 mg	22 lb	1 kg	1 day	= the maximum safe
kg/day		2.2/lb	3 doses (tid)	dosage tid is 20 mg

qid:

6 mg	22 lb	1 kg	1 day	= the maximum safe
kg/day		2.2/lb	4 doses (qid)	dosage tid is 15 mg

The only dosage that is safe for this child is 15 mg qid.

Content Area: *Pediatrics—Hematological*
Integrated Processes: *Nursing Process: Implementation*
Client Need: *Health Promotion and Maintenance: Pharmacological and Parenteral Therapies: Dosage Calculations*
Cognitive Level: *Synthesis*

3. **ANSWER: 6.8 mL**

TEST-TAKING TIP: The test taker must read carefully because the question asked the test taker to calculate the total amount of medication in milliliters that the child will consume each day.

Ratio and proportion method:

20 mg tid = 20 × 3 = 60 mg

Next, the test taker must calculate the quantity of elixir equal to the child's daily dosage.

60 mg/x mL = 44 mg/5 mL

44x = 300

x = 6.81, or rounded to the nearest tenth = 6.8 mL

Dimensional analysis method:

20 mg	3 doses (tid)	5 mL	= 6.81, or rounded to the
tid		44 mg	nearest tenth = 6.8 mL

Content Area: *Pediatrics—Hematological*
Integrated Processes: *Nursing Process: Implementation*
Client Need: *Health Promotion and Maintenance: Pharmacological and Parenteral Therapies: Dosage Calculations*
Cognitive Level: *Synthesis*

4. **ANSWER: 3**

Rationale:

1. It is possible that the child could have SCA, but only if both parents carry a sickle cell gene.
2. This statement is incorrect. SCA is an autosomal recessive illness, not an autosomal dominant illness.
3. **This statement is correct. The baby could only have sickle cell anemia if both the woman and the baby's father carry a sickle cell gene.**
4. This statement is incorrect. SCA is an autosomal recessive illness, not an X-linked recessive illness.

TEST-TAKING TIP: Test takers should be familiar with the inheritance patterns of common genetic illnesses such as the autosomal recessive inheritance of SCA. Those with the disease must carry affected genes on both of their chromosomes. Those with the carrier state have an affected gene on one of their chromosomes and a normal gene on their other chromosome.

Content Area: *Pediatrics—Hematological*
Integrated Processes: *Nursing Process: Implementation; Teaching/Learning*
Client Need: *Health Promotion and Maintenance: Health Screening*
Cognitive Level: *Application*

5. ANSWER: 2

Rationale:

1. Administering the narcotic is an important action but not the priority action.
2. Infusing IV fluids is the priority action.
3. Administering oxygen is an important action but not the priority action.
4. Obtaining and assessing the arterial blood gases are important actions but not the priority action.

TEST-TAKING TIP: When determining the priority action, nurses must consider which of the actions will be most apt to improve their client's condition. The pathology of a vaso-occlusive crisis results in clumping of the RBCs and poor blood flow. The only action that will improve circulation is the IV infusion that will increase the child's blood volume.

Content Area: *Pediatrics—Hematological*
Integrated Processes: *Nursing Process: Implementation*
Client Need: *Safe and Effective Care Environment: Management of Care: Establishing Priorities*
Cognitive Level: *Analysis*

6. ANSWER: 4

Rationale:

1. It is unlikely that acting in the school play would precipitate a vaso-occlusive crisis.
2. It is unlikely that playing the violin would precipitate a vaso-occlusive crisis.
3. It is unlikely that painting would precipitate a vaso-occlusive crisis.
4. Wrestling most likely would precipitate a vaso-occlusive crisis.

TEST-TAKING TIP: Vaso-occlusive crises occur when children are dehydrated, hypoxic, and/or acidotic. The child could become hot and sweaty while wrestling, which could lead to dehydration, hypoxia, and acidosis. The child would need to drink quantities of fluid in excess of his maintenance needs and take frequent rest breaks during wrestling practice.

Content Area: *Pediatrics—Hematological*
Integrated Processes: *Nursing Process: Implementation*
Client Need: *Physiological Integrity: Reduction of Risk Potential: Potential for Alterations in Body Systems*
Cognitive Level: *Analysis*

7. ANSWER: 1,718 mL

TEST-TAKING TIP: A child's maintenance fluid needs are calculated as follows:
100 mL/kg for the first 10 kg
50 mL/kg for the second 10 kg
20 mL/kg for weight above 20 kg
First, the child's weight in pounds must be converted to kg.

$$2.2 \text{ lb}/1 \text{ kg} = 68 \text{ lb}/x \text{ kg}$$

$$2.2x = 68$$

$$x = 30.909 = 30.9 \text{ (nearest tenth)}$$

Next, the child's fluid needs must be determined in relation to his weight, as noted above.
First 10 kg (30.9 − 10 = 20.9) × 100 mL = 1,000 mL
Second 10 kg (20.9 − 10 = 10.9) × 50 mL = 500 mL
Remaining weight 10.9 kg × 20 mL = 218 mL
Total maintenance fluid needs = 1,718 mL

Content Area: *Pediatrics—Hematological*
Integrated Processes: *Nursing Process: Analysis*
Client Need: *Physiological Integrity: Reduction of Risk Potential: Potential for Alterations in Body Systems*
Cognitive Level: *Synthesis*

8. ANSWER: 1, 3, and 4

Rationale:

1. Priapism is symptom seen in males during a vaso-occlusive crisis.
2. The pain level is much higher during a vaso-occlusive crisis, often rated at 9/10 or 10/10 on a numeric pain rating scale.
3. Hematuria is a symptom seen during a vaso-occlusive crisis.
4. Elevated liver enzymes are seen during a vaso-occlusive crisis.
5. The nurse would expect to see a low hematocrit in a child with SCA.

TEST-TAKING TIP: To remember signs and symptoms seen during vaso-occlusive crises, the test taker should remember the pathology of the attack (i.e., sickling and clumping of RBCs). Vascular organs, therefore, are most affected by the crisis. The blood becomes trapped in the vessels of the penis, resulting in a painful erection. The kidneys become ischemic, resulting in the loss of blood into the urine. The liver becomes ischemic, resulting in elevated liver enzymes. Patients in vaso-occlusive crisis experience severe pain.

Content Area: *Pediatrics—Hematological*
Integrated Processes: *Nursing Process: Assessment*
Client Need: *Physiological Integrity: Physiological Adaptation: Alterations in Body Systems*
Cognitive Level: *Application*

9. ANSWER: 3

Rationale:

1. Leukocyte count should be within normal limits. The child does not have an infection.
2. The child's platelet count should be within normal limits.
3. The nurse would expect the PTT to be prolonged.
4. The nurse would expect the child's PT to be within normal limits.

TEST-TAKING TIP: Hemophilia A is characterized by a deficiency in or altered functioning of factor VIII. PTT is prolonged in those with factor VIII deficiency. Hemophilia A is not characterized by a change in platelet number. PT is prolonged when other clotting factors are deficient but not factor VIII. Also, if the PT were affected, it would be prolonged, not shorter.

Content Area: *Pediatrics—Hematological*
Integrated Processes: *Nursing Process: Assessment*
Client Need: *Physiological Integrity: Physiological Adaptation: Alterations in Body Systems*
Cognitive Level: *Application*

10. ANSWER: 1
Rationale:
1. Hemophilia B, an X-linked disease, is carried on the X chromosome. Sons would exhibit the disease, while daughters would carry the affected gene but not exhibit the illness.
2. Prenatal testing can diagnose whether a fetus has hemophilia.
3. The expressivity of hemophilia is variable. Some children with hemophilia have worse bleeding problems than other children with the same genetics.
4. Children with hemophilia B are lacking one of the important factors—factor IX—that is needed to clot blood.
TEST-TAKING TIP: X-linked recessive diseases are carried on the X chromosome. Because males have only one X chromosome, they will exhibit the disease. For females to exhibit the disease, they must receive an affected X from both their father and their mother. This is extremely rare.
Content Area: *Pediatrics—Hematological*
Integrated Processes: *Nursing Process: Implementation*
Client Need: *Health Promotion and Maintenance: Health Promotion/Disease Prevention*
Cognitive Level: *Application*

11. ANSWER: 2
Rationale:
1. This young man is 16 years old. He should be administering his own factor replacement.
2. Before the young man begins the procedure, he should wash his hands carefully and put on sterile gloves.
3. Hemophilic factors are infused two to three times a week, and they are usually administered via IV push.
4. Antifibrinolytic medication is administered after injuries or before surgeries.
TEST-TAKING TIP: Not only is this question asking the test taker regarding the actual procedure involved in the administration of factor replacement, but also asking the test taker regarding expected actions based on a patient's growth and development. This young man is old enough to be engaged in complete self-care.
Content Area: *Pediatrics—Hematological*
Integrated Processes: *Nursing Process: Assessment*
Client Need: *Physiological Integrity: Pharmacological and Parenteral Therapies: Medication Administration*
Cognitive Level: *Application*

12. ANSWER: 1
Rationale:
1. The nurse should assess for signs and symptoms of osteoarthritis.
2. Hemophiliacs are not especially at high risk for diabetes mellitus.
3. Hemophiliacs are not especially at high risk for asthma.
4. Hemophiliacs are not especially at high risk for hypothyroidism.
TEST-TAKING TIP: With recurrent bleeding into the joints (hemarthrosis), hemophiliacs are at high risk for bone destruction, joint damage, and osteoarthritis.
Content Area: *Pediatrics—Hematological*
Integrated Processes: *Nursing Process: Assessment*
Client Need: *Physiological Integrity: Physiological Adaptation: Alterations in Body Systems*
Cognitive Level: *Application*

13. ANSWER: 1 and 2
Rationale:
1. The child likely presented with bruising.
2. The child likely presented with lethargy.
3. Jaundice is not related to a diagnosis of ALL.
4. The child presented with leukocytosis, not leukopenia.
5. Erythema is not related to a diagnosis of ALL.
TEST-TAKING TIP: Children with ALL present with laboratory findings consistent with the following: anemia, thrombocytopenia, and leukocytosis. Lethargy is a symptom of anemia. Bruising is a symptom of thrombocytopenia. Although the children have markedly elevated white blood cell counts, the cells are immature and poorly functioning. The children, therefore, also present with a history of recurring infections and low-grade fevers.
Content Area: *Pediatrics—Hematological*
Integrated Processes: *Nursing Process: Assessment*
Client Need: *Physiological Integrity: Physiological Adaptation: Alterations in Body Systems*
Cognitive Level: *Application*

14. ANSWER: 1, 2, 4, and 5
Rationale:
1. Malaise is a side effect of chemotherapy.
2. Alopecia is a side effect of chemotherapy.
3. Priapism is not a side effect of chemotherapy.
4. Anorexia is a side effect of chemotherapy.
5. Epistaxis is a side effect of chemotherapy.
TEST-TAKING TIP: The therapeutic goal of chemotherapy is bone marrow suppression. Symptoms related to anemia and thrombocytopenia—malaise and epistaxis—would be expected. In addition, chemotherapeutic medications impede DNA synthesis, resulting in alopecia, and lead to serious gastric distress—nausea, vomiting, and anorexia.
Content Area: *Pediatrics—Hematological*
Integrated Processes: *Nursing Process: Implementation*
Client Need: *Physiological Integrity: Pharmacological and Parenteral Therapies: Adverse Effects/Contraindications/Side Effects/Interactions*
Cognitive Level: *Application*

15. ANSWER: 4
Rationale:
1. Orange juice would not be recommended for children with stomatitis.
2. Whole-grain crackers would not be recommended for children with stomatitis.
3. Dried apple chips would not be recommended for children with stomatitis.
4. A milkshake would be appropriate for a child with stomatitis.

TEST-TAKING TIP: Stomatitis refers to painful ulcerations in the mouth. Foods that are acidic, such as orange juice, or irritating, such as chips and crackers, increase the stomatitis pain. Cold, nonirritating foods are consumed most readily. Milkshakes also are recommended because they are both sweet and nutritious.
Content Area: *Pediatrics—Hematological*
Integrated Processes: *Nursing Process: Implementation*
Client Need: *Physiological Integrity: Basic Care and Comfort: Nutrition and Oral Hydration*
Cognitive Level: *Application*

16. ANSWER: 4
Rationale:
1. Var (varicella) administration is contraindicated.
2. MMR (measles, mumps, rubella) administration is contraindicated.
3. LAIV (live attenuated influenza vaccine) administration is contraindicated.
4. PCV (pneumococcal) should be administered.
TEST-TAKING TIP: Children undergoing chemotherapy become immunosuppressed. They are unable, therefore, to tolerate live, attenuated vaccinations. Var, MMR, and LAIV are all live, attenuated vaccines. PCV is a dead vaccine that protects the children from pneumococcal infections. It should be administered.
Content Area: *Pediatrics—Hematological*
Integrated Processes: *Nursing Process: Implementation*
Client Need: *Physiological Integrity: Pharmacological and Parenteral Therapies: Adverse Effects/Contraindications/Side Effects/Interactions*
Cognitive Level: *Application*

17. ANSWER: 4
Rationale:
1. Therapeutic touch would be an appropriate complementary therapy.
2. Healing meals would be an appropriate complementary therapy.
3. Pet therapy would be an appropriate complementary therapy.
4. Folic acid supplements would be inappropriate to administer to a child undergoing chemotherapy.
TEST-TAKING TIP: Complementary therapies should enhance traditional therapies. They should not be in conflict with the traditional therapies. High doses of folic acid, taken to promote DNA synthesis, can interfere with the action of some chemotherapeutic agents (i.e., DNA suppression).
Content Area: *Pediatrics—Hematological*
Integrated Processes: *Nursing Process: Implementation*
Client Need: *Physiological Integrity: Reduction of Risk Potential: Potential for Alterations in Body Systems*
Cognitive Level: *Application*

Chapter 19

Nursing Care of the Child With Integumentary System Disorders

KEY TERMS

Atopic dermatitis (eczema)—An inflammatory response secondary to the release of high levels of histamine.
Candidiasis—An infection caused by the fungus *Candida albicans* that is frequently transferred from the mother to her baby during a vaginal delivery.
Cellulitis—Bacterial infection of the lower layers of the skin.
Dermatophytosis—Ringworm or tinea infection.
Erythematous—Reddish inflammation of the skin.
Impetigo—Lesions progressing to a blister-like rash that are caused by a bacterial infection.
Maculopapular rash—A rash characterized by flat discolorations (macules) and small raised bumps (papules).
Methicillin-resistant Staphylococcus aureus (MRSA)—An *S. aureus* bacterium that has mutated and become resistant to all of the most commonly prescribed antibiotics.
Pediculosis—Lice.
Scabies—Inflammatory response to burrowing mites and their feces.
Thrush—White patches, on an erythematous base, on the tongue, gingiva, and buccal mucosa caused by *C. albicans*.
Vesicular rash—A rash characterized by blister-like sacs or pustules.

I. Description

The integumentary system (i.e., the skin) is the largest organ system of the body. It is comprised of three layers: the epidermis, or the outer layer; the dermis, which is underneath the epidermis; and a layer of subcutaneous fat below the dermis. The skin is responsible for a number of functions.

- Protects the body from infection.
- Helps to maintain the body's temperature.
- Excretes fluid in the form of perspiration.
- Aids in the production of vitamin D.
- Protects the body through the sensation of touch.

A number of integumentary illnesses are commonly seen in the pediatric population.

II. Diaper Rash

This rash, which is seen in the perineal area of babies, is a form of contact dermatitis. In other words, the baby's skin is reacting to an irritant.

A. Incidence.
1. At least 1 out of every 10 children will develop a diaper rash. In some populations, the incidence is much higher.
2. Diaper rashes are most common in babies during the latter half of their first year.

B. Etiology.
1. The baby's skin reacts to an irritant that is in direct contact with the skin.
2. The most common irritant is ammonia in the baby's urine in conjunction with fecal enzymes.
3. Babies also develop diaper rashes from pathogens (e.g., *Candida albicans*) (See "Neonatal Candidiasis").
4. Some babies' skin reacts to the chemicals in paper diapers and/or commercial diaper wipes.

C. Pathophysiology.
1. The epidermal layer that is in contact with the irritant becomes **erythematous**, or reddish in color. If the irritant is not removed, the rash may develop into a **maculopapular rash**, characterized by flat discolorations (macules) and small raised bumps (papules).
2. Rashes from *C. albicans* have a distinct, bright-red appearance and are quite painful.

D. Diagnosis.
1. Clinical picture.

E. Treatment.
1. Prevention.
   a. Frequent diaper changes so that the baby does not sit in a soiled and wet diaper for an extended period of time.
   b. Application of an ointment barrier at each diaper change (e.g., petroleum jelly, zinc oxide, vitamin-based ointment).
      i. Because some substances migrate through the skin, it is important that the parents make sure that the ointment is safe for use with babies.
   c. The diaper area should be cleansed with mild soap and water or commercial diaper wipes at each diaper change.
      i. Many commercial wipes, however, contain alcohol that can be irritating to the baby's tissue.
   d. Diapers should be removed and the skin exposed to the air for a few minutes each day.
2. Intervention—when a rash is present.
   a. A number of interventions may be used, including steroid creams.
   b. Antifungal medications may be prescribed if the rash is caused by *C. albicans*.

F. Nursing considerations.
1. Impaired Skin Integrity/Risk for Infection/Risk for Acute Pain/Deficient Knowledge.
   a. Parents should be taught proper diapering practices, including:
      i. Changing the baby's diaper after each voiding/defecation.
      ii. Using preventative ointment (e.g., petroleum jelly, zinc oxide, or vitamin-based ointment) at each diaper change.
   b. Parents should be advised periodically to expose the diaper area to the air as preventative and/or to treat a rash.
   c. Because they prevent air from penetrating the material, parents should be advised to refrain from using rubber pants to cover their baby's diaper.
   d. If a rash or irritation develops:
      i. Parents should be taught to cleanse the skin with mild soap and rinse thoroughly.
      ii. The nurse should suggest that the parents change the brand and/or stop using disposable diapers and/or baby wipes if irritation develops.
         (1) If parents use cloth diapers, they must be advised to wash and rinse them thoroughly to remove all irritants.

III. Neonatal Candidiasis

A. Incidence.
1. No clear numbers are available regarding the incidence of neonatal **candidiasis**.

B. Etiology.
1. Babies usually become infected during delivery.
   a. The vagina is often colonized with *C. albicans*. When the baby passes through the birth canal during delivery, he or she may become infected.
2. The organism may also be transmitted from mother to baby via poorly washed hands.

C. Pathophysiology.
1. Begins as **thrush**, or white patches, on an erythematous base, on the tongue, gingiva, and buccal mucosa.
2. Progresses to a severe diaper rash.
   a. Bright-red, contiguous lesions in the diaper area (Fig. 19.1).

D. Diagnosis.
1. Clinical picture.

E. Treatment.
1. Oral and/or topical antifungal medication, e.g., nystatin or fluconazole (Diflucan).
2. If the mother is breastfeeding, it is essential that the medication be administered to both the mother and the baby for 2 full weeks to eradicate the infection.

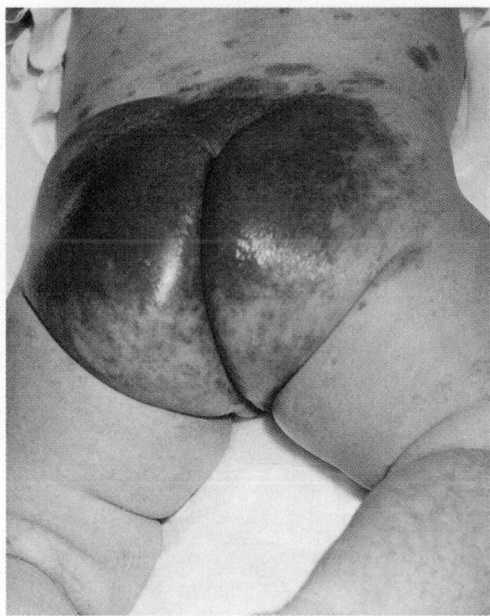

Fig 19.1 Candidiasis diaper rash.

MAKING THE CONNECTION

Women often carry *C. albicans* in their vaginas. During birthing, babies can develop thrush, or oral candidiasis, from being exposed to the fungus. They can also become infected if mothers fail to wash their hands well after toileting. In either case, the fungus can lead to a severe diaper rash in the baby and, if the baby is breastfed, a very painful infection of the mother's breasts. Nurses must educate the mothers to wash their hands well to prevent this and other infections in their babies. If treatment is needed, babies are usually prescribed oral anti-fungal medication, and mothers are advised to apply the same medication to their nipples and areolae. To prevent a reinfestation, the medication must be administered to both the mother and the baby for a minimum of 2 weeks.

F. Nursing considerations.
1. Impaired Skin Integrity/Acute Pain/Deficient Knowledge.
   a. Educate the parents regarding the importance of meticulous handwashing.
   b. Educate the parents regarding actions to prevent and to treat, if indicated, diaper rash (see above).
   c. Educate the parents regarding safe medication dosage and proper medication administration, to baby and to mother, if prescribed.
   d. Advise the parents periodically to expose the diaper area to the air.
   e. If indicated, educate the parents regarding the importance of cleaning bottles and/or pacifiers as well as toys that have been placed in the baby's mouth.

IV. Atopic Dermatitis (eczema)

A. Incidence.
1. **Atopic dermatitis (eczema)** is frequently seen in infants.
2. The incidence of eczema decreases as children age.

B. Etiology.
1. Eczema is an inherited illness in which the child exhibits an allergic response to an environmental stimulus.
   a. The child's allergy may be caused by a number of items including foods, detergents, soaps, shampoos, or fabrics.
2. A number of factors have been shown to intensify a child's symptoms, e.g., warm, ambient environment; woolen fabric; and dry skin.

C. Pathophysiology.
1. The child mounts an allergic, inflammatory response secondary to high levels of histamine release, resulting in patches of skin that are reddened, edematous, and highly pruritic.
2. Signs and symptoms.
   a. Red, edematous, and itchy areas that eventually weep and crust.
      i. Lesions usually are bilateral.
      ii. Lesions most commonly are seen on the cheeks and distal surfaces of the arms and legs.
   b. As the child scratches the area, often by rubbing against the bed sheets, the itching intensifies.
      i. The itching often results in skin breakdown (i.e., skin abrasions).
   c. Secondary infections may develop in the excoriated areas.

D. Diagnosis.
1. Clinical picture.

E. Treatment.
1. Prevention.
   a. Exclusive breastfeeding has been shown to provide a protective effect (Gdalevich, Mimouni, David, and Mimouni, 2001).
   b. Parents should avoid dressing their child to the point of overheating.
   c. Unless medically indicated, infants should not be started on solid foods until they are at least 6 months of age.
   d. All irritants that have been found to trigger the allergic response should be avoided (e.g., foods that are known to have precipitated an outbreak).

e. Other irritants that may exacerbate the adverse response should also be avoided (e.g., perfumed soaps, wool clothing, fluffy toys).

2. Treatment.
   a. Several different medications may be used.
      i. Oral and/or topical antihistamines as preventatives.
      ii. Topical corticosteroids to treat flare-ups.
      iii. Antibiotics to treat a secondary infection.
      iv. Oral steroids, although these are prescribed with caution.
   b. Skin hydration is promoted through a variety of means (e.g., frequent bathing in tepid baths and the application of emollients or wet dressings after bathing).
      i. After the bath, the child should be dressed in soft, cotton clothing.

F. Nursing considerations.
1. Impaired Skin Integrity/Risk for Acute Pain/Risk for Infection/Deficient Knowledge.
   a. Educate the parents and child, if appropriate, to:
      i. Investigate what substances trigger outbreaks, and to eliminate the triggers from the child's environment and/or diet.
      ii. Follow the therapeutic regimen.
      iii. Remove wool and other known irritating items from the child's environment (e.g., fuzzy toys, blankets).
      iv. Refrain from overheating the child.
      v. Refrain from using such products as perfumed/dyed soaps, detergents, and laundry softeners in child's bath or when washing the child's clothing.
      vi. Dress the child in lightweight, cotton clothing.
      vii. Keep fingernails short, and dress the child in clothing that prevents direct itching of irritated areas.
      viii. Monitor for skin breakdown/infected skin, and report to the health-care provider.
2. Risk for Altered Coping/Risk for Altered Family Process.
   a. Allow the parents and child, if appropriate, to discuss their frustrations/concerns regarding the diagnosis, symptoms, and/or treatments.
   b. Provide the parents and child, if appropriate, with stress reduction techniques.

V. Impetigo

A. Incidence.
1. **Impetigo** is seen in children at any age, but most frequently in toddlers and preschoolers.
2. Primarily seen during the summer months.

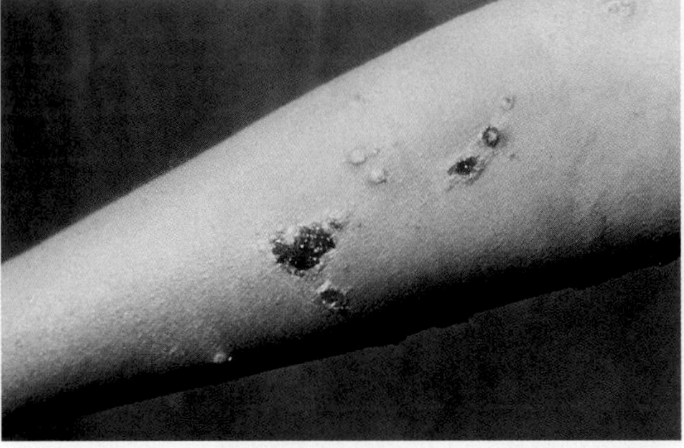

Fig 19.2 Impetigo.

3. Most frequently seen in children in environments where they are in close proximity with each other.

B. Etiology.
1. Highly contagious bacterial infection.
   a. Most frequently caused by *S. aureus*.
   b. May also be caused by *Streptococcus pyogenes* (i.e., group A strep).

C. Pathophysiology (Fig. 19.2).
1. Lesions, which are frequently pruritic, usually begin as a macular rash and progress to a **vesicular**, or blister-like rash.
2. Vesicles eventually rupture and ooze.
   a. Vesicular discharge eventually dries into a honey-colored crust.
   b. Discharge can contaminate and infect adjacent areas of the skin as well as direct contacts.

D. Diagnosis.
1. Clinical picture and culture of the lesion.

E. Treatment.
1. Frequent removal of the crusted lesions.
2. Oral and/or topical antibiotics.

F. Nursing considerations.
1. Impaired Skin Integrity/Infection/Deficient Knowledge.
   a. Maintain contact isolation, including no school, camp, or swimming, until the child is on antibiotics for a full 24 hr.
   b. Educate the parents and child, if appropriate, to:
      i. Practice meticulous handwashing.
      ii. Follow the therapeutic regimen carefully and to complete the full course of medication.
      iii. Employ contact precautions.
      iv. Cleanse the lesions and remove the crusts several times a day.
      v. Always bathe the child alone with antibacterial soap and to use a clean wash cloth and towel for each bath.
      vi. Make sure the child sleeps alone.

vii. Have the child change into clean clothes and, if needed, to wash the child's bedding each day.

viii. Avoid the spread of the infection to another surface, such as refraining from:

(1) Scratching the lesions and touching another surface of the body.

(2) Using a towel or touching another vector that has been in contact with the affected body part.

VI. Cellulitis

A. Incidence.

1. **Cellulitis** is seen in children of all ages.

B. Etiology.

1. Bacterial infection of the lower layers of the skin that is caused most frequently by *S. aureus* or group A streptococci. In some instances, community-associated MRSA (methicillin-resistant *S. aureus*) has been found to be the pathogen causing cellulitis (see "Pustules or Boils").
2. Bacteria usually enter the body through a puncture wound, scratch, abrasion, or other break in the epidermis.
3. Cellulitis also can develop after a serious upper respiratory infection, dental infection, or otitis media.

C. Pathophysiology (Fig. 19.3).

1. Cellulitis usually begins as an inflammatory response but, as bacteria proliferate, develops into a full-blown infection that migrates throughout the subcutaneous layer of the skin.
2. Unless a pustule develops, the infection is not contagious.
3. Signs and symptoms.
   a. Classic inflammatory signs and symptoms, i.e., redness, edema, warmth, and pain.
   b. The inflammatory responses often are accompanied by elevated temperature, malaise, lymphadenopathy, and induration.
   c. If the cellulitis is periorbital, the tissues surrounding the eye may appear bluish in color.

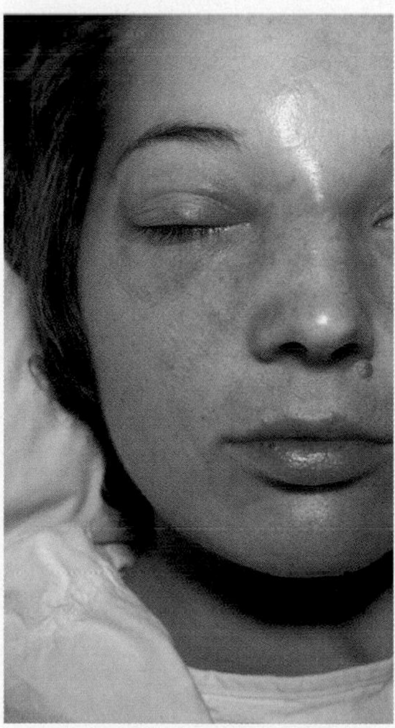

Fig 19.3 Periorbital cellulitis.

D. Diagnosis.

1. Clinical picture.
2. Culturing of the discharge, if present.
   a. If discharge is not present, a culture of an aspirate of the area may be performed.
3. Blood cultures, if indicated.
4. Complete blood count (CBC).

E. Treatment.

1. Intramuscular (IM), IV, and/or oral antibiotics.
   a. If the child is infected with MRSA, antibiotics specifically shown to be effective against the bacteria must be administered.
2. Acetaminophen or ibuprofen is prescribed for the pain.
3. Warm soaks are applied to the area to promote circulation and to reduce discomfort.
4. Excision and drainage of the wound may be required.

F. Nursing considerations.

1. Impaired Skin Integrity/Infection/Deficient Knowledge.
   a. If the child is hospitalized, a safe dosage of IM or IV antibiotics, employing the five rights, will likely be administered.
   b. If the child is treated at home, educate the parents and child, if appropriate, to:
      i. Practice meticulous handwashing.
      ii. Follow the therapeutic regimen carefully and to complete the full course of medication.
      iii. Apply warm soaks to the area—usually every 4 hr.
      iv. Monitor the child carefully for early signs of inflammation in the future and to report signs to the primary health-care provider in a timely manner.
2. Pain.
   a. Assess the child's pain level using an age-appropriate pain scale.
   b. If hospitalized, administer safe dosages of pain medication, as prescribed and as needed.
   c. If treated at home, educate the parents regarding the safe dosage and administration of pain medication.

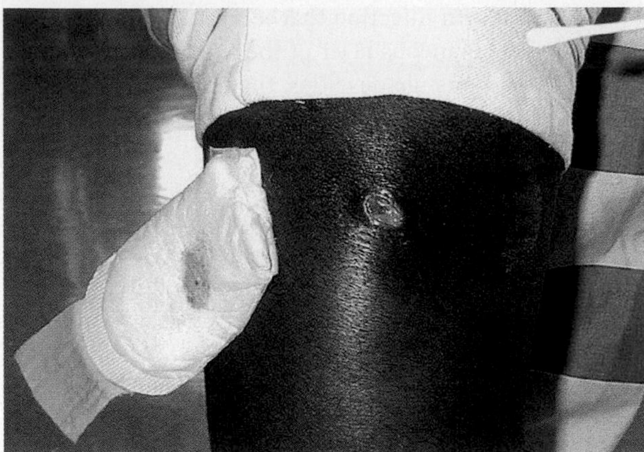

Fig 19.4 Cutaneous abscess caused by CA-MRSA.

d. Employ nonpharmacological pain reduction strategies, as needed.

VII. Pustules or Boils

Skin infections that ooze pus are called pustules, or boils. They often begin as what appears to be an insect bite or bump but quickly develop into purulent lesions. The most serious form of these infections is caused by community-associated **methicillin-resistant** ***S. aureus*** (Fig. 19.4). The remainder of this section of the chapter, therefore, is devoted to this infection.

A. Incidence.

1. Approximately one out of every three individuals carries CA-MRSA on his or her skin or in the nasal passages, but the majority of the individuals do not become infected by the bacteria.
2. The exact number of children who become infected is currently unknown, but the incidence is increasing.

B. Etiology.

1. MRSA is a *Staphylococcus aureus* bacterium that has mutated and become resistant to all of the most commonly prescribed antibiotics. When MRSA is contracted in the health-care environment (HA-MRSA), it usually causes serious invasive infections, for example, of the blood or of prostheses. Community-acquired MRSA (CA-MRSA) is spread skin-to-skin and most commonly causes pustules or boils.
2. The bacterial mutation has resulted from the indiscriminate and/or inappropriate use of antibiotics, i.e., prescribed to treat viral illnesses, such as the common cold, and many acute ear infections.

C. Pathophysiology.

1. A small injury to the skin, either via an abrasion, a cut, or other wound, becomes a portal for bacteria to enter the body.
2. CA-MRSA proliferates at the site.
3. The wound develops into a pus-filled lesion.
4. CA-MRSA infections can be life threatening when the bacteria spread into the blood or other areas of the body.

D. Diagnosis.

1. Clinical picture.
2. Culture and sensitivity of the purulent discharge.

E. Treatment.

1. Prevention.
   a. The Centers for Disease Control and Prevention (CDC) have developed an extensive procedure for such places as day-care centers, schools, and athletic facilities to maintain and clean their environs, including the following procedures: (For a full discussion, please see the CDC's "General Information About MRSA in the Community" [2013].)
      i. Meticulous handwashing.
      ii. Wearing clothing that protects the skin from punctures and abrasions.
      iii. Not sharing personal items, such as towels, razors, and clothing.
      iv. Thoroughly cleaning environmental surfaces.
   b. Parents should be advised to monitor their children's skin for bumps or lesions and, if any injuries fail to heal, to seek medical attention in a timely fashion.
2. Treatment.
   a. The CDC (2013) and the Infection Disease Society (Liu, et al, 2011) have developed an algorithm that practitioners are recommended to follow when an infection caused by CA-MRSA is suspected or confirmed.
      i. The treatment protocol includes excising and draining the lesion followed by keeping the area covered at all times.
      ii. If the injury fails to heal, antibiotics are administered.
         (1) Only antibiotics that have been shown to be effective against the infection are prescribed (see Table 19.1 for a list of the antibiotics that have been most effective).

F. Nursing considerations.

1. Risk for Infection/Deficient Knowledge.
   a. Parents must be educated regarding the possibility of severe infections developing from a small bite or skin lesion.
   b. Parents must be educated to:
      i. Practice meticulous handwashing.
      ii. Monitor their children's skin daily.

Table 19.1 Antibiotics Used to Treat CA-MRSA

Antibiotic	Important Information Relating to the Use in Children
clindamycin (Cleocin)	Has resulted in several severe cases of *Clostridium difficile* diarrhea.
tetracycline doxycycline (Vibramycin) minocycline (Minocin)	Tetracycline antibiotics are contraindicated for children under 8 years of age because the medication causes permanent staining of the secondary teeth.
trimethoprim-sulfamethoxazole (Bactrim)	Not recommended for children under 2 months of age.
rifampin (Rifadin)	Only administered with other medications, but drug-drug interactions are common.
linezolid (Zyvox)	Only administered in extreme cases because of the seriousness of medication side effects, including immunosuppression.

iii. Carefully cleanse and cover all small lesions on the skin.
iv. Seek medical assistance whenever signs of inflammation develop (i.e., warmth, redness, pain, swelling, and, especially, if pus is noted).

2. Impaired Skin Integrity/Infection/Deficient Knowledge if CA-MRSA is diagnosed.
   a. Educate the parents regarding the therapeutic regimen and, if antibiotics are prescribed, the importance of taking the correct dosages of the medications at prescribed times and until all medication has been taken.
   b. Educate the parents and child, if appropriate, regarding actions to prevent transmitting the infections to others, including:
      i. Practicing meticulous handwashing.
      ii. Keeping the lesion covered at all times.
         (1) Only if the drainage cannot be contained should the child be isolated and kept out of school.
      iii. Sharing no personal items, such as towels, sheets, and clothing, with others.
      iv. Wearing clean, washed attire each day.
         (1) All articles should be washed, as recommended by the manufacturer, with detergent and dried in a dryer.
3. Risk for Altered Coping/Anxiety if CA-MRSA is diagnosed.
   a. Allow the parents and child, if appropriate, to express fear, guilt, and concern over being diagnosed with a serious infection.

VIII. Dermatophytoses (also called Ringworm and Tinea Infections)

Even though the term *ringworm* is used to describe **dermatophytoses**, the infections are not caused by a worm or by any other insect. They are caused by a number of different fungi. The fungi live on top of (rather than in) the skin of humans; some also live on animal skin. In addition, the fungi can survive on inanimate surfaces (e.g., towels, bedding, floors) from which humans can become infected.

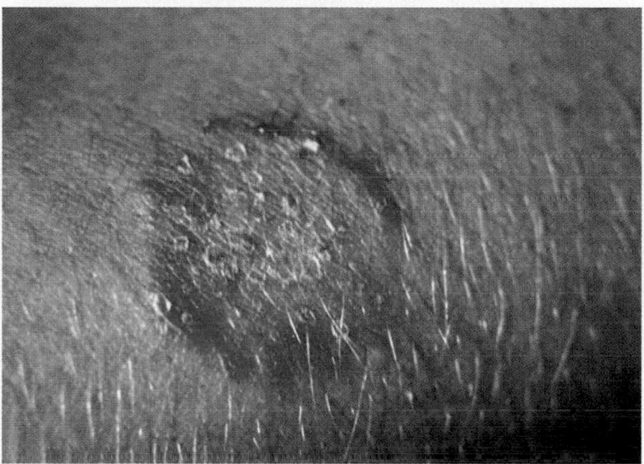

Fig 19.5 Tinea corporis, ringworm on the body.

A. Incidence: dependent on the type of dermatophyte.
1. Tinea capitis (i.e., ringworm of the head and scalp).
   a. Seen in children of all ages, but children with allergies are more susceptible to the infection than are others.
2. Tinea corporis (i.e., ringworm on body surfaces) (Fig. 19.5).
   a. Seen in children of all ages.
3. Tinea cruris (i.e., jock itch).
   a. Most commonly seen in adolescents, especially those involved in sports.
4. Tinea pedis (i.e., athlete's foot).
   a. Most frequently seen in teenagers, although it has been seen in younger children, especially those who wear rubber or plastic footwear.

B. Etiology.
1. There are several different fungi that can infect the child at each region of the body.

2. Two of the more common dermatophytes—*Trichophyton rubrum* and *Trichophyton tonsurans*—usually are transmitted from person to person. Other types are transmitted from animal to human or from inanimate object to human.

C. Pathophysiology.
1. The fungus, which resides on dead skin cells, usually is transmitted during direct contact.
2. Signs and symptoms.
   a. Skin, which is highly pruritic, appears reddened, dry, and scaly, and a distinct rash ring may be present.
   b. Patches of hair may fall out if the scalp or bearded areas of the body are infected.
   c. If the infection is not treated, cellulitis may result.

D. Diagnosis.
1. Clinical picture is highly suggestive.
2. Scrapings of the skin may be sent for fungal culture.

E. Treatment.
1. Oral or topical antifungal medications.
   a. Scalp infections usually require oral medications.
2. Complete eradication of the fungi may require many weeks of therapy.

F. Nursing considerations.
1. Impaired Skin Integrity/ Infection/ Deficient Knowledge.
   a. Educate the parents and child, if appropriate, regarding prevention strategies, including:
      i. Practicing frequent handwashing.
      ii. Refraining from sharing hairbrushes, caps, hats, and unwashed clothing.
      iii. Inspecting pets for signs of tinea infections.
      iv. Refraining from walking on damp, communal surfaces on which fungi may reside (e.g., near pools and in locker rooms).
   b. If child is infected, educate the parents and child, if appropriate, regarding treatment strategies, including:
      i. Maintaining excellent hygiene and handwashing practices.
      ii. Only using his or her own personal items, including towels, hair supplies, and caps.
      iii. Carefully following the prescribed treatment regimen and reporting any side effects of the medication to the primary health-care provider
      iv. If infected with tinea cruris, taking soothing sitz baths (i.e., plain water hip baths).
      v. If infected with tinea pedis, wearing light-colored socks and shoes that promote air exchange.

IX. Acne

A. Incidence.
1. Most frequently seen in adolescents, with a higher incidence in males.

B. Etiology.
1. Acne can be caused by many things, including bacterial invasion, stress, hormonal secretion, and heredity.

C. Pathophysiology.
1. Sebum is secreted resulting in a blockage of the sebaceous glands and proliferation of *Propionibacterium acnes* bacteria.
   a. For example, it is secreted during adolescence as a result of the increased hormone production.
2. If blockage is not reversed, black heads, white heads, and/or pustules develop.
3. A rupturing of the sebaceous gland blockage may result in scar formation.

D. Diagnosis.
1. Clinical picture.

E. Treatment.
1. Depends on the precise form that the acne has taken.
   a. Topical medications.
      i. Including benzoyl peroxide and tretinoin (Retin-A) to prevent the development of the acne lesions.
      ii. Antibiotics to reduce the *P. acnes* colonization levels.
   b. Oral medications are prescribed in severe cases.
   c. Additional topical therapies to remedy skin lesions (e.g., dermabrasion).

F. Nursing considerations.
1. Impaired Skin Integrity/Risk for Infection/ Deficient Knowledge.
   a. Educate the parents and teen regarding the etiology of acne.
   b. Educate the patient regarding the individualized treatment regimen, including washing the face twice daily with antibacterial soap and washing the hair daily.
   c. Advise the teen to refrain from injuring the face by overscrubbing or picking at lesions.
   d. Encourage the teen to use water-based cosmetics only.
   e. Reinforce the importance of eating a nutritious diet and living a healthy lifestyle.

2. Risk for Altered Coping/Risk for Disturbed Body Image.
   a. Encourage the teen to discuss concerns regarding the diagnosis and treatment regimen.
   b. Listen carefully to the teen's comments for signs of altered coping or disturbed body image.
   c. Encourage the parents to provide the teen with words of encouragement to promote his or her self-image and self-esteem.

X. Pediculosis (Lice)

A. Incidence.
1. **Pediculosis (lice)** are prevalent in children, especially in preschoolers and school-age children, with girls being affected more frequently than boys.

B. Etiology.
1. Small insects that survive by sucking human blood.
   a. Pediculosis capitis: head lice.
   b. Pediculosis corporis: body lice.
   c. Pediculosis pubis: pubic lice or "crabs."
2. Acquired through direct contact.
   a. Pubic lice are contracted during sexual activity.

C. Pathophysiology.
1. Head lice.
   a. Lice rarely are visible because they scurry to evade light, but the child experiences marked pruritus from the movement of the lice.
      i. Lesions, seen predominantly on the neck and behind the ears, develop from recurrent itching.
   b. Nits (i.e., lice eggs) are seen on the shaft of the hair.

DID YOU KNOW?
You can easily differentiate nits from dandruff. Nits are difficult to remove because of the "lice glue" holding them in place, while dandruff is easily brushed from the hair.

2. Body lice (Fig. 19.6).
   a. Pruritus and lesions of affected areas.
3. Pubic lice.
   a. Itching in the genital area.
   b. May see blue spots on the thighs.

D. Diagnosis.
1. Clinical picture.

E. Treatment.
1. Prevention.
   a. Children should be encouraged to avoid using others' combs and brushes and wearing others' hats.

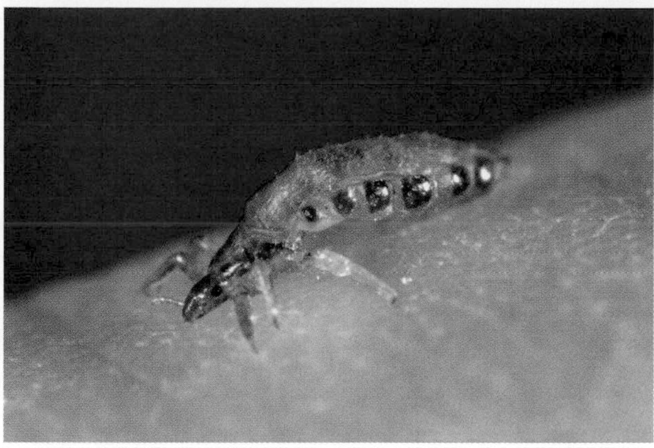

Fig 19.6 A female body louse.

   b. Sexually active individuals should be encouraged to engage only in monogamous relations, carefully examine the genitalia of their sexual partners and, if infested, to avoid all sexual contact until they have been treated.
2. Treatment: the goal of treatment is to kill both the insects and the eggs.
   a. Over-the-counter pediculicides, such as permethrin (e.g., Nix) or pyrethrins (e.g., Rid and Triple X) are the primary treatment.
      i. All persons who have had intimate contact with the infected person should be treated at the same time to prevent reinfestation.
      ii. All clothing that has been in contact with the infected site should be removed.
      iii. The area of infestation should be washed well with regular shampoo and dried.
         (1) Hair conditioner should not be used.
      iv. The medication should be applied to the affected area and, as stated on the label, removed after having been left in place for the allotted time.
         (1) If after 8 to 12 hr the lice are still as active as before the treatment, the primary health-care practitioner should be notified because a prescription medication may be required (e.g., lindane).
      v. The nits, or lice eggs, should be removed from the shafts of the hair with a fine-toothed comb.
         (1) The hair should be inspected each day following treatment and, if the nits reappear, they should be removed with the fine-toothed comb.

vi. Following the treatment, the child should don clean clothing that has been washed in water at least 130°F and dried in a hot dryer.

vii. Because any remaining eggs will hatch in 7 to 10 days, it is recommended that the site be retreated with the same medication approximately 1 week after the first administration.

3. As an alternate treatment, sitting under a commercial hair dryer for 30 min has shown some promise in killing lice.
4. To prevent reinfestation:
   a. All washable items (e.g., clothing, bedding, towels) that have been in contact with the child should be washed in water that is at least 130°F and dried on high heat for at least 20 min.
   b. Other items should be treated in the following manner:
      i. Either dry-cleaned or enclosed in an airtight, plastic bag for 2 weeks.
      ii. All hair products (i.e., brushes and combs) placed in hot water, 130°F or higher, for at least 10 min before reuse.
      iii. The entire living area vacuumed well, and the vacuum bag carefully disposed of.
   c. It is not recommended that the home be sprayed and fogged.

F. Nursing considerations.

1. Risk for Situational Low Self-Esteem/Deficient Knowledge.
   a. Reinforce the fact that pediculosis can happen to anyone; it is acquired from physical contact, not from poor hygiene.
   b. Educate the parents and children, if applicable, to refrain from using other children's personal items.
2. Impaired Skin Integrity/Infection.
   a. Maintain contact isolation in school, camp, or other similar environments until the child has been treated.
      i. Once treated, the child may return to school or other activities the next day.
   b. Educate the parents regarding the need for all members of the family who have had direct contact with the child (e.g., slept in same bed, shared hair products, shared hats) to be treated at the same time as the infected child.
   c. Educate the parents to follow the directions of the pediculicide carefully and to reapply in 7 to 10 days from first application.
   d. Following the application of the pediculicide, teach parents to remove the nits by carefully combing the hair using a fine-toothed comb (usually supplied with the pediculicide).
   e. Educate the parents regarding the need to perform delousing of the environment, as stated earlier.

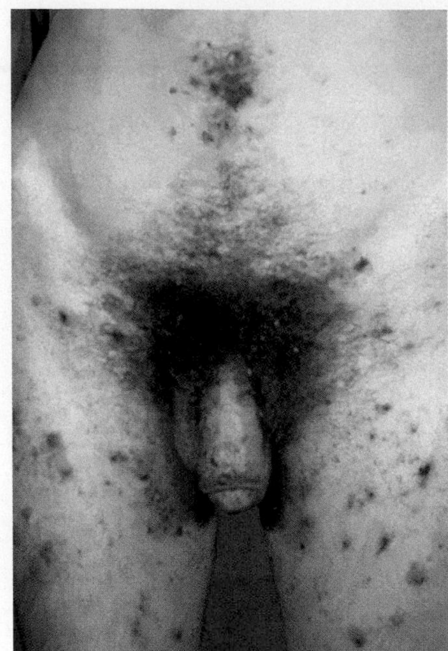

Fig 19.7 A patient with scabies.

XI. Scabies

A. Incidence.

1. **Scabies** (Fig. 19.7) is seen in children of all ages.
2. Most prevalent in areas where children are in close contact with each other.

B. Etiology.

1. Infecting agents are small mites.
2. Transmission occurs when a child is in direct contact with another individual who is infected with the mites.

C. Pathophysiology.

1. Mites crawl on the skin, and infestation occurs when female mites burrow under the skin and lay their eggs.
2. Eggs hatch, and mites crawl to the skin surface.
3. Intense itching results from an inflammatory response to the mites and their feces.
   a. Itching rarely is significant until the child has been infected for 2 or 3 weeks, but the child is communicable during that time.
   b. Itching usually persists for 2 to 4 weeks following treatment.

D. Diagnosis.
1. Visual evidence of the burrows is seen on the skin with a magnifying glass.

E. Treatment.
1. All persons who have had intimate contact with the infected person should be treated at the same time to prevent reinfestation.
2. Topical medications are obtainable only by prescription, such as:
   a. Permethrin cream 5% (Elimite): usually the first medication administered.
      i. Approved for use for anyone over the age of 2 months.
      ii. To kill both the mites and the eggs, two applications are required, 1 week apart.
      iii. Application.
         (1) The child should shower or bathe before treatment.
         (2) In older children and adolescents, the medicine should be spread over the entire body from the neck down, including the feet and toes, and left in place for the time recommended in the medication flyer, usually at least 8 hr.
         (3) For infants and young children, medication should also be applied to the scalp, face, and neck because scabies often affect those parts of their bodies.
         (4) After treatment, the child showers to remove the medicine and dons clean clothing.
   b. Lindane lotion 1%: should be used only if permethrin is ineffective.
      i. Should be used only on adolescents who weigh over 110 lb.
      ii. Should not be used if a teen is pregnant or lactating.
   c. Crotamiton lotion 10% and Crotamiton cream 10% (Eurax; Crotan).
      i. This medication has not been approved for use in children, and its failure rate is high.
   d. Ivermectin (Stromectol).
      i. Oral medication primarily is used to treat parasite infestation but has been seen to be effective against scabies.
      ii. This medication has not been approved for use in children or pregnant women.
3. Treatment of clothing and the environment (see "Pediculosis").
   a. Items that cannot be washed need only be in an airtight bag for 72 hr.

F. Nursing considerations (see "Pediculosis").

XII. Burns

A. Incidence.
1. Highest incidence is seen in preschoolers and young school-age children because of their inquisitiveness and increasing physical abilities.

B. Etiology.
1. Accidental.
   a. Playing with matches, candles, and other sources of open flame.
   b. Playing with electrical cords, sockets, and other sources of electricity.
   c. Playing with hot water faucets, pots and pans on the stove, hot coffee cups, and other sources of hot liquids.
2. Intentional (child abuse) accounts for about 6% of burns (see "Child Abuse and Neglect" in Chapter 23, "Nursing Care of the Child With Psychosocial Disorders").
   a. Cigarette burns.
   b. Emersion burns.
   c. Burns from irons, coffee, and boiling water.
3. The severity of the burn often is the determining factor in the potential for a positive outcome.

C. Pathophysiology.
1. Because of cell damage, intracellular fluid loss results in serious fluid volume and electrolyte shifts.
2. Portal of entry for bacteria places the child at high risk for infection.
3. Tissue damage, if extensive, can result in scarring and permanent disfigurement.

D. Diagnosis: the diagnosis of burns is dependent on a combination of two factors: the depth of the burn (i.e., how many layers of skin are affected), and the extent of the burn (i.e., how much of the child's skin has been burned).
1. The depth of the burn is classified as either first, second, or third degree (see Fig. 19.8 and Table 19.2).
2. Extent of the burn (Fig. 19.9).
   a. To determine the extent of the burn (i.e., how much of the body surface area has been affected), percentages of the body have been established:
      i. The rule of 9s has been developed to estimate the extent of burns for anyone over the age of 10.
      ii. Other percentage estimates have been developed for children from infancy through to 5 years of age and from 5 to 9 years of age.

Table 19.2 Burn Degrees and Characteristics

Burn Degree	Layers of Skin Affected	Characteristics
First Degree	Epidermal layer only is affected.	No blisters are seen, but the skin is reddened and painful.
Second Degree	Epidermal and dermal layers are affected.	Deep blistering is seen, and the area is very painful.
Third Degree	Deep tissue damage, including nerves.	Charred appearance, and sensory nerves are damaged.

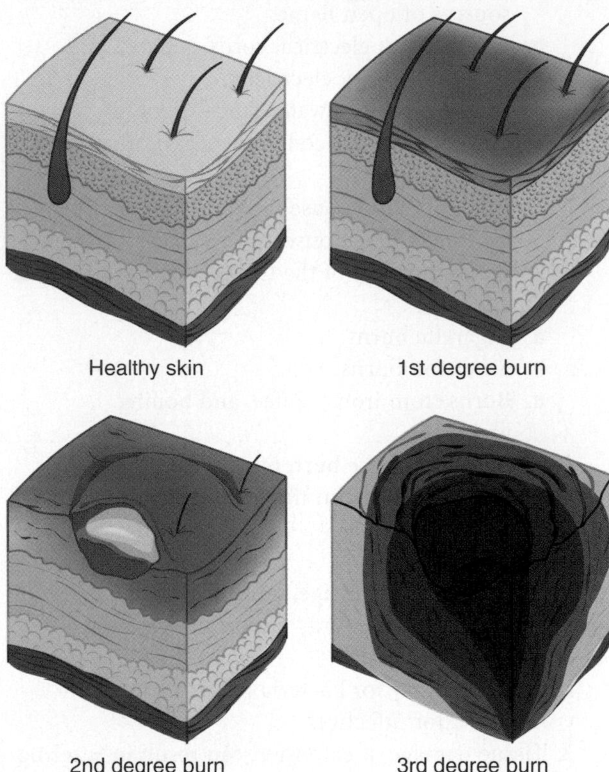

Fig 19.8 Degree of burn injury.

E. Treatment.

1. Prevention:
   a. It is essential to provide parent education regarding activities that place children at high risk for burns (see "Nursing considerations").
2. Dependent on the severity of the burn.
   a. Primary intervention, when indicated.
      i. Reverse fluid imbalance by administering IV fluids (see Chapter 13, "Nursing Care of the Child With Fluid and Electrolyte Alterations").
         (1) Lactated Ringer's solution often is ordered.
      ii. Assess serum electrolytes, and replace electrolytes, as needed.
         (1) With cell wall damage, shifts in electrolytes often are seen.
3. If first-degree burn.
   a. Cool down the site with a cool washcloth and cool water.
      i. Ice **should not be used for first-degree burns** because it may result in additional injury to the flesh.
      ii. Apply soothing lotions.
4. If second-degree burn.
   a. Cool down the site, as with first-degree burns.
   b. Unless the burn is extensive, usually the child will be cared for as an outpatient.
      i. Site is cleansed daily using aseptic technique.
      ii. Tetanus booster is administered if it has been more than 5 years since the last injection.
         (1) Burn sites are easy portals of entry to tetanus bacteria.
5. If third-degree burn: hospitalization is likely.
   a. Care as discussed for second-degree burns, plus:
   b. Debridement of the wound, which entails removing the eschar or dead tissue.
   c. Application of antibiotic dressings and ointments.
      i. Silvadene (silver sulfadiazine cream) is most commonly used.

F. Nursing considerations.

1. Deficient Knowledge regarding the potential for accidental burns.
   a. Children should be kept out of direct sunlight, especially between 10 a.m. and 4 p.m., unless they are covered with sun protection lotion. The lotions should:
      i. Contain both UVA and UVB protectant.
      ii. Be applied at least every 2 hr and reapplied whenever the child gets wet.

DID YOU KNOW?

The Food and Drug Administration (FDA) has established strict guidelines for the contents and labeling of sunscreen products. For specific information, see the FDA's Web site: www.fda.gov/ForConsumers/ConsumerUpdates/ucm258416.htm.

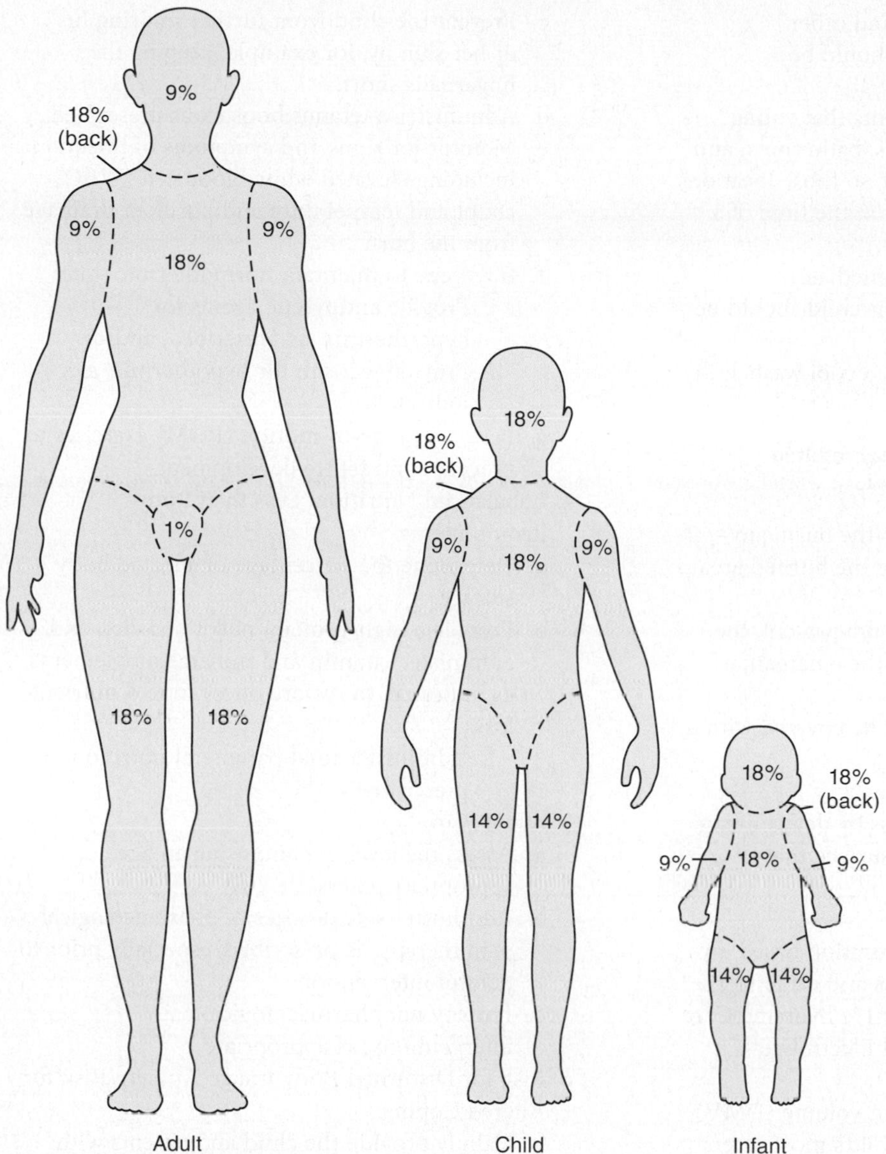

Fig 19.9 Extent of burn injury.

b. Fire and smoke alarms should be installed throughout the home, and batteries should be changed yearly.

DID YOU KNOW?

In order to help parents to remember to replace the fire and smoke alarm batteries, they can be taught to change the batteries at the same time each year (e.g., every spring when the time changes or every year on a specific holiday).

c. Have fire drills for home safety, including teaching children to "stop, drop, and roll."

d. Dangerous items (e.g., matches, electrical cords, electrical sockets) should be kept out of reach of young children.

e. The hot water heater should be set no higher than 120°F.

f. Pots should be placed on the back burners of the stove, and the handles should face toward the wall.

g. Stove knobs should be covered with childproof covers.

h. Children should be kept at a distance from hot foods, drinks, and other hot substances.

i. Grills, fireplaces, radiators, and other such heat-producing items should be gated off.
j. It is important to teach parents that young children often hide in closets, bathrooms, and under beds when frightened, so those locations should be searched carefully at the time of a fire.
k. Parents should be taught immediate intervention measures if their child should be burned.
   i. Cool down the site with a cool washcloth or cool water.

Ice should not be used because it may result in additional injury to the flesh.

   ii. Unless it has adhered to the burn, any clothing that is touching the burned area should be removed.
   iii. If blistering or charring are present, the child should be seen in the emergency department.
   iv. The burned area should be covered with a clean sheet.

2. Risk for Deficient Fluid Volume.
   a. Assess the extent of fluid loss by determining the percentage of the body surface that is affected.
   b. Weigh the child daily.
   c. Determine the level of dehydration based on the percentage of weight loss and other signs of dehydration (see Chapter 13, "Nursing Care of the Child With Fluid and Electrolyte Alterations").
   d. Calculate the daily minimum volume (DMV) for the child based on the child's most recent weight (See Chapter 13).
      i. The child's fluid needs will markedly exceed his or her DMV.
   e. Administer safe dosages of IV medications employing the five rights of medication administration, as needed and as prescribed.
   f. Carefully monitor strict intake and output (I&O).
   g. Monitor laboratory values, especially serum electrolytes, renal function studies, and complete blood count (CBC).
3. Risk for Infection/Impaired Skin Integrity.
   a. Gently clean the burn, and debride the wound, as needed.
   b. Maintain aseptic technique.
      i. Admit to the burn unit, and maintain reverse isolation.
      ii. Perform meticulous handwashing.
   c. Prevent the child from further injuring his or her skin by, for example, keeping the fingernails short.
   d. Administer a tetanus booster, as prescribed.
   e. Monitor for signs and symptoms of infection, including elevated white blood cell (WBC) count and temperature and purulent drainage from the burn.
   f. Intervene to maintain normothermic state.
      i. Provide antipyretic agents for hyperthermia, as prescribed, and/or:
      ii. Provide warmth for hypothermia, as indicated.
   g. Perform range-of-motion (ROM) exercises to prevent contracture development.
4. Imbalanced Nutrition: Less than Body Requirements.
   a. Determine the percentage of affected body surface.
   b. Provide a high-protein, nutritious diet, and administer vitamin and mineral supplements, as indicated, to restore nitrogen and nutrient loss.
      i. Administer total parenteral nutrition, if prescribed.
5. Acute Pain.
   a. Assess the level of pain, using an age-appropriate pain scale.
   b. Administer safe dosages of pharmacological pain therapy, as prescribed, especially prior to painful interventions.
   c. Employ nonpharmacological pain interventions, as appropriate.
6. Risk for Disturbed Body Image/Anxiety/Risk for Altered Coping.
   a. Calmly provide the child and parents with information regarding burn care, employing simple and concise language.
   b. Provide opportunities for the child and parents to express fears, concerns, and guilt.
   c. Refer the family, as needed, to social services and/or child protective services.
   d. Encourage the family, if appropriate, to seek spiritual guidance from a clergyperson.
   e. Assist the family to identify support systems and coping strategies.
   f. Allow the parents and child to express concerns/fears regarding the child's future appearance.
   g. Provide the child and family with honest answers regarding care and prognosis.
   h. Provide grief counseling, as needed.

CASE STUDY: Putting It All Together

An 8 year old girl

Subjective Data

- Mother calls her 8-year-old child's primary health-care provider and states,
  - "I just picked my daughter up from school because the school nurse says that my daughter has lice. That can't be. I wash my daughter's hair every night."

Objective Data

Nursing Assessment (performed via telephone)

- Nurse states,
  - "I am so sorry to hear that. It is possible for clean, healthy children to become infected with lice."
  - "While I am on the phone, I want you to check your child's hair. What do you see?"
- Mother responds,
  - "It looks like my daughter has dandruff."
- Nurse states,
  - "Are you able to brush the dandruff off from your child's hair?"
- Mother responds,
  - "No. It is really sticking to the hair! Oh, and my daughter says that her head itches really bad. In fact, I see scratch marks all along her neck and behind her ears."
- Nurse states,
  - "I am afraid that the school nurse is correct. Your child does have lice."
  - "I am sorry, I know that this is distressing. Please know, however, that it is not your or your child's fault. Lice are very small insects that can walk from one child to another very easily. Or, your child may have borrowed a hat or hair brush from another child. This does not, in any way, mean that your child is poorly cared for."
  - "The doctor has a standard care plan for children with lice and their families. Do you have an e-mail address where I can send the instructions? If you have any questions, please don't hesitate to call me. And please also note, the doctor does recommend that you and anyone else living in the home be treated at the same time. We also recommend that you notify the parents of your child's best friends so that they are informed."
- Mother responds with her e-mail address and thanks the nurse.

Health-Care Provider's Protocol for Lice Infestation (sent to the child's mother via e-mail)

- Purchase enough pediculicide to treat the entire family, such as permethrin (e.g., Nix) or pyrethrin (e.g., Rid and Triple X).
- Treatment procedure:
  - Remove all clothing from the child that is in contact with the hair.
  - Wash hair well with regular shampoo and dry.
    - Do NOT use hair conditioner after shampooing.
  - Apply medication as stated on the medication label, wait the allotted time, and remove the medication as stated on the label.
  - After removing the medication, carefully comb through the hair using the fine-toothed comb provided in the medication box to remove the eggs (nits) from the hair shafts.
  - After treatment, dress your child in clean clothes that have been washed in hot water and dried on high heat.
  - Check the hair 12 hr after the treatment is completed. If any lice are seen, notify the office for an appointment. A prescription medication may be required (e.g., lindane).
  - Inspect the hair daily following the treatment and remove any nits with the fine-toothed comb.
  - Retreat with the same medication in 7 to 10 days to kill lice newly hatched from eggs, and, again, comb the hair with the fine-toothed comb.
  - Follow the same directions as above for yourself and for anyone else living in the home who has had direct contact with the child, e.g., slept in the same bed, shared the child's hats or hair products, etc.
- Additional actions that should be taken:
  - Wash all washable items (e.g., clothing, bedding, towels) that have been in contact with the child in hot water, and dry the items on high heat for at least 20 min.
  - For any items that may not be washed (e.g., stuffed animals, wool coats), either dry-clean or enclose them in an airtight, plastic bag for 2 full weeks.
  - Place all hair products (e.g., brushes, combs, hair clips) in hot water for at least 10 min before reusing.
  - Vacuum the entire living area of the home well, and carefully dispose of the vacuum bag.
  - It is NOT recommended to spray and/or fog the home.

Continued

CASE STUDY: Putting It All Together *cont'd*

Case Study Questions

A. What *subjective* assessments indicate that this client is experiencing a health alteration?

1. ______
2. ______
3. ______

B. What *objective* assessments indicate that this client is experiencing a health alteration?

1. ______

C. After analyzing the data that has been collected, what **primary** nursing diagnosis should the nurse assign to this client?

1. ______

D. What interventions should the nurse plan and/or implement to meet this child's and her family's needs?

1. ______
2. ______
3. ______

E. What client outcomes should the nurse evaluate regarding the effectiveness of the nursing interventions?

1. ______

F. What physiological characteristics should the child exhibit after treatment?

1. ______

G. What subjective characteristics should the child exhibit after treatment?

1. ______

REVIEW QUESTIONS

1. A breastfed baby has thrush and a bright-red diaper rash. The baby's mother is complaining of severe pain each time the baby feeds. The nurse suspects that which of the following organisms is likely responsible for these complaints?
   1. *Staphylococcus aureus*
   2. *Candida albicans*
   3. *Streptococcus pyogenes*
   4. *Herpes simplex*

2. A mother telephones her 8-month-old baby's primary health-care provider and informs the triage nurse, "My baby has a diaper rash. I have been putting baby powder on the rash, but it doesn't seem to be getting any better. What should I do?" Which of the following responses by the nurse is most appropriate?
   1. "It is important that you stop using the powder. If the baby breathes it in, it will make the baby very sick."
   2. "Exposing the rash to the air often helps. I would suggest leaving the baby's diaper off for ten minutes every few hours. That should help."
   3. "I would suggest that you switch to cornstarch from the powder. The natural properties in the cornstarch are healing."
   4. "I am making an appointment for the baby to be seen. It is very rare for babies to develop diaper rashes when they are at your baby's age."

3. The nurse has provided teaching to a mother whose 5-month-old has been diagnosed with atopic dermatitis (eczema). Which of the following statements by the mother indicates that teaching was successful?
   1. "I make sure that my baby is clothed warmly each day."
   2. "My baby's favorite toy is a fuzzy teddy bear."
   3. "Today, my baby is wearing a hand-knit wool sweater that my mother knit."
   4. "Tomorrow, I plan to dress my baby in a cute cotton shirt and denim jeans."

4. To determine whether a baby is allergic to foods, the nurse should educate parents to feed their babies employing which of the following procedures?
   1. Babies' first foods should be either pureed apples or peaches.
   2. The first time babies are fed solid foods, the babies should be at least 8 months of age.
   3. Babies' first foods should be fed one at a time for 4 to 7 days each.
   4. The first time babies are fed solid foods, the foods should be mixed with apple juice.

5. A baby has been diagnosed with atopic dermatitis (eczema). Which of the following signs/symptoms would the nurse expect to see?
   1. Macular rash on the baby's back and shoulders.
   2. Vesicular rash over the baby's abdomen and perineum.
   3. Weepy rash over both of the baby's forearms and cheeks.
   4. Scaly rash on the baby's scalp and forehead.

6. The lesion on a child's face has been diagnosed as impetigo. Which of the following information should the nurse educate the parents in relation to this problem? **Select all that apply.**
   1. Child should refrain from bathing until the lesions are completely healed.
   2. Crusts should be removed several times each day using contact precautions.
   3. Child must be on antibiotics for at least twenty-four hours before returning to school.
   4. Meticulous handwashing must be maintained to prevent transmission to others in the family.
   5. Safe dosage of Benadryl (diphenhydramine) should be administered at bedtime until the lesions resolve.

7. A child has been diagnosed with periorbital cellulitis. For which of the following signs/symptoms should the nurse assess?
   1. Subconjunctival hemorrhages
   2. Yellow-tinged sclerae
   3. Bluish streaks in tissues surrounding the eye
   4. Absence of the red reflex during eye examination

8. A 10-year-old child has cellulitis of the calf. Which of the following interventions should the nurse educate the parents to implement?
   1. Have the child use crutches when ambulating.
   2. Apply warm compresses to the inflamed area.
   3. Measure the depth of edema each day the child is on antibiotics.
   4. Locate and culture the item that punctured the child's skin.

9. A 12-year-old child has been diagnosed with athlete's foot. Which of the following information should the nurse include in the patient education regarding the disease?
   1. The anaerobic bacteria that cause the infection must be treated with intravenous antibiotics.
   2. Eradication of the infection can take many weeks of treatment.
   3. Transmission of the mites is by direct, person-to-person contact.
   4. The child must deprive the causative organism of oxygen by wearing shoes that are fully enclosed.

10. A 17-year-old young woman is being seen in the primary health-care provider's office for a chief complaint of acne. Which of the following diagnoses would be appropriate for the nurse to include in the client's plan of care?
1. Powerlessness
2. Risk for Ineffective Coping
3. Risk for Self-mutilation
4. Self-neglect

11. The school nurse notifies the mother of a 7-year-old girl that her child has head lice (*pediculosis capitis*). Which of the following information should the nurse advise the mother regarding the problem?
1. "I strongly suggest that you cut your child's hair short before using the lice medicine, and keep it short from now on."
2. "Your child will need to be kept at home until she has received the second treatment, one week after the first."
3. "After using the lice medicine, you will need to comb your child's hair with a fine-toothed comb."
4. "For up to three weeks after being treated with the lice medicine, your child may complain of itching."

12. The clinic nurse is educating the parents of a 10-year-old child with scabies regarding medication administration. Which of the following information should the nurse include in the teaching?
1. The child should have been bathed at least 24 hours prior to the administration of the medication.
2. The oral medication must be administered on an empty stomach.
3. The topical medication must remain on the skin for 8 full hours.
4. The parent should readminister the medication in one week if the child continues to complain of itching.

13. A 5-year-old child who was playing with matches is admitted to the pediatric emergency department. The child has blistered burns covering both anterior thighs. Which of the following responses is consistent with the child's presentation?

The depth and extent of the burns are:
1. Depth: 1°; extent: 10%
2. Depth: 2°; extent: 7%
3. Depth: 2°; extent: 18%
4. Depth: 3°; extent: 3%

14. An 8-year-old child is admitted to the emergency department with burns over 30% of the body. Which of the following orders is highest priority for the nurse to perform?
1. Injection of tetanus booster
2. Debridement of the burns
3. Application of Silvadene ointment
4. Administration of intravenous fluids

15. A mother telephones the nurse at her child's primary health-care provider and states, "My child spilled my coffee on her arm. About one-half of the forearm is red, and there are 2 or 3 blisters that have developed. What should I do?" Which of the following is the best response for the nurse to give?
1. "Run cool water over the burned area and then call me back."
2. "Apply ice to the blisters for ten minutes on and ten minutes off."
3. "Proceed to the emergency department for a complete assessment."
4. "Cover the burned area with petroleum jelly and sterile bandages."

16. The mother of a 10-year-old child telephones the child's primary health-care provider's office. The mother informs the nurse, "A spider bit my daughter a couple of days ago, and today it is looking really bad. The bite is oozing, and the skin around the bite is red and painful." Which of the following statements by the nurse is appropriate at this time?
1. "I bet the bite is infected with a dangerous bacteria. She must be seen immediately, so that we can start her on antibiotics."
2. "I would like her to be seen today. Please cover the bite, and bring her in for an appointment."
3. "Spider bites are notorious for getting worse before they get better. It should clear up in a couple of days."
4. "It sounds like the bite has been inflamed. I want you to put warm compresses on it three times a day until it gets better."

REVIEW ANSWERS

1. ANSWER: 2

Rationale:

1. Although *S. aureus* can cause skin infections, the signs and symptoms of the baby and the mother are not consistent with an infection from *S. aureus*.

2. *C. albicans* causes thrush and bright-red diaper rashes in neonates. Breastfeeding mothers whose nipples are infected with *C. albicans* complain of severe pain while feeding.

3. Although *S. pyogenes* can cause skin infections, the signs and symptoms of the baby and the mother are not consistent with an infection from *S. pyogenes*.

4. Although *H. simplex* can cause skin infections, the signs and symptoms of the baby and the mother are not consistent with a herpes infection.

TEST-TAKING TIP: When a mother and her breastfed baby are infected with *C. albicans*, it is important for them both to be treated for at least 2 weeks. If either is treated independently, or if the length of treatment is less than 2 weeks, it is likely that the infection will continue.

Content Area: *Pediatrics—Infant*
Integrated Processes: *Nursing Process: Analysis*
Client Need: *Physiological Integrity: Physiological Adaptation: Pathophysiology*
Cognitive Level: *Application*

2. ANSWER: 2

Rationale:

1. This information is important to provide the mother, but the nurse should state the information using gentler language.

2. This is the appropriate response.

3. It is recommended that cornstarch be used rather than powder. It does not, however, have healing properties.

4. Babies develop diaper rash more frequently after they reach 6 months of age.

TEST-TAKING TIP: Diaper rashes usually develop from the combination of exposure to the baby's urine and fecal enzymes. Changing the diaper as soon as the child wets or soils the diaper and exposing the baby's bottom to the air for a few minutes after each diaper change help to prevent and to treat diaper rash.

Content Area: *Pediatrics—Infant*
Integrated Processes: *Nursing Process: Implementation; Teaching/Learning*
Client Need: *Physiological Integrity: Reduction of Risk Potential: Therapeutic Procedures*
Cognitive Level: *Application*

3. ANSWER: 4

Rationale:

1. This mother needs additional education. Babies who are too warmly dressed often exhibit worsening symptoms.

2. This mother needs additional education. Fuzzy toys often exacerbate symptoms.

3. This mother needs additional education. Wool often exacerbates symptoms.

4. It is recommended that babies with eczema be dressed in cotton clothing.

TEST-TAKING TIP: Food allergies often precipitate atopic dermatitis (eczema). When a baby suffers from eczema, parents should be taught that warm environments, wool fabrics, dry skin, and perfumed soaps often intensify the symptoms.

Content Area: *Pediatrics*
Integrated Processes: *Nursing Process: Evaluation*
Client Need: *Physiological Integrity: Reduction of Risk Potential: Potential for Alterations in Body Systems*
Cognitive Level: *Application*

4. ANSWER: 3

Rationale:

1. Babies' first foods should be nonallergenic cereals (e.g., rice cereal).

2. The American Academy of Pediatrics recommends that solids be introduced into infants' diets at approximately 6 months of age.

3. Babies' first foods should be fed one at a time for 4 to 7 days each. This statement is true.

4. The first time babies are fed solid foods, the foods should be mixed with formula or breast milk.

TEST-TAKING TIP: Parents should be taught to monitor their children for signs of atopic dermatitis after a new food is introduced into their infants' diet. If symptoms appear, the food should be eliminated from the diet until the child is older.

Content Area: *Pediatrics—Infant*
Integrated Processes: *Nursing Process: Implementation; Teaching/Learning*
Client Need: *Physiological Integrity: Reduction of Risk Potential: Potential for Alterations in Body Systems*
Cognitive Level: *Application*

5. ANSWER: 3

Rationale:

1. The red, weepy rash usually is seen over both of the baby's forearms and cheeks.

2. The red, weepy rash usually is seen over both of the baby's forearms and cheeks.

3. The red, weepy rash usually is seen over both of the baby's forearms and cheeks.

4. The red, weepy rash usually is seen over both of the baby's forearms and cheeks.

TEST-TAKING TIP: The nurse would expect to see the rash bilaterally. It most frequently appears on the baby's cheeks and on the forearms. The more the baby scratches the lesions, usually by rubbing them against the bedclothes, the worse the symptoms become.

Content Area: *Pediatrics*
Integrated Processes: *Nursing Process: Assessment*
Client Need: *Physiological Integrity: Physiological Adaptation: Alterations in Body Systems*
Cognitive Level: *Application*

6. **ANSWER: 2, 3, and 4**

Rationale:

1. This statement is false. The child should bathe regularly, albeit the child should always bathe alone.
2. **This statement is correct. The crusts, caused by the oozing of vesicular fluid, should be removed when they form. Contact precautions should be maintained to prevent transmission.**
3. **This statement is correct. After antibiotics have been taken for 24 hr, the child can return to school or camp.**
4. **This statement is correct. Meticulous handwashing must be maintained to prevent transmission to others in the family.**
5. Although the lesions are pruritic, Benadryl (diphenhydramine) usually is not prescribed.

TEST-TAKING TIP: Impetigo, caused by *S. aureus* or group A streptococci, is very contagious. To prevent transmission, the parents should be counseled that their child should bathe and sleep alone and have his or her own towel, clothing, and other personal items separate from those of others in the family.

Content Area: *Pediatrics*
Integrated Processes: *Nursing Process: Implementation; Teaching/Learning*
Client Need: *Physiological Integrity: Reduction of Risk Potential: Therapeutic Procedures*
Cognitive Level: *Application*

7. **ANSWER: 3**

Rationale:

1. Subconjunctival hemorrhages are not related to periorbital cellulitis.
2. Yellow-tinged sclerae are not related to periorbital cellulitis.
3. **Bluish streaks in tissues surrounding the eye are seen in children with periorbital cellulitis.**
4. Absence of the red reflex during eye examination is not related to periorbital cellulitis.

TEST-TAKING TIP: Cellulitis is characterized by an infection of the lower layers of the skin. In addition to the inflammatory signs and symptoms, when cellulitis surrounds the eye, bluish streaks often appear.

Content Area: *Pediatrics*
Integrated Processes: *Nursing Process: Assessment*
Client Need: *Physiological Integrity: Physiological Adaptation: Alterations in Body Systems*
Cognitive Level: *Application*

8. **ANSWER: 2**

Rationale:

1. The child may ambulate normally.
2. **Warm compresses promote circulation to the area.**
3. Some edema is noted, but it is not necessary to measure the depth of edema each day.
4. The object that punctured the skin may not be known, and, even if it is, it is rarely cultured.

TEST-TAKING TIP: In addition to warm compresses to the area, the child will be treated either with oral or IV antibiotics.

Content Area: *Pediatrics*
Integrated Processes: *Nursing Process: Implementation; Teaching/Learning*
Client Need: *Physiological Integrity: Physiological Adaptation: Illness Management*
Cognitive Level: *Application*

9. **ANSWER: 2**

Rationale:

1. The child will be prescribed either a topical or oral antifungal medication.
2. **This statement is correct. Eradication of the infection can take many weeks of treatment.**
3. Although the infection is transmitted by direct, person-to-person contact, the causative organism is one of a number of fungi.
4. The child should wear light-colored socks and shoes that provide good ventilation.

TEST-TAKING TIP: Athlete's foot, a form of ringworm, is caused by one of a number of fungi. The transmission usually occurs from walking on floors contaminated with the fungi. In addition, the fungi may be transmitted from person to person, or from pets to human.

Content Area: *Pediatrics*
Integrated Processes: *Nursing Process: Implementation; Teaching/Learning*
Client Need: *Physiological Integrity: Physiological Adaptation: Alterations in Body Systems*
Cognitive Level: *Application*

10. **ANSWER: 2**

Rationale:

1. This young woman has taken the initiative to be seen by a health-care practitioner for her acne. That action is not consistent with a nursing diagnosis of powerlessness.
2. **The young woman is at risk for ineffective coping. Acne can be disfiguring, adversely affecting one's self-esteem.**
3. Although some patients do try to rupture the blemishes, that action is not consistent with a nursing diagnosis of self-mutilation.
4. The young woman has taken the initiative to be seen by a health-care provider for her acne. That action is not consistent with a nursing diagnosis of self-neglect.

TEST-TAKING TIP: When young men and women with acne attempt to rupture their skin blemishes, they may injure or even scar their skin. The nurse must provide the patients with understanding and strongly encourage them not to try to remove the blemishes by scrubbing or pinching their skin.

Content Area: *Pediatrics*
Integrated Processes: *Nursing Process: Analysis*
Client Need: *Psychosocial Integrity: Mental Health Concepts*
Cognitive Level: *Application*

11. **ANSWER: 3**

Rationale:

1. It is not recommended that the child's hair be cut.
2. This is not true. The child may return to school or camp once he or she has had one treatment.

3. This is correct. After the treatment, the nits must be removed using a fine-toothed comb.
4. The child should not complain of itching once he or she has been treated.

TEST-TAKING TIP: Some parents have the incorrect assumption that short hair will prevent a lice infestation. This is not true. In addition, cutting the child's hair can be traumatic for the child.
Content Area: *Pediatrics*
Integrated Processes: *Nursing Process: Implementation*
Client Need: *Physiological Integrity: Physiological Adaptation: Illness Management*
Cognitive Level: *Application*

12. ANSWER: 3
Rationale:
1. The child should bathe and thoroughly dry himself or herself shortly before the medication is administered.
2. Topical medication is applied to the skin.
3. This statement is correct. The topical medication must remain on the skin for 8 full hours.
4. This statement is incorrect. It is common for the itching to persist for 2 to 4 weeks after treatment.

TEST-TAKING TIP: The inflammatory response causes the itching. Even after the mites are killed, the inflammation often persists for up to 4 weeks.
Content Area: *Pediatrics*
Integrated Processes: *Nursing Process: Evaluation*
Client Need: *Physiological Integrity: Reduction of Risk Potential: Potential for Alterations in Body Systems*
Cognitive Level: *Application*

13. ANSWER: 2
Rationale:
1. The child has a second-degree burn over approximately 7% of the body.
2. The child has a second-degree burn over approximately 7% of the body.
3. The child has a second-degree burn over approximately 7% of the body.
4. The child has a second-degree burn over approximately 7% of the body.

TEST-TAKING TIP: Depth: second-degree burns are characterized by blistering. Extent (Fig. 19.9): the child is almost 5 years of age. The anterior portion of both of the child's thighs are burned. Each leg accounts for approximately 14% of the child's body surface area. The anterior portion of the thigh of each leg, therefore, accounts for approximately 3.5% of the child's body surface area. (The entire anterior of the leg equals 7%; the anterior thigh of the leg equals 3.5%.) The total portion of the child's body that has been burned, therefore, is approximately 7%.
Content Area: *Pediatrics*
Integrated Processes: *Nursing Process: Analysis*
Client Need: *Physiological Integrity: Physiological Adaptation: Alterations in Body Systems*
Cognitive Level: *Application*

14. ANSWER: 4
Rationale:
1. This is important, but it is not the priority action.
2. This is important, but it is not the priority action.
3. This is important, but it is not the priority action.
4. Administration of IV fluids is the priority action.

TEST-TAKING TIP: Fluid and electrolyte balance is the child's highest priority. A large extent of the child's body is affected. The intracellular fluid loss, therefore, is extensive. The nurse should administer the IV fluids before performing any other action.
Content Area: *Pediatrics*
Integrated Processes: *Nursing Process: Implementation*
Client Need: *Physiological Integrity: Physiological Adaptation: Illness Management*
Cognitive Level: *Analysis*

15. ANSWER: 1
Rationale:
1. The skin should be cooled as soon as possible by running cool water over the burned area.
2. Ice should not be applied to burned skin. The ice can cause further damage to the skin.
3. The child will likely be treated as an outpatient by the primary health care provider. The nurse should, however, advise the parent to transport the child to the health-care provider's office after the burn has been cooled.
4. Petroleum jelly should not be applied to burned skin.

TEST-TAKING TIP: If a medication is needed, Silvadene or an antibiotic ointment will be applied to the burn.
Content Area: *Pediatrics*
Integrated Processes: *Nursing Process: Implementation*
Client Need: *Physiological Integrity: Physiological Adaptation: Illness Management*
Cognitive Level: *Application*

16. ANSWER: 2
Rationale:
1. The bite may be infected with community-associated methicillin-resistant *S. aureus* (CA-MRSA). It is inappropriate, however, for the nurse to make frightening statements to the child's parent.
2. This is the appropriate statement for the nurse to make. The lesion should be covered, and the child should be seen.
3. The bite may be infected with CA-MRSA. The child should be seen.
4. The health-care provider may order warm compresses to the area, but the child should be seen.

TEST-TAKING TIP: The CDC and the Infectious Disease Society have developed guidelines for the treatment of lesions infected with CA-MRSA. Although antibiotics may ultimately be prescribed, the first intervention usually is excision and drainage of the wound.
Content Area: *Pediatrics*
Integrated Processes: *Nursing Process: Implementation*
Client Need: *Physiological Integrity: Physiological Adaptation: Alterations in Body Systems*
Cognitive Level: *Application*

Nursing Care of the Child With Musculoskeletal Disorders

KEY TERMS

Clubfoot—A congenitally deformed foot. *Talipes equinovarus*, the most common form of club foot, is pointed inward and plantar flexed.
Developmental dysplasia of the hip (DDH)—Instability of the hip joint secondary to a laxity of the ligaments of the hip.
Duchenne muscular dystrophy (DMD)—An X-linked genetic disorder in which the cells in the muscles of the body are replaced by fat cells.
Ecchymosis—Bruising.
Gower's sign—Characterized by the need to push oneself to the standing position by holding onto furniture or using one's hands to "walk up" the body.
Legg-Calve-Perthes (LCP)—A temporary drop in the blood supply to the head of the femur and, in some circumstances, to the acetabulum as well, resulting in an aseptic necrosis of the bones.
Osteomyelitis—A bacterial infection of the bone.
Scoliometer—A device placed on the back of the child as he or she bends from the waist to measure the degree of the child's scoliotic curvature.
Scoliosis—A lateral curvature and rotation of the spine.
Slipped capital femoral epiphysis (SCFE)—A disorder in which the head of the femur, the epiphysis, separates from the rest of the femur at the site of the growth plate, frequently resulting in necrosis of the femur.

I. Description

The musculoskeletal system is comprised of the bones, joints, muscles, ligaments, and tendons. The terms ligaments and tendons often are used interchangeably, but they actually are different structures in the body: ligaments are fibrous tissues that attach bones to other bones, while tendons are fibrous tissues that attach muscles to bones. Because of the magnitude of the system, a number of musculoskeletal problems are seen during childhood. First, because more accidents are seen in the children than in adults, many of those accidents result in broken bones and/or soft tissue injuries. In addition, there are a number of congenital pathologies as well as illnesses of older children that affect musculoskeletal structures.

II. Soft Tissue Injuries

The scope of soft tissue injuries is quite large and includes sprains, strains, dislocations, and contusions.

A. Incidence.
   1. Soft tissue injuries are common in the pediatric population, especially in the teenage years.

B. Etiology.
   1. Injuries from such events as falls, automobile accidents, and athletic pursuits.

2. Intentional injury (i.e., child abuse) by a parent or guardian may also result in a soft tissue injury.

C. Pathology: there are many types of soft tissue injuries, most commonly:
1. Sprain: a twisting of a joint that results in damage to the ligaments and/or blood vessels. The most common site of a sprain is the ankle. Signs and symptoms of inflammation are seen, i.e., edema, pain, heat, and redness, as well as **ecchymosis** (the escape of blood from blood vessels into subcutaneous tissue [i.e., bruising]).
2. Strain: the tearing or pulling of a muscle that also often includes damage to the tendon. The most common site of a strain is the back. Signs and symptoms of inflammation as well as ecchymosis are seen.
3. Dislocations: the bones of a joint are no longer in correct alignment. In other, more basic terms, the long bone is no longer positioned in the joint socket. Joint dislocations occur most frequently in the shoulder joint. Tendon strains often accompany dislocations. Signs and symptoms of inflammation are seen, and the range of motion of the dislocated joint is markedly affected.
4. Contusions: contusions are very serious bruises of a muscle. Signs and symptoms of inflammation are seen.

D. Diagnosis:
1. X-ray—Because it is impossible to determine whether a bone is broken or whether soft tissue damage has occurred, an x-ray should be performed.
2. CT scans, MRIs, ultrasounds, and, in rare cases, bone scans also may be performed.

E. Treatment.
1. RICE, i.e., rest, ice, compression, and elevation (see "Making the Connection").
2. Safe dosages of NSAIDS are often prescribed to reduce swelling.
3. Physical therapy, if needed.
4. Surgery may be required, if the injury is severe.

F. Nursing considerations.
1. Injury/Pain/Knowledge Deficit.
   a. Assess the injury utilizing the five Ps of extremity injury assessment (Box 20.1).

DID YOU KNOW?

The five Ps of extremity injury assessment provide the nurse with valuable information regarding a child's injury. The nurse must remember, however, that the severity of the injury cannot be determined conclusively by the presence or absence of one or more of the factors. Indeed, if after performing the assessment the nurse is still unsure of the extent of the injury, the child should be seen by a primary health-care provider, and the nurse should request that the injured site be x-rayed.

   b. If the injury appears severe (i.e., signs and symptoms of inflammation are present) and the child indicates a specific location of the pain, the child should be seen by a primary health-care provider who will be able to order an x-ray and make a definitive diagnosis.
   c. If a soft tissue injury is diagnosed, educate the parents and child, if appropriate, regarding RICE and the safe dosage and method of NSAID administration.
   d. Refer the child to a physical therapist:
      i. Educate the parents and child, if appropriate, regarding the need to restrict activities for the prescribed period of time.

MAKING THE CONNECTION

The acronym **RICE** is an excellent way to remember common treatments for musculoskeletal injuries.

R—Rest: treatment—bedrest, slings, and/or crutch walking; casting, if needed.

I—Ice: treatment—to prevent further injury to the skin, ice should never be applied directly to the skin. It should be wrapped in a thin cloth or towel. The recommended length of time ice should be applied varies, but experts in ligamental injuries "instruct[] their patients to use ice on the affected area 3 to 5 times a day, for 20 minutes each application" (Pires Prado and others, 2014).

C—Compression: treatment—if the injury is on an extremity, an ace bandage should be applied to the site.

E—Elevation: treatment—elevation of the injured site above the level of the heart.

Box 20.1 The Five Ps of Extremity Injury Assessment

Pain
- *Assess using an age-appropriate pain scale.*
- *If the child is 3 years of age or older, ask the child regarding the precise location of the pain.*

Pulses
- *Assess and compare pulses distal to the injury to check whether circulation is still intact.*

Pallor
- *Assess and compare the color of the limbs distal to the injury as a means of checking whether circulation is still intact.*

Paresthesia (unusual sensation, such as tingling or burning)
- *Ask the child whether he or she feels an odd sensation distal to the injury as one means of assessing whether nerve damage has occurred.*

Paralysis
- *Assess and compare for the ability to move the limbs distal to the injury as one means of assessing whether nerve damage has occurred.*

ii. Educate the parents and child, if appropriate, regarding any prescribed exercises.

III. Fractures

Fractured bones may be simple or open (compound) fractures. Simple fractures are fractures that are enclosed in intact skin, while compound fractures are broken bones that have punctured the skin.

A. Incidence.
1. Commonly seen in children, especially children in the school-age population.

B. Etiology.
1. Accidents and falls related to immature motor skills (e.g., playing on a rollerblade, playing on a playground, and skiing).
2. Motor accidents (e.g., accidents that occur while moving in a car, riding on a bicycle, walking as a pedestrian).
3. Accidents resulting from risk-taking behaviors (e.g., jumping from a high location, falling while climbing a tall tree).

C. Pathophysiology: there are a number of fractures commonly seen in children (Table 20.1).
1. Signs and symptoms.
   a. Signs of inflammation, bruising or pallor, as well as limited range of motion (ROM).
      i. A fracture should be suspected if a young child refuses to crawl or walk.

D. Diagnosis.
1. X-ray, CT, MRI, ultrasound, and/or bone scan.

E. Treatment.
1. Casting (i.e., immobilizing the extremity within a rigid device).
   a. Types include air casts, fiberglass casts, and plaster of Paris casts.
   b. Before a cast is applied, the extremity is covered in a protective, cotton padding.
   c. The primary practitioner exerts manual traction to the distal end of the limb and moves the limb into proper alignment before applying the cast (see following information).
2. Traction.
   a. Traction usually is employed when the fractured bone cannot be moved into alignment manually.
      i. In a traction apparatus, a weight is suspended from the fractured limb.
      ii. The weight that exerts the traction fatigues the muscles surrounding the bone and pulls the distal end of the bone until it is in direct alignment with the proximal portion of the bone.
      iii. For traction to work, there must be a force or weight that is exerted in the opposite direction from the weight of the traction.
         (1) The child's body weight usually acts as the counterweight.
         (2) Additional weights may need to be added if the child is very small.
   b. Types of traction.
      i. Manual traction is achieved when an individual pulls on the end of the bone during the casting procedure.

Table 20.1 Types of Fractures Most Commonly Seen in Children

Name of Fracture	Characteristics	
Greenstick, or Incomplete, Fracture	Named after the kind of break seen when one attempts to break a healthy twig off from a tree. Commonly seen in children because their bones are soft and healthy.	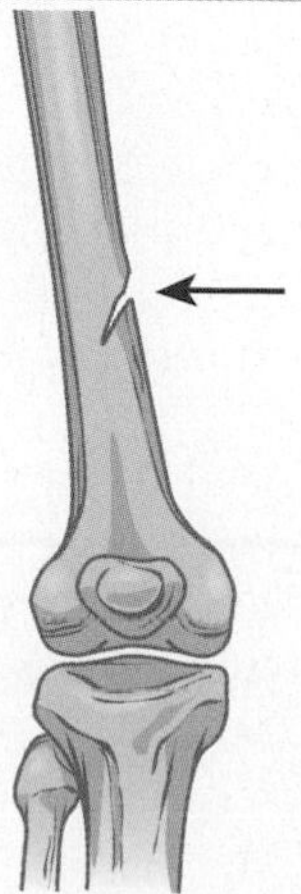

Continued

Table 20.1 Types of Fractures Most Commonly Seen in Children *cont'd*

Name of Fracture	Characteristics	
Buckle, or Torus, Fracture	This is a type of incomplete fracture that is characterized by compression of one side of the bone, causing the other side to bulge. Commonly seen in young children because their bones are soft and healthy.	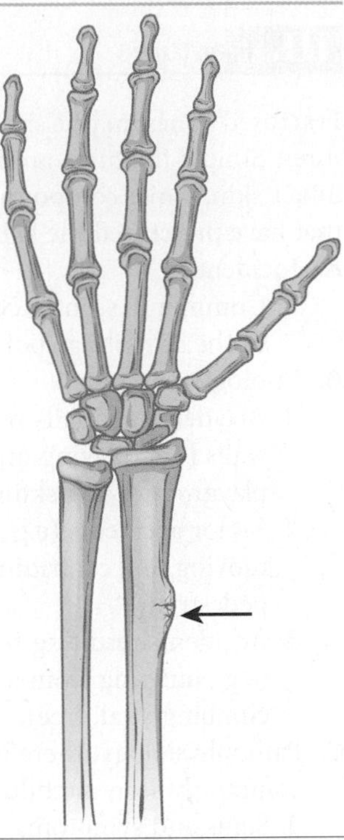
Bone Bend	The bone in this type of "fracture" actually does not break but rather bends into a curve. Commonly seen in young children because their bones are soft and healthy.	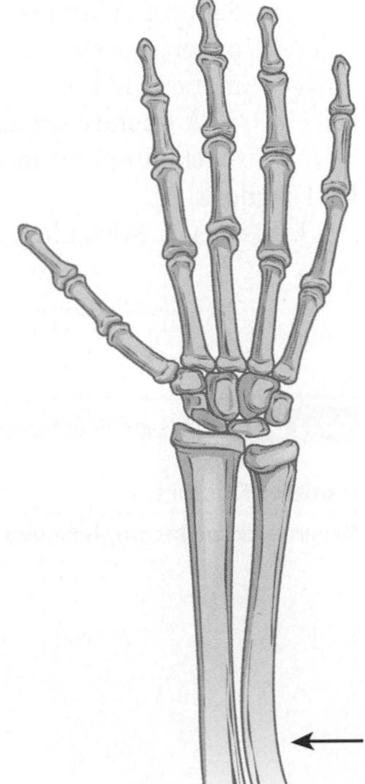

Table 20.1 Types of Fractures Most Commonly Seen in Children *cont'd*

Name of Fracture	Characteristics
Epiphyseal Fracture	A fracture that affects the child's epiphyseal or growth plate.
Spiral Fracture	Rarely seen as a result of an accident, spiral fractures are most often seen as a result of child abuse.

ii. Skin traction (Fig. 20.1) is achieved when the force is applied to an ace bandage, or other material, that has been placed on the skin surrounding the break.
   (1) Most common traction used on young children.
   (2) Not appropriate when the child has sustained an open fracture.
   (3) The most serious complications related to skin tractions are impaired skin integrity and neurovascular damage.

iii. Skeletal traction (Fig. 20.2): instead of the traction being exerted onto the skin, in skeletal traction a pin is inserted through the skin and the bone so that the traction can be applied directly to the bone.
   (1) Can usually be tolerated for longer periods of time than skin traction.
   (2) The most serious complication is osteomyelitis, a bone infection.

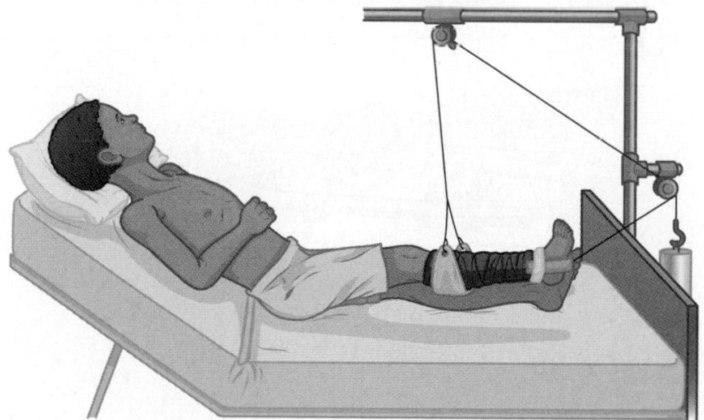

Fig 20.1 Skin traction.

3. External fixation devices (EFD): these devices act in a similar fashion to skeletal traction, but the child is not immobilized (i.e., the bone is maintained in alignment exclusively because of the action of the device). No weight is required. (Fig. 20.3) Osteomyelitis is a complication of EFD.

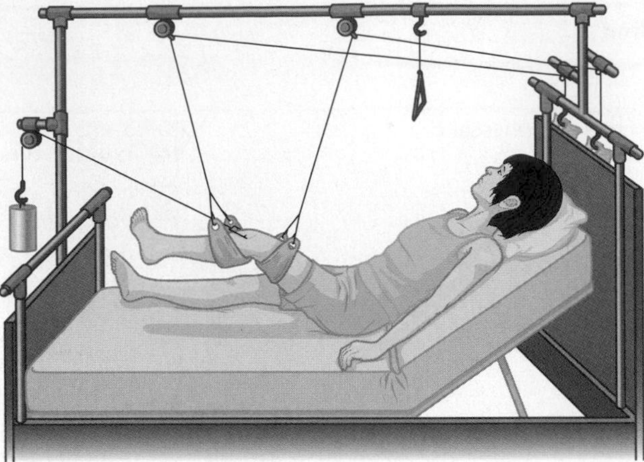

Fig 20.2 Skeletal traction.

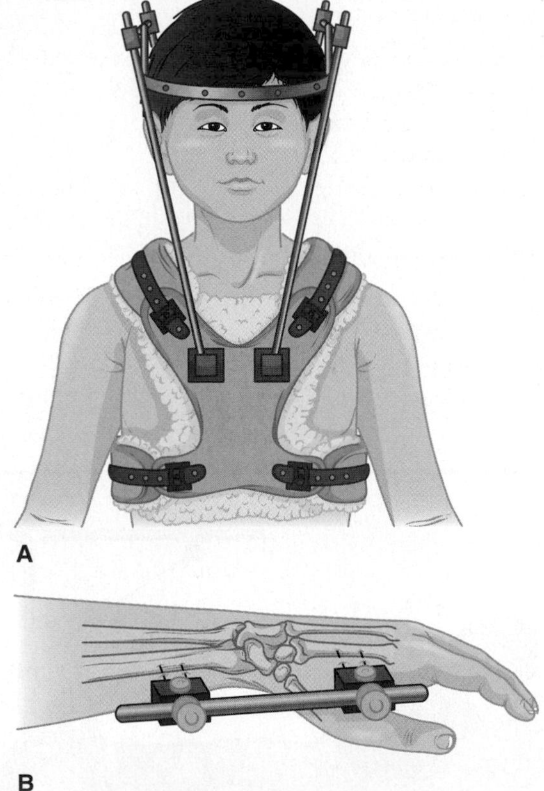

Fig 20.3 External fixation device (EFD).

F. Nursing considerations.

1. Injury/Pain/Knowledge Deficit following the initial injury.
    a. Assess the injury utilizing the five Ps of extremity injury assessment (Box 20.1).
    b. If the injury appears severe (i.e., signs and symptoms of inflammation are present) and/or the child indicates a specific location of the pain, the child should be seen by a primary health-care provider who will be able to make a definitive diagnosis.
    c. Educate the parents and child, if appropriate, regarding RICE and the safe dosage and method of NSAID administration.
    d. Refer the child to a physical therapist:
        i. Educate the parents and child, if appropriate, regarding the need to restrict activities for the prescribed period of time.
        ii. Educate the parents and child, if appropriate, regarding any prescribed.
2. Pain/Risk for Injury resulting from the treatment method.
    a. Assess neurovascular status every 2 hr for the first 48 hr.
        i. Must be especially vigilant if the patient is a young child because of the child's rapid growth.
            (1) The child's limb can become dangerously constricted during periods of rapid growth.
        ii. Assess the status of the injured limb in relation to that of the uninjured limb, that is:
            (1) Compare the temperature, capillary refill, pulses, and movement as well as the sensation and edema of the affected extremity distal to the injury with that of the unaffected extremity.
            (2) If the assessments reflect diminished neurovascular status in the affected extremity, immediately report the finding to the primary health-care provider.
    b. Elevate the extremity above the heart, and apply ice to reduce swelling.
    c. Monitor for signs of fat embolism and compartment syndrome.
        i. Common symptoms of fat emboli: shortness of breath and other signs of respiratory distress, change in sensorium, and petechiae.
        ii. Common symptoms of compartment syndrome: a persistent ache deep in the bone and/or a pain level that is markedly higher than expected from the injury.
    d. Administer safe dosages of analgesics, as prescribed.
        i. If moderate to severe pain, narcotics should be administered.
        ii. For mild pain, the administration of NSAIDS is usually appropriate.
        iii. If the child is discharged, educate the parents and child, if appropriate, regarding the safe administration of the analgesics.

e. Provide non-pharmacological pain interventions, as needed.
f. Apply restraints, as ordered.
   i. Jacket restraints may be needed when young children are on bedrest with casts or traction.
   ii. Communicate to the child that the restraint is not meant as disciplinary action but rather is important in order to get him or her better.
g. If limb is casted:
   i. Assist the child to reposition every 2 hr.
   ii. If plaster of Paris cast:
      (1) The cast should be held by the palms of the hands rather than the tips of fingers to minimize the potential for pressure points.
h. If child is in traction:
   i. Maintain weight alignment per order and maintain countertraction.
      (1) It is especially important to prevent the weight from swinging and/or the weight becoming attached to the frame of the child's bed when transporting the child to and from radiology, the playroom, and/or any other location.

It is essential that traction be maintained as prescribed at all times. First, it is critical that the therapeutic effect of fatiguing the muscle in order to realign the bone be constant. The weight, therefore, must hang freely and not be allowed to rest on the frame of the bed or on any other surface. As important, however, the weight must not be allowed to swing like a pendulum. The stress that a swaying weight can produce can be both injurious and painful.

i. If the child is discharged home, educate the parents and child, if appropriate, regarding all facets of the child's care.

3. Risk for Infection.
   a. From pin insertion in skeletal traction or EFD.
      i. Monitor insertion site carefully for REEDA (redness, edema, ecchymosis, discharge, and approximation).
         (1) If any signs appear, report immediately.
      ii. Monitor the child's temperature, pulse, and respiratory rate for elevations.
      iii. Monitor the child's laboratory results for an increase in the white blood cell (WBC) count.
      iv. Administer safe dosages of antibiotics, if prescribed.
   b. From casting.
      i. If a plaster of Paris cast:
         (1) Allow the cast to dry slowly.
            (a) A fan may be used, but heat from a hair dryer or other source is contraindicated.
            (b) When a cast dries too rapidly, the outer portion of the cast dries quickly while the cast closest to the skin remains wet. The wet skin can become macerated and infected.
      ii. Assess entire cast for warm areas and/or signs of discharge, which may indicate infected areas.
         (1) Compound fractures are especially high risk for infection.
      iii. Monitor for rise in vital signs and/or WBC count.
      iv. Administer safe dosages of antibiotics, as prescribed.
4. Risk for Impaired Breathing Patterns/Impaired Gas Exchange resulting from bedrest.
   a. Monitor respiratory rate.
   b. Monitor lung sounds.
   c. Encourage deep breathing and coughing and/or incentive spirometry every 2 hr.

DID YOU KNOW?

The nurse can use games to encourage children to perform deep breathing exercises. Blowing bubbles, raising the ball on an incentive spirometer, or twirling a pinwheel will all help to encourage deep breathing.

5. Risk for Impaired Skin Integrity related to the injury, treatment, and/or bedrest.
   a. Assess the skin for signs of breakdown.
   b. If on bedrest, place the child on a soft surface (e.g., lambskin).
   c. Gently cleanse, dry, and massage the skin, especially areas in communication with the surface of the bed.
   d. If the child has yet to be toilet trained, change diapers frequently.
   e. Reposition the child every 2 hr, if appropriate.
6. Risk for Constipation resulting from bedrest and/or narcotic ingestion.
   a. Monitor bowel sounds and stooling patterns.
   b. Provide a diet that is high in fluids, fresh fruits, vegetables, and whole grains.
   c. Administer stool softeners, as prescribed and as needed.
7. Risk for Impaired Physical Mobility resulting from injury and/or bedrest.
   a. Encourage active ROM exercises of unaffected limbs.

b. Assist with passive ROM exercises of joints distal to the injury on the affected extremity, if permitted.
c. Provide and encourage participation in age-appropriate activities that encourage appropriate movement.

8. Powerlessness/Risk for Ineffective Coping/Risk for Altered Growth and Development/Anger.
a. Provide the child and parents opportunities to verbalize anger and frustration.
b. Explain all interventions in age-appropriate language.
c. Provide opportunities for therapeutic play.

The child should be moved to the playroom for play as often as possible, but if in traction, weight alignment must be maintained. Many play activities can be used to dispel the anger children may feel from long-term confinement. For example, throwing bean bags at a target and hammering pegs into holes in a thick board are therapeutic actions that can help children to release their anger in socially acceptable ways.

d. Allow regression early in the hospitalization, but foster growth, as appropriate, if hospitalized for an extended period of time. For example, set limits, allow appropriate decision making, and allow personal food and clothing choices.
e. Encourage the child to complete schoolwork provided by tutors and home school teachers, as appropriate.
f. Provide toys and activities that are compatible with the child's therapy and that promote fine and gross motor development.

IV. Clubfoot

A. Incidence.
1. **Clubfoot** affects boys more frequently than girls.
2. Defect often accompanies other defects (e.g., spina bifida).
3. Clubfoot may be unilateral or bilateral.

B. Etiology.
1. There is increased incidence in some families, but no genetic markers have been identified.
2. Some cases of clubfoot appear to result from fetal malposition while in utero and/or intrauterine restriction resulting from oligohydramnios.

C. Pathophysiology (Fig. 20.4).
1. Over 90% of cases of clubfoot are classified as *talipes equinovarus*, a foot that is plantar flexed and pointed inward. The remaining 10% are classified as:
a. *Talipes equinovalgus*: plantar flexed and pointed outward.

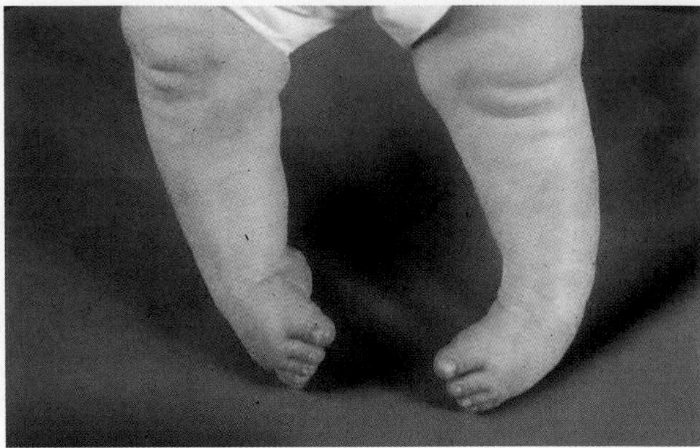

Fig 20.4 Clubfoot.

b. *Talipes calcaneovarus*: dorsiflexed and pointed inward.
c. *Talipes calcaneovalgus*: dorsiflexed and pointed outward.

2. Although many neonates' feet appear malaligned, clubfoot is only diagnosed when the feet resist being moved into proper alignment.

D. Diagnosis.
1. Clinical picture, i.e., the inability to move the neonate's foot into correct alignment is suggestive.
2. Definitive diagnosis is determined by x-ray and/or ultrasound.

E. Treatment.
1. Serial casting.
a. Every 1 to 2 weeks beginning shortly after birth, casts are applied to the affected foot, incrementally moving the foot into proper alignment.
i. Casts must be removed and reapplied frequently because of the rapid growth of the neonate.
ii. The goal of the serial casts is to stretch ligaments and tendons on the inner aspect of the foot.
b. Bracing often follows casting.
2. Surgery may be needed if correction is not achieved through casting.
3. Physical therapy may be prescribed.

F. Nursing considerations (see "Casting").
1. Risk for Injury/Pain related to cast compression.
a. Educate the parents regarding the importance of monitoring the child who has been casted for signs of neurovascular compromise (see the following "Making the Connection" box).
b. Educate the parents regarding age-appropriate pain assessment.
c. Administer a safe dosage of an appropriate analgesic, as needed.

MAKING THE CONNECTION

After casts are applied, babies with club feet will be discharged home. It is critically important for the nurse to educate the parents regarding assessing the child for neurovascular compromise at least once each day and immediately to report any deviations from normal. Because babies grow so rapidly during the first weeks of life, the cast can become too tight very quickly. The parents must assess for the:

- Presence of pain, which is usually exhibited in neonates as crying.
- Presence of pedal pulses bilaterally.
- Color of the feet, which should be pink bilaterally.
- Spontaneous movements of both feet.
- Temperature of both feet. Although babies' feet are often cool to the touch, the temperature of both feet should be the same.
- Presence of edema.
- Capillary refill.

d. If surgery is performed, monitor surgical site for REEDA, and report abnormal findings.

2. Knowledge Deficit/Risk for Ineffective Coping of parents.
   a. Provide parents the opportunity to verbalize grief, anger, and frustration over birthing a child with a physical defect.
   b. Carefully explain to the parents the rationale for each treatment method.

V. Developmental Dysplasia of the Hip

A. Incidence.
1. **Developmental dysplasia of the hip** (DDH) is seen seven times more frequently in girls than in boys.
2. Higher incidence in breech babies.
3. Frequently seen in conjunction with other defects (e.g., spina bifida).

B. Etiology.
1. There is increased incidence in families, but no genetic evidence has been found.
2. Most commonly associated with fetal positioning and in conjunction with other defects.

C. Pathophysiology (Fig. 20.5).
1. Instability of the hip joint secondary to a laxity of the ligaments of the hip.
2. The severity of the defect—subluxation to complete dislocation—is dependent on the extent of the dysplasia.
3. Signs and symptoms.
   a. Positive Ortolani's sign (see Box 20.2).
   b. Positive Barlow's sign (see Box 20.3).
   c. Limited abduction of one or both legs.

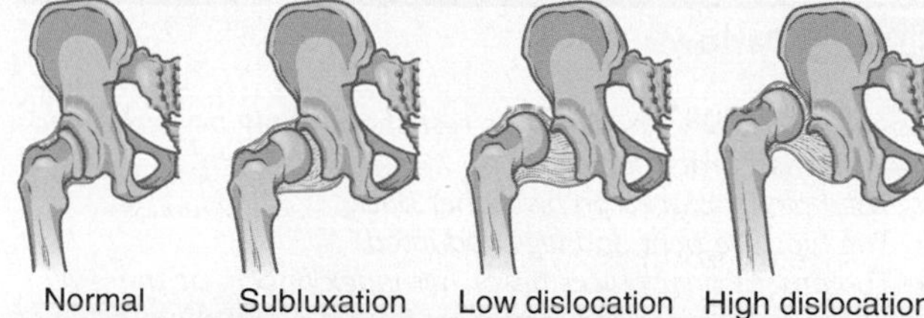

Fig 20.5 Developmental dysplasia of the hip.

   d. Asymmetry of skin folds on the anterior and posterior surfaces of the thigh.
   e. Asymmetry of femur lengths.

D. Diagnosis.
1. Clinical findings are suggestive, and assessments should be performed at each well-baby visit.
   a. Ortolani's test (Box 20.2).
   b. Barlow's test (Box 20.3).
2. Definitive diagnosis is determined by x-ray and/or ultrasound.

E. Treatment.
1. To prevent permanent damage, it is important that treatment be instituted before the child starts to creep and crawl.
2. Pavlik harness: if the child is less than 6 months of age, the Pavlik harness is the classic treatment (Fig. 20.6).

Box 20.2 Ortolani's Test

To prevent injury, Ortolani's test should only be performed by a trained practitioner.
- *The baby is placed on his or her back.*
- *The knees and hips are bent at right angles.*
- *The practitioner places his or her index fingers at the level of the trochanter and remaining fingers along the outside of the legs.*
- *The thumbs are placed on the inner aspects of the thighs.*
- *The practitioner internally and externally rotates the legs.*
- *If instability is felt, DDH is suspected.*

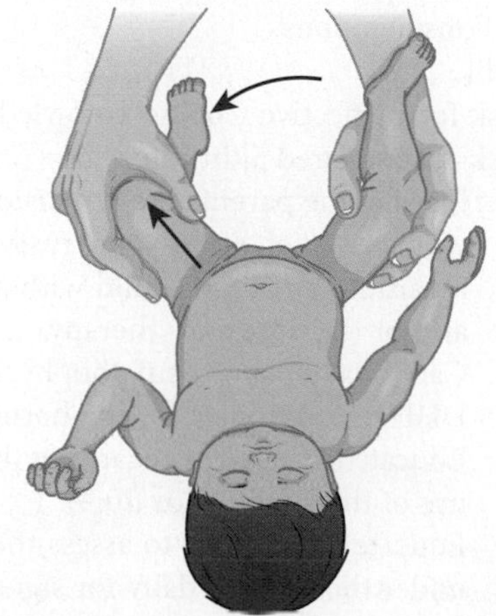

Box 20.3 Barlow's Test

To prevent injury, the Barlow's test should only be performed by a trained practitioner.

- *The baby is placed on his or her back.*
- *The hips are bent and legs abducted.*
- *The practitioner places his or her index fingers at the level of the trochanter and remaining fingers along the outside of the legs.*
- *The thumbs are placed on the inner aspects of the thighs.*
- *The practitioner pushes the legs posteriorly, and DDH is suspected if a slippage of the hip is felt.*

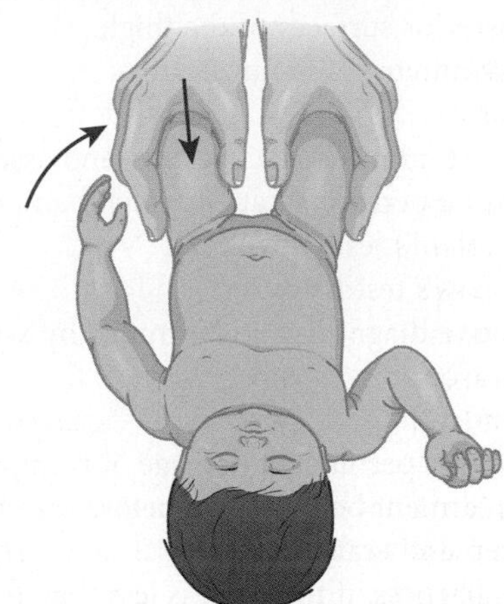

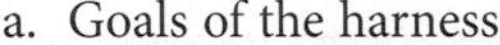

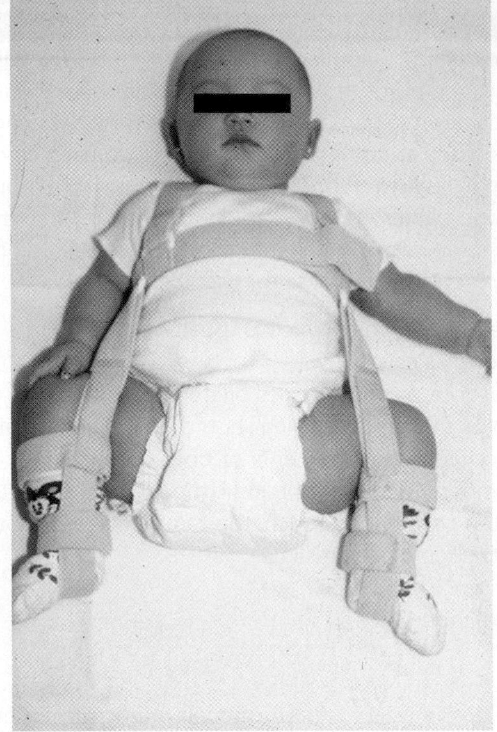

Fig 20.6 Pavlik harness.

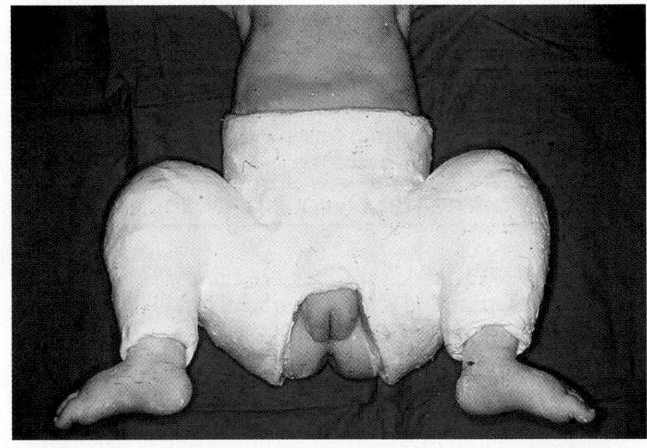

Fig 20.7 Spica cast.

a. Goals of the harness.
    i. Keep the legs abducted.
    ii. Keep the trochanter positioned in the acetabulum.
    iii. Enable the hip ligaments to mature and strengthen.

3. If the child is older than 6 months or if the Pavlik was not effective:
    a. Invasive procedures may be performed (e.g., traction; surgery; spica casting [Fig. 20.7], in which the trunk as well as one or more limbs is enclosed in a cast).

F. Nursing considerations.

1. If Pavlik:
    a. Risk for Ineffective Coping/Knowledge Deficit/Risk for Impaired Skin Integrity.
        i. Provide the parents the opportunity to verbalize grief, anger, and frustration regarding birthing a child with a defect and/or the necessary therapy.
        ii. Carefully explain the pathophysiology of DDH and rationale for the harness.
        iii. Educate the parents regarding the proper use of the Pavlik (Box 20.4).
        iv. Educate the parents to assess the skin under the harness daily for signs of skin breakdown.
        v. Because car seats adduct the legs, parents should be advised to avoid long trips in the car.
2. If spica cast:
    a. See "Casting."
    b. Risk for Impaired Skin Integrity.
        i. Advise the parents to use disposable diapers and sanitary pads to prevent urine and feces from soiling the cast.
    c. Risk for Injury.
        i. Advise the parents to monitor for signs of neurovascular compromise (see earlier).

Box 20.4 Parent Education for Use of the Pavlik Harness

- *The harness must be worn 23 to 24 hr per day, as prescribed.*
  - *If the primary health-care provider states that the harness may be removed, the parents must be taught how to reapply it correctly.*
- *The parents must be advised to return to the primary healthcare provider on a regular basis to have the length of the straps adjusted to accommodate the baby's rapid growth.*
- *The harness will keep the baby's hips bent and abducted, but the baby should show no signs of discomfort.*
- *To maintain proper positioning, the diaper must be put on under the harness and all outer clothing must fit loosely over the lower extremities.*
- *To protect the skin, a tee shirt should be worn by the baby under the harness.*
  - *To prevent pressure points from developing, the parents should be advised to check for wrinkles in the shirt.*

ii. Advise the parents to support all extremities with pillows and/or blankets.
iii. Advise the parents to perform safe position changes throughout the day.
iv. Advise the parents to exercise care in carrying and traveling with the child.
v. Advise the parents never to leave the child unattended.
(1) Even children who have been casted may learn to move independently.

d. Risk for Impaired Breathing Patterns/Risk for Impaired Gas Exchange.
i. Educate the parents to monitor the child's respiratory effort and breathing patterns each day and to report any deviations from normal.

e. Risk for Altered Growth and Development.
i. Provide toys and activities that are compatible with the child's therapy and that promote fine and gross motor development.

VI. Legg-Calve-Perthes

A. Incidence.
1. **Legg-Calve-Perthes (LCP)** can be seen in children from toddlerhood through the end of the school-age period but is most commonly seen in children aged 4 to 8 years of age.
2. It is most commonly seen in boys and in Caucasian children.

B. Etiology.
1. The etiology of LCP is unknown.

C. Pathophysiology.
1. A temporary drop in the blood supply to the head of the femur and, in some circumstances, to the acetabulum as well, resulting in an aseptic necrosis of the bones.
2. Eventually, the blood supply returns to normal and the bone regenerates, but the ischemia may last for months or years.
3. The resultant bone may be normal or may be markedly deformed.
4. Signs and symptoms:
a. Pain
b. Limp that increases as the child's activity level increases.

D. Diagnosis.
1. Clinical picture is suspicious.
2. Definitive diagnosis is made with x-ray, bone scan, and/or MRI.
3. Early diagnosis is essential in order to prevent permanent damage.

E. Treatment.
1. Anti-inflammatory medications and non-weight bearing.
a. Non-weight bearing may be achieved with crutch walking.
b. If pain is severe, bedrest may be needed.
2. Casting and/or surgical intervention may be necessary.

F. Nursing considerations.
1. Risk for Ineffective Coping/Pain/Knowledge Deficit/Risk for Altered Growth and Development.
a. Provide the parents and children, if appropriate, the opportunity to verbalize anger and frustration with the diagnosis and treatment plan.
b. Carefully explain the pathophysiology of the disease and the rationale for therapy.
c. Advise the parents to provide the child with age-appropriate activities to maintain and promote fine and gross motor development.
d. Advise the child and parents that the child is able to and should go to school but must refrain from engaging in activities that will interfere with the treatment.
e. Emphasize the importance of non-weight bearing to prevent further injury to the joint.
i. If prescribed, reinforce education by the physical therapist (PT), or, if PT is unavailable, educate the child regarding safe crutch walking (Box 20.5).
f. Educate the parents and child, if appropriate, regarding the safe administration of anti-inflammatory medications.
g. Educate parents and child, if appropriate, regarding the safe administration of analgesics and regarding appropriate nonpharmacological pain interventions, as needed.

Box 20.5 How to Use Crutches

1. *Standing with the unaffected foot on the floor:*
   - *The elbows should be slightly bent.*
   - *The hands should grip the hand supports.*
   - *When moving, the axilla should be placed over the underarm suports but not touching the underarm supports.*
2. *While continuing to stand on the unaffected foot:*
   - *The crutches should be moved forward slightly.*
   - *While continuing to keep a space between the underarm supports and the axilla, the patient should push down on the hand grips.*
3. *Last, the body should swing to meet the placement of the crutches.*

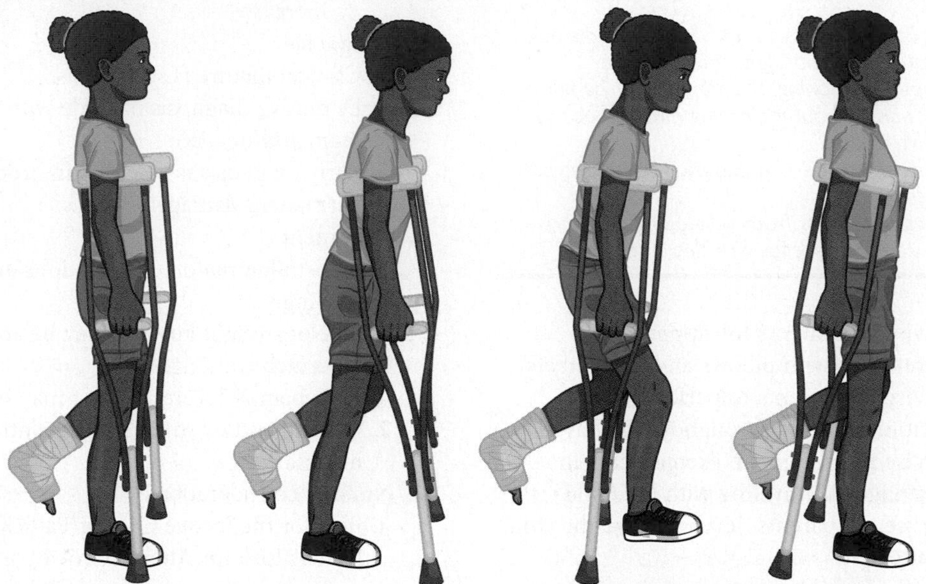

VII. Slipped Capital Femoral Epiphysis

A. Incidence.
1. **Slipped capital femoral epiphysis** (SCFE) is seen in children during the pubertal growth spurt.
2. Most commonly seen in males and obese children.

B. Etiology.
1. The cause of SCFE is unknown; however, obesity is presumed to be a significant risk factor, if not a cause; the vast majority of children who develop the problem are in the top 10th percentile for weight.
2. SCFE is also associated with other diseases (e.g., endocrine disorders), and, because of its proximity to the adolescent growth spurt, hormonal changes likely factor into its development.
3. There is increased incidence in some families, although a direct genetic link has not been identified.

C. Pathophysiology (Fig. 20.8).
1. The head of the femur separates from the rest of the femur at the site of the growth, or epiphyseal, plate.
2. Blood supply to the femoral head is disrupted and frequently results in necrosis of the bone.

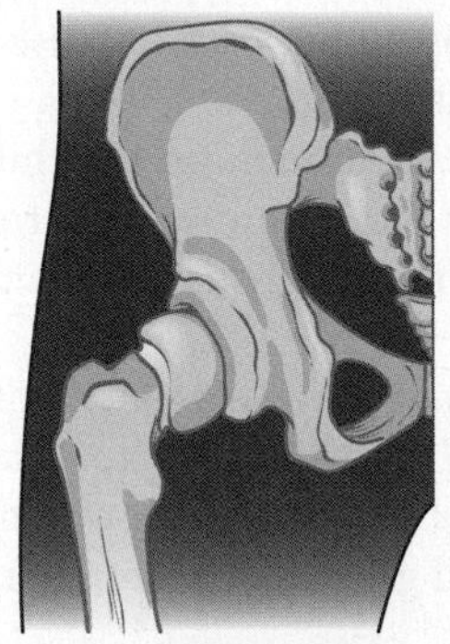

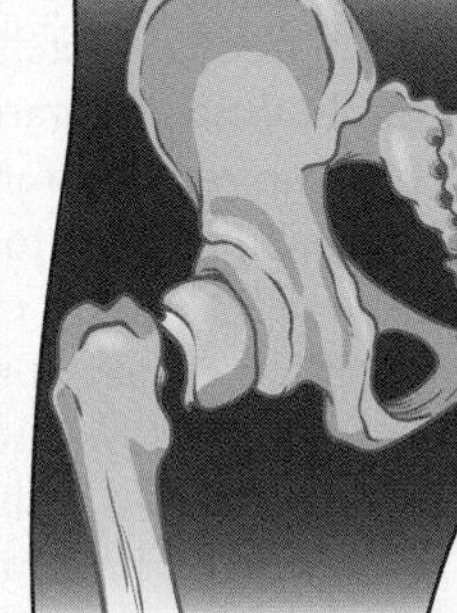

Fig 20.8 Slipped capital femoral epiphysis.

3. Signs and symptoms.
   a. Hip tenderness or pain.
   b. Decreased hip flexion.
   c. Limp.
   d. Increased pain when the toes are turned inward.

D. Diagnosis.
1. The clinical picture of an obese preteen with a painful limp is highly suggestive.
2. Definitive diagnosis is made by x-ray.

E. Treatment.
1. Surgery usually is performed as soon as the diagnosis is made.

a. The sooner interventions are instituted, the less likely the child will experience permanent damage.
b. Traction often is instituted following surgery.

2. Immobility of the joint, including bedrest and/or crutch walking, both before and following surgery is usually prescribed.

F. Nursing considerations: (see "Traction Care").

1. Pain/Deficient Knowledge.
   a. Carefully explain the pathophysiology of the disease and rationale for therapy.
   b. If prescribed, reinforce education by the physical therapist (PT), or, if PT is unavailable, educate the child regarding safe crutch walking (Box 20.5).
   c. Administer safe dosages of analgesics, as prescribed.
      i. If moderate to severe pain, narcotics should be administered.
         (1) Patient-controlled analgesia is an excellent mode of medication administration for this age patient.
      ii. For mild pain, NSAIDS should be administered.
      iii. When the child is discharged, educate the parents and child, if appropriate, regarding the safe administration of analgesics.
   d. Provide nonpharmacological pain interventions, as needed.
2. Risk for Ineffective Coping/Risk for Altered Growth and Development.
   a. Provide the parents and child the opportunity to verbalize anger and frustration with the diagnosis and treatment plan.
   b. Strongly encourage the child to continue close relationships with friends and to invite friends to visit when in the hospital or confined to the home.
   c. Advise the child and parents that the child is able to and should keep up with schoolwork.
3. Readiness for Enhanced Self-Health Maintenance.
   a. Encourage the primary health-care provider to refer the child and family for nutrition counseling.
   b. Support the education provided during nutrition counseling.
   c. Provide positive reinforcement for dietary changes made.
   d. Following convalescence, strongly encourage the child to begin a wellness exercise program.

VIII. Scoliosis

A. Incidence.

1. Although **scoliosis** is seen in other children, including neonates, by far the highest incidence of the disease is seen in adolescent girls during their pubertal growth spurt.

B. Etiology.

1. In the vast majority of cases, there is no apparent cause.
2. There is a rare autosomal dominant form of the disease.
   a. A genetic test is available for the small, at-risk population.
3. Scoliosis is also seen in conjunction with other diseases (e.g., cerebral palsy, muscular dystrophy).
4. It is believed that scoliosis is neither caused by nor worsened by carrying heavy backpacks and/or by engaging in sports.

C. Pathophysiology (Fig. 6.4).

1. Scoliosis is characterized by a lateral curvature and rotation of the spine, defined in terms of degrees of curvature.
   a. A deviation of greater than 10 degrees is diagnostic.
2. The rotation of the spine is related to weakness in muscles and ligaments on the opposite side of the body.
3. Signs and symptoms.
   a. Uneven posture with:
      i. One scapula protruding farther than the other.
      ii. Uneven shoulder and waist heights.
      iii. Hip and rib asymmetry.
      iv. In severe cases, respiratory and cardiac compromise because of thoracic compression.

D. Diagnosis.

1. Clinical picture is suggestive.
   i. Deviation and asymmetries are seen when the child bends at the waist and allows his or her arms to fall freely (Fig. 20.9).

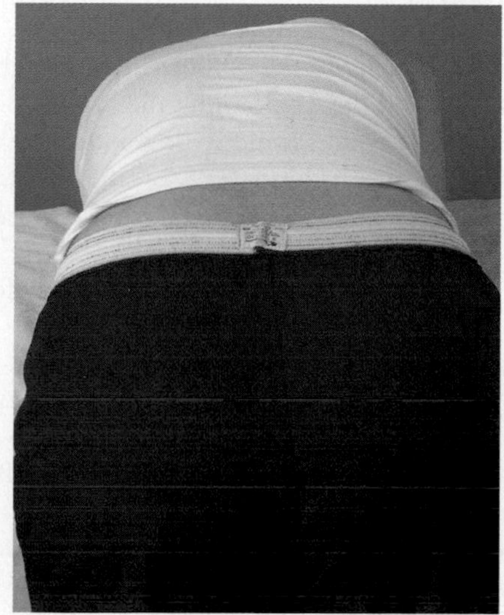

Fig 20.9 Adolescent with scoliosis.

ii. **Scoliometer** is a device placed on the back of the child as he or she bends from the waist to measure the curvature of the spine.

2. Definitive diagnosis is made by x-ray.

E. Treatment.

1. Mode of treatment is dependent on many factors, including the extent of the deviation and the age of the child.
2. Bracing usually is the treatment of choice for relatively minor deviations.
   a. It is important to realize that bracing is not curative; braces merely help to prevent any further deviation.
   b. It is not uncommon for children to refuse to wear the braces. Therefore, to promote compliance:
      i. Most braces currently used are small enough to hide under one's clothing.
      ii. Some braces are designed only to be worn while sleeping.
3. Exercises often are employed in conjunction with bracing, but exercises alone are not effective.
4. In severe cases and when bracing fails to prevent further injury, surgery is performed.
   a. Most frequently, one or more rods are inserted adjacent to and wired to the spine.
   b. Bone grafts from the child's hip or other site are used to fuse and/or stabilize the vertebrae.
   c. Renal and/or neurological damage, as well as extensive blood loss, are possible complications from the surgery.
   d. Following surgery, the child will usually be required to wear a brace until the site is fully healed.

F. Nursing considerations.

1. If bracing:
   a. Risk for Impaired Skin Integrity.
      i. The child's skin should be thoroughly dried before donning the brace.
      ii. The child should wear a cotton tee shirt under the brace.
         (1) Care should be taken to eliminate all wrinkles in the shirt.
      iii. The skin should be assessed daily for signs of breakdown.
      iv. The use of lotions and powders on the skin under the brace should be avoided.
   b. Risk for Ineffective Coping/Deficient Knowledge/Anger/Risk for Disturbed Body Image.
      i. Carefully explain to the parents and child the pathophysiology of the disease and the rationale for therapy.
      ii. Educate the parents and child regarding the importance of wearing the brace to prevent further deviation.
      iii. Allow the parents and child to express anger and frustration over the need to wear a brace and, if required, the need to refrain from normal physical activities.
      iv. Educate the parents and child regarding how to put on the brace in order to prevent complications.
      v. Consider introducing the child to a child of the same age and gender who is compliant with the therapy.
      vi. Provide the child with consistent encouragement and positive reinforcement when complying with therapy.
      vii. Introduce the child and family to relevant community organizations (e.g., National Scoliosis Foundation).
2. If surgery:
   a. Risk for Anxiety/Fear/Anger/Deficient Knowledge.
      i. Allow the child and parents to express their anxieties, fears, and anger regarding the need for surgery.
      ii. Provide the child and parents with comprehensive education regarding the surgical procedures as well as preoperative and postoperative care.
      iii. Parents should be advised that the child may regress during the surgical period, for example:
         (1) The child may wish to hold a favorite toy or other possession from when he or she was younger while in the hospital.
         (2) The child will likely request his or her parents to stay with him or her immediately pre- and postsurgery and throughout the remainder of the hospitalization.
   b. Risk for Impaired Mobility/Risk for Injury.
      i. Immediately following surgery, log rolling should be performed when changing the child's position to prevent injury to the surgical site.
      ii. Provide needed assistance for the application of the postoperative brace and educate the parents to do the same.
      iii. Assist with physical therapy interventions, as prescribed.
      iv. Carefully monitor for postoperative complications and report any adverse findings.
         (1) Because the spinal column is manipulated during surgery, thorough

neurological assessments must be performed.
(2) Assess lung fields and encourage use of the incentive spirometer.
(3) Assess bowel sounds and monitor for return of bowel movements.

c. Risk for Deficient Fluid Volume because surgical blood loss may be excessive.
  i. Monitor vital signs and report to the healthcare provider evidence of tachycardia and/or hypotension.
  ii. Maintain strict intake and output (I&O).
  iii. Monitor laboratory values (e.g., hematocrit and hemoglobin, electrolytes, renal function tests) and report significant changes.
  iv. Employing protocols, administer IV therapy and/or blood replacement products, as prescribed.

d. Pain.
  i. Assess pain using an age-appropriate pain rating scale.
  ii. Administer safe dosages of analgesics utilizing appropriate technique, as prescribed.
    (1) Narcotic analgesics are essential during the immediate postoperative period.
    (2) Patient-controlled analgesia is an excellent mode of medication administration for teenage patients.
  iii. Prior to discharge, educate the parents and child, if appropriate, regarding the safe administration of analgesics.
  iv. Provide nonpharmacological pain interventions, as needed.
  v. Assess the response to pain intervention methods and intervene, as needed.

IX. Muscular Dystrophies

There are a number of progressively debilitating hereditary diseases that adversely affect muscular function and result in impaired, or a total loss of, mobility. The most severe and most common form, **Duchenne muscular dystrophy (DMD)**, is presented as an exemplar in this chapter.

A. Incidence.
1. Approximately 1 of every 3,500 males is diagnosed with DMD.

B. Etiology: all muscular dystrophies have a genetic etiology. Some are X-linked, others are autosomal dominant, and others are autosomal recessive.
1. Classically, DMD is a single gene, X-linked recessive disease.
2. Many cases of DMD, however, are found to be caused by spontaneous genetic mutations.

C. Pathophysiology.
1. Children with DMD have a genetic defect that results in the inability to produce the protein, dystrophin, which is essential for maintaining the health and well-being of muscle tissue.
2. Slowly over time, the cells of the muscles of the body are replaced by fat cells.
3. Initially, the long muscles of the legs and the muscles in the pelvic area are affected, but eventually all muscle is replaced by fat, including the muscles of the respiratory and cardiac systems.
4. Characteristically, the fatal illness ends in death from respiratory infection or cardiac failure when the men reach their late teens or early twenties.
5. Signs and symptoms.
  a. The growth and development of children with DMD usually are within normal limits for the first few years of life.
  b. At approximately age 3, gross motor development stalls and begins to decline (i.e., the child never is able to ride a tricycle and starts to have difficulty running and climbing stairs).
  c. Slowly over time, gross motor skills become more and more difficult, and the child develops:
    i. Lordosis (concave curvature of the back, commonly called sway back).
    ii. Waddling gait.
    iii. **Gower's sign** (Fig. 20.10), characterized by the need to push oneself to the standing position by holding onto furniture or using one's hands to "walk up" the body.
      (1) Usually seen during the school-age period.
    iv. By the time the children become teenagers, they usually are wheelchair bound.

D. Diagnosis.
1. Suggestive from clinical picture, that is:
  a. Normal growth and development from birth through toddlerhood.
  b. Slow regression of motor function after age 3.
  c. Gower's sign beginning at approximately age 7.
  d. Elevated serum creatine kinase levels, indicating that muscle cells have been damaged.
2. Definitive diagnosis.
  a. Muscle biopsy showing fat infiltrates in the muscle tissue.
  b. DNA analysis.

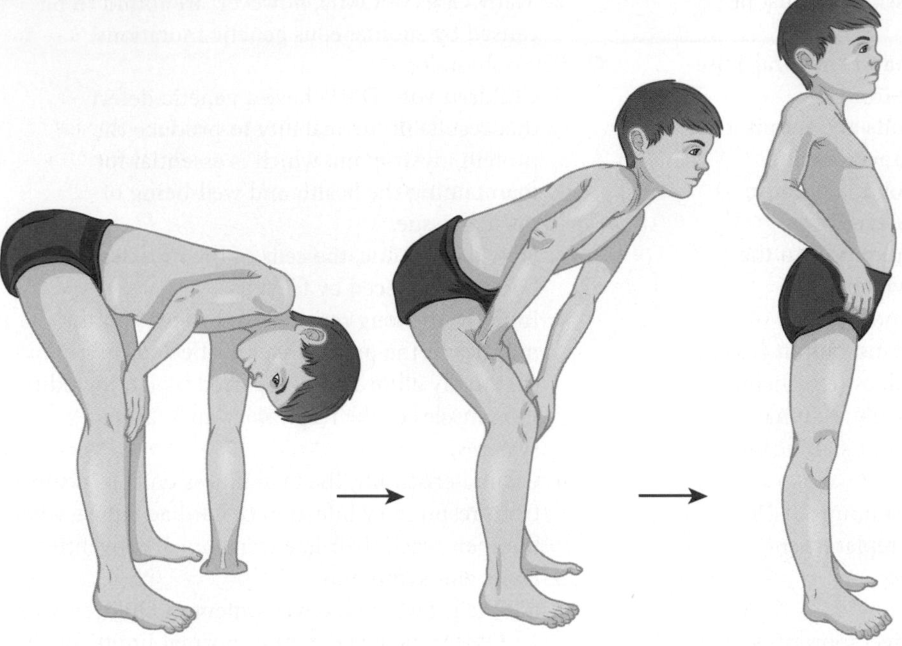

Fig 20.10 Gower's sign.

E. Treatment.

1. There is no cure for DMD; the goal of the treatment for DMD is to maintain ambulatory and vital organ function for as long as possible.
   a. Preventing obesity and preventing the development of contractures help the children to prolong their mobility.
   b. When needed, additional interventions are instituted, including bracing, PT, and crutch walking.
   c. Those who engage in vigorous exercise programs have been shown to prolong their mobility longer than those who live a more sedentary lifestyle.
2. Corticosteroids have been administered and have slowed the progression of the illness in some cases.
3. Prophylactic antibiotics, respiratory physical therapy, and aggressive intervention for all upper respiratory infections and symptoms related to cardiac failure help to maintain function of the vital organs.

F. Nursing considerations.

1. Knowledge Deficit.
   a. Provide the parents and child, when appropriate, with comprehensive education regarding the etiology and pathophysiology of the disease.
   b. Refer the family to a genetic counselor for comprehensive, familial genetic analysis.
2. Risk for Impaired Coping/Anxiety/Fear/Anger/Grieving.
   a. Allow the parents and child to express concerns, anxiety, and fears regarding the diagnosis, including the knowledge and fear of eventual death.
   b. Allow the teen to express anger at his or her physical restrictions and increasing dependency related to the progression of disease.
   c. Encourage the family to join supportive community organizations (e.g., Muscular Dystrophy Association).
   d. Be prepared to assist the child and family with grief work.
3. Impaired Physical Mobility/Risk for Impaired Skin Integrity.
   a. Reinforce education by the physical therapist (PT), or, if PT is unavailable, educate the child and family regarding safe crutch walking and/or wheelchair use.
   b. Assist the child to maintain activity levels as long as possible by incorporating a structured exercise routine into the daily plan of care.
   c. If wheelchair bound, educate the parents and child to monitor for signs of skin breakdown.
   d. Because maintaining optimal body weight enables affected children to maintain ambulation longer, refer the family to a registered dietitian and reinforce nutrition counseling.
4. Risk for Infection/Risk for Impaired Gas Exchange/Risk for Impaired Breathing Patterns as the child's muscular function deteriorates.
   a. Educate the parents to perform daily respiratory PT.
   b. Educate the parents to assess the child's respiratory function daily (see Chapter 16,

"Nursing Care of the Child With Respiratory Illnesses").
   c. Educate the parents to protect the child from others with active infection.
   d. Educate the parents immediately to seek medical care whenever the child exhibits signs of respiratory infection.
   e. Educate the parents and child regarding signs and symptoms of congestive heart failure and immediately to seek medical care if signs and symptoms appear (See Chapter 17, "Nursing Care of the Child With Cardiovascular Illnesses").
5. Risk for Injury/Impaired Urinary and Bowel Elimination.
   a. Educate the parents and child to monitor daily I&O.
   b. Educate the parents regarding the child's DMV needs.
   c. Encourage the parents to provide the child with a high-fiber diet.
   d. Administer stool softeners/laxatives, as needed.

X. Osteomyelitis

A. Incidence.
1. **Osteomyelitis** most frequently affects children in the late toddler and preschool period.
2. Boys are more frequently affected than are girls.

B. Etiology.
1. Bacterial invasion into the bone occurs either indirectly via the vascular system or directly as a result of a break in the skin.
2. The most common pathogen is *Staphylococcus aureus*. Other responsible bacteria are *Escherichia coli, Haemophilus influenzae*, and *Streptococcus pyogenes*. In addition, pathogens found in the soil (e.g., *Pseudomonas aeruginosa*) also are seen.

C. Pathophysiology.
1. Either via the vascular tree or directly via a break in the skin, bacteria enter the bone, most commonly the epiphyseal plate.
2. Pus develops in the area but, because the pus is unable to be evacuated from the site, abscesses often develop.
3. Over time, the blood supply to the area is adversely affected.
4. If unsuccessfully treated, an acute or subacute form of the disease can result in a chronic disease.
5. Signs and symptoms.
   a. In infants and young toddlers: nonspecific signs and symptoms:
      i. Elevated temperature, irritability, poor feeding, and lethargy.
   b. Older children exhibit more specific symptoms.
      i. Signs of inflammation (e.g., redness, warmth, swelling, pain) over the site of the infection.
      ii. Limping, if the child is ambulatory.
      iii. Children sometimes complain of pain in a nearby joint, even though the joint is unlikely the site of the infection.

D. Diagnosis.
1. The clinical picture is suggestive, including the characteristic signs and symptoms plus:
   a. Laboratory evidence, including elevated WBC count, elevated erythrocyte sedimentation rate (ESR), and/or positive blood cultures.
2. Definitive diagnosis is made from:
   a. X-ray, MRI, CT scans, and/or bone scans.
   b. Culture and sensitivity of the aspirate from the bone.

E. Treatment.
1. High-dose, IV antibiotics, including aminoglycosides, which must often be administered for 6 weeks or more.
2. Surgery is often required when:
   a. An abscess is present and/or the infection is not treated effectively by the antibiotics.
   b. Bone necrosis has occurred.

F. Nursing considerations.
1. Knowledge Deficit/Risk for Impaired Coping/Anxiety/Fear/Anger.
   a. An excellent nursing history must be conducted in an attempt to determine how the bacteria entered the child's body.
   b. Once a correct diagnosis is made, educate the parents and child, if appropriate, regarding the etiology and pathophysiology of the disease.
   c. Allow the parents and child, if appropriate, to express concerns, anxiety, and fears regarding the disease and treatment plan.
   d. Allow the child to express, in his or her own way, anger at the requisite physical restrictions.
2. Pain.
   a. Assess pain using an age-appropriate pain rating scale.
   b. Administer safe dosages of analgesics utilizing appropriate technique, as prescribed.
   c. Prior to discharge, educate the parents and child, if appropriate, regarding the safe administration of analgesics.
   d. Provide nonpharmacological pain interventions, as needed.
3. Risk for Injury that may develop from prolonged use of antibiotics.
   a. Administer safe dosages of antibiotics using the five rights of medication administration.
   b. Monitor the IV site for signs and symptoms of phlebitis and/or infiltration of the IV (see

Chapter 9, "Pediatric Medication Administration").

c. Recommend to the primary health-care provider that a peripherally inserted central catheter (PICC) or other central line be inserted to preclude the child from having multiple IV insertions.
   i. If a PICC line is in place, the child must be monitored carefully for complications, including air emboli, infection, phlebitis, and thrombi.

d. Carefully monitor the child for signs and symptoms of side effects to the antibiotics (e.g., diarrhea, ototoxicity, nephrotoxicity, rash, respiratory complications, adverse laboratory values).

e. Use necessary restraint systems in order to prevent the child from removing the IV catheter (e.g., arm board, elbow restraints).

4. Infection.
   a. If wound care is needed, maintain standard precautions during dressing changes.
      i. If the hospitalized child is young and unreliable, or if the infection is caused by a resistant organism, consider placing the child in a private room on contact isolation.

5. Imbalanced Nutrition: Less than Body Requirements/Risk for Altered Growth and Development.
   a. Encourage the parents to provide the child with a high-protein, high-calorie diet to promote resolution of the infection.
   b. Encourage the parents to offer the child small, frequent servings of foods that are favored by the child.
   c. Encourage the parents to provide the child with age-appropriate activities that are consistent with the treatment plan.
   d. To prevent complications, if the child is required to remain immobile, monitor respiratory and bowel function and perform prescribed active and passive ROM exercises.

CASE STUDY: Putting It All Together

Young man, accompanied by his parents, arrives in the emergency department via ambulance

Subjective Data
- 17-year-old male with DMD
- Paramedic, who is wheeling the patient into the ED on a stretcher, states,
  - "History of muscular dystrophy."
  - "Dyspnea and hyperthermia secondary to an upper respiratory infection."
  - "Temperature of 102.4 °F, heart rate of 154 bpm, and a respiratory rate of 60 rpm."
  - "Oxygen administered at 2 L/min while on route."
- Mother states,
  - "He needs immediate help. He must have pneumonia. Notify his pulmonologist now!"
- Young man states, with marked difficulty,
  - "I don't want any treatment. I am ready to die."

Vital Signs	
Temperature:	102.4 °F
Heart rate:	154 bpm
Respiratory rate:	60 rpm

Objective Data

Nursing Assessment
- Unmarried, 17-year-old Caucasian male
- Gasping for breath
- Respiratory assessment
  - Rales bilaterally
  - Minimal intercostal retractions
  - Poor aeration to the bases
- Physical findings
  - Marked muscular wasting
  - Edema of the feet and lower legs

Health-Care Provider's Orders
- Admit to emergency department
- Head of bed elevated 60 degrees
- Oxygen via face mask at 2 L/min
- Ethics conference between parents, patient, and hospital ethics committee

CASE STUDY: Putting It All Together

cont'd

Case Study Questions

A. What *subjective* assessments indicate that this client is experiencing a health alteration?

1. ______
2. ______
3. ______

B. What *objective* assessments indicate that this client is experiencing a health alteration?

1. ______
2. ______
3. ______
4. ______
5. ______
6. ______
7. ______

C. After analyzing the data that has been collected, what **primary** nursing diagnosis should the nurse assign to this client?

1. ______

D. What interventions should the nurse plan and/or implement to meet this child's and his family's needs?

1. ______
2. ______
3. ______
4. ______
5. ______

E. What client outcomes should the nurse evaluate regarding the effectiveness of the nursing interventions?

1. ______
2. ______

F. What physiological characteristics should the child exhibit before being discharged from the emergency department?

1. ______
2. ______

G. What subjective characteristics should the child exhibit before being discharged from the emergency department?

1. ______
2. ______

REVIEW QUESTIONS

1. A 16-year-old gymnast falls from the uneven parallel bars onto her right arm. The school nurse is called to the scene. The young woman points to her right forearm and states, "It really hurts there." Which of the following actions should the nurse perform at this time? **Select all that apply.**
   1. Apply pressure to the site of point tenderness.
   2. Ask the young woman to move the fingers of her right hand.
   3. Compare the radial pulses on the right wrist to those on the left wrist.
   4. Compare the range of motion of the right wrist to that of the left wrist.
   5. Ask the young woman whether her right hand and arm feel differently from the left hand and arm.

2. A school-age child has been diagnosed with a right ankle sprain. Which of the following actions should the nurse advise the child and parents to perform?
   1. Surround the ankle in a heating pad at moderate heat.
   2. Position the ankle at a level below that of the heart.
   3. Wrap the ankle in an ace bandage or an ankle brace.
   4. Practice range of motion exercises until the pain is resolved.

3. A 5-year-old child, diagnosed with a greenstick fracture of the left ulna, is being discharged home from the emergency department in a fiberglass cast. Which of the following actions should the nurse make at this time?
   1. Inform the parents to use a hair dryer to facilitate the drying of the cast.
   2. Report the suspected child abuse case to the local child abuse agency.
   3. Refer the family to a specialist to investigate the etiology for the unusual break.
   4. Educate the parents to monitor the temperature and color of the child's left hand.

4. A 9-year-old child is in the hospital in skin traction after sustaining a simple fracture of the femur. Which of the following assessments should the nurse make during rounds with the child's orthopedist? The nurse should assess the: **(Select all that apply.)**
   1. child's level of pain.
   2. child's bowel sounds.
   3. capillary refill of the child's toes.
   4. skin under the ace bandage for signs of skin breakdown.
   5. wound for signs of redness, edema, ecchymosis, drainage, and approximation.

5. A 3-year-old child is admitted to the pediatric unit in skeletal traction after fracturing the femur. Which of the following orders should the nurse request from the child's primary health-care practitioner?
   1. Jacket restraint when not accompanied by parent
   2. Liquid diet
   3. Active range of motion exercises of lower extremities
   4. Foley catheter

6. A neonate, who was delivered by Cesarean section for a breech presentation, is being examined in the neonatal nursery. For which of the following complications should the nurse carefully assess the baby?
   1. Developmental dysplasia of the hips (DDH)
   2. Legg-Calve-Perthes (LCP)
   3. Duchenne muscular dystrophy (DMD)
   4. Slipped capital femoral epiphysis (SCFE)

7. The nurse is assessing a 3-month-old during a well-baby visit. Which of the following findings would warrant the nurse to recommend that the baby have an ultrasound for a possible diagnosis of developmental dysplasia of the hip (DDH)?
   1. Bilateral plantar flexion
   2. Unequal knee heights
   3. Bilateral polydactyly
   4. Positive Babinski test

8. The nurse is teaching the parents of a child with developmental dysplasia of the hip (DDH) regarding the application of the Pavlik harness. Which of the following information should the nurse include in the teaching?
   1. Three diapers should be worn at all times under the harness.
   2. Harness should be removed for ten minutes every hour.
   3. Harness should always keep the legs fully adducted.
   4. Clothing should always fit loosely over the harness.

9. An 8-year-old child has been diagnosed with Legg-Calve-Perthes disease. Which of the following information should the nurse include in the patient teaching regarding the illness?
   1. "You will have to stay home from school and learn from a tutor until you get better."
   2. "The infection in your bone will be treated with a special medicine that you will receive through your vein."
   3. "You will have to use crutches and be allowed only to walk on your healthy leg until your bones are all better."
   4. "The cast must stay on your ankle and calf for a few weeks until they are fully healed."

10. A nurse who works with overweight children monitors them carefully for signs and symptoms of which of the following musculoskeletal illnesses?
   1. Scoliosis
   2. Legg-Calve-Perthes
   3. Slipped capital femoral epiphysis
   4. Duchenne muscular dystrophy

11. A nurse is observing a child with a leg cast who is learning how to crutch walk. Which of the following assessments would lead the nurse to identify deficient knowledge as a priority nursing diagnosis for the child? While using the crutches, the child:
   1. bends her elbows at all times.
   2. swings her legs forward before moving the crutches.
   3. keeps a space between her axillae and the underarm supports.
   4. moves both crutches forward at the same time.

12. A 13-year-old girl, who has been diagnosed with scoliosis, has been ordered to wear a therapeutic brace for 20 hours each day. The nurse identifies which of the following nursing diagnoses for this child?
   1. Risk for Disturbed Body Image
   2. Bathing Self-care Deficit
   3. Risk for Impaired Urinary Elimination
   4. Ineffective Breathing Pattern

13. An adolescent is being admitted to the pediatric intensive care unit following rod placement for a diagnosis of scoliosis. Which of the following assessments is highest priority for the nurse to perform?
   1. Pain level
   2. Intravenous flow rate
   3. Blood loss
   4. Electrolyte values

14. A nurse must change the position of an adolescent who is 2 hours' post-op rod placement for a diagnosis of scoliosis. Which of the following actions should the nurse perform?
   1. Elevate the head of the bed to thirty degrees.
   2. Lower the bed into the Trendelenburg position.
   3. Turn the child while keeping the child's spine straight.
   4. Place a pillow under the knees and keep the child supine.

15. A nurse is reviewing the results of a genetic analysis performed on a child with Duchenne muscular dystrophy (DMD). Which of the following results would the nurse expect to see?
   1. 46 XY, X linked recessive inheritance
   2. 46 XX, autosomal dominant inheritance
   3. 46 XY, autosomal recessive inheritance
   4. 46 XX, mitochondrial inheritance

16. The nurse is educating the parents of a child with Duchenne muscular dystrophy (DMD) regarding priority actions that they should take when caring for their child. Which of the following actions should the nurse include during the teaching session? Immediately report to the child's primary health-care provider if the child:
   1. has diarrhea.
   2. refuses to eat.
   3. develops an upper respiratory infection.
   4. complains of pain in any limbs.

17. An ambulatory 11-month-old child has been diagnosed with osteomyelitis. Which of the following signs/symptoms would the nurse expect to see?
1. Feeding problems
2. Pain
3. Warmth at the site
4. Limp

18. A child with osteomyelitis is receiving IV gentamycin. The nurse should monitor which of the child's laboratory values to assess for possible toxicity from the medication?
1. Hematocrit
2. Platelet count
3. Serum sodium
4. Blood urea nitrogen

19. An 8-year-old child diagnosed with osteomyelitis is being cared for at home with IV antibiotics that are being administered by a home-care nurse via a peripheral intravenous central catheter (PICC). The home-care nurse should immediately call the emergency contact number if the child exhibits which of the following signs/symptoms? **Select all that apply.**
1. Dyspnea
2. Chest pain
3. Tachycardia
4. Hypertension
5. Hyperthermia

REVIEW ANSWERS

1. ANSWER: 2, 3, 4, and 5

Rationale:

1. It would be inappropriate to apply pressure to the site of point tenderness.
2. **The nurse should assess the young woman's ability to move the fingers of her right hand.**
3. **The nurse should compare the radial pulses on the right wrist to those on the left wrist.**
4. **The nurse should compare the ROM of the right wrist to that of the left wrist.**
5. **The nurse should ask the young woman whether her right hand and arm feel differently from the left hand and arm.**

TEST-TAKING TIP: After a patient is injured, the nurse should attempt to evaluate the severity of the injury by assessing for the five Ps: severity of the pain, including a specific point of tenderness; pulse distal to the injury; pallor or loss of color distal to the injury; presence of paresthesias distal to the injury; and paralysis of movement distal to the injury.

Content Area: *Pediatrics—Neuromuscular*
Integrated Processes: *Nursing Process: Assessment*
Client Need: *Health Promotion and Maintenance: Techniques of Physical Assessment*
Cognitive Level: *Application*

2. ANSWER: 3

Rationale:

1. An ice pack should be applied to the ankle.
2. The ankle should be elevated above the level of the heart.
3. **The ankle should be wrapped in an ace bandage or an ankle brace.**
4. The child should not move the ankle or place weight on the ankle.

TEST-TAKING TIP: When an extremity has suffered a soft tissue injury, the actions summarized in the acronym RICE should be instituted: rest, ice, compression, and elevation.

Content Area: *Pediatrics—Neuromuscular*
Integrated Processes: *Nursing Process: Implementation*
Client Need: *Physiological Integrity: Physiological Adaptation: Alterations in Body Systems*
Cognitive Level: *Application*

3. ANSWER: 4

Rationale:

1. A hair dryer should not be used to dry a cast.
2. Unless the parents' explanation for the child's injury is questionable, a greenstick fracture should not trigger the nurse to suspect that the child has been physically abused.
3. Greenstick fractures commonly are seen in children.
4. **The parents should be taught to monitor the temperature and color of the child's left hand.**

TEST-TAKING TIP: After a cast has been applied, a patient's caregivers should carefully assess the neurovascular status of the extremity distal to the cast.

Content Area: *Pediatrics—Neuromuscular*
Integrated Processes: *Nursing Process: Implementation*
Client Need: *Physiological Integrity: Reduction of Risk Potential: Potential for Complications of Diagnostic Test/Treatments/Procedures*
Cognitive Level: *Application*

4. ANSWER: 1, 2, 3, and 4

Rationale:

1. **The nurse should assess the child's level of pain.**
2. **The nurse should assess the child's bowel sounds.**
3. **The nurse should assess the capillary refill of the child's toes.**
4. **The nurse should assess the skin under the ace bandages for signs of skin breakdown.**
5. There is no wound for the nurse to assess.

TEST-TAKING TIP: A simple fracture is an internal fracture that is enclosed in intact skin. Skin traction is applied directly to the skin using ace bandages or other external devices. One of the complications of skin traction is impaired skin integrity. Children who are in traction are confined to the bed. A complication of immobility is impaired elimination secondary to decrease in peristalsis.

Content Area: *Pediatrics—Neuromuscular*
Integrated Processes: *Nursing Process: Implementation*
Client Need: *Physiological Integrity: Reduction of Risk Potential: Potential for Complications of Diagnostic Test/Treatments/Procedures*
Cognitive Level: *Application*

5. ANSWER: 1

Rationale:

1. **The nurse should request an order for a jacket restraint when the child is not accompanied by a parent.**
2. To prevent constipation, the child should consume a high-fiber diet.
3. The child should not perform active ROM exercises of the knee or hip of the affected leg.
4. The child would be able to urinate.

TEST-TAKING TIP: Three-year-old children do not understand the rationale for bedrest and traction following a serious fracture. They often will attempt to get out of bed in order to walk and run. They may also attempt to twist and turn to get out of the traction. A jacket restraint will help to keep the child in the appropriate position in the bed. However, it should never be used as punishment.

Content Area: *Pediatrics—Neuromuscular*
Integrated Processes: *Nursing Process: Implementation*
Client Need: *Physiological Integrity: Reduction of Risk Potential: Potential for Complications of Diagnostic Test/Treatments/Procedures*
Cognitive Level: *Application*

6. ANSWER: 1

Rationale:

1. **Neonates should be assessed in the neonatal nursery for DDH.**
2. LCP affects children from 4 to 8 years of age.
3. DMD is a hereditary illness that is diagnosed when children fail to achieve growth and development milestones.

4. SCFE affects children who are in their pubertal growth period.

TEST-TAKING TIP: If he or she has been taught, the nurse should perform Ortolani's and Barlow's tests during the newborn assessment to check for the presence of hip dysplasia. If the nurse has not received training, to prevent injury, the baby's primary health-care practitioner should perform the assessments.

Content Area: *Pediatrics—Neuromuscular*
Integrated Processes: *Nursing Process: Assessment*
Client Need: *Health Promotion and Maintenance: Ante/Intra/Postpartum and Newborn Care*
Cognitive Level: *Comprehension*

7. ANSWER: 2

Rationale:

1. Bilateral plantar flexion is a sign of clubfoot, not DDH.
2. **Unequal knee heights is a sign of DDH.**
3. Extra digits on the hands and/or toes is a common, benign, birth anomaly.
4. Positive Babinski test is normal in infants.

TEST-TAKING TIP: Signs and symptoms of DDH may appear after the neonatal period. Infants at each well-baby check, therefore, should be assessed for the problem. In addition to Ortolani's and Barlow's tests being performed, the nurse should assess for unequal knee heights and unequal anterior and posterior thigh folds.

Content Area: *Pediatrics—Neuromuscular*
Integrated Processes: *Nursing Process: Assessment*
Client Need: *Health Promotion and Maintenance: Techniques of Physical Assessment*
Cognitive Level: *Comprehension*

8. ANSWER: 4

Rationale:

1. Triple diapering is not employed in conjunction with the Pavlik harness. Some practitioners still recommend triple diapering in lieu of the Pavlik, but the practice is not as therapeutic as wearing the harness 23 to 24 hr each day.
2. If allowed, the harness should only be removed for bathing.
3. The harness should always keep the legs fully abducted, not adducted.
4. **Clothing should always fit loosely over the harness.**

TEST-TAKING TIP: In order for the Pavlik to maintain the child's legs in abduction, nothing should restrict the harness. Diapers, therefore, should always be applied under the harness, and clothing should always fit loosely over the harness.

Content Area: *Pediatrics—Neuromuscular*
Integrated Processes: *Nursing Process: Implementation; Teaching/Learning*
Client Need: *Physiological Integrity: Reduction of Risk Potential: Potential for Complications of Diagnostic Tests/Treatments/Procedures*
Cognitive Level: *Comprehension*

9. ANSWER: 3

Rationale:

1. This statement is inappropriate. The child will be able to attend school.
2. LCP is not characterized by a bone infection.
3. **This statement is correct. The child will have to use crutches and only walk on the healthy leg until the bones have healed.**
4. The pathology of LCP is in the head of the femur.

TEST-TAKING TIP: To prevent permanent damage, it is important for the child to bear no weight on the affected joint. This can be difficult for an active school-age child. Alternate activities must be provided to the child in order to promote continued gross and fine motor development.

Content Area: *Pediatrics—Neuromuscular*
Integrated Processes: *Nursing Process: Implementation; Teaching/Learning*
Client Need: *Physiological Integrity: Reduction of Risk Potential: Potential for Complications of Diagnostic Tests/Treatments/Procedures*
Cognitive Level: *Application*

10. ANSWER: 3

Rationale:

1. Scoliosis is seen more frequently in girls than in boys, but it is not seen more frequently in obese children.
2. There is no known high-risk group for LCP.
3. **Slipped capital femoral epiphysis is seen more frequently in obese children.**
4. Muscular dystrophy is caused by a genetic defect.

TEST-TAKING TIP: School nurses should monitor obese children for the characteristic signs and symptoms of slipped capital femoral epiphysis: hip tenderness or pain, decreased hip flexion, limp, and increased pain when the toes are turned inward.

Content Area: *Pediatrics—Neuromuscular*
Integrated Processes: *Nursing Process: Assessment*
Client Need: *Health Promotion and Maintenance: Health Screening*
Cognitive Level: *Comprehension*

11. ANSWER: 2

Rationale:

1. The child should bend her elbows at all times.
2. **The crutches should be placed forward, then the legs should swing forward to meet the crutch location.**
3. The crutch walker should keep a space between her axillae and the underarm supports.
4. Both crutches should be moved forward at the same time.

TEST-TAKING TIP: When crutches are used incorrectly, injuries can occur. The nurse should carefully assess the child's crutch walking prior to discharge to make sure that they are being used correctly.

Content Area: *Pediatrics—Neuromuscular*
Integrated Processes: *Nursing Process: Analysis*
Client Need: *Physiological Integrity: Reduction of Risk Potential: Potential for Complications of Diagnostic Tests/Treatments/Procedures*
Cognitive Level: *Comprehension*

12. ANSWER: 1
Rationale:
1. Risk for Disturbed Body Image is an appropriate nursing diagnosis for the nurse to identify.
2. The girl should have no difficulty bathing.
3. The girl is not at high risk for Impaired Urinary Elimination.
4. The girl is not at high risk for Ineffective Breathing Pattern.
TEST-TAKING TIP: Adolescent girls are concerned about their bodies and how they appear to others, especially their peers. As a result, many refuse to comply with wearing their braces, especially when they are asked to wear the braces to school.
Content Area: *Pediatrics—Neuromuscular*
Integrated Processes: *Nursing Process: Analysis*
Client Need: *Physiological Integrity: Reduction of Risk Potential: Potential for Complications of Diagnostic Tests/Treatments/Procedures*
Cognitive Level: *Application*

13. ANSWER: 3
Rationale:
1. Pain assessment is important, but it is not the highest priority.
2. The assessment of the IV flow rate is important, but it is not the highest priority.
3. Assessment of blood loss is the highest priority.
4. The assessment of the child's electrolyte values is important, but it is not the highest priority.
TEST-TAKING TIP: Blood loss during rod placement for scoliosis can be extensive and can result in impaired perfusion to vital organs (e.g., kidneys).
Content Area: *Pediatrics—Neuromuscular*
Integrated Processes: *Nursing Process: Assessment*
Client Need: *Safe and Effective Care Environment: Management of Care: Establishing Priorities*
Cognitive Level: *Analysis*

14. ANSWER: 3
Rationale:
1. The bed should remain flat.
2. The bed should remain flat.
3. The child should be turned while keeping the child's spine straight.
4. The child should be kept flat but should be moved from side to side.
TEST-TAKING TIP: To prevent damage to the child's surgical site and spinal cord following rod placement for scoliosis, the child should be log rolled. It usually requires more than one nurse to roll a patient like a log and to keep from bending the child's spine.
Content Area: *Pediatrics—Neuromuscular*
Integrated Processes: *Nursing Process: Implementation*
Client Need: *Physiological Integrity: Reduction of Risk Potential: Potential Complications From Surgical Procedures and Health Alterations*
Cognitive Level: *Application*

15. ANSWER: 1
Rationale:
1. The results of a genetic analysis of a child with DMD will state that the child has 46 chromosomes, is male, and does have an X-linked recessive disease.
2. The results of a genetic analysis of a child with DMD will state that the child has 46 chromosomes, is male, and does have an X-linked recessive disease.
3. The results of a genetic analysis of a child with DMD will state that the child has 46 chromosomes, is male, and does have an X-linked recessive disease.
4. The results of a genetic analysis of a child with DMD will state that the child has 46 chromosomes, is male, and does have an X-linked recessive disease.
TEST-TAKING TIP: DMD is a single gene genetic disease that is carried on the X chromosome. As a result, women carry the gene that can then be inherited by their children. Because women carry two X chromosomes, they do not exhibit the disease. Only men, who carry only one X chromosome, exhibit the fatal disease.
Content Area: *Pediatrics—Neuromuscular*
Integrated Processes: *Nursing Process: Assessment*
Client Need: *Physiological Integrity: Physiological Adaptation: Pathophysiology*
Cognitive Level: *Application*

16. ANSWER 3
Rationale:
1. Although persistent diarrhea can be problematic, it is no more dangerous in children with DMD than in other children.
2. Although refusing to eat can be problematic, it is no more dangerous in children with DMD than in other children.
3. The parents must report immediately if their child with DMD develops an upper respiratory infection.
4. Although complaints of pain can be problematic, it is no more dangerous in children with DMD than in other children.
TEST-TAKING TIP: As the child's muscle fibers are replaced by fat cells, he is less and less able to fight upper respiratory infections. The child must be seen by a health-care practitioner so that an aggressive therapy can be instituted.
Content Area: *Pediatrics—Neuromuscular*
Integrated Processes: *Nursing Process: Implementation; Teaching/Learning*
Client Need: *Physiological Integrity: Physiological Adaptation: Alteration in Body Systems*
Cognitive Level: *Application*

17. ANSWER: 1
Rationale:
1. The nurse would expect to see feeding problems.
2. The child may or may not exhibit pain.
3. The site may or may not feel warm to the nurse.
4. The child may or may not limp when walking.
TEST-TAKING TIP: When they are infected, infants and young toddlers usually exhibit generalized, systemic symptoms rather than specific, localized symptoms.

Anorexia is one of the more frequent systemic symptoms seen.
Content Area: Pediatrics—Neuromuscular
Integrated Processes: Nursing Process: Assessment
Client Need: Physiological Integrity: Physiological Adaptation: Alteration in Body Systems
Cognitive Level: Application

18. ANSWER: 4
Rationale:
1. A child's hematocrit is unrelated to whether he or she is developing gentamycin toxicity.
2. A child's platelet count is unrelated to whether he or she is developing gentamycin toxicity.
3. A child's serum sodium is unrelated to whether he or she is developing gentamycin toxicity.
4. A child's blood urea nitrogen (BUN) levels should be monitored when he or she receives an aminoglycoside antibiotic.
TEST-TAKING TIP: Gentamycin, an aminoglycoside, can cause nephrotoxicity. BUN is one of the renal function tests that should be monitored by the nurse.
Content Area: Pediatrics—Neuromuscular
Integrated Processes: Nursing Process: Evaluation
Client Need: Physiological Integrity: Pharmacological and Parenteral Therapies: Adverse Effects/Contraindications/Side Effects/Interactions
Cognitive Level: Application

19. ANSWER: 1, 2, 3, and 5
Rationale:
1. The nurse should monitor the child for dyspnea.
2. The nurse should monitor the child for chest pain.
3. The nurse should monitor the child for tachycardia.
4. The nurse should monitor the child for hypotension. Hypertension is not related to an adverse reaction to a PICC line.
5. The nurse should monitor the child for hyperthermia.
TEST-TAKING TIP: Two of the serious complications that can develop when a child has a PICC line in place are air embolism and infection. Dyspnea, chest pain, and hypotension are all symptoms of an air embolism. Tachycardia and hyperthermia are both symptoms of an infection.
Content Area: Pediatrics—Medication
Integrated Processes: Nursing Process: Implementation
Client Need: Physiological Integrity: Pharmacological and Parenteral Therapies: Adverse Effects/Contraindications/Side Effects/Interactions
Cognitive Level: Application

Nursing Care of the Child With Endocrine Disorders

KEY TERMS

Acanthosis nigricans—Darkening of the skin, especially around the neck.
Catabolism—The metabolic process of breaking down molecules to release energy.
Congenital hypothyroidism (CHT)—A dysfunction of the thyroid gland in which the hormone thyroxin (T4) is not produced.
Glucagon—A hormone that stimulates the release of glucose from the liver.
Growth hormone deficiency (GHD)—Reduction in human growth hormone, resulting in slowed growth (below the 5th percentile for height), delayed puberty, poor muscle mass, small penis, and hypoglycemia.
Kussmaul respirations—A deep and labored respiratory pattern.
Phenylketonuria (PKU)—The inability of the liver to break down the amino acid phenylalanine.
Precocious puberty—The onset of physical sexual development at an earlier age than normal.
Spasticity—Stiff, tight, or rigid muscles.
Thyroid-stimulating hormone (TSH)—A hormone produced by the anterior pituitary gland that signals the thyroid gland to produce thyroxine (T4).
Thyroxine (T4)—A hormone required by the body to produce proteins and enable the cells to utilize oxygen.

I. Description

The endocrine system is classically defined as the glandular tissues of the body in which hormones are produced. This chapter, however, begins with a discussion of **phenylketonuria** (PKU) that results because of the inability of the liver to produce an enzyme to break down an essential amino acid—phenylalanine. The chapter continues with a discussion of the more common endocrine disorders seen in children and the glands in which the hormones are produced.

II. Phenylketonuria

A. Incidence.
1. The disease is seen in about 1 in 15,000 live births.

B. Etiology.
1. PKU is an autosomal recessive disease. A child must carry both affected alleles to exhibit the disease.

DID YOU KNOW?

Newborn screening tests are conducted in all 50 of the United States. All states are mandated to screen for 21 disorders, including PKU, while some states screen for many more. In other words, each state decides whether to screen for a number of additional diseases. To learn more about newborn screening and/or to determine which diseases are tested in each state, parents and nurses can visit the following Web sites: Genetics Home Reference (http://ghr.nlm.nih.gov/nbs) and National Newborn Screening and Global Resource Center (http://genes-r-us.uthscsa.edu/).

C. Pathophysiology.
1. A mutation in a gene on chromosome 12 results in the inability of the liver to metabolize phenylalanine, an essential amino acid.
2. If the child's diet is not modified, the child:
   a. Will develop profound cognitive deficits.
   b. Will exhibit physiological signs/symptoms, including vomiting, musty-smelling urine, **spasticity** (stiff, tight, or rigid muscles), and hyperactive behavior.

D. Diagnosis.
1. Newborn screening test is performed in all 50 states.
   a. For accurate results, the test must be performed after the child has consumed protein for at least 24 hr.

DID YOU KNOW?

The test for PKU is conducted on newborns' blood from a heel stick on day 2 of life. Because phenylalanine is present in animal proteins, until the baby consumes the proteins in breast milk or formula, undigested phenylalanine will not be present in the bloodstream. The blood, therefore, should not be collected until the child is at least 24 hr old.

2. If the screening test is positive, elevated blood levels of phenylalanine are confirmatory.

E. Treatment.
1. Immediate and continual dietary modification. However, because phenylalanine is an essential amino acid, low levels of phenylalanine must be consumed.
2. In infancy.
   a. Babies with PKU are either placed on a formula that contains low levels of phenylalanine or are breastfed.
      i. Breast milk contains relatively low levels of the amino acid.
3. When the children begin to eat solids:
   a. They must avoid consuming all animal protein, including milk, fish, eggs, and meats.
   b. Some grains also contain phenylalanine.
   c. The foods that are safe for children with PKU to eat are vegetables, fruits, and starches.
4. Monitoring of serum phenylalanine levels is essential throughout childhood.
5. Whether to continue the diet into adulthood is controversial, but it is essential that pregnant women with PKU maintain a strict low-phenylalanine diet because the fetus will become seriously affected if the mother has high levels in her serum.
   a. The newborn will be born with one or more serious complications, including intellectual disability, microcephaly, and/or seizures.

F. Nursing considerations.
1. Deficient Knowledge/Risk for Altered Family Process/Anxiety/Grieving.
   a. Educate parents regarding newborn screening tests.
   b. If the child is diagnosed with PKU, provide the parents with an explanation of the child's disease.
   c. Allow the parents to express grief and loss of the perfect child.
   d. Enable the parents to discuss concerns regarding the child's diet and future health.
   e. Refer the parents to a dietician for diet counseling.
   f. Refer the parents to community resources (e.g., National PKU Alliance).
   g. Refer the parents for genetic counseling to determine the potential for delivering another child with PKU.
   h. Educate the parents regarding the need for regular testing of the child's serum.
      i. Because the child must consume some phenylalanine for growth and development, the child's serum levels must be monitored on a regular basis.
2. Risk for Impaired Growth and Development (see Chapter 24, "Nursing Care of the Child With Intellectual and Developmental Disabilities").
   a. At each well-child visit, assess the child for achievement of normal growth and development milestones.
      i. Even with dietary alteration, biological growth and cognitive development may be adversely affected.
   b. If indicated, refer the child to programs that provide early educational intervention.
   c. Depending on additional deficits exhibited by the child, refer the family for specialized care, e.g., occupational therapy, physical therapy.

III. Congenital Hypothyroidism

The thyroid gland has been labeled the energy center of the body. **Thyroxine (T4)** is produced by the thyroid in response to **thyroid-stimulating hormone** (TSH) that is produced by the anterior pituitary gland. The hormone, T4, is required by the body for growth and development; the tissues of the body respond to T4 by producing proteins and enabling the cells to utilize oxygen.

A. Incidence.

1. Approximately 1 out of every 4,000 neonates is diagnosed with **congenital hypothyroidism** (CHT).

B. Etiology.

1. In rare cases, the disease runs in families, but the majority of cases have no known cause.

C. Pathophysiology.

1. Either the anterior pituitary fails to send TSH to the thyroid, or the thyroid gland fails to develop in utero.
   a. In either case, T4 is not produced.
2. Sign and symptoms (Fig. 21.1).
   a. Large fontanelles.
   b. Protruding tongue.
   c. Umbilical hernia.
   d. Constipation.
   e. Lethargy.
   f. Prolonged jaundice.
   g. Most concerning: if left untreated, the child will develop profound cognitive deficits.

D. Diagnosis.

1. Clinical picture is suggestive of the disorder.

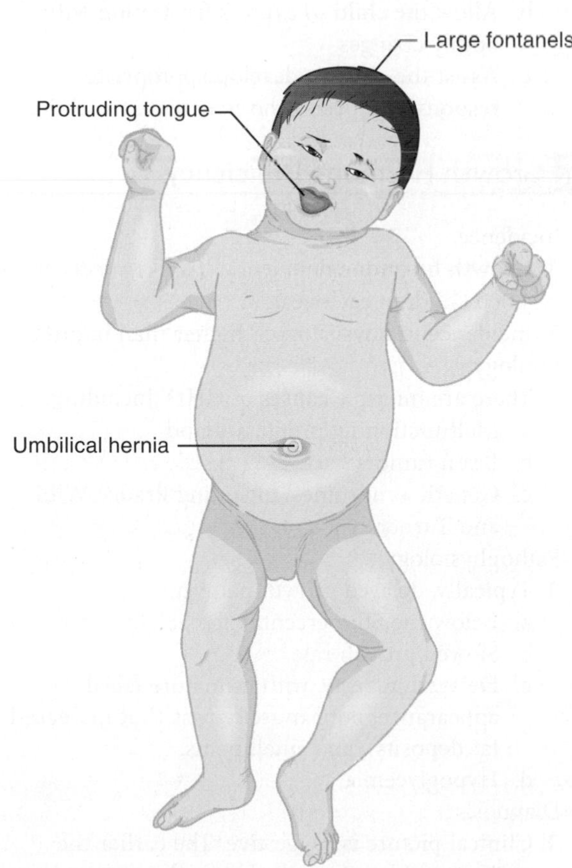

Fig 21.1 Congenital hypothyroidism.

2. Newborn screening is performed in all 50 states.
   a. Because a false negative result may be reported, the screen should not be performed before the baby is 24 hr old.

DID YOU KNOW?

Newborn screening for congenital hypothyroidism is similar to that for PKU. The testing is performed in all 50 states, and, because of the possibility of false negatives, the blood for the test should not be collected until the baby is at least 24 hr old.

3. If the newborn screening is positive, thyroid scans provide a definitive diagnosis.

E. Treatment.

1. Daily oral dosage of Synthroid (levothyroxine)—based on the child's age and weight—begun as soon as hypothyroidism is diagnosed and to be taken daily for the rest of the child's life.

F. Nursing considerations.

1. Deficient Knowledge/Risk for Altered Family Process/Anxiety/Grieving.
   a. Provide the parents with an explanation of the child's disease.
   b. Allow the parents to express grief and loss of the perfect child.
   c. Educate the parents regarding the importance of administering the levothyroxine supplements to prevent signs and symptoms of hypothyroidism and potentially irreversible developmental disabilities.
   d. Provide opportunities for the parents to discuss their concerns regarding the child's medication needs.
      i. Educate the parents (and remind teens with CHT) regarding the importance of taking the medication each day.
      ii. Explain that the dosage of Synthroid will increase as the child ages and gains weight.
         (1) Explain that the signs and symptoms of hypothyroidism, e.g., constipation, lethargy, dry skin, and weight gain, may begin to appear as the child grows and his or her medication dosage is no longer adequate.
      iii. Educate the parents regarding the signs of hyperthyroidism, including tachycardia, weight loss, and sleeplessness, in case of levothyroxine overmedication.

(!) It is important to advise the parents that, until the correct dosage of the medication for their baby is determined, the baby may exhibit signs of hypo- or hyperthyroidism. They should be aware of the signs and symptoms and notify the child's primary health-care provider in either case.

e. Educate the parents that the child will likely need serum testing of T4 levels at each well-child visit.
f. Refer the parents to outside resources (e.g., American Thyroid Association).
2. Risk for Delayed Growth and Development.
a. Educate the parents regarding the need for frequent health maintenance assessments to monitor the child's growth and development.

IV. Precocious Puberty

As stated in Chapter 6, "Normal Growth and Development: Adolescence," girls begin sexual maturation at about 9 years of age, with some girls showing signs of puberty as early as 7 years and others as late as 11 years. Boys, on the other hand, usually begin to show pubertal changes between 9½ and 15 years of age. Some children who experience **precocious puberty**, however, begin their physical sexual development much earlier. Although they are physically advanced, they rarely exhibit precocious sexual behaviors.

A. Incidence.
1. About 1 out of every 5,000 children will experience precocious puberty.
2. Girls outnumber boys by a ratio of 10 to 1.

B. Etiology.
1. In the vast majority of cases, there is no known cause.
2. Obesity, heredity, stress, and/or environmental exposures have been cited as possible causes.
3. Adrenal tumors, central nervous system tumors, and tumors of the gonads have also resulted in precocious puberty.

C. Pathophysiology.
1. Early signs of puberty.
a. In girls.
i. Appearance of secondary sex characteristics (e.g., breast development, pubic and axillary hair growth, growth spurt).
ii. Vaginal changes and early menarche.
b. In boys.
i. Appearance of secondary sex characteristics (e.g., pubic and axillary hair growth, vocal changes).
ii. Testicular enlargement, penile growth, and ejaculation.
2. Early bone fusion often resulting in short adult stature.

D. Diagnosis.
1. Clinical signs are suggestive.
2. Hormonal blood tests (e.g., LH, FSH, testosterone, and estrogen).
3. X-rays of the wrists to determine bone growth.
4. Thorough medical examination to rule out the presence of tumors.

E. Treatment.
1. The most common therapy is the administration of a medication (e.g., leuprolide acetate [Eligard, Lupron]) to inhibit the release of gonadotropin-releasing hormone (GnRH) from the hypothalamus, which then results in reduction in pituitary hormone production.

F. Nursing considerations.
1. Deficient Knowledge.
a. Educate the parents and child regarding the disease process.
b. Remind the parents that, although the child appears older than his or her years, the child is still young and should be parented accordingly.
c. Educate the parents regarding the medication regimen, including injection procedure, if prescribed.
i. Medications usually are administered monthly by intramuscular (IM) injection.
d. If needed, educate the parents and child regarding care of the body during menstruation.
2. Risk for Disturbed Body Image/Impaired Social Interaction.
a. Encourage the parents to dress the child in age-appropriate attire.
b. Allow the child to express frustration with bodily changes.
c. Assist the child to develop appropriate responses to peers who may tease the child.

V. Growth Hormone Deficiency

A. Incidence.
1. **Growth hormone deficiency** (GHD) affects about 4,000 children each year.
2. Incidence in boys is much higher than in girls.

B. Etiology.
1. There are multiple causes of GHD, including:
a. Malfunctioning pituitary gland.
b. Brain tumors.
c. Genetic syndromes, including Prader-Willi and Turner syndrome.

C. Pathophysiology.
1. Typically, delayed growth pattern.
a. Below the 5th percentile for height.
b. Slowed growth rate.
c. Delayed puberty, with immature facial appearance, poor muscle mass (but increased fat deposits), and small penis.
d. Hypoglycemia.

D. Diagnosis.
1. Clinical picture is suggestive. The earlier the problem is identified, the better the outcome. Children considered at risk of GHD should be referred to an endocrinologist.

a. Any girl 10 to 13 years of age or boy 12 to 16 years of age growing less than 5 cm per year, and/or:
b. When there is a marked flattening of the child's normal growth curve; or when the child's height falls below the 5th percentile.

2. Thorough examination, including laboratory data and x-rays of the growth plates of the wrist.
3. Hormonal studies.
   a. To assess the child for other hormonal deficiencies because many hormones work together to enhance maturation (i.e., thyroid studies and sex hormones).
4. Definitive diagnosis.
   a. Growth hormone (GH) levels assessed.
      i. The hormone is naturally secreted during the night, so the pituitary is stimulated to produce GH during the day.
         (1) Examples of stimulating medications: insulin, clonidine hydrochloride (Catapres, Duraclon).
      ii. GH levels less than 10 ng/mL, on two separate occasions, are diagnostic.

E. Medical management.
1. Administration of synthetic GH.
   a. Administered subcutaneously at bedtime six to seven times/week.
      i. Expect 2 cm/yr growth over pretherapy growth.
      ii. Given until the child reaches desired height or until the growth plates close.
   b. Child's growth monitored closely.

F. Nursing considerations.
1. Delayed Growth and Development/Risk for Situation Low Self-Esteem/Risk for Altered Coping/Risk for Disturbed Body Image.
   a. Allow the child and the parents to express their concerns, fears, and/or anger.
   b. If appropriate, reassure the child and parents that the injections will help.
      i. It is important, however, not to provide false hope because the child may not reach the full desired height.
   c. While the child is receiving GH, carefully measure the child's growth on growth charts.
2. Deficient Knowledge.
   a. Educate the parents and child, if appropriate, regarding reconstituting the medication and injection technique.
   b. Educate the parents and child regarding the use of growth charts.

VI. Type 1 Diabetes Mellitus

Diabetes in children is the same disease that is seen in adults. Because of the growth patterns and activity patterns of children, however, the care and monitoring of children must be vigilant. Initially, parents must assume the majority of the management of the disease, but, because of the chronic nature of the disease, the child must take on more responsibility as he or she grows older. This disease will be subdivided into type 1 and type 2 diabetes.

A. Incidence.
1. The risk of developing type 1 diabetes mellitus (DM) is higher than virtually all other chronic diseases of childhood.
2. Peak ages at time of diagnosis are: 5 to 7 years of age and at puberty.
3. Rarely seen in children younger than 2 years of age but type 1 DM has been seen in infants.

B. Etiology.
1. Multiple genetic predisposition loci are present in the genome, but no absolute genetic inheritance pattern has been identified.
2. Likely multifactorial etiology.

C. Pathophysiology.
1. Autoimmune inflammatory process, resulting in destruction of beta cells in the islets of Langerhans.
2. No insulin is produced, therefore the cells of the body are unable to utilize glucose, resulting in:
   a. Excess circulating glucose, eventually spilling into the urine.
   b. The body compensating for lost fuel by the **catabolism** (breaking down) of fats and proteins.
      i. Ketones are formed, resulting in metabolic acidosis.
3. Signs and symptoms.
   a. Hyperglycemia.
   b. The three "polys":
      i. Polyuria.
      ii. Polydipsia.
      iii. Polyphagia.
   c. Weight loss.
   d. Blurred vision.
   e. Fatigue.
   f. Headache.

DID YOU KNOW?

Diabetes mellitus in children often is not suspected until a child develops ketoacidosis and exhibits marked confusion or, in some cases, coma. Only then do parents recognize that the child is seriously ill. Once the child is admitted into the emergency department, the child's serum laboratory values are analyzed, and a clear diagnosis of type 1 diabetes is made.

4. Ketoacidosis, coma, and death may result if insulin is not administered. Ketoacidosis is a medical emergency.

a. Signs and symptoms.
   i. Glucose greater than 300 mg/dL.
   ii. Serum pH less than 7.25.
   iii. Markedly elevated urine ketones.
   iv. Nausea and vomiting.
   v. Abdominal pain.
   vi. Extreme weakness and fatigue.
   vii. Dry, itchy skin.
   viii. "Fruity" breath.
   ix. **Kussmaul respirations**, that is, a deep and labored respiratory pattern.
   x. Altered sensorium.
b. Intensive care is required with fluid replacement, IV insulin, and potassium monitoring and replacement, if needed.

(!) Diabetic ketoacidosis (DKA), seen most frequently in newly diagnosed children, is a life-threatening condition. When the body is unable to utilize glucose because of the lack of insulin production, the body will go into fat catabolism. A marked rise in circulating ketones and a large urinary output follow. Ultimately, the child becomes severely dehydrated, acidotic, and his or her electrolytes shift, especially potassium. Cerebral edema is a potentially serious complication of DKA.

D. Diagnosis.
1. Glycosuria with signs and symptoms of diabetes are suggestive of the disease.
2. Definitive diagnosis is made based on the results of any of the following (Chang et al., 2014):
   a. Hemoglobin A1C greater than or equal to 6.5%.

DID YOU KNOW?

Hemoglobin A1C, or glycosylated hemoglobin, is a compound molecule of hemoglobin and glucose. The higher the glucose level in the bloodstream, the higher the percentage of red blood cells that will become glycosylated. Hemoglobin A1C test results provide health-care providers with an approximation of a patient's average blood glucose level over the preceding 2 or 3 months.

   b. Fasting blood glucose level greater than or equal to 126 mg/dL.
   c. A 2-hr, 75-g, oral glucose tolerance test result of 200 mg/ dL or higher.
   d. An incidental blood glucose of 200 mg/dL or higher, if signs and symptoms of diabetes are present.

E. Treatment: multidisciplinary approach.
1. Insulin via subcutaneous injections or insulin pump.
   a. Must be titrated to each individual's lifestyle, usually a combination of fast-acting and intermediate or no peak types.

MAKING THE CONNECTION

When injecting insulin, the nurse, parents, and child, if appropriate, must follow important principles.

1. If fast-acting insulin is being administered, the child ideally should eat within 5 min of the injection.
2. If two types of insulin are to be injected at the same time, carefully read whether they are compatible in the same syringe.
3. If two types of insulin are compatible, regular insulin should always be drawn up first and intermediate-acting insulin drawn up second.
4. Injection sites should be rotated around the body. The recommended sites for insulin injections are, in order of more rapid to less rapid absorption: abdomen, upper arms, hips, thighs. (Keeping track of injection sites is an excellent task for the young child to take responsibility for.)

(!) Only fast-acting insulins are used in insulin pumps. The principle of insulin pump administration is to cover continuous insulin needs. No intermediate or long-acting insulin should ever be placed in an insulin pump.

   b. Types of insulins (Table 21.1).
2. Regular blood glucose testing determines insulin dosages.
   a. Usually performed at least before meals and before bedtime snack.
      i. May need to be performed more frequently depending on glucose control.
   b. Before meal glucose goals are individualized.
      i. Goals set for infants and toddlers are often higher than for older children because hypoglycemic episodes are most common in young children.
   c. Hemoglobin A1C goals: less than 7.5.
3. Regular urine testing.
4. Diabetic diet.
   a. Tailored to the child's food preferences.
      i. Personal likes versus dislikes.
      ii. Cultural norms.
   b. Aimed at maintaining a consistent pattern of food intake.
5. Daily exercise is recommended to promote optimal glucose usage by cells.
6. If hypoglycemia develops, immediate ingestion of a simple sugar (e.g., packet of sugar, hard candy) is required (see "Making the Connection" on p. 396).
   a. If the child is unconscious or incoherent and is unable to consume a simple sugar, an emergency injection of glucagon should be administered.

Table 21.1 Types of Insulins

	Type	Onset	Peak	Duration	Notes
Fast-Acting Insulins	Aspart (Novolog)	Less than 15 min	1–3 hr	3–5 hr	May mix with NPH in same syringe, but it is not to be mixed with other insulins in the pump
	Lispro (Humalog)	Less than 30 min	30–90 min	Less than 6 hr	Not to be mixed with other insulins in the pump
	Glulisine (Apidra)	Less than 30 min	30–90 min	Less than 6 hr	May be mixed with NPH in same syringe, but it is not to be mixed with other insulins in the pump
	Regular (Humulin R)	0.5–1 hr	2–4 hr	6–12 hr	
Intermediate-Acting and No True Peak Insulins	**Type**	**Onset**	**Peak**	**Duration**	**Notes**
	Detemir (Levemir)	1 hr	No true peak	6–23 hr	
	Glargine (Lantus)	1 hr	No true peak	24 hr	Do not mix with other insulins in the same syringe
	NPH (Humulin N)	1–2 hr	4–14 hr	10–greater than 24 hr	

i. **Glucagon**, which is administered via injection, is a hormone that stimulates the release of glucose from the liver.
ii. Emergency glucagon kits, available by prescription only, should be prescribed for any child with type 1 DM.
iii. Glucagon must be mixed in the syringe immediately before administering. It may be injected into any muscle in the body.
iv. Common side effects of glucagon are:
(1) Nausea and vomiting; therefore, the child should be positioned on his or her side to prevent aspiration of any vomitus.
(2) Hyperglycemia; therefore, the child's glucose levels should be closely monitored following the injection.
v. It is essential that the child's parents, teachers, sports coaches, and other pertinent individuals be educated regarding how to administer an emergency glucagon injection.

F. Nursing considerations.

1. Risk for Injury from hyperglycemia.
a. Educate the parents, child, school officials, and others regarding the signs and symptoms of hyperglycemia (see earlier "Signs and symptoms").
b. Instruct the parents and child, if appropriate, regarding the need for blood glucose testing throughout the day.
c. Educate the parents and child, if appropriate, regarding insulin administration, including rotation of injection sites and the principles of injecting different types of insulin.
d. Refer the parents and child to diabetic and nutrition counselors.
e. Assist the parents and child on ways to prevent hyperglycemic episodes, including diet counseling and exercise routines.
f. Educate the parents and child regarding the potential for hyperglycemia during times of illness.
g. Inform the primary health-care provider if the child repeatedly experiences hyperglycemic episodes.

2. Risk for Injury from hypoglycemia.
a. Educate the parents, child, school officials, and others regarding the signs and symptoms of hypoglycemia, including:
i. Tachycardia, clammy skin, irritability, slurred speech, and loss of consciousness.
(1) Hypoglycemia may be mistaken for temper tantrums in young children.
ii. If uncertain whether the child is hypo- or hyperglycemic, one should always assume hypoglycemia.
iii. Educate the parents, child, school officials, and others regarding the need to treat hypoglycemia immediately with:
(1) Simple sugars (including juice, candies, and soda) if the child is alert and can swallow.
(2) Glucagon injection, if unable to swallow.
iv. Educate the parents, child, school officials, and others regarding the need to recheck the blood glucose level after he or she has consumed the simple sugar.

MAKING THE CONNECTION

In general, hypoglycemia is much more dangerous for children with DM than is hyperglycemia. When a child becomes hypoglycemic, the child has insufficient circulating glucose for the cells of the body, especially the brain cells. Hypoglycemia is a life-threatening state. The nurse, therefore, must teach the parents a number of principles to follow when caring for their diabetic child.

1. Very young children are at especially high risk for hypoglycemia because of their high activity levels. Their target preprandial glucose levels, therefore, are usually higher than those for older children.
2. If parents are unable to determine whether their child is hyper- or hypoglycemic, they should assume that the child is hypoglycemic and give their child a simple sugar.
3. The parents and child, if appropriate, should carry easily digested, simple sugars at all times.
   - Breast milk, formula, and juice for babies.
   - Packs of sugar, candy bars, hard candies, and juice for older children.
   - Emergency glucagon injection to be administered if the child is unresponsive.
4. Oral sugars should only be administered if there is no concern that the child will choke.
5. Many children, often by preschool age, are aware of themselves becoming hypoglycemic. The parents and children should decide on a code word that the child will say to signal the parents to intervene.
6. After a hypoglycemic child has consumed a simple sugar, the child's glucose level should be rechecked.
7. Once a child's glucose level returns to normal and he or she becomes alert, the child should consume a protein source that will help to maintain the normal blood glucose level.
8. Teach children, when age appropriate, always to consume a snack before high-energy activities (e.g., athletic practice, playground recess) in order to maintain adequate serum glucose levels.

v. Once the child's glucose level returns to normal and the child is alert, educate the parents, child, school officials, and others to have the child consume a protein source in order to maintain the normal glucose level.

vi. Inform the primary health-care practitioner if the child repeatedly experiences hypoglycemic episodes.

3. Imbalanced Nutrition: Less than Body Requirements.
   a. Educate the parents and child, if appropriate, regarding the interaction between food intake and insulin needs.
   b. Assist the parents and child to develop a plan to manage food intake, blood glucose testing, and exercise.
   c. Assist the parents and child to develop a diet that includes food preferences but also meets the medical needs of the child.
4. Anxiety/Risk for Altered Coping.
   a. Allow the family and child to express anger, frustration, and guilt regarding the genetic predisposition and the chronic nature of the disease.
   b. Encourage the parents to join a support group (e.g., American Diabetes Association).
   c. Introduce the child and family to other children with the disease.
   d. Encourage the parents to allow the child to engage in age-appropriate activities.
5. Deficient Knowledge.
   a. Help the parents to identify age-appropriate skills their child can perform in relation to the illness, such as:
      i. Toddler and preschooler: choose location for glucose testing, choose and monitor rotation of insulin injection sites.
      ii. School-ager: perform glucose testing, push syringe plunger, or, if capable, administer insulin after the parent has drawn up a dosage.
      iii. Adolescent: independent care but with oversight by the parent to make sure that he or she is following the prescribed health-care plan.
   b. Forewarn parents of adolescents regarding the potential for the child to become noncompliant with his or her diabetes management (see Chapter 6, "Normal Growth and Development: Adolescence," for information regarding risk-taking behavior and possible concerns about peer acceptance).

VII. Type 2 DM

A. Incidence.
1. Up to 45% of new cases of DM in children.
2. Primarily diagnosed during adolescence.
3. Highest incidence in African American, Native American, Hispanic American, and Asian-Pacific Islander populations.

B. Etiology.
1. Type 2 DM is not an autoimmune disease.
2. Primarily seen in children who are obese and who are sedentary.

C. Pathophysiology.
1. Reduced insulin secretion and/or cellular resistance to the utilization of insulin.

a. Although the pancreas produces insulin, the cells are unable to utilize the glucose.

2. Signs and symptoms. Most common include:
   a. The three "polys": polyphagia, polydipsia, and polyuria.
   b. Hyperglycemia.
   c. Fatigue.
   d. **Acanthosis nigricans:** darkening of the skin, often around the neck.
      i. Sign of insulin resistance syndrome.
   e. Ketoacidosis rarely is seen.

D. Diagnosis.
1. Same as type 1 (see earlier).

E. Treatment.
1. Blood glucose monitoring: at least once per day.
2. Weight control regimen with physical exercise.
3. Oral hypoglycemic agents or, if needed, injectable insulin.
   a. Metformin (Glucophage) is often the first drug of choice.

F. Nursing considerations.
1. See earlier type 1 DM nursing considerations and modify accordingly.
2. Deficient Knowledge.
   a. Educate the parents regarding the potential for type 2 DM in children.
      i. Especially parents of high-risk children.
   b. Encourage the parents and children to participate in weight management programs and healthful diet choices as a means of preventing the illness.
      i. Family-centered dietary changes should be encouraged because:
         (1) Dietary patterns usually are learned at home; therefore, additional family members may also be at risk of poor health, including the child's parents and siblings.
         (2) Dietary changes, when family based, often are better received because the child feels less like he or she is being singled out or punished.
   c. Encourage children to engage in daily exercise of their choice.
      i. If the child is reluctant to begin an exercise routine, family-centered exercise programs can also be encouraged because:
         (1) Other family members may also be exhibiting sedentary lifestyles.
         (2) They often are better received because the child feels less like he or she is being singled out.

CASE STUDY: Putting It All Together

The parents of an 8-year-old boy enter the emergency department shortly after the child arrives via ambulance from school.

Subjective Data
- The parents state,
  - "Where is our son? We received a telephone call from the school nurse that our child collapsed in his classroom and that he was immediately transported to the hospital via ambulance."
  - "He is a good boy. We know that he didn't take anything that he shouldn't."
  - "Please, we must see him to let him know that we love him and want him to get better."
  - "He has had a bad cold for the past couple of days, but that's it."
- After a brief interview with the nurse, the parents state,
  - "He has been drinking and eating a lot lately, but we just thought that he was an active, growing boy."
  - "We'll be honest with you, we don't pay too much attention to how often he goes to the bathroom. He is a very private boy."

Vital Signs

Temperature:	99.8 °F
Heart rate:	130 bpm
Respiratory rate:	32 rpm, deep
Blood pressure:	95/56 mm Hg
O_2 saturation:	96%
Current weight:	86 lb/8.1% weight loss (7 lb less than his last well-child check when he was at the 50th percentile for height and weight)

Objective Data
- Glasgow Coma score: 11/15 (see Glasgow coma scales in Chapter 22, "Nursing Care of the Child With Neurological Problems")
  - Eye opening: opens eyes in response to speech, 3
  - Motor response: makes localized movements in response to painful stimuli, 5
  - Verbal responses: responds with inappropriate words, 3
- Other assessments
  - Dry mucous membranes
  - Skin tenting

Continued

CASE STUDY: Putting It All Together *cont'd*

Lab Results

Complete blood count	
Red blood cell count:	5.5 million cells/mm^3
Hematocrit:	48%
Hemoglobin:	16 G/dL
Platelets:	180,000 cells/mm^3
White blood cell count:	8,300 cells/mm^3
• Serum glucose:	325 mg/dL
• Serum potassium:	2.5 mEq/L
• Hemoglobin:	A1C 12%
• pH:	7.0

Health-Care Provider's Orders

- Admit to pediatric intensive care unit
- Complete bedrest
- NPO
- IV NS 400 mL over one hour, 20 mL/kg thereafter
- Insulin drip at 0.05 units/kg/hr
- Perform serum glucose assessments every 15 min and report to primary health-care provider
- Repeat hourly potassium levels and report to primary health-care provider
- Monitor Glasgow findings every 15 min. If the level drops below 11, notify the primary health-care provider immediately

(Potassium replacement and additional insulin administration to be determined based on laboratory data.)

Case Study Questions

A. What *subjective* assessments indicate that this client is experiencing a health alteration?

1. __________
2. __________
3. __________
4. __________
5. __________

B. What *objective* assessments indicate that this client is experiencing a health alteration?

1. __________
2. __________
3. __________
4. __________
5. __________
6. __________
7. __________
8. __________

C. After analyzing the data that has been collected, what **primary** nursing diagnosis should the nurse assign to this client?

1. __________

CASE STUDY: Putting It All Together *cont'd*

Case Study Questions

D. What interventions should the nurse plan and/or implement to meet this child's and his family's needs?

1. ___
2. ___
3. ___
4. ___
5. ___
6. ___

E. What client outcomes should the nurse evaluate regarding the effectiveness of the nursing interventions?

1. ___
2. ___
3. ___
4. ___
5. ___
6. ___
7. ___

F. What physiological characteristics should the child exhibit before being discharged home?

1. ___
2. ___
3. ___
4. ___
5. ___
6. ___
7. ___

G. What psychological characteristics should the child and family exhibit before being discharged home?

1. ___
2. ___
3. ___
4. ___
5. ___

REVIEW QUESTIONS

1. A school-age child with phenylketonuria is eating lunch. The child has the following foods on the lunch plate. Which of the food choices should the nurse question the child for choosing?
   1. Buttered baked potato
   2. Salted stringed beans
   3. Stewed Bing cherries
   4. Fried chicken legs

2. A nurse is performing the newborn screen for phenylketonuria. Which of the following actions is the nurse performing?
   1. Sending cord blood from delivery to the hospital laboratory
   2. Collecting blood from a heel stick on a two-day-old baby
   3. Placing a urine collection bag on the one-day-old baby
   4. Analyzing a baby's meconium stool under the microscope

3. A neonate, 3,377 grams, has been diagnosed with congenital hypothyroidism. The neonatologist has ordered Synthroid (levothyroxine sodium) to be administered orally once each day beginning today. The recommended dosage of the medication is: *infants and neonates birth to 3 months:* 10 to 15 mcg/kg PO daily. Please calculate the safe maximum dosage of the medication for this neonate. **If rounding is needed, please round to the nearest hundredths place.**

   ________ mcg PO daily.

4. A nurse is admitting a baby to the newborn nursery who the nurse suspects may have congenital hypothyroidism. Which of the following findings has the nurse observed? **Select all that apply.**
   1. Clubfeet
   2. Cleft palate
   3. Protruding tongue
   4. Umbilical hernia
   5. Imperforate anus

5. The nurse notes that a girl, 8 years old, is exhibiting signs of precocious puberty. If left untreated, the nurse is aware that the young girl is at high risk for which of the following complications?
   1. Plagiocephaly
   2. Short stature
   3. Infertility
   4. Endometriosis

6. A young girl is experiencing precocious puberty. Which of the following patient-care goals would be appropriate for the nurse to include in the child's plan of care? The young girl will: **Select all that apply.**
   1. Wear age-appropriate attire.
   2. Shave axillary hair, as needed.
   3. Not menstruate before age nine.
   4. Have normal hormonal levels while receiving medication.
   5. State an understanding of the need for daily oral medications.

7. A young boy who has been diagnosed with growth hormone deficiency is to receive synthetic growth hormone. When providing medication teaching to the boy and his parents, which of the following information should the nurse include?
   1. Educate the boy and his parents regarding the rationale for the administration of the subcutaneous injections.
   2. Advise the boy to immediately report signs and symptoms of gynecomastia.
   3. Advise the boy that he will reach his desired height if he takes the medication as ordered.
   4. Educate the boy that to maintain his height, he will have to take the medication for the rest of his life.

8. A nurse is educating a young boy about the assessments required to make a diagnosis of growth hormone deficiency. Which of the following information should the nurse include in his or her teaching?
   1. A biopsy of the child's testes will be conducted.
   2. An x-ray of the child's wrists will be performed.
   3. The child will have an MRI of his hypothalamus.
   4. The child will receive IV dye for an adrenal fluoroscopy.

9. A child with type 1 diabetes mellitus has been diagnosed with ketoacidosis. Which of the following laboratory findings is consistent with the diagnosis?
   1. Hemoglobin A1C: 5.5%
   2. Fasting blood glucose: 124 mg/dL
   3. Serum pH: 7.24
   4. Potassium level: 3.9 mEq/L

10. A 2-year-old child has just been diagnosed with type 1 diabetes. The nurse is providing education to the parents regarding signs of hypoglycemia. Which of the following information should the nurse include in her teaching session?
   1. Child's breath will smell like fruit.
   2. Child will complain of excessive thirst.
   3. Child will complain of sleepiness and will appear fatigued.
   4. Child's behavior will resemble a burst of anger or a temper tantrum.

11. A nurse is providing education to 4 sets of parents whose children have been diagnosed with type 1 diabetes. The nurse should provide follow-up education to the parents who state that they will perform which of the following actions?
   1. Parents of a 2-year-old: "We will have our daughter prick her finger for each glucose testing."
   2. Parents of a 5-year-old: "We will give our daughter a code word that she will say when she feels a hypoglycemic episode developing."
   3. Parents of a 9-year-old: "We will monitor our daughter as she draws up and administers her insulin injections."
   4. Parents of a 17-year-old: "We will allow our daughter to take responsibility for all of her own diabetic care."

12. The nurse advises the parents of a 1½-year-old who is newly diagnosed with type 1 diabetes that the child's blood glucose level before dinner should be between 90 and 140 mg/dL. The mother states, "But that is much higher than I read on an Internet Web site." Which of the following responses by the nurse is appropriate?
   1. "I am sorry, I was thinking of the level for after dinner. The correct before dinner level is 70 to 110 mg/dL."
   2. "The level is higher than what you will usually see because young children's diets are not as predictable as the diets of older children and adults."
   3. "The level before breakfast should be 70 to 100 mg/dL, but the before dinner level should be a higher level."
   4. "You will find that your primary health-care provider will change the level at each visit. The goal starts at a high level and drops as your child responds to the insulin."

13. The school nurse is responsible for caring for a number of school children with type 1 diabetes. Before which of the following activities should the nurse make sure a child consumes a snack? The child who:
   1. sculpts in art class.
   2. plays in the band.
   3. acts in the school play.
   4. plays on the soccer team.

14. A child has recently been diagnosed with type 1 diabetes mellitus. Which of the following factors in his medical and family histories would the nurse expect to see?
   1. Child's grandfather has been diabetic since childhood.
   2. Child's body mass index is 30.
   3. Child rarely engages in aerobic activities.
   4. Child has recently gained 15 pounds.

15. A teenage child has been diagnosed with type 2 diabetes. The nurse determines that the child will likely be administered which of the following medications?
   1. Metformin (Glucophage)
   2. Aspart (Novolog)
   3. Detemir (Levemir)
   4. Glargine (Lantus)

16. Four sick children with type 1 diabetes have been admitted to the hospital. Which child is most at risk of developing hypoglycemia? The child with:
   1. bacterial sepsis.
   2. intussusception.
   3. jaundice.
   4. chickenpox.

REVIEW ANSWERS

1. ANSWER: 4

Rationale:

1. Children with PKU may eat starches and fats.
2. Children with PKU may eat vegetables.
3. Children with PKU may eat fruits.
4. **Children with PKU may not consume animal proteins.**

TEST-TAKING TIP: Children with PKU are unable to digest phenylalanine, an essential amino acid. The amino acid primarily is found in animal protein. Because the amino acid is essential, the children must consume some phenylalanine, but the children's serum levels are monitored to make sure that the levels do not become dangerous. If children's levels do exceed safe levels, the children would experience cognitive deficits as well as other signs/symptoms.

Content Area: *Pediatrics*

Integrated Processes: *Nursing Process: Implementation*

Client Need: *Physiological Integrity: Reduction of Risk Potential: Potential for Alterations in Body Systems*

Cognitive Level: *Application*

2. ANSWER: 2

Rationale:

1. Cord blood is sent for blood typing and Coombs' testing. It should not, however, be sent for newborn screening.
2. **Blood collected by heel stick on a 2-day-old baby would be sent for newborn screening.**
3. Urine may be collected to assess for pathology in the baby (e.g., the presence of toxic substances). Urine is not sent for newborn screening.
4. Meconium is not sent for newborn screening.

TEST-TAKING TIP: Blood is sent for newborn screening in all 50 states, although the list of diseases assessed is not consistent from state to state. One disease that newborn blood is assessed for in all states is PKU. Because a child with PKU does not possess the enzyme needed to digest phenylalanine, the amino acid remains in the baby's bloodstream. The amino acid is found in formula and in breast milk. In order for the test to be accurate, the baby must have consumed the protein for 24 hr. Babies should, therefore, be at least 24 hr old before their blood is sent for analysis.

Content Area: *Child Health*

Integrated Processes: *Nursing Process: Implementation*

Client Need: *Health Promotion and Maintenance: Health Screening*

Cognitive Level: *Application*

3. ANSWER: 50.66 mcg PO daily

Rationale:

Ratio and proportion method:

3,377 grams equals 3.377 kg because:

$$1 \text{ kg}:1{,}000 \text{ g} = x \text{ kg}:3{,}377 \text{ g}$$

$$x = 3.377$$

If the maximum safe dosage of Synthroid is 15 mcg/kg/day, then a baby whose weight is 3.377 kg would require a medicine that is 15 times the baby's weight = 50.655.

$$15 \text{ mcg}/1 \text{ kg} = x \text{ mcg}/3.377 \text{ kg}$$

$$x = 50.655 \text{ mcg}$$

When rounded to the second place to the right of the decimal, the maximum safe dosage becomes 50.66 mcg PO daily.

Dimensional analysis method:

$$\frac{15 \text{ mcg}}{1 \text{ kg/day}} \times \frac{1 \text{ kg}}{1{,}000 \text{ g}} \times 3{,}377 \text{ g} = 50.655, \text{ or } 50.66 \text{ mcg/day}$$

TEST-TAKING TIP: The recommended safe dosage for this medication is quoted as a range—from 10 to 15 mcg/kg. Because the question asked for the "safe maximum dosage," only the higher recommended dosage needs to be calculated.

Content Area: *Pediatrics*

Integrated Processes: *Nursing Process: Implementation*

Client Need: *Physiological Integrity: Pharmacological and Parenteral Therapies: Dosage Calculation*

Cognitive Level: *Synthesis*

4. ANSWER: 3 and 4

Rationale:

1. Clubfeet are not associated with congenital hypothyroidism (CHT).
2. Cleft palate is not associated with CHT.
3. **Protruding tongue is associated with CHT.**
4. **Umbilical hernia is associated with CHT.**
5. Imperforate anus is not associated with CHT.

TEST-TAKING TIP: The appearance of newborns with CHT is quite distinctive: large fontanels, protruding tongue, and umbilical hernia. In addition, the nurse will likely note a baby who eats very poorly because of marked lethargy and a baby with jaundice that lasts longer than expected.

Content Area: *Pediatrics*

Integrated Processes: *Nursing Process: Assessment*

Client Need: *Physiological Integrity: Physiological Adaptation: Alterations in Body Systems*

Cognitive Level: *Application*

5. ANSWER: 2

Rationale:

1. Plagiocephaly, or flat head syndrome, is seen in neonates who are placed on their backs all day as well as for sleep.
2. **Short stature is seen in children with precocious puberty.**
3. Infertility is not associated with precocious puberty.
4. Endometriosis is not associated with precocious puberty.

TEST-TAKING TIP: When children mature early, their growth plates will close prematurely. As a result, their statures are lower than their genetically expected height.

Content Area: *Pediatrics*

Integrated Processes: *Nursing Process: Analysis*

Client Need: *Physiological Integrity: Reduction of Risk Potential: Potential for Alterations in Body Systems*
Cognitive Level: *Application*

6. ANSWER: 1, 3, and 4
Rationale:
1. The nurse would expect the child to wear age-appropriate attire.
2. The nurse would not expect the child to shave her axillary hair.
3. The nurse would expect the child not to menstruate before age 9.
4. The nurse would expect the child to have normal hormonal levels while receiving medication.
5. The medications are administered intramuscularly, usually once per month.
TEST-TAKING TIP: Girls who are experiencing precocious puberty are maturing much earlier than expected. Even though the girls may appear to be older than their years, they are still young children. The nurse, therefore, would expect the children's behavior to be consistent with their age.
Content Area: *Pediatrics*
Integrated Processes: *Nursing Process: Planning*
Client Need: *Physiological Integrity: Reduction of Risk Potential: Potential for Alterations in Body Systems*
Cognitive Level: *Application*

7. ANSWER: 1
Rationale:
1. This statement is correct. The child will receive growth hormone (GH) subcutaneous injections at bedtime six to seven times each week.
2. Gynecomastia is not seen with GH injections.
3. This statement is untrue. Even with the injections, the boy may not reach his desired height.
4. The medication is taken until either the child reaches his desired height or the growth plates fuse.
TEST-TAKING TIP: Because GH is naturally produced by the anterior pituitary gland during periods of sleep, the injections of GH for those children who produce deficient supplies is administered at bedtime. The vast majority of children who are treated for GH deficiency are male.
Content Area: *Pediatrics*
Integrated Processes: *Nursing Process: Implementation*
Client Need: *Physiological Integrity: Pharmacological and Parenteral Therapies: Expected Actions/Outcomes*
Cognitive Level: *Application*

8. ANSWER: 2
Rationale:
1. A biopsy of the child's testes is not conducted.
2. An x-ray of the child's wrists will be performed.
3. An MRI of the hypothalamus will not be performed.
4. An adrenal fluoroscopy will not be performed.
TEST-TAKING TIP: To determine whether the child's growth is complete, the endocrinologist will x-ray the child's wrists. The growth plate will be measured to determine whether the child has reached his or her maximum height.
Content Area: *Pediatrics*
Integrated Processes: *Nursing Process: Implementation; Teaching/Learning*
Client Need: *Physiological Integrity: Reduction of Risk Potential: Diagnostic Tests*
Cognitive Level: *Application*

9. ANSWER: 3
Rationale:
1. Hemoglobin A1C of 5.5% is a normal finding.
2. Fasting blood glucose of 124 mg/dL is a normal finding.
3. Serum pH of 7.24 is indicative of ketoacidosis.
4. Potassium of 3.9 mEq/L is a normal finding.
TEST-TAKING TIP: Ketoacidosis results when the body is devoid of circulating glucose and, as a result, goes into fat catabolism. When ketones, the by-product of fat catabolism, rise in the bloodstream, the pH of the blood drops precipitously.
Content Area: *Pediatrics*
Integrated Processes: *Nursing Process: Assessment*
Client Need: *Physiological Integrity: Physiological Alterations: Alterations in Body Systems*
Cognitive Level: *Application*

10. ANSWER: 4
Rationale:
1. The child's breath will smell like fruit if the child is hyperglycemic.
2. The child will complain of excessive thirst if the child is hyperglycemic.
3. The child will complain of sleepiness and will appear fatigued if he or she is hyperglycemic.
4. The child's behavior will resemble a burst of anger or a temper tantrum if the child is hypoglycemic.
TEST-TAKING TIP: Caring for toddlers with type 1 diabetes can be difficult because the children's daily behaviors often mimic signs of hypoglycemia. For that reason, parents must be forewarned to consider hypoglycemia as the reason for a child's aberrant behavior rather than simply as a "phase that the child is going through."
Content Area: *Pediatrics*
Integrated Processes: *Nursing Process: Implementation; Teaching/Learning*
Client Need: *Physiological Integrity: Physiological Alterations: Alterations in Body Systems*
Cognitive Level: *Application*

11. ANSWER: 1
Rationale:
1. Two-year-old children are too young to prick their own fingers for glucose testing.
2. This statement is appropriate. Five-year-old children often are able to predict a hypoglycemic episode. To assist the child to communicate the information to his or her parents, a short code word should be decided on.
3. This statement is appropriate. Nine-year-old children are able to draw up and inject their own insulin. The procedure, however, should be monitored by the parents.

4. This statement is appropriate. Although 17-year-old children may not be 100% reliable, by the time they are that age, they should be fully responsible for their own diabetic care.

TEST-TAKING TIP: Even though the disease state referenced in this question is diabetes mellitus, the question really relates to growth and development issues. The nurse should be familiar with the abilities of children at different ages.

Content Area: *Pediatrics*

Integrated Processes: *Nursing Process: Implementation; Teaching/Learning*

Client Need: *Physiological Integrity: Reduction of Risk Potential: Potential for Complications of Diagnostic Tests/Treatments/Procedures*

Cognitive Level: *Application*

12. ANSWER: 2

Rationale:

1. This statement is false.

2. This statement is correct. Toddlers often go through a stage when they are finicky eaters. They are, therefore, at high risk for becoming hypoglycemic. The higher preprandial blood glucose level helps to reduce the risk of developing low blood glucose levels.

3. This statement is false.

4. This statement is false. Each child's therapeutic regimen is individualized to his or her physiological condition and response.

TEST-TAKING TIP: If a child's glucose levels are markedly elevated over a number of days, the parents should be advised to report the results to the child's diabetic care provider. In response, it is likely that the practitioner will increase the child's insulin dosages.

Content Area: *Pediatrics*

Integrated Processes: *Nursing Process: Implementation*

Client Need: *Physiological Integrity: Reduction of Risk Potential: System Specific Assessments*

Cognitive Level: *Application*

13. ANSWER: 4

Rationale:

1. The child will likely not need an extra snack before sculpting in art class.

2. The child will likely not need an extra snack before playing in the band.

3. The child will likely not need an extra snack before acting in the school play.

4. The child will need an extra snack before playing on the soccer team.

TEST-TAKING TIP: Aerobic exercise improves the utilization of glucose by the cells of the body. As a result, during active exercise, children's insulin needs drop. To compensate for the reduced insulin demand, the child should consume an extra snack.

Content Area: *Pediatrics*

Integrated Processes: *Nursing Process: Implementation*

Client Need: *Physiological Integrity: Reduction of Risk Potential: Potential for Alterations in Body Systems*

Cognitive Level: *Application*

14. ANSWER: 1

Rationale:

1. The nurse would expect to see that the child has a direct relative who is (or was) a type 1 diabetic.

2. Children with a variety of body structures develop type 1 diabetes.

3. Both active and sedentary children develop type 1 diabetes.

4. Type 1 diabetes may occur after a recent weight loss or when the child's weight is stable.

TEST-TAKING TIP: Type 1 diabetes is an autoimmune disease with a strong genetic etiology. Although no direct genetic inheritance has been identified, the influence of a variety of factors, one of which is genetics, is known to be the etiology of the disease.

Content Area: *Pediatrics*

Integrated Processes: *Nursing Process: Assessment*

Client Need: *Physiological Integrity: Physiological Adaptation: Alterations in Body Systems*

Cognitive Level: *Application*

15. ANSWER: 1

Rationale:

1. Metformin (Glucophage) is usually the first-line drug for patients with type 2 diabetes.

2. Aspart (Novolog) is an injectable, short-acting insulin. It is administered to those with type 1 diabetes.

3. Detemir (Levemir) is an injectable, intermediate-acting insulin. It is administered to those with type 1 diabetes.

4. Glargine (Lantus) is an injectable, intermediate-acting insulin. It is administered to those with type 1 diabetes.

TEST-TAKING TIP: The nurse must be familiar with the medications administered to those with diabetes. Because those with type 1 diabetes secrete no insulin, and because insulin is digested when taken orally, type 1 diabetics must receive injectable insulin. In contrast, those with type 2 diabetes do produce insulin, but their bodies utilize the insulin poorly. They usually are controlled while taking an oral hypoglycemic agent.

Content Area: *Pediatrics*

Integrated Processes: *Nursing Process: Analysis*

Client Need: *Physiological Integrity: Pharmacological and Parenteral Therapies: Expected Actions/Outcomes*

Cognitive Level: *Application*

16. ANSWER: 1

Rationale:

1. The child with bacterial sepsis is most at high risk for developing hypoglycemia.

2. The child with intussusception is not especially at high risk for developing hypoglycemia.

3. The child with jaundice is not especially at high risk for developing hypoglycemia.

4. The child with chickenpox is not especially at high risk for developing hypoglycemia.

TEST-TAKING TIP: Those with bacterial sepsis have bacteria in their bloodstream. Most bacteria utilize glucose for fuel. Because the bacteria would be consuming much of the glucose in the child's bloodstream, he or she would be at most high risk for developing hypoglycemia.

Content Area: *Pediatrics*
Integrated Processes: *Nursing Process: Implementation*
Client Need: *Physiological Integrity: Reduction of Risk Potential: Potential for Alterations in Body Systems*
Cognitive Level: *Analysis*

Chapter 22

Nursing Care of the Child With Neurological Problems

KEY TERMS

Brudzinski sign—Pain and hip flexion when chin is flexed onto chest.

Cerebral palsy (CP)—Disorder caused by a hypoxic insult to the brain prenatally or during or after delivery, resulting in permanent motor disability.

Decerebrate posturing—Body positioning in which the arms and legs are rigid, with toes pointed inward, and head and neck held stiffly backward.

Decorticate posturing—Body rigidity in which the arms are bent toward the body with hands in tight fists and legs held stiffly straight.

Hydrocephalus—An imbalance in either the production or absorption of cerebrospinal fluid, leading to increased fluid in the ventricles of the brain.

Increased intracranial pressure (ICP)—A rise in the pressure of the cerebral spinal fluid.

Kernig sign—Pain when the leg and knee are elevated and extended.

Meningitis—A viral or bacterial infection of the meninges.

Papilledema—Swelling of the optic disk due to increased intracranial pressure.

Reye syndrome—Brain damage and impaired liver function seen in children who had been given aspirin following viral illnesses, most notably varicella (chickenpox) and influenza.

Spina bifida—Birth defect in which the neural tube fails to completely close during fetal development.

Tonic-clonic seizure—A type of seizure consisting of a period of muscle stiffening (the tonic phase) followed by shaking or jerking movements (the clonic phase).

Ventriculoperitoneal (VP) shunting—Procedure used to relieve intracranial pressure resulting from excess cerebrospinal fluid.

I. Description

The neurological system, or central nervous system (CNS), is comprised of the brain, spinal cord, and peripheral nerves. There are three distinct sections of the brain: the cerebrum, or the intelligence/thought center of the brain; the cerebellum, or the section of the brain that coordinates motor function, including balance and coordination; and the brain stem, which connects the cerebrum with the spinal cord and coordinates many vital functions, including breathing and blood pressure. The spinal cord is also divided into sections, corresponding to the adjacent vertebrae: cervical, thoracic, lumbar, and sacral. The skull and vertebrae along with the cerebral spinal fluid (CSF) protect the brain and spinal cord from injury. The meninges surround the brain and spinal cord.

II. Increased Intracranial Pressure

Increased intracranial pressure (ICP) is, by far, the most common finding seen in illnesses of the CNS. Because the CNS is a closed, nonelastic system, whenever a growth or inflammation develops, pressures rise in the system. As a result, patients develop characteristic signs and symptoms. Before discussing the main illnesses of the CNS, therefore, it is important to understand the processes involved when a child develops increased ICP.

A. Incidence.
  1. Most common finding seen in illnesses of the CNS.

B. Etiology.
  1. Develops as a result of a number of conditions (e.g., head injury, CNS infection, tumor, excess cerebral spinal fluid).

C. Pathophysiology.
  1. Directly related to the etiology, for example:
    a. If a head injury is sustained, the brain swells, leading to increased pressures in the brain.
    b. If quantities of CSF increase, pressures in the brain will increase.
  2. If the physiological abnormality is not corrected, herniation of the brain may occur.
  3. Signs and symptoms: dependent on the age of the child.
    a. Infants, because their skulls are still unfused, usually exhibit nonspecific symptoms: poor feeding, vomiting, irritability, lethargy, **plus** signs of an enlarging head:
      i. Increased head circumference.
      ii. Separated sutures.
      iii. Bulging and enlarged fontanels.
      iv. Frontal bossing.
      v. Setting sun sign.
      vi. Shrill cry.
      vii. Seizures.
        (1) Seizures that babies frequently exhibit, called focal seizures, are much less organized than those of older children and are often difficult to identify.
        (2) Neonates who are exhibiting focal seizures may simply seem to be staring into space or may have repetitive movements of one or two extremities.
        (3) It is important for the health-care staff to be vigilant in monitoring babies for atypical movements that may actually be seizure activity.
    b. Older children: after fusion of the sutures, children exhibit more characteristic symptoms of increased ICP.
      i. Headache.
      ii. Visual disturbances.
      iii. Behavioral changes/altered consciousness.
        (1) Irritability and agitation to
        (2) Mild disorientation to
        (3) Lethargy and nonresponsiveness.
      iv. **Papilledema** (swelling of the optic disk).
      v. Nausea and vomiting.
      vi. Abnormal posturing (see decerebrate and decortical posturing in the following "Seizures" section).
      vii. Seizures.
      viii. Vital sign changes.
        (1) Elevated temperature.
        (2) Elevated blood pressure.
        (3) Bradycardia, which is a late sign.

D. Diagnosis: common diagnostic tests include:
  1. Children's Glasgow Scale assessment.
    a. The correct scale, dependent on the age of the child, must be used (Table 22.1).
  2. X-ray, MRI, and/or CT scan.
  3. Lumbar puncture.
  4. Serum laboratory data, including:
    a. Complete blood count (CBC).
    b. Serum electrolytes.
    c. Blood gases.

E. Treatment: treatment is dependent on the exact etiology of the elevated cerebral spinal fluid pressure (see following illnesses).
  1. Antiseizure medications: following is a sample list of medications (with a partial list of considerations/adverse reactions).
    a. Tegretol (carbamazepine): for focal or generalized seizures.
      i. Adverse reactions.
        (1) Child may exhibit behavioral changes while on the medication.
          (a) Poor performance in school.
          (b) Confusion.
          (c) Drowsiness.
          (d) Impaired coordination.
        (2) Serious reactions.
          (a) Carriers of HLA-B*1502 allele are at very high risk for Stevens-Johnson syndrome.
            (i) Child should be screened before medication is administered.
          (b) Aplastic anemia.
            (i) CBC should be carefully monitored.
      ii. Additional considerations.
        (1) Should **not** be taken with erythromycin.
          (a) The drug levels of Tegretol increase.

Table 22.1 Glasgow Coma Scales for Children Under 2, Children Aged 2 to 5, and Children Aged 6 and Over

	Score	Children Under 2	Children (Aged 2–5)	Children (Aged 6 and Over)
Eye Opening	4	Spontaneous	Spontaneous	Spontaneous
	3	To verbal stimuli	To verbal stimuli	To verbal stimuli
	2	To pain	To pain	To pain
	1	No response	No response	No response
Verbal Response	5	Coos and babbles	Oriented, speaks, interacts	Oriented to time, place, and person; uses appropriate words and phrases
	4	Irritable and cries but is consolable	Confused and disoriented but consolable	Confused
	3	Cries persistently to pain	Inappropriate words or verbal response, inconsolable	Inappropriate words or verbal response
	2	Moans to pain	Incomprehensible, agitated	Incomprehensible
	1	No response	No response	No response
Motor Response	6	Normal, spontaneous movement	Normal, spontaneous movement	Obeys commands
	5	Withdraws to touch	Localizes pain	Localizes pain
	4	Withdraws to pain	Withdraws to pain	Withdraws to pain
	3	Flexion to pain (decorticate)*	Flexion to pain (decorticate)	Flexion to pain (decorticate)
	2	Extension to pain (decerebrate)*	Extension to pain (decerebrate)	Extension to pain (decerebrate)
	1	No response	No response	No response

From Teasdale, G., & Jennett, B. (1974). Assessment of coma and impaired consciousness. *The Lancet*, 304(7872), 81–84.
*For illustrations of decorticate and decerebrate posturing, see Figures 22.3 and 22.4, p. 419.

b. Felbatol (felbamate): for focal or generalized seizures.
   i. Adverse reactions.
      (1) Behavioral changes.
         (a) Agitation.
         (b) Aggression.
      (2) Gastrointestinal symptoms.
         (a) Anorexia.
         (b) Nausea and vomiting.
      (3) Serious reactions.
         (a) Aplastic anemia.
            (i) CBC should be carefully monitored.
         (b) Liver failure.
            (i) Liver function tests should be carefully monitored.
   ii. Additional considerations.
      (1) The oral suspension must be shaken well.

c. Dilantin (phenytoin): for focal or generalized seizures.
   i. Adverse reactions.
      (1) Behavioral changes.
         (a) Drowsiness.
         (b) Confusion.
      (2) Tremors.
      (3) Slurred speech.
      (4) Serious reactions.
         (a) If administered via IV rapidly, severe cardiac arrhythmias and hypotension may result.
   ii. Additional considerations.
      (1) Medication often results in hypertrophy of the gingiva.
         (a) The parents and child must be taught to perform excellent oral care routinely.

d. Depakene (valproic acid): for all types of seizures.
   i. Adverse reactions: multiple reactions, including:
      (1) Behavioral changes.
         (a) Nervousness.
         (b) Depression.
         (c) Labile moods.
      (2) Alopecia.
      (3) Gastrointestinal symptoms.
         (a) Abdominal pain.
         (b) Nausea and vomiting.
         (c) Gastritis.
      (4) Serious reactions.
         (a) Liver failure.
            (i) Liver function tests should be carefully monitored.

(b) Teratogenesis.
(i) Pregnant women should take care not to consume the medication.
(c) Pancreatitis.
(i) Children should be monitored carefully for signs and symptoms.

2. Other medications.
   a. Antibiotics: for infections.
   b. Osmitrol (mannitol): diuretic.
      i. To increase urinary output and decrease cerebral edema.
   c. Sedatives.
   d. Insertion of an intraventricular catheter: usually via burr hole.

DID YOU KNOW?

A burr hole is a hole drilled through the skull. The hole provides health-care practitioners access to the ventricles of the brain. Subdural screws or bolts, epidural sensors, or catheters may be inserted through burr holes in order to measure intracranial pressures.

F. Nursing considerations.
1. Risk for Injury.
   a. Place the child on seizure precautions.
      i. Pad the crib or bed.
      ii. Maintain access to suction and oxygen at the bedside and administer, as needed.
      iii. Note, document, and report any seizure activity, including specific physiological changes (e.g., breathing pattern, length of seizure, focal versus tonic/clonic movements, skin color).
   b. Monitor vital signs.
   c. Monitor level of consciousness, using the appropriate Glasgow Scale.
   d. Monitor cerebral spinal fluid pressures via bolt or intraventricular catheter, if present.
   e. Monitor for signs of infection.
      i. Infection may be the cause of increased ICP (see "Meningitis" below).
   f. Maintain head of bed at about a 30-degree elevation.
      i. Gravity helps the CSF to descend from the brain when the head is elevated.
   g. Administer safe doses of medications, as prescribed.
      i. Antiseizure medications.
      ii. Antibiotics.
      iii. Mannitol.
      iv. Sedatives.

III. Spina Bifida

There are three forms of **spina bifida**, a defect present at birth: spina bifida occulta, meningocele, and meningomyelocele (also called myelomeningocele). The differences between the forms lie in how severely the nerves have been impacted by the defect (see the following "Pathophysiology" section).

A. Incidence.
1. The incidence is variable, but about 1 in 4,000 children will be born with myelomeningocele each year.

B. Etiology.
1. The exact cause of spina bifida is unknown, but it is known to have both environmental and genetic triggers.
   a. There is an increased incidence of spina bifida in families.
   b. Folic acid deficiency has been shown to result in the failure of the neural tube to close during fetal development.

C. Pathophysiology (Fig. 22.1).
1. The neural tube fails to close completely during fetal development, resulting in one of three major defects (in order of severity).
   a. Spina bifida occulta.
      i. Posterior vertebral arches are unclosed.
      ii. No herniation of the spinal cord is present.
      iii. The defect is not visible externally, although a tuft of hair may be present at the point of the defect.
   b. Meningocele.
      i. Saclike cyst of meninges filled with spinal fluid protrudes through the skin in the lumbar, lumbosacral, or sacral area.
      ii. There is no herniation of the spinal cord into the sac.
   c. Myelomeningocele (meningomyelocele).
      i. Saclike cyst of meninges, spinal fluid, and spinal cord nerves protrude through

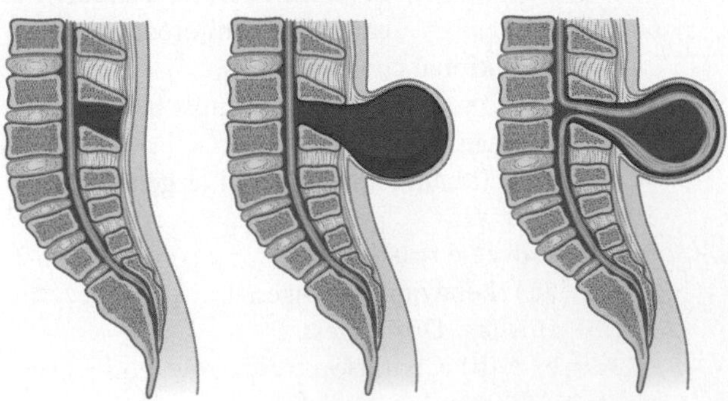

Fig 22.1 Forms of spina bifida.

the skin of the lumbar, lumbosacral, or sacral area.

2. Degree of neurological dysfunction.
   a. Related to the anatomic level of the defect and whether spinal nerves are involved.
3. **Hydrocephalus** (see the following "Hydrocephalus" section).
   a. Present in 90% to 95% of children with spina bifida.
4. Children with spina bifida are at high risk of developing an allergy to latex.
   a. Symptoms of the allergy can range from urticaria, watery eyes, wheezing, and rales to a full anaphylactic response.
5. Signs and symptoms: dependent on the degree and level of the defect but include:
   a. Spina bifida occulta.
      i. Tuft of hair at base of spine.
      ii. Dimpling at base of spine.
   b. Meningocele and/or meningomyelocele.
      i. No control over bladder and/or bowel function.
      ii. Diminished or absent sensation distal to the defect.
      iii. Partial or complete paralysis of the lower limbs.
      iv. Increased ICP.

D. Diagnosis.

1. Prenatally.
   a. Screening: indicates possible presence of the defect.
      i. Elevated alpha-fetoprotein levels.
         (1) May be obtained either via serum or amniotic fluid testing.
      ii. Ultrasound visualization confirms the diagnosis.
2. Newborn: direct visualization.
   a. X-ray, ultrasound, MRI, and/or CT scan are used to determine the severity of the defect.

E. Treatment.

1. Prevention.
   a. Folic acid supplementation preconceptually and throughout pregnancy (see "Making the Connection").
2. Treatment.
   a. Surgical closure: prenatally or after delivery.
      i. When surgery is performed prenatally, fewer physical deficits may be present.
      ii. If surgery is performed after delivery, it is usually completed within 48 hr of delivery.
   b. Extensive physical therapy is often required to enable the child to reach his or her optimal level of functioning.
      i. Depends on the level of the defect.
      ii. May be taught to walk with braces or crutches, or the child may be wheelchair-bound.
      iii. May need bowel training and/or repeated urinary catheterizations.

DID YOU KNOW?

In some cases, when the defect is diagnosed prenatally, corrective surgery can be performed on the fetus in utero. Babies who have been repaired as fetuses have been born with minimal permanent injury and normal growth and development, including the ability to walk, urinate, and stool normally (The Children's Hospital of Philadelphia, 2011).

F. Nursing considerations.

1. Prevention:
   a. Deficient Knowledge.
      i. Provide preconception counseling to women of childbearing age regarding the importance of taking a multivitamin supplement including folic acid from the cessation of use of birth control until the birth of the baby.
2. Treatment:
   a. Deficient Knowledge/Risk for Altered Coping/Anger/Anxiety/Fear/Grieving.
      i. Allow the parents to express grief over the loss of the perfect child.
      ii. Explain the pathophysiology and rationale for care to the parents and child, if appropriate.

MAKING THE CONNECTION

Although not totally preventable, folic acid intake during pregnancy does significantly reduce the probability of delivering a baby with spina bifida. Mothers are strongly encouraged to take a folic acid supplement and to consume foods high in folic acid to prevent neural tube defects. It is important that the mothers be advised that they should begin folic acid intake before trying to become pregnant so that the vitamin is present in the system during the entire organogenic period of the first trimester of pregnancy.

Foods that are high in folic acid are dark-green, leafy vegetables; most fruits, including oranges and bananas; potatoes; and, beginning in 2005, grain products in the United States have been enriched with folic acid.

The dosage of folic acid for women with no family or personal history of spina bifida is 400 mcg per day. However, the recommended dosage is increased tenfold for those women who have a family or personal history to 4 mg per day.

iii. Encourage the family and child to discuss their concerns and guilt regarding the diagnosis.
iv. Help the parents to develop realistic goals for the child's growth and development and to provide toys and activities that will maximize the child's growth and development.
v. Consider introducing the parents to other parents with children with spina bifida.
vi. Encourage the parents to join a supportive organization (e.g., Spina Bifida Association).

3. Preoperative considerations.
   a. Risk for Infection/Impaired Skin Integrity.
      i. Practice meticulous handwashing.
      ii. Prevent the sac from drying out.
         (1) Maintain moist, sterile dressings over the defect using aseptic technique.
         (2) Reinforce moist dressings with a dry, sterile dressing to prevent bacteria from entering the sac via the moist dressings.
      iii. Monitor for signs of infection, including elevated WBC, hyperthermia, and redness or purulent discharge at the site.
      iv. Monitor the sac for signs of rupture, CSF leakage, or drying.
      v. Place the child in the prone position to prevent damage to the exposed sac.
      vi. Change soiled diapers and underpads immediately to prevent contamination of the site.
      vii. Monitor for signs of pressure points on dependent surfaces.
   b. Hypothermia.
      i. Monitor for drop in temperature.
      ii. If needed, place the baby in a warmer or Isolette, but ensure that the dressing remains moist and intact.
   c. Risk for Injury.
      i. Monitor for signs of hydrocephalus (see the following "Hydrocephalus" section).
      ii. Assess for additional defects (e.g., developmental dysplasia of the hip, clubfoot) (see Chapter 20, "Nursing Care of the Child With Musculoskeletal Disorders).
         (1) Musculoskeletal defects are commonly seen in children with spina bifida.
      iii. Avoid unnecessarily exposing the child to products that contain latex.
         (1) Administer antihistamines and steroids, as prescribed and as needed.
            (a) The medications are often administered before and after surgical procedures to prevent allergic symptoms.

4. Postoperative considerations.
   a. Risk for Infection.
      i. Perform meticulous handwashing.
      ii. Monitor the surgical site for complications, including performing the REEDA (redness, edema, ecchymosis, discharge, approximation) assessment, and report any deviations from normal.
      iii. Change diapers and underpads, as needed, to prevent contamination of the site.
   b. Risk for Injury/Risk for Altered Development/Pain.
      i. Monitor for signs of increased ICP.
      ii. Maintain prone position until the surgical site is completely healed.
      iii. Monitor vital signs and intake and output (I&O).
      iv. Maintain body temperature.
      v. Provide tactile stimulation.
         (1) Place the baby on the parent's lap, and encourage the parents to stroke and caress the baby.
      vi. Provide visual and auditory stimulation, including drawings, music, and mobiles.
      vii. Assess pain level using an age-appropriate pain rating scale.
      viii. Provide safe dosages of pharmacological pain management, employing professional guidelines.
      ix. Provide nourishment, as prescribed.

5. Long-term considerations.
   a. Risk for Ineffective Self-Health Management/Risk for Impaired Mobility/Risk for Impaired Elimination/Deficient Knowledge.
      i. At each well-child visit, growth and development milestones must be assessed carefully.
      ii. Assess for the level of the disorder to determine the potential motor dysfunction.
         (1) May be paralysis or spasticity (e.g., hip flexors, and adductors [innervated by L1 to L3]) and extensors and abductors [innervated by L5 to S1]).
         (2) May exhibit complete incontinence of stool.
         (3) May exhibit complete incontinence of urine or bladder spasticity.
      iii. Perform range-of-motion exercises to help to prevent contractures.

iv. Educate the parents and child, when appropriate, regarding the level of the defect and the potential for motor and elimination dysfunction.
(1) Refer the child to physical therapy, occupational therapy, and orthopedic management, as prescribed
(a) Therapy will likely be a long, continuous process.
(2) Apply braces or other assistive devices, when needed, to facilitate mobility.

b. Impaired Urinary Elimination/Risk for Infection (urinary).
i. Educate the parents to monitor urinary output and signs of urinary tract infection.
ii. Educate the parents and child, frequently at about 6 years of age, to perform intermittent catheterizations, if needed.
iii. Educate the parents to administer antispasmodic medications to reduce bladder spasms, if prescribed.

c. Bowel incontinence.
i. Provide support to the parents and child, if appropriate, regarding the prolonged period of bowel training.
ii. Refer the child to an occupational therapist for assistance with bowel training, if needed.
iii. Educate the parents and child, when appropriate, regarding diet and medications (to prevent constipation and diarrhea) (e.g., high-fiber foods, supplements, laxatives, suppositories).
iv. Educate the parents and child regarding the necessity for regular toileting.

d. Risk for Altered Development.
i. Encourage age-appropriate tasks to maximize abilities.
(1) If no paralysis:
(a) Place toys and other interesting objects just out of the baby's reach.
(b) Praise the baby for attempts at obtaining the desired object.
(2) If paralysis:
(a) Provide toys to foster upper-body development.
(b) Praise the baby for successfully achieving upper-body function.

IV. Hydrocephalus

In the healthy brain, CSF is produced by the choroid plexus in the lateral ventricles, circulates throughout the ventricular system, and finally is absorbed into the subarachnoid space. In **hydrocephalus**, however, there is either an imbalance in the production or the absorption of CSF. The imbalance leads to an accumulation of fluid in the ventricles of the brain.

A. Incidence.
1. Occurs in about 1 of every 500 children.
2. If left untreated, 50% to 60% of the children will die and less than 10% of the survivors will achieve normal intelligence.
3. If treated, there is an 80% survival rate, with the surviving children exhibiting varying levels of intelligence.

B. Etiology.
1. May be congenital or may develop as a result of such things as CNS infections and tumors.
2. The vast majority of children with spina bifida (see earlier) also have hydrocephalus.

C. Pathophysiology: two main forms of hydrocephalus.
1. Communicating hydrocephalus: impaired absorption of CSF into the subarachnoid space.
2. Noncommunicating hydrocephalus: obstruction of the flow of CSF within the ventricles (most common form in children).
a. When seen in infancy, hydrocephalus is usually either congenital or secondary to an infection or perinatal hemorrhage.
b. When seen in older children, the pathology is usually secondary to the presence of a tumor.

D. Diagnosis.
1. Clinical picture is suggestive.
a. Presence of spina bifida, and/or
b. Signs of increased ICP.
2. Definitive diagnosis is made by CT and/or MRI.

E. Treatment.
1. **Ventriculoperitoneal (VP) shunt** insertion: to drain excess fluid from the ventricles (Fig. 22.2).

DID YOU KNOW?

VP shunt catheters are placed in the ventricles of the brain. They are then threaded under the skin via the neck and thorax, finally ending in the peritoneal cavity. Extra tubing, to allow for growth of the child, is positioned in the peritoneal cavity.

a. Shunts often become obstructed and need to be revised or replaced.

F. Nursing considerations.
1. Preoperative VP shunt insertion.
a. Risk for Injury.
i. Monitor vital signs.
ii. Monitor for signs of increased ICP (see earlier).
(1) *If infants,* mark the exact point on the head where the head circumference is measured.

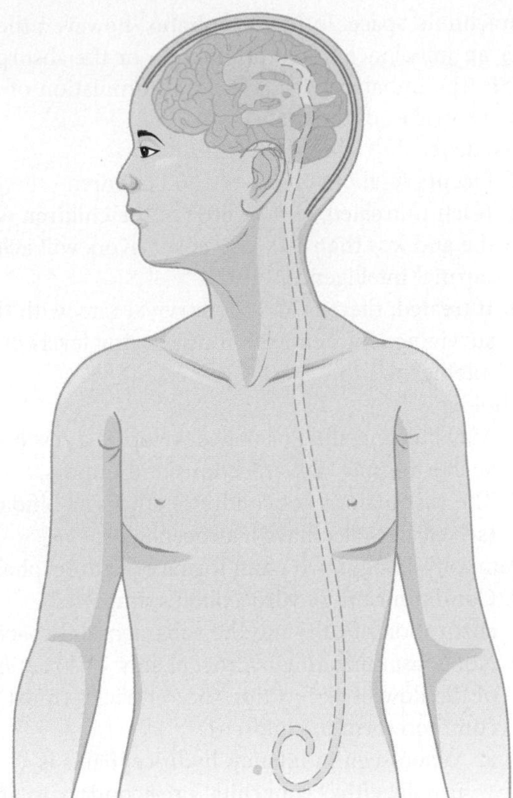

Fig 22.2 Ventriculoperitoneal (VP) shunt insertion.

iii. Position the crib or bed at 30-degree elevation.
iv. Maintain seizure precautions.
    (1) Pad the crib or bed.
    (2) Maintain access to suction and oxygen at the bedside and administer, as needed.
v. Note, document, and report any seizure activity, including specific physiological changes (e.g., breathing pattern, length of seizure, focal versus tonic/clonic movements, skin color).
vi. When holding the baby, carefully support the enlarged head.

b. Risk for Imbalanced Nutrition: Less than Body Requirements/Risk for Injury.
   i. Small, frequent feedings to decrease the potential for vomiting.
   ii. Carefully support the head and neck during feedings.

c. Risk for Impaired Skin Integrity.
   i. Frequent position changes—every 1 to 2 hr.
   ii. Range-of-motion exercises of all extremities.

2. Postoperative VP shunt insertion.
   a. Risk for Infection.
      i. Perform meticulous handwashing and aseptic technique.
      ii. Assess the surgical site for complications (see earlier) and report any deviations from normal.
      iii. Monitor temperature and vital signs.
      iv. Monitor CBC for elevated leukocyte count.
   b. Risk for Injury.
      i. Assess surgical site for leakage of CSF.
      ii. Position the child flat on his or her nonsurgical side.
         (1) The child is slowly elevated over time, per neurosurgeon's orders, until pressures are equalized.

(!) After a VP shunt insertion, the nurse must carefully follow the guidelines set by the neurosurgeon regarding when to change the child's position. If the child is elevated too rapidly, the CSF will drain too quickly. As a result, the child's brain may be injured.

      iii. Monitor for signs of increased ICP.
      iv. Monitor for abdominal distension.
         (1) Because the CSF is draining into the peritoneal cavity, the abdomen may distend.
   c. Deficient Knowledge.
      i. Educate the parents regarding signs of increased ICP.
         (1) Because VP shunts may become obstructed, the parents must be prepared to note the signs of increased ICP.
      ii. Educate the parents regarding signs of infection.
         (1) If a VP shunt becomes infected the shunt may become obstructed.
      iii. Advise the parents to inform their primary health-care provider immediately if any adverse signs appear.
   d. Risk for Ineffective Coping/Anxiety/Fear/Anger/Grieving.
      i. Allow the parents to express grief over the loss of the perfect child.
      ii. Carefully explain the pathophysiology and rationale for the therapeutic regimen to the parents and child, if appropriate.
      iii. Encourage the family and child, if appropriate, to discuss their concerns and anxieties regarding the diagnosis.
      iv. Help the parents to develop realistic goals for the child, and to provide toys and activities to maximize the child's growth and development.

V. Cerebral Palsy

Cerebral palsy (CP), a nonprogressive, permanent condition, is the most common disability of childhood affecting movement. The vast majority of children with CP are diagnosed in the first year of life. CP can develop later in life, however, if a child experiences a period of prolonged hypoxia.

A. Incidence.
  1. Two to 4 per 1,000 children.

B. Etiology.
  1. Hypoxic insult to the brain.
  2. The hypoxia may occur at any point in the pregnancy cycle: prenatally, during delivery, or after delivery or may occur later in the child's life.
    a. The vast majority of children with CP were born prematurely.

C. Pathophysiology.
  1. Hypoxic insult to the motor centers of the brain.
  2. Severity of the disability is directly related to the location and severity of the insult.
  3. CNS comorbidities are common, including seizures, sensory defects, and cognitive deficits.
    a. Comorbidities are also related to hypoxia of the brain.
  4. Signs and symptoms: depend on the location and severity of the insult.
    a. There are three main types of CP as well as a mixed form when a child exhibits signs and symptoms of two or more of the three main forms.
      i. Spastic: characterized by hyperreflexia with hypertonia and spasticity of muscles.
        (1) Signs and symptoms include:
          (a) Prolongation of neonatal reflexes.
          (b) Scissoring of the legs.
          (c) Toe walking.
          (d) Jerky movements.
      ii. Dyskinetic: characterized by almost constant wormlike, writhing movements.
        (1) Children with the dyskinetic form may have difficulty speaking as well as difficulty chewing and swallowing.
      iii. Ataxic: characterized by uncoordinated and/or unbalanced movements.

D. Diagnosis.
  1. Clinical picture: usually diagnosed in infancy and toddlerhood when the child fails to achieve expected milestones.
  2. Gross Motor Function Classification System (GMFCS) (Palisano et al, 1997) is a diagnostic tool that may be used to determine the extent of the child's condition.
  3. The child should have a complete medical work-up to rule out any other medical problems that may be responsible for the child's motor impairments.

E. Treatment.
  1. There is no cure.
  2. Multidisciplinary interventions related to the child's motor dysfunction include therapies that are developed and modified to maximize the child's growth and development potential.
    a. Physical and occupational therapy.
      i. Specialized equipment specific to the child's needs is often required, including braces, crutches, and splints.
    b. Orthopedic surgeries may be performed to improve the movement of muscles and joints.
    c. Muscle relaxants and antianxiety medications may be administered to facilitate the child's movements.
  3. Additional therapies are often needed to treat the child's comorbidities, such as:
    a. Antiseizure medications for seizure disorders (see earlier).
    b. Sensory-assistive devices for hearing and/or vision deficits (see Chapter 25, "Nursing Care of the Child With Sensory Problems").
    c. Early intervention for cognitive deficits (see Chapter 24, "Nursing Care of the Child With Intellectual and Developmental Disabilities").

F. Nursing considerations.
  1. Delayed Growth and Development.
    a. At each well-child visit, growth and development milestones must be assessed carefully.
      i. If the child is delayed in acquisition of milestones or in any aspect of motor development, referral for accurate diagnosis is essential.
    b. Expect behaviors at the child's functional age and ability rather than his or her chronological age.
  2. Risk for Injury/Deficient Knowledge.
    a. Educate the family regarding the need to provide a safe environment for the child.
    b. Provide access to child protective equipment, if needed (e.g., helmet, knee, elbow and wrist pads).
    c. Educate the family to provide the child with safe toys that foster growth and development.
    d. To prevent aspiration, educate the family regarding the need to position the child upright during feeding and following meals.
  3. Impaired Physical Mobility/Pain.
    a. Refer the child and family for physical and occupational therapy and for needed specialized equipment.

b. Monitor the child's pain level during physical therapy and occupational therapy sessions, following surgeries, and during and after any other painful experiences.
c. Provide nonpharmacological and safe dosages of pharmacological pain interventions, as needed.

4. Anxiety/Fear/Anger/Grieving/Risk for Ineffective Coping.
   a. Allow the parents to express grief over the loss of the perfect child.
   b. Carefully explain the pathophysiology and rationale for care to the parents and child, if appropriate.
   c. Encourage the family and child, if appropriate, to discuss their concerns, frustrations, and guilt regarding the diagnosis and therapy.
   d. Help the parents to develop realistic goals for the child's growth and development.
   e. Consider introducing the child and family to another family with a child with CP.
   f. Refer the child and family to community resources (e.g., United Cerebral Palsy).

VI. Head Injury

Severe head injuries are also referred to as total brain injuries (TBIs).

A. Incidence.
1. Leading cause of death in children over 1 year of age in the United States.

B. Etiology.
1. Babies under 1 year of age.
   a. Trauma sustained during automobile accidents.
   b. Trauma sustained as a result of shaken baby syndrome (SBS).
2. Older children.
   a. Trauma sustained from automobile, bicycle, skate boarding, skiing, and other such accidents.
   b. Trauma sustained during sporting events (e.g., hockey, football, soccer).

DID YOU KNOW?

Prevention is the key. To prevent SBS, all parents should be educated regarding the potential for serious injury that can result from shaking an infant. Many hospitals are requiring new parents to view videos on SBS prior to being discharged from the postpartum unit. All children should be in age-appropriate restraint devices when riding in automobiles, and children should be seated in the back seat of the car until at least age 12. In addition, children's heads must be protected with helmets when they are engaged in potentially dangerous activities (e.g., bicycling, skiing, skateboarding, as well as when playing contact sports like football, hockey, and soccer).

C. Pathophysiology.
1. Dependent on extent of injury.
   a. Fractures of the skull.
   b. Contusions, i.e., bruises of the brain.
   c. Concussion, i.e., a brain injury defined as "a complex pathophysiological process affecting the brain, induced by biochemical forces" (McCrory et al, 2013).
      i. Concussion can result from a direct hit to the head or from an impact sustained in another part of the body that results in brain injury.
         (1) All contact sports place children at high risk for a concussion.
         (2) Females are at higher risk than are males.
      ii. Concussions, although serious, usually resolve in time. If more than one concussion occurs within a short period of time, however, the length of time needed to recover increases dramatically.
      iii. Concussions may or may not result in loss of consciousness.
      iv. A lengthy list of signs and symptoms has been developed by an international panel of experts on concussions and the sequelae that can develop as a result of concussive injuries (McCrory and Colleagues, 2013).
   d. Intracranial hemorrhage.
      i. Epidural hemorrhage, or bleeding above the dura, usually results in rapid onset of symptoms.
      ii. Subdural hemorrhage, or bleeding below the dura, may be difficult to diagnose because physiological changes often develop slowly.
2. Signs and symptoms of a TBI are dependent on the extent of the injury but frequently mimic those of increased ICP (see earlier).

D. Diagnosis.
1. History of injury.
2. Clinical picture is suggestive (see signs and symptoms of increased ICP).
   a. Comprehensive diagnostic assessments have been developed by an international panel of experts for use by health-care providers. All are available online in the *British Journal of Sports Medicine*.
      i. Sport Concussion Assessment Tool–3rd Edition (SCAT3) (http://bjsm.bmj.com/content/47/5/259.full.pdf): to be used for anyone over the age of 12.

ii. Child-SCAT3 (http://bjsm.bmj.com/content/47/5/263.full.pdf): to be used for children from 5 to 12 years of age.
iii. Pocket Concussion Recognition Tool (http://bjsm.bmj.com/content/47/5/267.full.pdf): can be used to assess for a concussion in individuals of all ages.

3. X-ray, CT, and/or MRI.

E. Treatment.

1. Initial care.
   a. Emergency management must be instituted, if needed, following the American Heart Association's CAB (circulation, airway, breathing) guidelines (see Chapter 10, "Pediatric Emergencies").
2. Follow-up care is dependent on the extent of the injury.
   a. Any child who has sustained a serious head injury should be thoroughly evaluated by a qualified health-care provider before resuming the activity.
   b. The child may require extensive recuperative time before it is safe to resume the activity.
      i. If the child has a concussion, a minimum of 1 week's rest is recommended before the child is allowed to resume normal activities (see following).
   c. If multiple injuries have been sustained over a period of time:
      i. The child may be strongly encouraged to retire from the offending activity.
      ii. Permanent damage to the brain may have occurred.

F. Nursing considerations.

1. Prevention.
   a. Deficient Knowledge.
      i. Educate the parents and child, if appropriate, regarding the potential for injury and prevention strategies related to activities, including:
         (1) Importance of not vigorously shaking infants and young toddlers.
         (2) Importance of children sitting in a recommended child protective restraint system when riding in an automobile.
         (3) Importance of children wearing head protection when engaging in potentially dangerous activities.
2. Treatment.
   a. Risk for Injury/Deficient Knowledge
      i. Perform a primary assessment, CAB, and intervene, if needed.
         (1) Even if vitals are normal immediately following the injury, frequent assessments should be performed during the next 24 to 48 hr.
            (a) Signs and symptoms of increased ICP can develop slowly, especially if a subdural hematoma is present.
      ii. If possible, take an excellent history of the accident.
      iii. Immobilize the neck until a neck injury has been ruled out.
      iv. Assess the ears and nose for bleeding and for leakage of CSF.
      v. Assess level of consciousness using the age-appropriate Glasgow coma scale (Table 22.1).
      vi. Assess for presence of concussion using SCAT3 or Child-SCAT3 and/or Pocket Concussion Recognition Tool.
      vii. Monitor for signs of increased ICP.
      viii. Place the child on seizure precautions.
      ix. If a concussion is present, a "graduated return to play protocol" (McCrory et al, 2013) is recommended that includes:
         (1) An initial full rest period of 24 to 48 hr followed by:
         (2) Slow progression, as long as symptoms are subsiding, beginning with light activity and ending, only if all symptoms have disappeared, with resumption of full activity approximately 1 week later.

VII. Seizures

Children may develop chronic seizure disorders but, for the purposes of this text, febrile seizures are used as the exemplar. They are almost always benign in origin, but injury prevention strategies used during the seizures are the same as those used during any seizure.

A. Incidence.

1. Febrile seizures are usually only seen in young children.
   a. Most children outgrow febrile seizures by the time they enter elementary school.
2. Febrile seizures are more commonly seen in boys than girls.

B. Etiology.

1. Appear to have a strong genetic link.
   a. Sons of fathers who had febrile seizures are likely also to have febrile seizures.
2. Seizures occur as the child's temperature is rising—usually above 100.4°F.
   a. Seizures rarely develop once the temperature has reached its highest level.

C. Pathophysiology.

1. Physiological immaturity, resulting in a number of neural impulses firing at the same time.

2. With physiological maturation, which usually occurs by the school-age period, the majority of children outgrow the disorder.
3. Although children who develop febrile seizures are slightly at higher risk for epilepsy, in the vast majority of cases, the children experience no long-term effects from the seizures.
4. Signs and symptoms.
   a. Loss of consciousness.
   b. Generalized, systemic **tonic-clonic** activity.
      i. The tonic portion consists of a period of muscle rigidity during which the child may stop breathing and become cyanotic.
      ii. The clonic portion is characterized by a shaking and jerking of both the arms and the legs.
      iii. The seizures may last up to 15 min.

D. Diagnosis.
1. Clinical evidence is suggestive. To distinguish febrile seizures from epilepsy, a thorough history of the seizure should be obtained from the parents.
2. Supportive evidence may be obtained from:
   a. Video recordings.
   b. Electroencephalogram.
   c. CT and/or MRI.
   d. Lumbar puncture.

E. Treatment.
1. Safe dosages of antipyretics are administered to prevent a rapid temperature rise.
   a. Administration of safe dosages of acetaminophen and ibuprofen are often alternated every 2 to 4 hr.
2. Unless a febrile seizure lasts longer than 15 min, it is rare for antiseizure medications to be ordered.
   a. Children should have an epilepsy work-up if the child exhibits atypical febrile seizures, e.g., seizure that lasts longer than 15 min, is focal in nature, and/or a family member has epilepsy.

F. Nursing considerations.
1. Risk for Injury/Deficient Knowledge.
   a. Prevention.
      i. Parents must learn to be proactive when they think that their child is ill, seeking medical care, as needed.
         (1) Any underlying illness (e.g., bacterial infection) should be treated.
      ii. Because the seizure usually occurs as the temperature is rising, the nurse should educate parents whose children have had febrile seizures to intervene early as a means of preventing future seizures.

! Safe dosages of antipyretics should be given *as the temperature is rising*. Parents should NOT wait until the temperature reaches its peak.

      iii. The child should be kept well hydrated and clothed in lightweight clothing.
      iv. Advise the parents that old remedies are no longer recommended.
         (1) Alcohol and/or tepid baths often result in the child becoming chilled.
            (a) Shivering results when one is chilled, resulting in the child's temperature rising rather than lowering.
   b. During a seizure:
      i. Protect the head from injury.
         (1) The remainder of the body should not be restrained.
      ii. Loosen any restrictive clothing, e.g., unbutton a shirt at the neck.
      iii. Document and report the characteristics of the seizure, including specific physiological changes (e.g., breathing pattern, length of seizure, focal versus tonic/clonic movements, skin color)
      iv. Institute CAB, as needed, following any seizure.

VIII. Reye Syndrome

Reye syndrome is a relatively rare, mainly preventable syndrome that follows viral illnesses, most notably varicella (chickenpox) and influenza.

A. Incidence.
1. May be seen at any age, although it is rare after 14 years of age.

B. Etiology.
1. Related to ingestion of aspirin during a viral episode (usually varicella or influenza).

C. Pathophysiology.
1. In some individuals, the viral illness, often in conjunction with the ingestion of aspirin, leads to a disruption in fat metabolism, most notably in the liver, kidneys, and brain.
2. Cytokines are released, resulting in serious changes in the affected organs.
3. Signs and symptoms.
   a. Elevated serum ammonia levels.
   b. Hypoglycemia.
   c. Signs and symptoms of increased ICP (see earlier).
4. The syndrome is staged based on signs and symptoms. Children who recover from the illness (reversal of symptoms can happen at any stage of the illness) may suffer permanent brain injury.

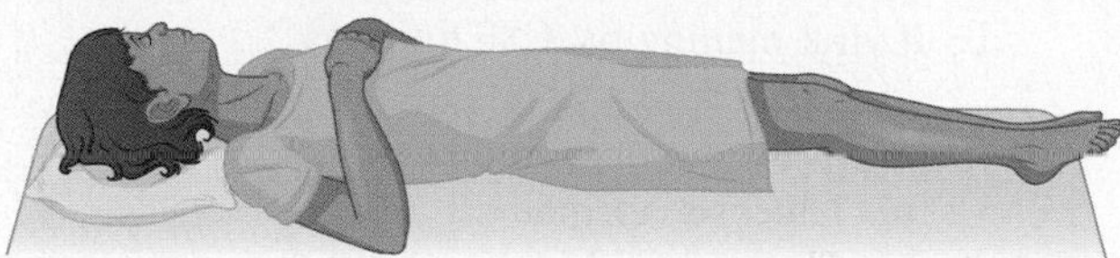

Fig 22.3 Decorticate posturing.

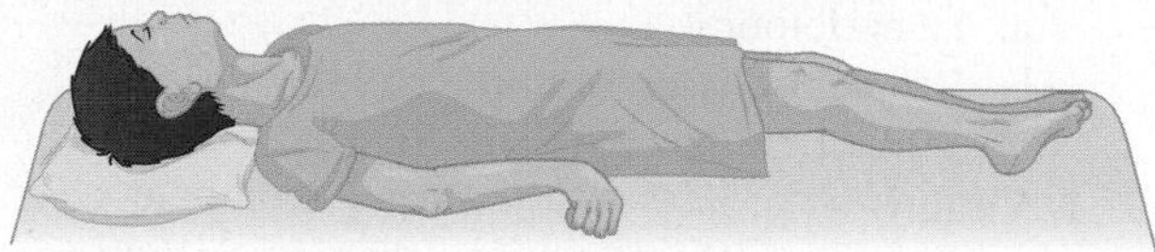

Fig 22.4 Decerebrate posturing.

a. Stage 1.
   i. Sleepiness with vomiting.
   ii. Tachypnea in some children.
b. Stage 2.
   i. Hyperreflexia and combative behavior.
   ii. Positive Babinski reflex.
   iii. Failure to respond to pain.
c. Stages 3 to 5.
   i. Children slowly deteriorate from **decorticate posturing** (arms bent toward the body, with hands in tight fists and legs held stiffly straight, as shown in Fig. 22.3).
   ii. To **decerebrate posturing** (rigid arms and legs, with toes pointed inward and head and neck held stiffly backward, as shown in Fig. 22.4).
   iii. To paralyzed posturing, and death, as they continue to seize.
d. Children who are unable to be staged correctly because they are on medications are classified as stage 6.

D. Diagnosis.
1. Clinical picture, i.e., severe illness characterized by lethargy and vomiting followed by agitation, combative behavior, and seizures, that develops about 1 week after a viral syndrome that was treated with aspirin.
2. Confirmatory findings include:
   a. Elevated AST and ALT.
   b. Elevated serum ammonia.

E. Treatment.
1. Palliative therapy because there is no specific cure.
   a. Oxygen and mechanical ventilation, if needed.
   b. IV therapy.
   c. Anticonvulsants for seizures.
   d. Diuretics for cerebral edema.
   e. Hemodialysis for markedly elevated ammonia levels.

F. Nursing considerations.
1. Deficient Knowledge.
   a. Educate the parents to medicate childrens' viral illnesses, especially varicella and influenza, only with acetaminophen or ibuprofen.
2. Risk for Injury
   a. Provide care, as cited earlier, for the client with increased ICP.
   b. Administer oxygen, as prescribed, and mechanical ventilation, if needed.
   c. Maintain IV therapy.
   d. Administer safe dosages of anticonvulsants, as prescribed.
   e. Administer safe dosages of diuretics, as prescribed.
   f. Provide hemodialysis, as prescribed.
3. Risk for Altered Coping/Grieving.
   a. Explain the pathophysiology and rationale for care to the parents and child, if appropriate.
   b. Encourage the family and child to discuss their concerns, guilt, and fear regarding the diagnosis and possible death.

IX. Meningitis

Meningitis is the most common infection of the central nervous system seen in children and is the exemplar presented in this chapter. Other infections of the CNS include encephalitis, infection of the brain, and myelitis, infection of the spinal cord. Encephalitis may develop from viral illnesses, including mumps and rubella and those transmitted by insect vectors. Myelitis may develop in a baby born with spina bifida.

A. Incidence.
1. Meningitis most commonly is seen in children less than 5 years of age, although meningococcal meningitis is seen in older children living in confined spaces (e.g., college dormitories).
2. The number of children diagnosed with meningitis has dropped significantly since the *Hemophilus influenzae* type b (Hib), pneumococcal, and meningococcal vaccinations have become routine.

B. Etiology: there are a number of causative organisms.
1. Bacteria.
   a. Infants aged 0 to 3 months old: most common organisms are *Escherichia coli* or group B strep.
   b. Children 3 months of age to 12 years: most common organisms.
      i. *Neisseria meningitides:* prevented by the meningococcal vaccine.
         (1) If *N. meningitides* enters the bloodstream, the child will develop

meningococcemia, a medical emergency.
(a) Characterized by petechiae covering the body.
ii. *Streptococcus pneumoniae:* prevented by the pneumococcal vaccine.
iii. *H. influenzae:* prevented by the Hib vaccine.
2. Viruses: many agents, including mumps and enteroviruses.
a. Viral meningitis is usually much less serious than the bacterial form.
3. Miscellaneous other pathogens.

C. Pathophysiology.
1. Inflammation of the meninges as a result of pathogenic invasion.
a. Increased ICP develops.
b. If inflammation persists, it may create an obstruction, resulting in hydrocephalus (see earlier).
2. Signs and symptoms: dependent on the age of the child.
a. Infants and young children:.
i. Usually exhibit nonspecific symptoms, including hyperthermia or hypothermia, poor feeding, irritability, nausea and vomiting, and seizures.
ii. See also signs and symptoms of increased ICP in infants (see earlier).
b. Older children exhibit signs of meningeal irritation.
i. **Kernig sign:** pain when the leg and knee are elevated and extended.
ii. **Brudzinski sign:** pain and hip flexion when the chin is flexed onto the chest.
iii. Late signs: seizures and behavioral changes.

D. Diagnosis.
1. Suggestive.
a. Clinical picture: see signs and symptoms.
b. Positive bacterial throat and nose cultures: the bacteria often enter the body via the respiratory tract.
c. Positive bacterial blood cultures: bacteria may enter the CNS via the vascular system.
2. Definitive diagnosis is made by lumbar puncture.
a. If bacterial meningitis, CSF findings:
i. Cloudy fluid.
ii. WBC count: more than 100 cells/mm^3 (normal is less than 5).
iii. Glucose: below 45 mg/dL (normal is 50 to 80 mg/dL).
iv. CSF pressure: above 15 mm Hg (normal is 8 to 15 mm Hg).
v. Positive bacterial culture.
b. If viral meningitis, CSF findings.
i. Clear fluid.
ii. WBC count: normal.
iii. Glucose: normal.
iv. Elevated CSF pressure.
v. Culture negative.

E. Treatment.
1. Bacterial.
a. IV antibiotics.
b. Droplet isolation until the child has been on antibiotics for a full 24 hr.
2. Viral.
a. Assume that the etiology is bacterial until proven otherwise; therefore isolation and antibiotic regimens are begun.
b. Once bacterial cultures are found to be negative, palliative care can be provided at home: bedrest, antipyretics.

F. Nursing considerations.
1. Prevention.
a. Deficient Knowledge.
i. Educate parents regarding the importance of having their children immunized per the ACIP vaccination schedule.
2. Treatment.
a. Infection.
i. Perform meticulous handwashing.
ii. Administer safe doses of IV antibiotics, as prescribed.
iii. Place child on droplet precautions and maintain precautions either until a negative CSF culture has been received and/or the child has been on antibiotics for a full 24 hr.
iv. Educate the family and other visitors regarding isolation protocols.
v. Inform the child that isolation precautions are not a punishment. They are needed to prevent others from also getting sick.
vi. Take an excellent history, including the child's.
(1) Immunization history.
(2) Recent contacts.
(i) Report information to the primary health-care provider.
(ii) Currently healthy contacts may need to receive prophylactic antibiotics.
b. Risk for Injury.
i. Monitor for and report to the primary health-care provider any signs of increased ICP (see earlier).
ii. Maintain seizure precautions.
(1) If the child seizes, immediately institute seizure care (see earlier).

c. Pain.
   i. If possible, avoid moving the child's head and neck.
      (1) An excellent way to maintain head stability is to place pillows on either side of the child's head.
   ii. Reduce auditory and visual stimulation in the child's room.
   iii. Assess pain using an age-appropriate pain rating scale.
   iv. Provide safe dosages of pharmacological pain medication, as prescribed and as needed.
   v. Provide nonpharmacological pain therapy, as needed.

d. Deficient Knowledge/Risk for Altered Coping.
   i Encourage the child and parents to express their concerns and fears regarding the symptoms and the disease process.
   ii. Inform the parents and child, if appropriate, regarding the disease process and therapy.
   iii. Encourage the parents to stay with the child during hospitalization.

X. Brain Tumors

A. Incidence.
   1. Brain tumors are the second most common type of cancer seen in children and the most common form of solid tumor seen in children.

B. Etiology.
   1. Approximately 5% of brain tumors are hereditary in nature.
   2. The cause of the remaining 95% is currently unknown.

C. Pathophysiology.
   1. There are a large number of different types of brain tumors and brain tumors can develop in a number of different locations in the brain. (For information regarding each of the specific types and locations, please consult a comprehensive pediatric textbook.)
      a. Brain tumors may be either benign or cancerous.
      b. The most common type of brain cancer seen in children from infancy through early adolescence is pliocytic astrocytoma (PA), a slow-growing cancer of the cerebellum.
      c. Teens over the age of 14 most commonly are diagnosed with either PAs or tumors of the pituitary gland.
   2. Signs and symptoms.
      a. Because brain tumors occupy space in the skull, the signs and symptoms are consistent with those of increased ICP.
      b. Depending on the location of the tumor, additional signs and symptoms may be exhibited, e.g.:
         i. Uncoordinated movements.
         ii. Paralysis of one side of the body.
         iii. Altered speech patterns.
         iv. Altered eye movements.
   3. The majority of children with brain tumors will survive the illness, but many of the survivors will experience long-term complications (e.g., hydrocephalus, cognitive deficits, seizure disorders).

D. Diagnosis—the presence of a brain tumor is a medical emergency. Ideally, diagnosis is made as swiftly as possible.
   1. Complete neurological assessment.
      a. Lumbar puncture may be contraindicated because of the potential for herniation of the brain.
   2. MRI/CT.

E. Treatment.
   1. Surgical removal of the entire tumor is ideal, although complete removal may not be feasible.
   2. Chemotherapy and/or radiation are often performed following surgery.
      a. See the discussion of acute lymphoblastic leukemia (ALL) in Chapter 18, "Care of the Child With Hematologic Illnesses" for information regarding chemotherapy.
   3. If hydrocephalus develops, a VP shunt may be inserted during the surgery (see "Hydrocephalus").

F. Nursing considerations.
   1. Preoperative.
      a. Anxiety/Fear/Anger/Grieving/Deficient Knowledge.
         i. Provide age-appropriate information to the parents and child, if appropriate, regarding the diagnosis and the surgery.
         ii. Allow the parents and child, if appropriate, to express anger, fears, and anxiety related to a life-threatening diagnosis.
         iii. Prepare the parents and child, if appropriate, regarding the need to shave the child's head and the size of the dressing that will cover the head following surgery.
      b. Risk for Injury.
         i. Perform complete age-appropriate neurological assessments, including Glasgow assessment, and immediately report any deterioration in status to the primary health-care provider.

2. Postoperative.
   a. Routine postoperative nursing care, including pain management, REEDA assessment, vital sign assessments, monitoring of gastrointestinal functioning, and bleeding potential.
   b. Risk for Injury.
      i. Perform complete age-appropriate neurological assessments including Glasgow assessments and immediately report any deviations from normal to the neurosurgeon.
         (1) Immediately report to the neurosurgeon any signs and symptoms of increased ICP that may develop as a result of bleeding into the brain, hydrocephalus, or swelling of the brain tissue.
      ii. Elevate the head of the bed, as prescribed.
         (1) To prevent worsening of the ICP, the bed should never be placed in the Trendelenburg position.
   c. Risk for Infection/Impaired Skin Integrity.
      i. Perform meticulous handwashing.
      ii. Use aseptic technique when performing dressing changes.
      iii. Monitor the child for signs of infection, at the surgical site as well as urinary and pulmonary infections, and monitor laboratory data.
   d. Risk for Imbalanced Fluid Volume.
      i. Strict I&O.
      ii. Report if the child is excreting below the minimum output for his or her weight.
      iii. Monitor the child's weight daily.
   e. Risk for Delayed Growth and Development/ Risk for Impaired Coping.
      i. Perform growth and development assessments to determine the extent of the child's disability.
      ii. Refer the child to programs that provide early educational intervention, if needed.
      iii. Depending on additional deficits exhibited by the child, refer the family for specialized care, e.g., occupational therapy, physical therapy, sensory assessments.
      iv. Provide children with clear, simple explanations of all tasks/treatments.
      v. Refer the family for counseling, if prescribed.

XI. Neuroblastoma

A. Incidence.
1. The most common malignancy in infants.
2. Over 15% of all children who die from cancer have been diagnosed with neuroblastoma.

B. Etiology.
1. Although the exact cause of the mutation is unknown, neuroblastoma is a cancer of the peripheral nervous system that originates from embryonic tissue.
2. A small number of neuroblastomas are hereditary.
3. Some neuroblastomas are environmental in origin; some of the parents of children with neuroblastoma have worked in industries that exposed them to cancer-causing chemicals.

C. Pathophysiology.
1. Neuroblastomas originate from embryonic tissue. Rather than developing into normal sympathetic nerve cells, some of the tissue mutates and develops into cancer cells.
2. Neuroblastomas may be relatively small, round tumors or may grow into more mature tumors.
3. Metastasis to other organs is common.

D. Diagnosis.
1. Diagnosis is often difficult because the signs and symptoms, depending on the location of the tumor(s), are similar to those of other diseases.
   a. Diagnosis is usually made with x-ray, MRI, and/or CT
   b. Once identified, the exact genetic mutation is determined. The clinical prognosis is often dependent upon the age of the child in conjunction with the genetics of the tumor.
   c. Once diagnosed, additional tests to determine the extent of metastasis may be performed.
2. Signs and symptoms of neuroblastoma range from a large abdominal mass, to hypertension, to marked sweating, to marked diarrhea, to signs and symptoms of spinal cord compression.
   a. Children often complain of pain related to the specific nerve involvement.

E. Treatment.
1. Surgical removal of the tumor.
2. Depending on the extent of tumor involvement, the genetics of the tumor and the child's age, surgery may be followed by chemotherapy and/or radiation.
   a. See the discussion of acute lymphoblastic leukemia (ALL) in Chapter 18, "Nursing Care of the Child with Hematologic Illnesses" for information regarding chemotherapy.

F. Nursing considerations.
1. Preoperative.
   a. Anxiety/Fear/Anger/Grieving/Deficient Knowledge/Pain.
      i. Provide age-appropriate information to the parents and child, if appropriate, regarding the diagnosis and the surgery.
      ii. Allow the parents and child, if appropriate, to express anger, fears, and anxiety related to a life-threatening diagnosis.

iii. Administer safe dosages of analgesics, as prescribed.
(1) If the pain is moderate to severe, narcotics may be needed.
iv. Provide nonpharmacological pain interventions, as needed.
b. Risk for Injury.
i. Perform complete age-appropriate neurological assessments including Glasgow assessment and immediately report any deterioration in status to the primary health-care provider.
2. Postoperative.
a. Routine postoperative nursing care, including pain management, REEDA assessment, vital signs assessment, monitoring of gastrointestinal functioning, and bleeding potential.
b. Risk for Injury/Pain.
i. Perform complete age-appropriate neurological assessments including Glasgow assessments and immediately report any deviations from normal to the neurosurgeon.
ii. Administer safe dosages of analgesics, as prescribed.
(1) If the pain is moderate to severe, narcotics may be needed.
iii. Provide nonpharmacological pain interventions, as needed.
c. Risk for Impaired Coping.
i. Consider introducing the family to another family with a child with neuroblastoma.
ii. Refer the family to a neuroblastoma association (e.g., The Neuroblastoma Children's Cancer Society, Children's Neuroblastoma Cancer Foundation).

CASE STUDY: Putting It All Together

Newborn with spina bifida seen on prenatal ultrasound delivered at 39 weeks' gestation via cesarean section

Subjective Data
- Mother states,
  - "My aunt is in a wheelchair. I am so sad that my baby will never walk."
  - "I eat hamburgers and French fries every day for lunch. Dinner is an on-the-go thing."

Objective Data

Nursing Assessment
- Unmarried, 17-year-old, Caucasian mother
- Late entry into prenatal care (26 weeks' gestation)
- Spina bifida noted on ultrasound
- Physical findings
  - Weight: 2,500 g
  - Apgar: 8/10
  - Open sac at base of spine in lumbosacral region
  - Constant dribbling of urine
  - Constant oozing of feces
  - Bilateral flaccid paralysis of both legs
  - Asymmetry of leg folds
  - Head circumference: 37 cm; chest circumference: 32 cm

Vital Signs	
Temperature:	97.7°F
Heart rate:	156 bpm
Respiratory rate:	58 rpm

Lab Results	
Coombs' test:	negative
Hematocrit:	52% (normal 48%–69%)
Hemoglobin:	17 g/dL (normal 14.5–22.5 g/dL)
White blood cell count:	15,000 cells/mm^3 (normal 9,000–30,000 cells/mm^3)

Health-Care Provider's Orders
- Admit to NICU
- Ultrasound of sacral sac
- Maintain in the prone position, even while feeding
- Cover sac with moist, sterile dressing
  - Maintain moisture with sterile saline
  - Reinforce moist dressing with a dry, sterile dressing
  - Keep feces and urine from contaminating sac
- Monitor vitals every 2 hr, and report any sign of infection
- Assess head circumference daily
- Prepare for surgery in AM

Continued

CASE STUDY: Putting It All Together *cont'd*

Case Study Questions

A. What *subjective* assessments indicate that this client is experiencing a health alteration?

1. ______
2. ______

B. What *objective* assessments indicate that this client is experiencing a health alteration?

1. ______
2. ______
3. ______
4. ______
5. ______
6. ______
7. ______
8. ______

C. After analyzing the data that has been collected, what **primary** nursing diagnosis should the nurse assign to this client?

1. ______

D. What interventions should the nurse plan and/or implement to meet this child's and his family's needs?

1. ______
2. ______
3. ______
4. ______
5. ______
6. ______
7. ______
8. ______
9. ______
10. ______
11. ______
12. ______
13. ______
14. ______
15. ______
16. ______

CASE STUDY: Putting It All Together *cont'd*

Case Study Questions

E. What client outcomes should the nurse evaluate regarding the effectiveness of the nursing interventions?

1. ______________________________
2. ______________________________
3. ______________________________
4. ______________________________
5. ______________________________

F. What physiological characteristics should the child exhibit before being discharged home?

1. ______________________________
2. ______________________________
3. ______________________________
4. ______________________________

G. What subjective characteristics should the child exhibit before being discharged home?

1. ______________________________

REVIEW QUESTIONS

1. The nurse, who is admitting a neonate into the well-baby nursery, assesses the following: widely separated sagittal suture and enlarged anterior and posterior fontanels. Which of the following follow-up assessments is most important for the nurse to perform at this time?
   1. Tonic neck reflex
   2. Head and chest circumferences
   3. Ortolani's sign
   4. Red reflexes of both eyes
2. A child has been prescribed Tegretol (carbamazepine) for a seizure disorder. Which of the following information in relation to this child is essential for the nurse to consider? **Select all that apply.**
   1. Gender
   2. Behavior
   3. Dental health
   4. Genetic profile
   5. Antibiotic prescriptions
3. A baby with myelomeningocele is admitted to the neonatal intensive care unit. Which of the following signs/symptoms would the nurse expect to see?
   1. Hyperreflexia
   2. Ptosis
   3. Bilateral lower limb paralysis
   4. Marked respiratory distress
4. The nurse is admitting a newly delivered neonate with meningocele into the nursery. Which of the following assessments is priority for the nurse to perform?
   1. Assessment of the red reflexes
   2. Hard palate assessment
   3. Trunk incurvation reflex
   4. Head and chest circumferences
5. A baby is preoperative for closure of a myelomeningocele. Which of the following is the baby's priority nursing diagnosis?
   1. Risk for Infection
   2. Impaired Physical Mobility
   3. Risk for Latex Allergy
   4. Bowel Incontinence
6. A baby is admitted to the neonatal intensive care unit following closure of a myelomeningocele. Which of the following patient care goals should the nurse include in the nursing care plan?
   The baby will:
   1. maintain supine positioning.
   2. have normal elimination patterns.
   3. exhibit a normal startle reflex.
   4. consume feedings and gain weight.
7. A 4-year-old child has had a ventriculoperitoneal shunt in place since birth. The parents called the triage nurse at the child's primary health-care provider and stated that when the child awoke, he complained of a "bad" headache, and he vomited shortly thereafter. Which of the following actions by the nurse is appropriate?
   1. Advise the parents to have the child seen in the emergency department.
   2. Make an afternoon appointment for the child to see the health-care provider.
   3. Tell the parents to give the child electrolyte replacement therapy instead of food.
   4. Inform the parents that they should call back if the child also develops diarrhea.
8. A 7-month-old child has been diagnosed with cerebral palsy (CP). Which of the following signs/symptoms would the nurse assess as consistent with the diagnosis?
   1. Positive grasp reflex
   2. Pigeon chest
   3. Harlequin sign
   4. Circumoral cyanosis
9. A pediatric nurse is having a discussion with a father whose child has recently been diagnosed with spastic cerebral palsy. Which of the following statements by the nurse is appropriate?
   1. "It must be very hard to know that your child's ability to move will decrease over time."
   2. "I am sure that it is hard for you to know that your child has this disease, but at least the medicine will treat the underlying problem."
   3. "The treatment plan for your child will focus on enabling him to have as normal movements as possible."
   4. "The nerve stimulation of your child's legs will enable him to walk on his own when he is older."
10. A child has been diagnosed with febrile seizures. Which of the following information should the nurse include in the parent teaching session?
    1. "Whenever your child develops a fever, place him in a warm bath and pour the water over his arms and legs."
    2. "Make sure to give your child high dosages of acetaminophen whenever his temperature goes above 104°F."
    3. "It is very important that your child have no more seizures to prevent him from experiencing permanent injury to his brain."
    4. "It should be comforting to know that most children outgrow the febrile seizures by the time they reach 6 years of age."

11. The nurse is educating the parents of a child who has been diagnosed with febrile seizures. Which of the following actions should the nurse advise the parents is important for them to perform if their child has another seizure?
1. Protect the child's head.
2. Restrain the child's arms and legs.
3. Place a tongue blade in the child's mouth.
4. Administer mouth-to-mouth resuscitation.

12. A nurse is providing health promotion/disease prevention education to a group of parents at a neighborhood clinic. Which of the following information should the nurse include in the teaching?
1. The rotavirus vaccine will protect their children from the infection that causes meningitis.
2. Aspirin should be administered to children who are sick with viral illnesses.
3. A well-padded helmet should be worn by any child who plays a contact sport or rides a bicycle.
4. The parent should carefully check the tongue for injury whenever a child experiences severe head trauma.

13. A 12-year-old child is being assessed in the emergency department for possible Reye syndrome. The child was diagnosed with influenza by a primary health care provider 2 weeks earlier. Which of the following findings would the nurse expect to see? **Select all that apply.**
1. Child's Babinski reflex is positive.
2. Child has had vomiting episodes for the past 24 hr.
3. Child's serum ammonia levels are markedly lower than normal.
4. Child was administered ibuprofen (Advil) when the child had the flu.
5. Child is unusually argumentative and aggressive.

14. A teenager has been in an automobile accident. The parents are advised that their child has experienced a cerebral contusion. When they ask what that means, the nurse should provide which of the following explanations?
1. "Your child has ruptured a blood vessel between the layers that protect the brain from injury."
2. "Your child has a bruise of the brain tissue."
3. "Your child has a fracture in one part of the skull."
4. "Your child has a great deal of swelling of the part of the brain that is called the brain stem."

15. A 7-year-old child has just had a lumbar puncture in the emergency department for complaints of elevated temperature and a stiff neck. Which of the following cerebral spinal fluid findings would indicate that this child has bacterial meningitis?
1. Markedly lower than normal pressure
2. Glucose 20 mg/dL
3. White blood cell count 3 cells/mm^3
4. Clear fluid

16. A child is admitted to the pediatric unit with a diagnosis of meningitis. Which of the following actions should the nurse perform? **Select all that apply.**
1. Raise the head of the bed.
2. Dim the lights in the room.
3. Place the child on droplet isolation.
4. Administer intravenous antibiotics, as prescribed.
5. Perform passive range-of-motion exercises of the neck.

17. A nurse is providing counseling to parents regarding an important action they can take to prevent their children from developing meningitis. Which of the following actions did the nurse suggest?
1. Have children sleep in separate beds during sleepover parties.
2. Have children receive all recommended immunizations.
3. Teach children to wash their hands after toileting and before eating.
4. Teach children to cover their faces with a tissue when they sneeze.

18. A child who is experiencing high fever and neck pain is diagnosed with viral meningitis. Which of the following should the nurse include in the discharge teaching?
1. Keep the child isolated until the temperature returns to normal.
2. Pad the child's bed headboard.
3. Rent a commode for the child to use at home.
4. Administer over-the-counter analgesics as needed.

19. The nurse has taken a health history from a school-age child who is being assessed 6 weeks' post-surgery for a benign brain tumor. The nurse should report which of the following findings to the health-care provider?

1. The child states that he fell at school three times last week.
2. The child states that he has had no headaches all week.
3. The child states that he did very well on yesterday's history test.
4. The child states that he has decided to join the school's swim team.

20. A nurse is admitting a 7-month-old infant with a diagnosis of neuroblastoma to the pediatric in-patient unit. The infant is the parents' third child. The infant's father asks, "The doctor keeps talking about the genetics of the tumor. What the heck does that mean?" Which of the following responses by the nurse is appropriate?

1. "The doctor wants to determine whether any of your other children is at high risk of developing a neuroblastoma."
2. "The doctor wants to determine whether the genetic code in your baby's tumor is different from the genetic code in the rest of the baby's cells."
3. "The doctor is mandated by law to report to the health department any genetic mutation that is caused by environmental contaminants."
4. "The doctor will be better able to determine how the baby's therapy will work once the exact genetic code of the tumor is identified."

REVIEW ANSWERS

1. ANSWER: 2

Rationale:

1. It is important to assess the tonic neck reflex, but another response is more important.

2. It would be most important for the nurse to assess the child's head and chest circumferences carefully.

3. It is important to assess Ortolani's sign, but another response is more important.

4. It is important to assess for the red reflex in both of the baby's eyes, but another response is more important.

TEST-TAKING TIP: Babies with widely separated sagittal sutures and enlarged fontanels may have heads that are larger than normal. The head circumference should be approximately 2 cm larger than the chest circumference. If it is markedly larger, the baby may be developing hydrocephalus.

Content Area: *Newborn-At-Risk*
Integrated Processes: *Nursing Process: Assessment*
Client Need: *Physiological Integrity: Physiological Adaptation: Alterations in Body Systems*
Cognitive Level: *Analysis*

2. ANSWER: 2, 4, and 5

Rationale:

1. Gender need not be considered when administering Tegretol. It is safe both for boys and for girls to take the medication.

2. It is important for the nurse to assess the behavior of children on Tegretol. While on the medication, children often become drowsy and confused. In addition, their schoolwork may be poorly completed, and they may exhibit impaired coordination.

3. Children on Dilantin (phenytoin) often experience hypertrophy of the gums. It would be important for the nurse to assess the child's dental health while on that medication rather than when on Tegretol.

4. Children who carry the HLA-B*1502 allele in their genomes and are being prescribed Tegretol are at high risk for Stevens-Johnson syndrome. Before administering the medication, the child should be HLA tested.

5. Children taking Tegretol should be prescribed erythromycin with extreme caution because the drug levels of Tegretol will increase while they are on the antibiotic.

TEST-TAKING TIP: Any time a medication is administered, the nurse should be completely knowledgeable of its actions and safe dosages as well as the drug's side effects. If the medication has been ordered and the nurse has concerns regarding its safety, he or she should question the primary health-care provider regarding the order.

Content Area: *Pediatrics—Neuromuscular*
Integrated Processes: *Nursing Process: Assessment*
Client Need: *Physiological Integrity: Pharmacological and Parenteral Therapies: Adverse Effects/Contraindications/Side Effects/Interaction*
Cognitive Level: *Application*

3. ANSWER: 3

Rationale:

1. The nurse would expect to see no reflex response in the lower limbs.

2. The nurse would not expect to see ptosis.

3. The nurse would expect to see bilateral lower limb paralysis.

4. The nurse would not expect to see signs of respiratory distress.

TEST-TAKING TIP: Babies with myelomeningocele are born with a sac of cerebral spinal fluid and nerves protruding through the skin in the lower back. The nerves to the upper body are unaffected, but the nerves to the lower body are adversely affected. The lower extremities of these babies often are paralyzed.

Content Area: *Newborn-At-Risk*
Integrated Processes: *Nursing Process: Assessment*
Client Need: *Physiological Integrity: Physiological Adaptation: Alterations in Body Systems*
Cognitive Level: *Application*

4. ANSWER: 4

Rationale:

1. Assessment of the red reflex is important, but it is not the priority assessment.

2. Hard palate assessment is important, but it is not the priority assessment.

3. Assessment of the trunk incurvation reflex is important, but it is not the priority assessment.

4. It is priority for the nurse to assess the baby's head and chest circumferences.

TEST-TAKING TIP: Over 90% of babies born with meningocele and myelomeningocele will also have hydrocephalus. It is priority, therefore, for the nurse to assess the circumferences to determine whether the baby is suffering from that complication.

Content Area: *Newborn-At-Risk*
Integrated Processes: *Nursing Process: Assessment*
Client Need: *Physiological Integrity: Physiological Adaptation: Alterations in Body Systems*
Cognitive Level: *Analysis*

5. ANSWER: 1

Rationale:

1. Risk for Infection is the baby's highest priority nursing diagnosis.

2. Impaired Physical Mobility is an appropriate nursing diagnosis, but it is not the priority diagnosis.

3. Risk for Latex Allergy is an appropriate nursing diagnosis, but it is not the priority diagnosis.

4. Bowel Incontinence is an appropriate nursing diagnosis, but it is not the priority diagnosis.

TEST-TAKING TIP: Although babies born with meningomyelocele are at risk for latex allergy and have both impaired physical mobility of their lower extremities and bowel incontinence, their most significant problem is their risk for infection. The exposed sac is a direct portal for bacterial invasion. The sac must be protected with moist, sterile dressings until it is surgically closed.

Content Area: *Newborn-At-Risk*
Integrated Processes: *Nursing Process: Analysis*
Client Need: *Physiological Integrity: Reduction of Risk Potential: Potential for Alterations in Body Systems*
Cognitive Level: *Analysis*

6. **ANSWER: 4**
Rationale:
1. The correct patient-care goal would be for the baby to maintain prone positioning.
2. Because of the defect, the baby will not have normal elimination patterns.
3. Because of the defect, the baby will not exhibit a normal startle reflex.
4. The baby would be expected to consume feedings and gain weight.
TEST-TAKING TIP: Patient-care goals are expectations of patients' behavior. A baby with a meningomyelocele would not be expected to have normal elimination patterns or a normal startle (Moro) reflex because of the nerve damage sustained from the defect. In addition, to prevent injury to the surgical site, the baby must be placed in the prone position. After surgery, the baby would be expected to feed and gain weight.
Content Area: *Newborn-At-Risk*
Integrated Processes: *Nursing Process: Planning*
Client Need: *Physiological Integrity: Reduction of Risk Potential: Potential for Alterations in Body Systems*
Cognitive Level: *Application*

7. **ANSWER: 1**
Rationale:
1. The child should be seen in the emergency department.
2. This child is exhibiting signs of increased ICP. The child needs to be seen as soon as possible.
3. The child is exhibiting signs of increased ICP.
4. This child is exhibiting signs of increased ICP. The child needs to be seen as soon as possible.
TEST-TAKING TIP: Ventriculoperitoneal (VP) shunts drain the cerebral spinal fluid from the ventricles of the brain in order to maintain normal intracranial pressures. When they malfunction, patients exhibit signs of increased ICP. The child needs to be assessed as an emergency so that the needed shunt revision can be scheduled and performed.
Content Area: *Pediatrics—Neuromuscular*
Integrated Processes: *Nursing Process: Implementation*
Client Need: *Physiological Integrity: Physiological Adaptation: Alternations in Body Systems*
Cognitive Level: *Application*

8. **ANSWER: 1**
Rationale:
1. Positive grasp reflex would be consistent with the diagnosis.
2. Pigeon chest is unrelated to a diagnosis of CP.
3. Harlequin sign is unrelated to a diagnosis of CP.
4. Circumoral cyanosis is unrelated to a diagnosis of CP.
TEST-TAKING TIP: In healthy babies, the neonatal grasp reflex begins to fade at about 3 months of age and is replaced by a voluntary grasp by about 5 months of age. A grasp reflex that does not fade is consistent with a diagnosis of CP.
Content Area: *Pediatrics—Neuromuscular*
Integrated Processes: *Nursing Process: Assessment*
Client Need: *Physiological Integrity: Physiological Adaptation: Alteration in Body Systems*
Cognitive Level: *Application*

9. **ANSWER: 3**
Rationale:
1. The symptoms of CP do not get worse over time.
2. Although medicines are available for some of the comorbidities associated with CP, there is no medication that treats the underlying cause of CP.
3. This statement is accurate.
4. This statement is false. The pathology of CP is in the brain.
TEST-TAKING TIP: The signs and symptoms of CP result from a hypoxic insult to the brain. The therapeutic interventions are aimed at enabling the child to reach his or her highest potential.
Content Area: *Pediatrics—Neuromuscular*
Integrated Processes: *Nursing Process: Implementation*
Client Need: *Physiological Integrity: Physiological Adaptation: Alterations in Body Systems*
Cognitive Level: *Application*

10. **ANSWER: 4**
Rationale:
1. Tepid baths are no longer recommended.
2. Antipyretics should be administered as soon as the child's temperature begins to rise. In addition, to prevent liver damage, only safe dosages of acetaminophen should be administered.
3. Children who experience febrile seizures rarely develop a permanent seizure disorder.
4. Most children do outgrow febrile seizures by the time they reach 6 years of age.
TEST-TAKING TIP: Febrile seizures usually occur as a child's temperature is rising. It is recommended, therefore, to administer antipyretics as soon as an elevation is noted. When placed in tepid baths, children usually shiver. Shivering actually stimulates the body to raise its temperature.
Content Area: *Pediatrics—Neuromuscular*
Integrated Processes: *Nursing Process: Implementation; Teaching/Learning*
Client Need: *Physiological Integrity: Physiological Adaptation: Alterations in Body Systems*
Cognitive Level: *Application*

11. **ANSWER: 1**
Rationale:
1. The parents should be taught to protect their child's head.
2. The child's arms and legs should not be restrained.
3. A tongue blade should not be inserted into the child's mouth.

4. Only if the child fails to start breathing after the seizure has stopped, which happens rarely, should CPR be instituted.

TEST-TAKING TIP: During tonic-clonic seizures, patients are unconscious and are thrashing indiscriminately. In order to prevent the child from experiencing a head injury, his or her head should be protected, but restraining a child's arms and legs may actually result in an injury.

Content Area: *Pediatrics—Neuromuscular*
Integrated Processes: *Nursing Process: Implementation; Teaching/Learning*
Client Need: *Physiological Integrity: Reduction of Risk Potential: Therapeutic Procedures*
Cognitive Level: *Application*

12. **ANSWER: 3**

Rationale:

1. The rotavirus vaccine protects children from an infection that causes severe gastrointestinal illness.
2. Aspirin should not be administered to children who are sick with viral illnesses.
3. **A well-padded helmet should be worn by any child who plays a contact sport or rides a bicycle.**
4. The ears and nose should be checked carefully for the leakage of blood or fluid whenever a child experiences severe head trauma.

TEST-TAKING TIP: Children can experience very serious head injuries, including contusions, concussions, fractures, and hematomas, when they fall or are hit while engaged in a variety of activities. Whenever possible, they should wear helmets for protection. Because of the potential for developing Reye syndrome, aspirin should not be administered to children suffering from a viral illness.

Content Area: *Child Health*
Integrated Processes: *Nursing Process: Implementation; Teaching/Learning*
Client Need: *Health Promotion and Maintenance: Health Promotion/Disease Prevention*
Cognitive Level: *Application*

13. **ANSWER: 1, 2, and 5**

Rationale:

1. **A positive Babinski reflex is seen in children with Reye syndrome.**
2. **Vomiting episodes are seen in children with Reye syndrome.**
3. Serum ammonia levels rise with Reye syndrome.
4. Aspirin is contraindicated when a child has the flu.
5. **Combative behavior, including being argumentative and aggressive, is seen in children with Reye syndrome.**

TEST-TAKING TIP: Reye syndrome is seen as a sequela to some viral illnesses, most notably varicella and influenza. It is more likely to occur if a child has received aspirin during the viral illness.

Content Area: *Pediatrics—Neuromuscular*
Integrated Processes: *Nursing Process: Assessment*
Client Need: *Physiological Integrity: Physiological Adaptation: Alterations in Body Systems*
Cognitive Level: *Application*

14. **ANSWER: 2**

Rationale:

1. This explanation is a subdural hematoma.
2. **A cerebral contusion is a brain bruise.**
3. This explanation simply is a fractured skull.
4. This child has severe increased ICP.

TEST-TAKING TIP: Although this question refers to a conversation between parents and a nurse, it simply is asking for the definition of a contusion.

Content Area: *Pediatrics—Neuromuscular*
Integrated Processes: *Nursing Process: Implementation*
Client Need: *Physiological Integrity: Physiological Adaptation: Pathophysiology*
Cognitive Level: *Comprehension*

15. **ANSWER: 2**

Rationale:

1. Cerebral spinal fluid pressures are elevated with a diagnosis of bacterial meningitis.
2. **Low glucose (below 45 mg/dL) is consistent with a diagnosis of bacterial meningitis.**
3. Elevated white blood cell counts are consistent with a diagnosis of bacterial meningitis (normal is less than 5 cells/mm^3).
4. Cerebral spinal fluid is cloudy with a diagnosis of bacterial meningitis.

TEST-TAKING TIP: When a child has bacterial meningitis, he or she has bacteria in the cerebral spinal fluid. The bacteria use the glucose for energy. As a result, glucose levels drop.

Content Area: *Pediatrics—Neuromuscular*
Integrated Processes: *Nursing Process: Assessment*
Client Need: *Physiological Integrity: Physiological Adaptation: Alterations in Body Systems*
Cognitive Level: *Application*

16. **ANSWER: 1, 2, 3, and 4**

Rationale:

1. **The head of the bed should be raised.**
2. **The room lights should be dimmed.**
3. **The child should be placed on droplet isolation.**
4. **The child will receive IV antibiotics.**
5. The nurse should refrain from moving the child's neck. The movement is very painful.

TEST-TAKING TIP: The bacteria that cause meningitis are transmitted via the respiratory route. The child, therefore, should be placed on droplet isolation. Once the child has been on antibiotics for a full 24 hr or if the culture report is negative for bacteria, he or she no longer needs to remain on isolation.

Content Area: *Pediatrics—Neuromuscular*
Integrated Processes: *Nursing Process: Implementation*
Client Need: *Physiological Integrity: Physiological Adaptation: Illness Management*
Cognitive Level: *Application*

17. **ANSWER: 2**

Rationale:

1. Sleeping in separate beds may help to prevent transmission if one child is harboring bacteria that cause meningitis, but it is not the best response.

2. Many of the vaccinations administered to children immunize children against bacteria that cause meningitis.
3. Teaching children to wash their hands after toileting and before eating helps to prevent many types of illnesses, most notably gastrointestinal illnesses.
4. Teaching children to cover their faces with a tissue when they sneeze helps to prevent the transmission of upper respiratory illnesses to other children.
TEST-TAKING TIP: Immunizations against *H. influenzae, N. meningitides,* and *S. pneumoniae* have prevented many children from developing meningitis.
Content Area: *Child Health*
Integrated Processes: *Nursing Process: Implementation; Teaching/Learning*
Client Need: *Health Promotion and Maintenance: Health Promotion/Disease Prevention*
Cognitive Level: *Analysis*

18. ANSWER: 4
Rationale:
1. It is unnecessary to be in isolation for viral meningitis.
2. It is rare for children with viral meningitis to seize.
3. The child will be able to walk to the bathroom. A commode will not be needed.
4. Children with meningitis often have headaches. Over-the-counter analgesics are administered for the pain.
TEST-TAKING TIP: Viral meningitis is much more benign than is the bacterial disease. Palliative care is provided to the child until the meningeal inflammation diminishes.
Content Area: *Pediatrics—Neuromuscular*
Integrated Processes: *Nursing Process: Implementation; Teaching/Learning*
Client Need: *Physiological Integrity: Physiological Adaptation: Illness Management*
Cognitive Level: *Application*

19. Answer: 1
Rationale:
1. The nurse should report that the child states that he fell at school three times last week.
2. The child should no longer suffer from headaches.
3. The nurse need not report that the child did well on a recent history test.
4. The nurse need not report that the child is joining the school's swim team.
TEST-TAKING TIP: The child has communicated that he has fallen, which likely is related to poor coordination. Even after a brain tumor has been removed, a number of children will experience long-term complications.
Content Area: *Pediatrics—Neuromuscular*
Integrated Processes: *Nursing Process: Implementation*
Client Need: *Physiological Integrity: Physiological Adaptation: Alterations in Body Systems*
Cognitive Level: *Application*

20. Answer: 4
Rationale:
1. Neuroblastoma develops from embryonic tissue. Because they are older, the parents' other children are unlikely to be at high risk for the disease.
2. All cancers are caused by mutated cells. The genetic code of the neuroblastoma, therefore, is different from the infant's other cells.
3. There is no law mandating the doctor to report the information to the health department.
4. This statement is true. The prognosis for children with neuroblastoma is dependent upon the child's age and the exact genetic mutation of the cancer.
TEST-TAKING TIP: Although the exact cause of the mutation is unknown, neuroblastoma is a cancer of the peripheral nervous system that originates from embryonic tissue. A small number of neuroblastomas are hereditary and some neuroblastomas are environmental in origin.
Content Area: *Pediatrics—Neuromuscular*
Integrated Processes: *Nursing Process: Implementation*
Client Need: *Physiological Integrity: Physiological Adaptation: Alterations in Body Systems*
Cognitive Level: *Application*

Chapter 23

Nursing Care of the Child With Psychosocial Disorders

KEY TERMS

Refeeding syndrome—A severe drop in serum phosphate, potassium, and magnesium levels as well as sodium and fluid retention when nutrition resumes after a period of starvation.

Russell's sign—Abrasions on the fingers and knuckles from induced vomiting in people with bulimia.

I. Description

As is true of all psychosocial problems, the major psychosocial problems seen in the pediatric population result from a combination of psychological and social factors. This chapter provides the nurse with foundational information on each of the illnesses, but if the nurse needs an in-depth analysis of the illnesses and/or the treatment plans for the disorders, he or she should consult the psychiatric literature.

II. Attention Deficit Hyperactivity Disorder

A. Incidence.
  1. Five to 10% of all children are diagnosed with attention deficit hyperactivity disorder (ADHD), with approximately twice as many boys diagnosed as girls.

B. Etiology.
  1. There is evidence of genetic, physiological, and environmental etiologies.
     a. Genetic etiology: there is a high incidence of ADHD among first-degree relatives.
     b. Environmental etiology: ADHD is seen in children diagnosed with lead toxicity.
     c. Physiological etiology: some children with ADHD are diagnosed with neurological abnormalities.

C. Pathophysiology.
  1. Weak signals in the prefrontal cortex of the brain.
  2. The prefrontal cortex is associated with the neurological regulation of behavior.

D. Diagnosis.
  1. Based on the clinical picture as defined by the American Psychiatric Association (APA) (2013) in the DSM-5:
     a. The young child must exhibit at least six of the following behaviors; the older child or teen must exhibit at least five. The child may exhibit only signs of inattention or hyperactivity or a combination of the two.
        i. Inattention: defined as, for example, poor listening, difficulty in following directions, distractibility, and carelessness.
        ii. Hyperactivity and impulsivity: defined as, for example, constantly talking when others are speaking, frequently interrupting,

moving when the child should be sitting still, and the inability to engage in individualized work.

b. The child's behaviors must:
   i. Have been evident by at least age 12.
   ii. Be evident in more than one social setting (e.g., school and church, school and work).
   iii. Not be explained by any other psychiatric diagnosis. (An exception to this statement is made in the case of autism spectrum disorder because the two problems are often seen in the same child. See Chapter 24, "Nursing Care of the Child With Intellectual Developmental Disabilities.")
   iv. Be negatively affecting the child's development (e.g., the child is not able to learn up to his or her potential).

E. Treatment.

1. Therapy or counseling, which may include behavioral modification, family therapy, and/or psychotherapy.
2. Medication, most notably stimulants, such as:
   a. Ritalin (methylphenidate), Adderall (dextroamphetamine/amphetamine), and Dexedrine (dextroamphetamine).
      i. Side effects related to these medications include drug dependence; arrhythmias; hypertension; and, when taken over long periods of time, growth suppression.

F. Nursing considerations.

1. Impaired Social Interaction/Risk for Injury/Impaired Coping/Deficient Knowledge.
   a. Assist with determining the diagnosis, employing the criteria published in the DSM-5.
   b. Enable family members to express their anger, frustration, and other feelings regarding the child's behavior and/or the child's diagnosis.
   c. Educate the family members regarding the diagnosis.
   d. Educate the family members on ways to positively reinforce appropriate behavior.
   e. Assist with implementing the prescribed therapy when the child is in the health-care environment and during school time.
   f. Educate the parents regarding the prescribed dosage, route, action, and side effects of medications. Important considerations include:
      i. Stimulants should not be administered to children with cardiac anomalies or other cardiac diseases.
         (1) Hypertension and cardiac arrhythmias are serious side effects.
      ii. Stimulants can adversely affect sleep; therefore, they should be administered early in the day.
      iii. Other medications should never be administered in conjunction with the stimulants unless approved by the primary health-care provider.
      iv. Medications are highly addictive and may be abused.
      v. Ritalin can delay physical growth, so the child's height should be carefully monitored on growth charts.
   g. Although there is little evidence of therapeutic value, discuss controversial alternative therapies with parents, including dietary changes (i.e., removing refined sugars and additives from the diet), hypnosis, exercise, vitamin supplementation, and metronome therapy.

III. Eating Disorders

A. Anorexia nervosa.

1. Incidence.
   a. Predominately in white, adolescent females from middle and upper socioeconomic strata, although seen in all groups of children.
   b. About 1 to 2 in 10 anorexics will succumb to the disease or to suicide.
   c. Only about 15% of anorexics fully recover.
2. Etiology.
   a. There is no known cause of anorexia, although the majority of patients have a pre-existing emotional illness (e.g., depression).
   b. The refusal to eat often begins with a perceived traumatic event (e.g., someone intimated that the young woman was overweight; a developmental change, like menarche; or a reprimand).
   c. Some attribute the disorder to an identity crisis for the child.
      i. Difficulty in making the transition from a child to a sexually mature young man or woman.
3. Pathophysiology.
   a. Refusal to eat related to a distorted view of one's weight and appearance.
      i. Self-imposed starvation: in essence, the patient is committing a slow suicide.
4. Diagnosis.
   a. As defined by the APA (2013) in the DSM-5:
      i. Weight is 15% or more below the minimum weight for the child's height.
      ii. Intense fear of gaining weight, even though the child is distinctly underweight.
      iii. Disturbed body image.

b. Signs and symptoms.
   i. Classic characteristics of the anorexic child.
      (1) The "good kid."
      (2) Perfectionist (e.g., high academic and/or athletic achiever).
   ii. Common behaviors exhibited by the child:
      (1) Eats alone but is preoccupied with food, including performing rituals around making and eating food.
      (2) Maintains an excessive exercise schedule.
      (3) Labels himself or herself as fat.
   iii. Physiological signs, in addition to those above.
      (1) Renal compromise.
         (a) High risk for urinary tract infections.
         (b) Protein and ketones in the urine that are related to protein and fat catabolism.
      (2) Vital sign instability.
         (a) Hypotension.
         (b) Dysrhythmias, leading to bradycardia.
         (c) Hypothermia.
      (3) Other.
         (a) Anemia.
         (b) Hair and bone loss.
         (c) Amenorrhea in women.
   iv. Psychological characteristics.
      (1) Disturbed body image.
         (a) Child perceives himself or herself as normal and believes that everyone is trying to make him or her fat.
      (2) Confused perception of inner stimuli.
         (a) Ignores hunger pangs.
         (b) Engages in excessive exercise even when exhausted.
      (3) Feelings of depression, self-doubt, and negative self-worth.

5. Treatment: see the following "Binge eating disorder" section.
6. Nursing considerations: see the following "Binge eating disorder" section.

B. Bulimia nervosa: often called the invisible eating disorder.

1. Incidence.
   a. Slightly more common than anorexia with 3% to 5% of teens diagnosed with the disorder.
   b. More common in females than in males.
2. Etiology.
   a. Similar etiology to anorexia (see earlier).
3. Pathophysiology.
   a. Characterized by binge eating—often of many thousands of calories—followed by alternating behaviors of purging and nonpurging.
      i. Purging: induced vomiting and/or taking large doses of laxatives.
      ii. Nonpurging: starving and/or excessive exercising.
4. Diagnosis.
   a. As defined by the APA (2013) in the DSM-5:
      i. Episodes of out-of-control binge eating accompanied by purging and nonpurging.
      ii. Engaging in the episodes at least once per week for at least the preceding 3 months.
      iii. Eating episodes are usually associated with a negative self-image.
   b. Signs and symptoms.
      i. Obsessed with food.
      ii. Often eat alone and in secret, hoarding food for future eating.
      iii. Physiological signs and symptoms.
         (1) Weight usually remains fairly stable.
         (2) Signs of purging.
            (a) Eroded enamel of the teeth from the repeated exposure to stomach acids.
            (b) Scars/abrasions on the fingers/knuckles, called **Russell's sign**, caused by induced vomiting.
            (c) Parotitis and/or an inflamed throat from the repeated exposure to stomach acids.
         (3) Severe complications that can result in death include:
            (a) Hypokalemia that can lead to arrhythmias and death.
            (b) Severe dehydration.
            (c) Esophagitis/esophageal erosion that can result in perforation and hemorrhage.
      iv. Psychological characteristics.
         (1) Feelings of depression, self-doubt, and negative self-worth.
5. Treatment: see the following "Treatment" section.
6. Nursing considerations: see the following "Nursing considerations" section.

C. Binge eating disorder: binge eating is similar to bulimia nervosa (see above), but the patient rarely engages in purging or nonpurging behaviors. The child's weight, therefore, increases accordingly.

1. Treatment.
   a. Children and adolescents with eating disorders are treated in accordance with the severity of their symptoms.

i. Those whose physiological condition is serious are treated in a hospital with constant cardiac monitoring, frequent laboratory assessments, and carefully titrated nutritional therapy.

ii. Those whose physiological condition is relatively stable are treated, as indicated, in either an inpatient psychiatric facility or on an outpatient basis.

b. Nutritional therapy.

i. Carefully monitored to prevent serious complications, e.g., **refeeding syndrome**, which can be fatal, characterized by a severe drop in serum phosphate, potassium, and magnesium levels as well as sodium and fluid retention.

ii. A dietitian works one-on-one with the patient and family once the child is reliably consuming oral foods.

c. Psychiatric therapy.

i. The type and frequency of therapy is dependent on the severity and the exact manifestations of the illness, but both individual and family therapies are usually employed.

ii. Through therapy, the patient is helped to develop a more realistic and positive body image.

d. Medications.

i. Selective serotonin reuptake inhibitor (SSRI) antidepressants and antianxiety medications are frequently used in conjunction with nutritional and psychiatric therapies.

(1) Because of an increase in suicidal ideations and suicide attempts by some children and adolescents, SSRI medications must be administered to that population very carefully.

2. Nursing considerations.

a. Imbalanced Nutrition: Less than Body Requirements/Deficient fluid Volume/Risk for Injury.

i. Closely monitor vital functions and the implementation of emergency medical intervention, when required.

ii. Assess, monitor, and replace, if needed, electrolytes, minerals, calories, and fluids.

(1) IV fluids, nasogastric feeding tubes, total parenteral nutrition, and other such means may be used to replace needed nutrients.

iii. Closely monitor serum electrolytes and complete blood counts (CBCs) for signs of refeeding syndrome and anemia.

iv. Administer safe dosages of prescribed medications employing the five rights of medication administration.

b. Ineffective Coping/Anxiety/Fear/Powerlessness.

i. Allow the child to express anger and other emotions regarding the forced feedings as well as the eventual need to consume maintenance meals.

ii. Monitor the child for signs of hoarding of food, purging, and other such dangerous behaviors.

iii. Assist with therapy to redirect the child's emotions toward healthier actions.

iv. If SSRI medications are prescribed, monitor the child carefully for signs of severe depression and/or suicidal behaviors.

c. Altered Family Processes.

i. Assist family members to express their feelings regarding the child's actions.

ii. Educate family members regarding the signs and symptoms of eating disorders.

iii. Assist with family therapy to redirect communication within the family toward healthier alternatives.

IV. Substance Abuse

Substance abuse in the pediatric setting refers to the use and misuse of a large number of substances, from legal substances (i.e., alcohol and cigarettes) to prescribed substances (e.g., oxycodone and hydrocodone) to illicit drugs (e.g., marijuana, heroin, and cocaine). This section does not include the specifics of the vast majority of these substances. For an in-depth discussion of the substances most commonly abused in the United States, see the National Institutes of Health's Web page, "National Institute on Drug Use" (www.drugabuse.gov/drugs-abuse).

A. Incidence.

1. Based on 2012 data obtained by the Substance Abuse and Mental Health Services Administration Center for Behavioral Health Statistics and Quality (2013):

a. "The rate of current alcohol use among youths aged 12 to 17 was 12.9 percent in 2012. Youth binge and heavy drinking rates in 2012 were 7.2 and 1.3 percent, respectively" (p. 3).

i. Binge drinking is defined as consuming greater than or equal to five drinks in one day.

ii. Heavy drinking is defined as binge drinking greater than or equal to five times during one month.

b. "In 2012, 7.2 percent of youths aged 12 to 17 were current users of marijuana, 2.8 percent were current nonmedical users of psychotherapeutic drugs, 0.8 percent were current users of inhalants, 0.6 percent were current users of hallucinogens, and 0.1 percent were current users of cocaine" (p. 19).

B. Etiology: many of those who abuse substances:
1. Are genetically predisposed.
2. Have been abused, sexually and/or physically.
3. Suffer from mental illnesses, especially depression.

C. Pathophysiology: dependent on the exact drug.
1. Drugs alter the chemical processes within the brain, especially dopamine, leading to a feeling of well-being (i.e., the "high").
2. Signs and symptoms of alcohol toxicity, included in the chapter as an exemplar.
   a. Disorientation.
   b. Nausea and vomiting.
   c. Seizures.
   d. Loss of consciousness.
   e. Slow and/or irregular respirations, eventually resulting in apnea.
3. Examples of behaviors exhibited by children and adolescents who are abusing substances. The child/teen:
   a. Does poorly in school.
   b. Is frequently late or absent from school.
   c. Often is discovered sleeping in class or in meetings.
   d. Takes on an untidy appearance and/or fails to maintain his or her personal hygiene.
   e. Wears dark glasses at all times, day and night.
   f. Exhibits increased disciplinary and/or behavioral problems.
   g. Changes his or her peer group and/or refuses to introduce new friends to the family.
   h. Steals money and other items of value.
   i. Becomes disinterested in previously important things, such as hobbies and sports.
   j. Locks his or her bedroom door and refuses to allow parents into the room.

D. Diagnosis.
1. Positive urine and/or blood test for the specific substance.

E. Treatment.
1. If overdose:
   a. Immediate, emergency management is required (see Chapter 10, "Pediatric Emergencies").
2. If dependency:
   a. In-depth therapy in a treatment center specifically aimed at substance abuse.
   b. Participation in a self-help organization (e.g., Alcoholics Anonymous).
   c. Relapse rate is fairly high.

F. Nursing considerations.
1. Risk for Injury.
   a. Monitor for signs of impending cardiopulmonary collapse.
      i. Begin CPR and call for emergency assistance, if needed.
   b. Assess for physical signs of abuse and intervene, as needed.
2. Ineffective Coping/Impaired Social Interaction/Low Self-Esteem.
   a. School nurse and other school personnel observe for behavioral signs of substance abuse (see above).
   b. Assist with the therapeutic treatment plan.
3. Risk for Altered Family Coping.
   a. Enable family members to express their feelings, including anger, regarding the child's behavior.
   b. Educate the parents regarding the behavioral signs of substance abuse.
   c. Educate the parents regarding the five A's of parenting (see Chapter 6, "Normal Growth and Development: Adolescence").

V. Suicide

A. Incidence.
1. According to the CDC (2014), suicide accounts for over 4,500 deaths each year for youths between 10 and 24 years of age and, statistically, ranks third on the list of causes of death in that population.
2. Many more young people attempt suicide and/or contemplate committing suicide than who actually die.

B. Etiology: there are no absolute causes of suicide, but there are many factors that place children at risk for suicide.
1. Depression or other pre-existing mental illnesses.
2. Substance abuse or other self-injurious behavior.
3. History of physical or sexual abuse.
4. Recent suicide of a loved one or friend.
5. Accessibility to a firearm.
6. Homosexuality.
7. Death of a parent when the child was young.
8. Very low self-concept, especially if he or she feels extremely guilty about something he or she has done.

C. Pathophysiology.
1. Warning signs that a child or teen may be considering suicide.
   a. Previous suicide attempts.
   b. Preoccupied with themes of death.

c. Talks about dying and the desire to die.
d. Gives away precious items (e.g., favorite hat, baseball cards).
e. Exhibits a sudden change in behavior in school and/or home or engages in illegal activity.
f. Runs away from home.
g. Exhibits a dramatic change in his or her appetite or sleep pattern.

2. Success rate.
a. Boys tend to be more successful at committing suicide because they tend to use instantaneously lethal means (e.g., self-inflicted gunshot, hanging, jumping in front of a train).
b. Girls tend to use means that kill over time (e.g., pills, slitting the wrists).

Even though girls are less successful than are boys, they are no less intent on committing suicide.

D. Treatment.
1. Prevention.
a. Educate parents and youths regarding risk factors and warning signs.
b. Council parents and youths to report anyone who exhibits any of the warning signs.
c. Assist children and teens to develop healthy problem-solving and coping skills.
d. Council youths to seek assistance when they are in need, such as:
i. Seeking help from a trusted adult.
ii. Telephoning a suicide prevention hotline.
e. Educate parents to lock away firearms, ammunition, prescription medications, and other such dangerous items.
f. Intervene immediately, using the SLAP acronym, when a youth manifests a believable threat of suicide (Box 23.1).
2. When an attempt has been made and the youth survives:
a. Immediately begin to perform CPR.
b. Once stabilized, mental health counseling in an inpatient facility under 24-hr observation.
3. When an attempt has been made and the youth dies:
a. Provide the survivors, especially classmates, close friends, and family of the victim, with grief and crisis counseling.

E. Nursing considerations.
1. Risk for or Actual Self-Directed Violence/Low Self-Esteem/Ineffective Coping.
a. School nurse and others monitor vigilantly to identify high-risk individuals.
b. Educate the parents to remove all potentially harmful objects from the child's environment, especially weapons.

Box 23.1 SLAP for Suicide Intervention

S—Specificity

- *Ask the question, "Are you having thoughts of suicide?" Individuals do not commit suicide because they were asked, but someone may be saved if he or she is asked.*
  - *If the answer to the question is "yes," the young man or woman should be asked, "Have you thought of how you plan to do it?"*
  - *If the answer to that question is "yes," the threat is very serious, and the individual should not be allowed to be alone.*

L—Lethality

- *Determine whether the plan is life threatening (e.g., hanging, self-inflicted gunshot, ingestion of lethal medications).*

A—Accessibility

- *Determine whether the plan is realistic (i.e., does the young man or woman have access to the method?).*

P—Proximity

- *Determine when the individual plans to execute the plan.*
  - *The answers to the questions are "yes," the information must be communicated to the child's parents and, if appropriate, to the child's primary health-care provider or other person of authority.*
  - *It is important to remember that confidentiality is waived when a life is in danger.*

c. Immediately report any child who expresses an interest in suicide to the child's parents and/or other responsible adults.
i. This is a time when confidentiality is **NOT** observed.
d. Refer the at-risk child or adolescent for professional intervention.
i. The individual should never be left alone.
2. Risk for Altered Family Processes/Grieving.
a. Refer the family for family therapy, especially if an attempt or a successful suicide has occurred.
b. Provide opportunity for all family members to express their grief.
i. Special attention should be paid to preschool children, who often believe that they were responsible for the victim's actions.

VI. Child Abuse and Neglect

One of the most important responsibilities of a nurse—working in any health-care setting—is to be observant for signs of child abuse and neglect. Children possess an inherent trust that their parents, legal guardians, teachers, and/or other responsible adults will care for them. Indeed, children's caregivers have an ethical and legal obligation to provide care that fosters health and well-being. When an adult ignores a child's basic needs, abuses a child emotionally, or, more seriously, physically or sexually injures a child, that adult must be identified and, when appropriate, punished. When interacting with children, nurses are legally obligated to identify characteristics of child abuse and neglect.

A. Incidence.
1. In 2011, 9.1 out of every 1,000 children were reported as victims of child abuse or neglect (U.S. Department of Health and Human Services, 2012).
   a. Each child was counted only once, even if he or she had been reported as maltreated more than once.
   b. Three times as many of the victims were neglected than were abused.
   c. Children under 3 years of age were maltreated more often than were older children.

B. Etiology.
1. A number of factors contribute to the eventual abuse or neglect of a child, but, in the vast majority of cases, the nurse will identify a family in which one or more of the members are dysfunctional. Examples of individual dysfunction that can lead to family dysfunction and child maltreatment include:
   a. Alcohol, drug, and/or partner abuse by one or both of the parents.
   b. The family is facing economic challenges, especially if the parents are unexpectedly unemployed.
   c. One or both of the parents are stressed at work.
   d. One or both of the parents misunderstand the behaviors and/or needs of a child with intellectual and developmental disabilities.
   e. When the parents, for example adolescent parents, misunderstand or are unfamiliar with the normal growth and development of children.
   f. One or both of the parents were maltreated or sexually assaulted as a child.

C. Pathophysiology.
1. Any child who is 18 years old or younger is a potential victim of child abuse and/or neglect.
2. Depending on the state and location, any adult who is cognitively and/or developmentally disabled is also a potential victim of child abuse and/or neglect.
3. The pathophysiology can be either physical, emotional, or sexual in nature.
4. The nurse must observe for and report signs of maltreatment.
   a. If the nurse has a strong suspicion of abuse, he or she should report it to the primary health-care provider as well as the appropriate child welfare agency.
   b. The nurse is not required to provide absolute proof that the child is being abused or neglected.

DID YOU KNOW?

The nurse should be especially suspicious of maltreatment when the parents' explanation for the child's behavior or injury is inconsistent with the evidence. For example, if a parent states that a 5-month-old infant broke his or her leg when the infant fell while crawling up the stairs, the nurse must conclude that the child was abused. Five-month-old infants are developmentally unable to crawl.

5. Signs and symptoms of child neglect.
   a. Examples of physical indicators of neglect. The child exhibits:
      i. Inadequate weight gain for age.
      ii. Poor growth patterns and failure to thrive.
      iii. Constant hunger.
      iv. Poor hygiene.
      v. Untreated illness.
      vi. Inappropriate attire for the weather.
      vii. Adult behavior (e.g., making all meals for the family, maintaining the home environment).
   b. Examples of behavioral indicators of neglect exhibited by the child.
      i. Begs or steals food.
      ii. Attends school inconsistently.
      iii. Arrives very early and/or stays very late at school.
      iv. Is constantly fatigued or listless in class.
   c. Examples of behavioral indicators of neglect exhibited by one or more parents.
      i. Are unresponsive when the child's appearance is discussed.
      ii. Fail to take the child to the physician or dentist for needed care.
      iii. Fail to give the child needed medication.
      iv. Fail to provide a safe place for the child to reside.
      v. Fail to require the child to attend school.
      vi. Leave the young child or children unattended.
6. Signs and symptoms of child emotional abuse.
   a. Examples of behavioral indicators of emotional abuse exhibited by the child.
      i. Emotional extremes (i.e., overly aggressive or overly passive).
      ii. Repetitive behaviors (e.g., hand banging, biting).
      iii. No apparent affection for the parent.
      iv. Suicidal ideations.

MAKING THE CONNECTION

Self-destructive behaviors, most commonly seen in preteens and teens, are often exhibited in response to being a victim of physical or sexual abuse. Examples of self-destructive behaviors include promiscuity and prostitution, delinquency, running away from home, suicide and attempted suicide, drug abuse, and theft.

It is important for health-care providers to query children who are exhibiting maladaptive behaviors regarding their familial history to determine whether child maltreatment may be the cause of the child's actions.

b. Examples of behavioral indicators of emotional abuse exhibited by the parents.
   i. Are overly critical of the child's behaviors.
   ii. Exhibit no physical or emotional support when the child is injured or in pain.

7. Signs and symptoms of child physical abuse.
   a. Examples of physical indicators of physical abuse.
      i. Bruises and welts in unexpected places (e.g., in nonraised surfaces, on the torso, on the undersurfaces of the arms) or that are present in clusters.
      ii. Fractures, especially spiral fractures, skull fractures, rib fractures, and fractures that are at different stages of healing.
      iii. Subdural/subarachnoid hemorrhages.
      iv. Missing patches of hair.
      v. Injuries that are inconsistent with the age and/or developmental level of the child (e.g., bruises on an infant).
      vi. Injuries that are in a distinct pattern (e.g., in the shape of a shoe print).
      vii. Unexplained burns, especially on the soles, palms, back, and buttocks.
         (1) Small, circular injuries are likely cigarette burns.
      viii. Found to have alcohol and/or drugs in his or her system.
      ix. Exhibiting signs of self-destructive behavior.
   b. Examples of behavioral indicators of physical abuse.
      i. Wary of any adult contact.
      ii. Apprehensive when other children cry.
      iii. Fearful of parents or of going home.
      iv. Extremely aggressive or markedly withdrawn with a vacant or frozen stare.
      v. Insistent on keeping his or her arms and legs covered.
         (1) The child is hiding his or her injuries.
      vi. Responding inappropriately to painful procedures (i.e., acts as if he or she has often experienced pain).
      vii. Is dressed with arms and legs completely covered or shirt buttoned to the top, especially in warm weather.
      viii. Exhibiting self-destructive behaviors.
   c. Examples of behavioral indicators of physical abuse exhibited by parents.
      i. Are evasive when asked about the injury.
      ii. Seek care at a health-care facility a long distance from the child's home.
      iii. Provide an explanation for the injury that is not credible.
      iv. Dominate the conversation when the child is being interviewed.
      v. Leave the child in an unoccupied automobile, especially in the summer months.

8. Signs and symptoms of child sexual abuse.
   a. Examples of physical indicators of sexual abuse exhibited by the child.
      i. Has difficulty walking or sitting.
      ii. Has torn, stained, or bloody underclothing.
      iii. Complains of pain, swelling, or itching of the genitalia.
      iv. Complains of pain on urination.
      v. Has bruising, bleeding, and/or lacerations involving the external genitalia, vagina, or anal area and/or vaginal or penile discharge.
      vi. Tests positive for a sexually transmitted infection.
   b. Examples of behavioral indicators of sexual abuse exhibited by the child.
      i. Unwilling to change clothes or participate in gym activities.
      ii. Unexpectedly withdrawn and/or exhibiting infantile behavior.
      iii. Exhibiting bizarre, sophisticated, and/or unusually sexual behavior or knowledge.
      iv. Abruptly developing an eating disorder.
      v. Performing self-destructive behaviors.
      vi. Masturbating excessively.
      vii. Unwilling to divulge the fact that they were abused and/or feeling ashamed of the abuse.
   c. Examples of behavioral indicators of sexual abuse exhibited by the perpetrators.
      i. Usually well known to the child.
      ii. Blame the child for the abuse (i.e., the child "came onto" the adult).
      iii. Often access and view child pornography.

D. Diagnosis.
1. Suspicion of neglect or maltreatment is based on the clinical picture.
2. Definitive diagnosis is made after an in-depth review of the child and family by child protective services workers as well as members of the health-care system.
3. Diagnostic tests include:
   a. X-rays.
   b. Photographs.
   c. Laboratory tests.
   d. Interviews of the child, responsible adults, and others living or working near the family.

E. Treatment.
1. First, and foremost, the abuse must be reported to the appropriate child protective services agency.
   a. Health-care providers must be familiar with the child abuse/neglect laws that govern their actions in the state and locality where they practice.
   b. If warranted, removal of the child from the offending environment.
2. Physical and/or psychological intervention that is appropriate to the child's injuries should be performed.

F. Nursing considerations.
1. Prevention: Deficient Knowledge/Risk for Impaired Parenting.
   a. Educate parents, especially teen parents, regarding normal growth and development.
      i. Because adolescents frequently have poor coping skills and lack knowledge needed, they are especially high risk for committing child abuse or neglect.
      ii. Deficient knowledge of normal developmental behaviors and milestones is a common cause of child abuse (e.g., incorrect belief that a 1-year-old child should be fully toilet trained).
   b. Educate parents, especially teen parents, regarding safe disciplinary practices.
      i. Physical punishment can be physically and emotionally injurious and often ineffective.
      ii. Verbal abuse can be emotionally injurious and often ineffective.
      iii. Shaking a baby or young toddler can result in a severe total brain injury, i.e., shaken baby syndrome (SBS) (see Chapter 22: "Nursing Care of the Child With Neurological Problems").
   c. Role model appropriate behavior when communicating to and touching the child.
      i. Always ask the child for permission before touching bodily surfaces.
      ii. Always speak to the child with respect.
   d. Educate the child regarding safe and appropriate touch and unsafe and inappropriate touch.
      i. Advise children that they should report immediately if someone touches them inappropriately.
2. Impaired Parenting/Compromised Family Coping/Injury/Deficient Knowledge.
   a. Carefully assess the child's physical condition at each nurse-child interaction.
      i. Any signs/symptoms of sexual behavior in a child under 16 years of age mandates further inquiry.
      ii. Any teenager 16 years old or older who is exhibiting signs/symptoms of sexual behavior should be questioned regarding whether the sexual contact was consensual.
   b. Perform assessments and/or interventions, as needed, for example:
      i. Initiate CPR and other prescribed interventions, when injuries are severe or potentially life-threatening.
      ii. Assist with diagnostic testing, including x-raying areas of injury, photographing injuries, and completing laboratory tests.
   c. Evaluate the explanation of an injury given by the child's caregivers in relation to the injury itself.
      i. If the explanation is inconsistent with the injury, further inquiry must be performed.
   d. Carefully assess the child's behavior with parents and with other adults during each nurse-child interaction.
   e. Assess family support systems and coping mechanisms.
      i. Ask the parents regarding their own family interactions and experiences, including the methods their parents used when they were disciplined.
   f. Query the child about his or her personal interactions with adults.
   g. Young children often communicate more effectively through play or by drawing pictures.
   h. Immediately report any suspicion of child abuse and/or neglect to the appropriate agency.

CASE STUDY: Putting It All Together

8-year-old girl, Caucasian

Subjective Data

- Third-grade school teacher asks the school nurse to assess the child. The teacher states,
  - "At the beginning of the year, she did very well on all of her assignments and was very outgoing and talkative."
  - "For the last week or so, she has been so withdrawn. She sits alone in the corner during recess and refuses to play with her friends."
  - "She hasn't turned in any homework all week."

Nursing Assessments

- The school nurse interviews the child in her office. The girl refuses to say anything except,
  - "I really hate it when Uncle Jack visits."
- The school nurse replies,
  - "Why do you hate it when Uncle Jack visits?"
- The young girl starts to cry and replies,
  - "I can't say. I will get into trouble."
- When the child sits,
  - Child winces and states,
  - "It hurts down there."

Vital Signs	
Temperature:	98.6°F
Heart rate:	94 bpm
Respiratory rate:	24 rpm

Objective Data (examination in school nurse's office)

Nursing Assessments

School Nurse's Actions

- The school nurse calls the child's parents and states,
  - "Your daughter's teacher and I are very worried about your daughter. Is she acting differently at home than she has in the past?"
- The mother states,
  - "She hasn't eaten very well for the past week, and she stays in her room a lot. We have sent her to school, though, because she doesn't really seem sick."
- The school nurse continues,
  - "I am concerned that something happened when her Uncle Jack visited your family."
  - "She is not interacting with the other children and has stopped doing her school work."
  - "She is reluctant to tell me what happened when she was with her Uncle Jack because she is afraid that she will get into trouble, and she was crying when she told me that."
  - "When she sits down she winces and states that she is in pain 'down there.'"
  - "I strongly advise you to have your child seen by her primary health-care provider to see if she has been injured."
- Telephones the hotline of the local office of child protective services, and makes a report of:
  - Suspected sexual abuse.

CASE STUDY: Putting It All Together *cont'd*

Case Study Questions

A. What *subjective* assessments indicate that this client is experiencing a health alteration?

1. __________
2. __________
3. __________
4. __________

B. What *objective* assessments indicate that this client is experiencing a health alteration?

1. __________

C. After analyzing the data that has been collected, what **primary** nursing diagnosis should the nurse assign to this client?

1. __________

D. What interventions should the nurse plan and/or implement to meet this child's and her family's needs?

1. __________
2. __________
3. __________

E. What client outcomes should the nurse evaluate regarding the effectiveness of the nursing interventions?

1. __________
2. __________

F. What physiological characteristics should the child exhibit before leaving the clinic?

1. __________

REVIEW QUESTIONS

1. A second-grade teacher and school nurse notify the parents of a 7-year-old child that the child is having difficulty sitting still in class, concentrating on his work, and is repeatedly interrupting the teacher. The nurse recommends that the parents ask the child's primary health-care provider to perform which of the following assessments?
   1. Denver Developmental Screening Test (DDST)
   2. Blood lead level
   3. Electroencephalogram
   4. Computed tomography (CT) of the skull

2. A child has been diagnosed with attention deficit hyperactivity disorder (ADHD). The nurse is concerned that the child has been misdiagnosed because of which of the following factors? The child is:
   1. ten years old.
   2. at the top of the class in reading and math.
   3. disruptive in church and in school.
   4. able to communicate effectively.

3. A child who has been diagnosed with attention deficit hyperactivity disorder (ADHD) has been prescribed Ritalin (methylphenidate). Which of the following assessments should the nurse monitor closely as long as the child is taking the medication? **Select all that apply.**
   1. Sleep patterns
   2. Bilirubin levels
   3. Blood pressure
   4. Growth patterns
   5. Blood urea nitrogen levels

4. A child has been diagnosed with attention deficit hyperactivity disorder (ADHD). Although highly recommended by the child's primary health-care provider, the parents refuse to administer stimulants to their child. Which of the following alternative therapies might the nurse suggest the parents employ? **Select all that apply.**
   1. Hypnotherapy
   2. Diet modification
   3. Vitamin supplementation
   4. Structured exercise regime
   5. Rigid disciplinary strategies

5. A clinic nurse reports to the primary health-care provider a suspicion that a 14-year-old girl has anorexia nervosa. Which of the following findings led to the nurse's conclusion? The girl:
   1. had her first period when she was 13½ years old and has yet to have another.
   2. is at the 80th percentile for height and the 25th percentile for weight.
   3. is a member of her school swim team as well as the soccer team.
   4. complains that she is taller than all of the boys in her class.

6. The parents of a 15-year-old girl are concerned about her health and well-being. The school nurse confirms that which of the following of the parents' comments is of great concern?
   1. "Our daughter cooks elaborate meals for us, but she never sits down to eat."
   2. "Our daughter has decided to become a vegetarian and only to eat low-fat foods."
   3. "Our daughter wants to go on a diet so that she can fit into a special prom dress."
   4. "Our daughter eats cereal for breakfast, but eats no other grains the rest of the day."

7. A school nurse is monitoring high school students while they consume their lunches. The nurse asks to speak in private with which of the following young women regarding her eating habits? The teenager who has:
   1. 3 new tattoos on her forearm.
   2. pierced eyebrow and a tongue ring.
   3. black eyeliner and all black outfit.
   4. scars on the top of 3 fingers of one hand.

8. An adolescent has been admitted into the pediatric unit with a diagnosis of bulimia nervosa. The nurse carefully monitors the child for which of the following complications?
   1. Cardiac arrhythmias
   2. Hyperproteinemia
   3. Polycythemia
   4. Excessive weight loss

9. A nurse suspects that an adolescent is purging after eating large quantities of food. Which of the following assessments would help to confirm that suspicion? **Select all that apply.**
   1. Teen complains of severe sore throat.
   2. Stools of the teen are black and tarry.
   3. Enamel on the teen's front teeth is eroding.
   4. Teen's serum potassium level is markedly elevated.
   5. Teen runs to the bathroom immediately after consuming a large lunch.

10. A nurse is giving a presentation to parents on behaviors that are characteristic of adolescents who are using alcohol or other substances. Which of the following information should the nurse include in the presentation?
1. Teen asks to have a body part pierced or tattooed.
2. Teen requests to be tutored in a course he or she is failing.
3. Teen stops participating in all extracurricular activities.
4. Teen asks parents to knock before entering his or her bedroom.

11. A nurse is giving a presentation to adolescents regarding actions they should take if they believe that a friend has consumed too much alcohol. Which of the following information should the nurse include in the presentation?
1. Have the friend take a cold shower.
2. Make the friend drink coffee.
3. Call for medical emergency care.
4. Put the friend to bed to sleep it off.

12. A nurse is giving a presentation to parents regarding characteristics that place children and adolescents at risk of attempting suicide. Which of the following characteristics should the nurse include in the presentation? **Select all that apply.**
1. Recent suicide of a friend
2. Ability easily to access a gun
3. Parent who is a gay or lesbian
4. Often talks about death or being dead
5. Parents who work long hours each day

13. During a discussion with the school nurse, a 13-year-old student states, "I hate myself. I just want to die." Which of the following responses should the nurse make?
1. "You don't really mean that."
2. "You are scaring me."
3. "You can't do that. Have you thought about how much that would affect your parents?"
4. "You say that you want to die. Do you have a plan about how you might end your life?"

14. During a discussion with a 13-year-old student, a school nurse believes that the student has a plan to commit suicide. Which of the following responses would be appropriate for the nurse to perform?
1. Try to talk the student out of the plan.
2. Ask the student if it would be acceptable to break confidentiality in this case.
3. Provide the student with the name of a psychologist.
4. Have someone chaperone the student and call the parents to notify them of the plan.

15. Four 8-year-old boys are seen in the pediatric clinic during one week. All of the parents accompanying the children state that their children were injured when they fell from a playground apparatus. The nurse reports a suspicion of child abuse to the primary health-care provider regarding the child who exhibited which of the following signs/symptoms?
1. Greenstick fracture of the right arm
2. Abrasions on both knees
3. Laceration of the right cheek
4. Bald area above the right ear

16. A school nurse is making rounds in the kindergarten classrooms of an elementary school. The nurse, who interviews 5 of the boys, suspects that which of the boys is a victim of child neglect? The child who: **Select all that apply.**
1. is wearing shorts and a tee shirt on a cold winter day.
2. steals some breakfast cereal from a closet in the nurse's office.
3. states that his mother is going to buy fast-food hamburgers for supper.
4. is upset because his parents will not let him learn how to play hockey.
5. states that his parents are waiting for the two teeth with cavities to fall out.

17. A nurse, working in a pediatric clinic, has assisted with the care of 4 toddlers, all of whom were accompanied by their parents. In which of the cases should the nurse examine the child carefully for signs of maltreatment?

1. The child cries when the parent attempts to pick the child up to go home after the examination is over.
2. The parent holds the child firmly when the child is receiving an injection.
3. The child kicks and screams when the healthcare provider enters the room.
4. The parent demands that the child be seen by a specialist for an illness that is unresolved after two weeks.

18. A nurse, working in an emergency department, suspects that a 16-year-old is a victim of physical abuse. The parents state, "Our girl is hurt. She needs to be fixed up." Which of the following findings are consistent with the nurse's conclusions? **Select all that apply.**

1. Teen states that she had a bad snowboarding accident.
2. Parents report that the girl has run away twice this year.
3. Teen has sustained open fractures of the right ulna and radius.
4. Family lives fifty miles away from the emergency department.
5. Parents interrupt the girl whenever she tries to give answers to the nurse's questions.

REVIEW ANSWERS

1. **ANSWER: 2**
   Rationale:
   1. It would be inappropriate to ask to have the Denver Developmental Screening Test (DDST) performed. It is only valid for children through the age of 6.
   2. A blood lead level should be drawn because children with lead poisoning often exhibit symptoms similar to those of attention deficit hyperactivity disorder (ADHD).
   3. The symptoms do not justify having an electroencephalogram performed.
   4. The symptoms do not justify having a CT of the skull performed.
   TEST-TAKING TIP: The symptoms exhibited by the child in the scenario are consistent with a diagnosis of ADHD. Before making that diagnosis, however, all other possible explanations for the symptoms should be explored. One possible explanation for the symptoms is lead toxicity.
   Content Area: *Pediatrics—ADHD*
   Integrated Processes: *Nursing Process: Implementation*
   Client Need: *Psychosocial Integrity: Mental Health Concepts*
   Cognitive Level: *Application*

2. **ANSWER: 2**
   Rationale:
   1. ADHD can be diagnosed in any child whose symptoms appeared earlier than 12 years of age.
   2. The symptoms of ADHD adversely affect learning. This child is at the top of the class in reading and math.
   3. Those with ADHD should exhibit symptoms in more than one setting. Being disruptive both in church and in school is consistent with the diagnosis.
   4. Children with ADHD are able to communicate effectively.
   TEST-TAKING TIP: ADHD is a serious diagnosis. Children with this diagnosis often are placed on strong, stimulant medications. The diagnosis should only be made when the child's symptoms are consistent with those cited in the DSM-5.
   Content Area: *Pediatrics—ADHD*
   Integrated Processes: *Nursing Process: Analysis*
   Client Need: *Psychosocial Integrity: Mental Health Concepts*
   Cognitive Level: *Application*

3. **ANSWER: 1, 3, and 4**
   Rationale:
   1. Children on Ritalin often exhibit altered sleep patterns.
   2. A change in bilirubin levels is not associated with receiving Ritalin.
   3. Children on Ritalin may exhibit changes in their blood pressure, most notably hypertension.
   4. Children on Ritalin may exhibit delayed growth patterns.
   5. A change in blood urea nitrogen levels is not associated with receiving Ritalin.
   TEST-TAKING TIP: Ritalin, a stimulant medication, is administered to children with ADHD. There are many side effects related to the administration of the medication. In addition to those cited above, Ritalin has been shown to be highly addictive and to cause serious cardiac arrhythmias in those with cardiac disease.
   Content Area: *Pediatrics—ADHD*
   Integrated Processes: *Nursing Process: Assessment*
   Client Need: *Physiological Integrity: Pharmacological and Parenteral Therapies: Adverse Effects/Contraindications/Side Effects/Interactions*
   Cognitive Level: *Application*

4. **ANSWER: 1, 2, 3, and 4**
   Rationale:
   1. Hypnotherapy has been employed as a therapy for children with ADHD.
   2. Diet modification has been employed as a therapy for children with ADHD.
   3. Vitamin supplementation has been employed as a therapy for children with ADHD.
   4. Structured exercise regime has been employed as a therapy for children with ADHD.
   5. A more relaxed style of discipline, rather than more rigid disciplinary strategies, is recommended when caring for children with ADHD.
   TEST-TAKING TIP: Some parents are unwilling to administer medications to a child with ADHD. Although no formal research has shown that alternative practices are effective interventions for the children, it is appropriate to provide parents with information, both positive and negative, that is available on alternative therapies.
   Content Area: *Pediatrics—ADHD*
   Integrated Processes: *Nursing Process: Assessment*
   Client Need: *Psychosocial Integrity: Mental Health Concepts*
   Cognitive Level: *Application*

5. **ANSWER: 2**
   Rationale:
   1. This situation is not abnormal. Young women often have very irregular menstrual cycles.
   2. These data are consistent with a diagnosis of anorexia nervosa. There is a marked disparity—more than a 15-percentile difference—between the young woman's height and her weight.
   3. Many young women participate in more than one sport.
   4. Boys usually experience their growth spurts later than girls and, therefore, are shorter than girls at 14 years of age.
   TEST-TAKING TIP: Although in the DSM-IV, a 3-month period of amenorrhea was a diagnostic criterion for anorexia nervosa, this has been deleted from the diagnostic criteria for the disease in the DSM-5.
   Content Area: *Mental Health—Eating Disorders*
   Integrated Processes: *Nursing Process: Analysis*
   Client Need: *Psychosocial Integrity: Mental Health Concepts*
   Cognitive Level: *Application*

6. ANSWER: 1

Rationale:

1. **This statement is of concern. Adolescents with eating disorders are often obsessed with the topic of food, but they eat alone.**
2. Being a vegetarian and eating low-fat foods are unharmful eating practices, but the teen should be referred to a registered dietitian for diet counseling.
3. In general, this statement is not of great concern. The nurse should, however, refer the young woman to a registered dietitian for assistance with the diet.
4. Although the nurse should recommend to the young woman that she increase her fiber intake, this statement is not of great concern.

TEST-TAKING TIP: Adolescents are often very concerned with their appearance. They will, therefore, experiment with ways to improve their body, including dieting. The nurse must be able to conclude which behaviors are within normal limits and which are of great concern. Teens who refuse to eat with their families may be engaging in a number of unhealthy activities, including binge eating and self-imposed starvation.

Content Area: *Mental Health—Eating Disorders*
Integrated Processes: *Nursing Process: Analysis*
Client Need: *Psychosocial Integrity: Mental Health Concepts*
Cognitive Level: *Application*

7. ANSWER: 4

Rationale:

1. Many adolescents have tattoos on their forearms.
2. Many adolescents have a pierced eyebrow and tongue ring.
3. Many adolescents wear black eyeliner and all black outfits.
4. **A teen who has scars on the top of three fingers of one hand may be purging.**

TEST-TAKING TIP: Russell's sign, or scarring on the top of the fingers, is very characteristic of bulimia nervosa. The child or teen eats large quantities of food and then forces his or herself to vomit by inserting the fingers into the back of the throat.

Content Area: *Mental Health—Eating Disorders*
Integrated Processes: *Nursing Process: Implementation*
Client Need: *Psychosocial Integrity: Mental Health Concepts*
Cognitive Level: *Application*

8. ANSWER: 1

Rationale:

1. **The nurse should monitor the teen for cardiac arrhythmias.**
2. The nurse should monitor the teen for hypoproteinemia.
3. The nurse should monitor the teen for anemia.
4. Those with bulimia usually are of normal weight.

TEST-TAKING TIP: Because of the excessive use of laxatives and repeated vomiting, those with bulimia are often hypokalemic. They are, therefore, at high risk for cardiac arrhythmias. The nurse should monitor all of the child's electrolytes because they all may be markedly altered.

Content Area: *Mental Health—Eating Disorders*
Integrated Processes: *Nursing Process: Implementation*
Client Need: *Psychosocial Integrity: Mental Health Concepts*
Cognitive Level: *Application*

9. ANSWER: 1, 2, 3, and 5

Rationale:

1. **Those with bulimia often do complain of a severe sore throat.**
2. **Because of bleeding of esophageal varices, the stools of bulimics may be black and tarry.**
3. **Those with bulimia often do exhibit enamel erosion of their teeth.**
4. The serum potassium level of those with bulimia is usually low.
5. **Those with bulimia often do run to the bathroom immediately after consuming a large lunch.**

TEST-TAKING TIP: The repeated vomiting performed by those with bulimia can lead to very serious complications, including markedly altered electrolytes, esophagitis, esophageal varices, parotitis, and pharyngitis.

Content Area: *Mental Health—Eating Disorders*
Integrated Processes: *Nursing Process: Assessment*
Client Need: *Psychosocial Integrity: Mental Health Concepts*
Cognitive Level: *Application*

10. ANSWER: 3

Rationale:

1. Although there are complications related to piercing and tattooing, they are not directly associated with using alcohol or other substances.
2. A teen who requests to be tutored in a course he or she is failing is concerned about his or her academic performance.
3. **It is of concern when a teen stops participating in all extracurricular activities.**
4. Parents should afford teens some privacy. It is appropriate for parents to knock before entering an adolescent's bedroom.

TEST-TAKING TIP: Although it is appropriate for parents to knock before entering their children's rooms, it is not appropriate for a child or teen to lock his or her door and tell the parents never to enter the room. That behavior is often consistent with a child or teen who is trying to hide inappropriate behavior (e.g., substance abuse).

Content Area: *Substance Abuse*
Integrated Processes: *Nursing Process: Implementation; Teaching/Learning*
Client Need: *Psychosocial Integrity: Mental Health Concepts*
Cognitive Level: *Application*

11. ANSWER: 3

Rationale:

1. It is inappropriate to have the friend take a cold shower.
2. It is inappropriate to make the friend drink coffee.
3. **The friends should call for medical emergency care.**
4. It is inappropriate to put the friend to bed to sleep it off.

TEST-TAKING TIP: Alcohol is a central nervous system depressant. When consumed in large quantities, alcohol can result in coma, respiratory depression, and death. Teens must be strongly encouraged not to consume alcohol until they are 21 years of age, but, if they do, and they are in the company of someone who has consumed excessive quantities of the substance, the teen must be prepared to call for medical assistance.
Content Area: *Substance Abuse*
Integrated Processes: *Nursing Process: Implementation; Teaching/Learning*
Client Need: *Physiological Integrity: Physiological Adaptation: Medical Emergencies*
Cognitive Level: *Application*

12. ANSWER: 1, 2, and 4
Rationale:
1. The recent suicide of a friend does place children and adolescents at risk of attempting suicide.
2. The ability to easily access a gun does place children and adolescents at risk of attempting suicide.
3. A parent who is gay or lesbian does not place a child or teen at risk of attempting suicide.
4. A teen or child who talks about death or being dead is at risk of attempting suicide.
5. A teen or child who lives with parents who work long hours each day is not necessarily at risk of attempting suicide.
TEST-TAKING TIP: There are a number of factors that place children and adolescents at high risk of attempting suicide. Adults who are in close contact with children and/or adolescents should monitor them carefully for behaviors that indicate that they are seriously contemplating suicide.
Content Area: *Mental Health—Suicide*
Integrated Processes: *Nursing Process: Implementation; Teaching/Learning*
Client Need: *Psychosocial Integrity: Mental Health Concepts*
Cognitive Level: *Application*

13. ANSWER: 4
Rationale:
1. This is an inappropriate statement. One must assume that students are contemplating suicide when they say that they want to die.
2. This may be true, but the statement is inappropriate. The nurse should focus on the student, not on him or herself.
3. This is not the best response. The nurse should assess the student's current intentions.
4. The nurse should ask the student whether he or she has a plan.
TEST-TAKING TIP: It can be a daunting task to ask a child or adolescent whether he or she has a plan to commit suicide. The nurse may fear that he or she will actually cause the child/teen to do so. That, however, is not the case. Rather, if the nurse queries the child/teen and learns that he or she has a plan, the nurse can then intervene by making sure that the child/teen is never left alone by notifying the child's/teen's parents of the intention and by referring the family to a mental health practitioner who can intervene.
Content Area: *Mental Health—Suicide*
Integrated Processes: *Nursing Process: Implementation*
Client Need: *Psychosocial Integrity: Mental Health Concepts*
Cognitive Level: *Application*

14. ANSWER: 4
Rationale:
1. It is not appropriate to try to talk the student out of the plan.
2. When a student is in imminent danger of harming him- or herself, confidentiality is no longer maintained.
3. Although a mental health professional should be contacted, it is inappropriate simply to provide the student with the name of a psychologist.
4. This action is appropriate. Someone should be with the student at all times to make sure that the student does not complete the plan, and the parents should be notified of the plan.
TEST-TAKING TIP: When a child/teen communicates that he or she has a plan to commit suicide, he or she is fully intending to execute that plan. It is very important, therefore, that the child/teen never be left alone.
Content Area: *Mental Health—Suicide*
Integrated Processes: *Nursing Process: Implementation*
Client Need: *Psychosocial Integrity: Mental Health Concepts*
Cognitive Level: *Application*

15. ANSWER: 4
Rationale:
1. Greenstick fractures are commonly seen in the pediatric population. A fracture of the right arm is consistent with the parent's story.
2. It is foreseeable that a child could sustain abrasions on both knees after falling from a playground apparatus.
3. It is foreseeable that a child could sustain a laceration of the right cheek during a fall from a playground apparatus.
4. It is unlikely that a child's hair would be pulled out during a fall from a playground apparatus.
TEST-TAKING TIP: Bald spots are often seen in children who have been abused. Parents, when angry, may grab the child's hair and pull it out from the scalp.
Content Area: *Child Health, Abuse*
Integrated Processes: *Nursing Process: Implementation*
Client Need: *Psychosocial Integrity: Abuse/Neglect*
Cognitive Level: *Application*

16. ANSWER: 1, 2, and 5
Rationale:
1. A child wearing clothing that is inappropriate to the weather is likely a victim of child neglect.
2. A child who has not been served breakfast by his parents is likely a victim of child neglect.
3. Although fast food is not the most nutritious food choice, serving fast food to one's child is not a form of child neglect.

4. Not allowing a child to participate in a sport is not a form of child neglect.
5. Parents who fail to provide a child with needed dental care are neglecting their child's needs.

TEST-TAKING TIP: When a child is being neglected, he or she is not having his or her basic needs met or is being placed in a situation that may be dangerous. The nurse should report children who meet those criteria to the local child protection agency.

Content Area: *Child Health*
Integrated Processes: *Nursing Process: Analysis*
Client Need: *Psychosocial Integrity: Abuse/Neglect*
Cognitive Level: *Application*

17. ANSWER: 1

Rationale:

1. The nurse should investigate further when a child cries when he or she is picked up by his or her parents.
2. A parent who holds the child firmly when the child is receiving an injection is providing therapeutic holding so that the child will not be injured by the procedure.
3. It is normal child behavior for toddlers to cry when a health-care provider enters the room.
4. It is normal behavior for a parent to be concerned about his or her child's health when an illness remains unresolved after a long period of time.

TEST-TAKING TIP: In a healthy parent-child relationship, children view their parents as protectors and, therefore, are comforted when picked up and consoled by the parents. Children who cry when their parents touch them are often communicating that they have been abused by their parents.

Content Area: *Child Health, Abuse*
Integrated Processes: *Nursing Process: Implementation*
Client Need: *Psychosocial Integrity: Abuse/Neglect*
Cognitive Level: *Application*

18. ANSWER: 2, 4, and 5

Rationale:

1. Teens who have been in bad snowboarding accidents may need to be seen for emergency care.
2. Many teens who run away from their homes have been abused.
3. A teen who has sustained open fractures should be seen in the emergency department (ED). The fractures are consistent with a bad snowboarding accident.
4. It is not uncommon for abusing parents to take their child to an ED a long distance from their home. The parents are afraid to return to the same ED on repeated visits because the health-care providers will realize that the child is being abused. As a result, they go to different EDs each time the child needs care.
5. The girl is 16 years old. She is able to respond to questioning herself. Parents who interrupt their children are often trying to prevent their children from communicating the truth about their home environment to the health-care professionals.

TEST-TAKING TIP: Adolescents who run away from home, who steal, and who abuse substances are often ridiculed for their behavior. It is important for health-care professionals to realize, however, that the teens may be exhibiting the inappropriate behaviors because they have been abused.

Content Area: *Child Health, Abuse*
Integrated Processes: *Nursing Process: Analysis*
Client Need: *Psychosocial Integrity: Abuse/Neglect*
Cognitive Level: *Application*

Nursing Care of the Child With Intellectual and Developmental Disabilities

KEY TERMS

Chromosomal mosaicism—A condition in which the cells of the body have different numbers of chromosomes.
Failure to thrive (FTT)—A child who is growing and developing much slower than would be expected.
Fragile X syndrome—A genetic condition linked to the X chromosome, causing physical, cognitive, and behavioral defects, seen most commonly and most severely in males.
Muscular hypotonia—Poor muscle tone throughout the body.
Simian creases—Unbroken "life lines" that stretch across the palm of the hand, associated with Down syndrome.
Trisomy 21—The occurrence of three number 21 chromosomes in the zygote; the most common cause of Down syndrome.

I. Intellectual Disability

Although intellectual disability (ID), formerly called mental retardation, is often thought of as strictly a cognitive disability, the definition of the concept has taken on a broader context in recent years. Rather than referring strictly to a child's thought-based abilities, experts refer also to the child's behavioral abilities. As a result, when a person with limited intelligence is able to function relatively normally, he or she should be seen in a different light from someone who has the same intelligence quotient (IQ) but who has a great deal of trouble functioning in society.

A. Incidence.
   1. The IQ of 1% to 3% of the population in the United States falls below 70, but up to 85% of that group is shown to have only a mild disability.

B. Etiology: there are both genetic and environmental causes of cognitive deficits.
   1. Environmental causes.
      a. Fetal alcohol syndrome is the number one preventable cause of ID in the United States.
      b. Lead exposure: may occur either prenatally and/or as a childhood exposure.
      c. Infectious diseases: may occur either prenatally and/or as a childhood exposure.

d. Poor or abusive parenting (e.g., shaken baby syndrome).
e. Perinatal hypoxia that occurs during pregnancy, labor, and/or delivery.
f. Hypoxia of a child that may occur post-delivery, most commonly in premature infants, or as a result of an accident (e.g., near drowning).

2. Genetic causes.
   a. Fragile X syndrome.
      i. Most common genetic cause of ID.
      ii. X-linked recessive syndrome (Fig. 24.1).
         (1) A Punnett square with an example of the inheritance pattern for fragile X syndrome is shown below. The mother is heterozygous for the disease (i.e., she carries one affected X chromosome ["x"X]), and the father is unaffected (XY).

	"x"	X
X	"x"X	XX
Y	"x"Y	XY

(a) If the offspring is female, there is a 50% probability of carrying an affected X and potential for exhibiting symptoms of the fragile X syndrome and a 50% probability of having a normal genotype.
(b) If the offspring is male, there is a 50% probability of having fragile X syndrome and a 50% probability of having a normal genotype.

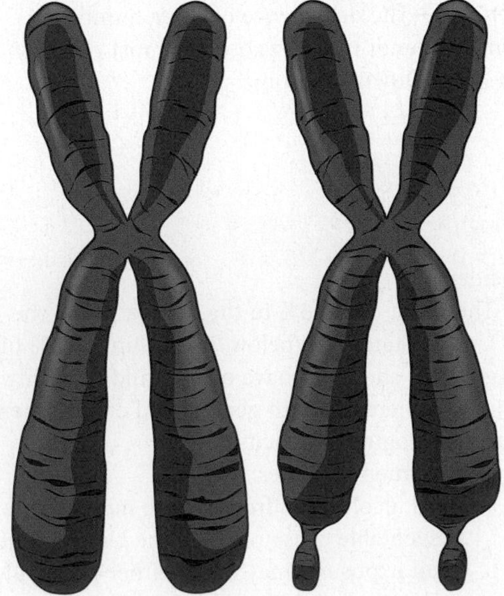

Fig 24.1 Fragile X chromosome.

   b. Down syndrome.
      i. Trisomy 21 is the most common Down syndrome genotype.

C. Pathophysiology.
1. Damage to the cognitive centers of the cerebrum of the brain that has occurred from one of many possible insults, including hypoxic injury, teratogenic insult, or genetic injury.

D. Diagnosis.
1. Prenatal screenings.
   a. May detect a fetus that is at high risk of a genetic syndrome.
   b. If the screening is positive, diagnostic tests (i.e., chorionic villus sampling or amniocentesis) may be performed.
2. Genetic diagnostic tests provide accurate diagnoses of genetic disorders.
3. Growth and development screenings (e.g., DDST, Ages and Stages) are performed during early childhood.
   a. When a child fails to achieve expected milestones, health-care practitioners should refer the child for additional, more sophisticated cognitive diagnostic testing.
4. Cognitive diagnosis tests include the Stanford-Binet Intelligence Scale (SB5), the Wechsler Preschool and Primary Scale of Intelligence (WPPSI-III), and the Wechsler Intelligence Scale for Children (WISC-III).
   a. SB5: for assessing age 2 through adulthood.
      i. Includes a comprehensive assessment of intelligence of the child.
   b. WPPSI-III: for assessing children 2 years 6 months to 7 years 3 months of age.
      i. Includes a number of subscales to provide a comprehensive assessment of intelligence of the young child.
   c. WISC-III: for assessing children over the age of 6.
      i. Includes 13 subscales for comprehensive assessment of intelligence.
   d. Tests for children under 2 are less predictive.
   e. Some children are not diagnosed until in school when they have difficulty in academic achievement.
   f. Signs and symptoms.
      i. To be identified as intellectually disabled, children must have exhibited cognitive impairment, with an IQ below 70, before the age of 18.

DID YOU KNOW?

IQ is a common way to measure an individual's cognitive ability. IQs are determined by the score persons receive on tests specifically designed to measure intelligence (e.g., SB5, WPPSI-III, WISC-III). The scores range from very low scores (below 20) for those who are profoundly disabled to scores above 145 for those who are considered to be geniuses. Those who receive an IQ of 100 are considered to be of average intelligence.

ii. Because of the multifactorial focus in relation to ID in recent years, to be labeled as having an intellectual deficit, a child not only must have a below 70 IQ but also must exhibit deficits in "adaptive behavior as expressed in conceptual, social, and practical adaptive skills" (AAIDD, 2013). In other words, the child must have difficulty in other aspects of his or her life (e.g., communicating with others, performing self-care skills, performing employable skills).

iii. Comorbidities are commonly seen in children with cognitive deficits, including sensory deficits, seizure disorders, behavioral problems, and psychological disorders.

iv. Because they are so vulnerable, children with cognitive deficits are at high risk for physical, emotional, and/or sexual abuse.

E. Treatment.

1. Repeated growth and development screenings.
2. Early intervention, especially educational stimulation programming, is key but is often dependent on the accessibility of resources.
3. Children with ID must be assessed for comorbidities, and, if they exist, they must also be treated (e.g., hearing aids, glasses).

F. Nursing considerations.

1. Deficient Knowledge.
   a. Preconception counseling is essential.
      i. Educate clients to avoid exposure to lead and alcohol before getting pregnant and throughout the pregnancy.
   b. Educate clients regarding lead poisoning prevention strategies for children after delivery (see Chapter 10, "Pediatric Emergencies").
   c. Prevent injury from shaken baby syndrome through education programs.
   d. Prevent injury from drowning by educating parents regarding the need for early child swim instruction.
   e. Refer couples at high risk for delivering a baby with a genetic defect for genetic counseling.
2. Risk for Altered Parenting/Grieving.
   a. Allow parents to express their grief, anger, and/or frustration regarding caring for a child with ID.
   b. Carefully assess parenting behaviors.
      i. Children with cognitive deficits are at very high risk for abuse and neglect.
   c. Refer the family to supportive organizations (e.g., National Down Syndrome Society, National Fragile X Foundation, American Association of Intellectual and Developmental Disabilities).
3. Many additional nursing diagnoses related to the cognitive deficit may be appropriate including Delayed Growth and Development, Deficient Knowledge, Impaired Coping, Self-Care Deficit, Impaired Memory, Risk for Injury, Risk for Self-Mutilation, and Impaired Verbal Communication.
   a. It is essential to assess growth and development, especially growth and development milestones, to determine the extent of the child's disability.
   b. It is very important to relate to the child at his or her functional level rather than the child's chronological age.
   c. Refer the child to programs that provide early educational intervention.
   d. Depending on additional deficits exhibited by the child, refer the family for specialized care, e.g., occupational therapy, physical therapy.
   e. Provide children with clear, simple explanations of all tasks/treatments.

MAKING THE CONNECTION

Although the probability of having a child with Down syndrome increases dramatically as a woman ages, because women in their twenties get pregnant more frequently than older women do, the majority of children with Down are birthed to younger women. As a result, it has become a standard of care to offer first-trimester screenings to all women who are pregnant. The screenings, which include blood testing and ultrasounding, are highly specific. To provide absolute diagnoses, however, those with positive screens are counseled regarding the availability of genetic diagnostic testing. If the genetic test is positive for Down syndrome, the couple is given the option of aborting the fetus.

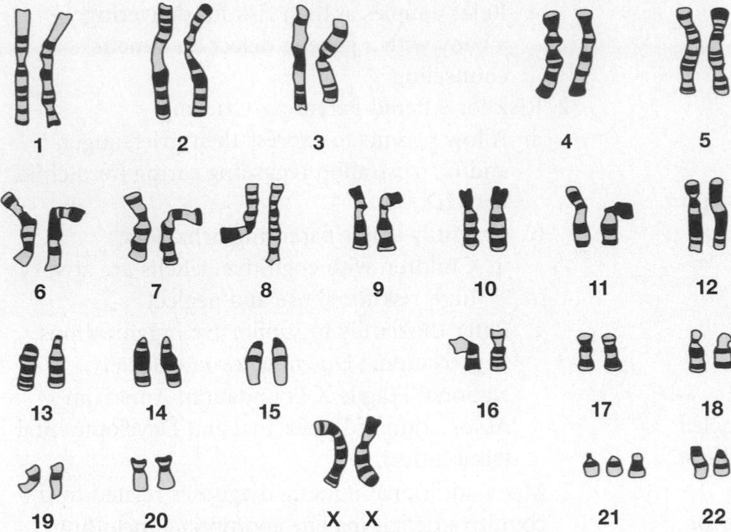

Fig 24.2 Down syndrome karyotype.

II. Down Syndrome

A. Incidence.

1. The risk of birthing a child with Down syndrome increases with maternal age. Probability:
   a. At age 25: 1/2,500 births.
   b. At age 30: 1/1,000.
   c. At age 40: 1/100.
   d. At age 49: 1/10.

B. Etiology.

1. The most common cause of Down syndrome is the nondisjunction of chromosome 21 during meiosis.
   a. Three number 21 chromosomes, called **trisomy 21**, end up in the nucleus of the zygote and in the growing embryo and fetus (Fig. 24.2).

DID YOU KNOW?

Nondisjunction (i.e., the failure of chromosome 21 pair to separate during meiotic division) results in the zygote receiving three, rather than two, number 21 chromosomes. The incidence of nondisjunction increases with maternal age; therefore, the probability of conceiving a child with Down syndrome increases as women age.

   b. The child, therefore, has a total of 47 chromosomes in the cells of his or her body.
2. Down syndrome may also occur as a result of a chromosomal translocation, including chromosome 21.

C. Pathophysiology.

1. Because of an excess of chromosome 21 genetic material, the characteristic features of Down appear as:

MAKING THE CONNECTION

It is important to note that there is a relatively high incidence of mosaicism in children with Down syndrome. **Chromosomal mosaicism** means that different cells of the body have different numbers of chromosomes. In Down syndrome mosaicism, some of the cells of the body have the characteristic Down syndrome trisomy 21 pattern and, therefore, a total of 47 chromosomes. Some of the cells of the body, however, have two number 21 chromosomes and, therefore, have the normal diploid number of 46 chromosomes. Children with mosaic Down syndrome usually have higher IQs than those children with a uniform genetic pattern.

   a. Cognitive deficits.
   b. Facial and cranial deformities (Fig. 24.3).
      i. Slanted eyes.
      ii. Wide, flat nasal bridge.
      iii. Protruding tongue.
      iv. Small, low-set ears.
   c. **Muscular hypotonia**, poor muscle tone throughout the body, often resulting in feeding difficulties, recurrent respiratory illnesses, obesity, and protruding abdomen.
   d. **Simian creases**: unbroken "life lines" that stretch across the palm of the hand (Fig. 24.4).
   e. Lax joints, often resulting in joint injuries.
   f. Also at high risk for:
      i. Cardiac and other congenital defects, including of the gastrointestinal and central nervous systems.

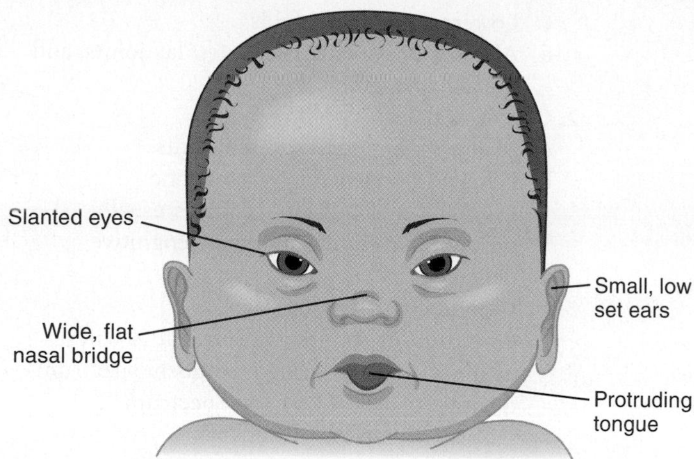

Fig 24.3 Down facial and cranial deformities.

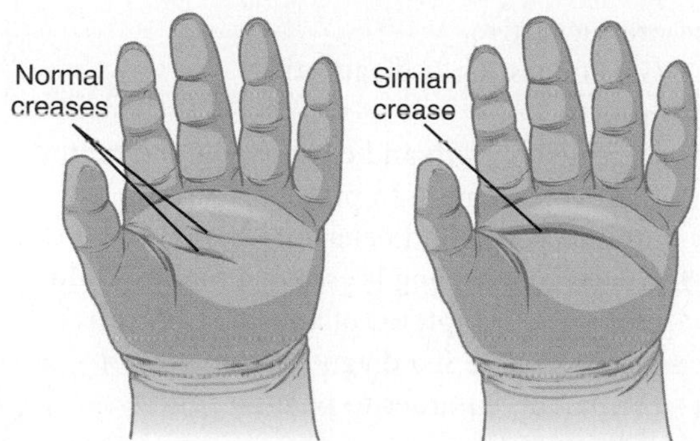

Fig 24.4 Simian creases.

  ii. Leukemia: 15 times the incidence of the general population.
  iii. Early onset Alzheimer's disease.

D. Diagnosis.
1. Prenatal.
   a. Prenatal screening provides fairly accurate probability of carrying a child with Down syndrome.
   b. Diagnostic testing is definitive.
      i. Genetic analysis: either via chorionic villus sampling (CVS) or amniocentesis.
2. Neonatal.
   a. Clinical picture is suggestive.
   b. Genetic analysis is diagnostic.

E. Treatment.
1. Surgery to correct any congenital defects.
2. Repeated growth and development screenings.
3. Early intervention to promote learning and optimal social and behavioral skills.
4. Genetic counseling to provide the couple with information regarding the probability of conceiving a Down syndrome baby in the future.

F. Nursing considerations: in addition to earlier information regarding the care of children with ID:
1. Deficient Knowledge/Risk for Caregiver Role Strain.
   a. Educate the parents regarding the genetic etiology of disease.
   b. Refer the parents for genetic counseling.
   c. Introduce the parents to another family with a Down syndrome child.
   d. Provide a referral to an appropriate organization (e.g., National Association for Down syndrome).
2. Risk for Imbalanced Nutrition: Less than Body Requirements (infancy)/More than Body Requirements (childhood).
   a. Educate the parents regarding the child's poor muscle tone.
   b. During infancy:
      i. Educate the parents regarding the need to feed the baby slowly (if bottle-fed) or refer the breastfeeding mother to an IBCLC (International Board Certified Lactation Consultant) for assistance with latch and milk transfer.
      ii. If bottlefed, the child may need specialized feeding devices (e.g., Haberman feeder) to facilitate feeding.
      iii. Refer the parents to an occupational therapist, if needed.
   c. As the child grows, to prevent obesity:
      i. Educate the parents to feed the child a diet with a minimal number of empty calories.
      ii. Educate the parents to encourage the child to engage in a daily exercise routine.

3. Risk for Altered Gas Exchange/Ineffective Airway Clearance.
   a. Educate the parents to seek medical care whenever the child develops an upper respiratory infection (URI).
   b. Educate the parents to perform respiratory PT to prevent URIs and pneumonia.
4. Risk for Injury.
   a. Refer the parents to a specialist to determine the potential for neck and joint injuries.
   b. Encourage the parents to have the child participate in safe physical activities in order to maximize muscle tone and joint health.

III. Fragile X Syndrome

A. Incidence.
1. **Fragile X syndrome** is the most common genetic form of ID.
2. Most commonly seen in boys, but girls do exhibit some characteristics of the syndrome.

B. Etiology.
1. X-linked recessive disease.
   a. Most severe form seen in males.
   b. Females are carriers of the syndrome and do exhibit some characteristics of the syndrome.

C. Pathophysiology.
1. Physical defects (Fig. 24.5) are often overlooked.
   a. Long, narrow face.
   b. Large ears.

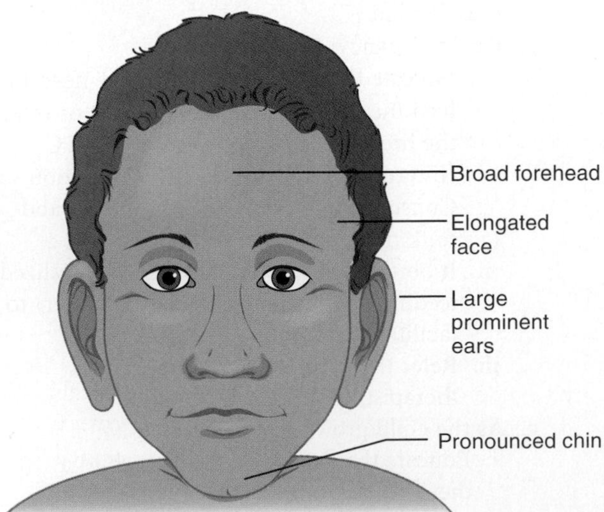

Fig 24.5 Discriminating characteristics of fragile X syndrome.

   c. Lowered epicanthal folds.
   d. Also may have enlarged testes, lax joints, and mitral valve prolapse.
2. Cognitive defect.
   a. Males: moderate to severe deficits.
   b. Females: because they possess one normal X chromosome, females usually only exhibit mild to moderate cognitive deficits.
3. Behavioral characteristics.
   a. One-third of children with fragile X will exhibit behaviors related to autism spectrum disorders (see the "Autism Spectrum Disorders" section).
   b. Aggression.
   c. Agitation.

D. Diagnosis: diagnosis is often missed, especially in girls.
1. Physical appearance and behavioral characteristics are suggestive.
2. Genetic testing is diagnostic.

E. Treatment.
1. Repeated growth and development screenings.
2. Early intervention to promote learning and optimal social and behavioral skills.
3. Genetic counseling is essential for any child exhibiting symptoms of autism spectrum disorders and, if a diagnosis is made, for the parents in order to plan for future pregnancies.

F. Nursing considerations: in addition to earlier information regarding the care of children with ID:
1. Deficient Knowledge.
   a. Educate the parents regarding the genetic etiology of the syndrome.
   b. Refer the parents for genetic counseling.
2. Caregiver Role Strain/Risk for Dysfunctional Family Processes/Risk for Injury/Risk for Self-Mutilation.
   a. Assess impact of the adverse behaviors on the family.
   b. Provide a referral to a facility where expert care/education is provided.
   c. Introduce the parents to another family with a child with fragile X syndrome.
   d. Provide a referral to an appropriate organization (e.g., National Fragile X Foundation, American Autism Association, American Autism Society).

IV. Fetal Alcohol Spectrum Disorders

Fetal alcohol spectrum disorders (FASD) are divided into three subcategories (Table 24.1).

Table 24.1 Fetal Alcohol Spectrum Disorders

Name	Defining Characteristics
Fetal alcohol syndrome	Most severe form of FASD, characterized by a wide range of signs and symptoms, including physical, intellectual, and behavioral problems.
Alcohol-related neurodevelopmental disorder	Characterized by cognitive and behavioral signs and symptoms.
Alcohol-related birth defects	Characterized by physiological alterations.

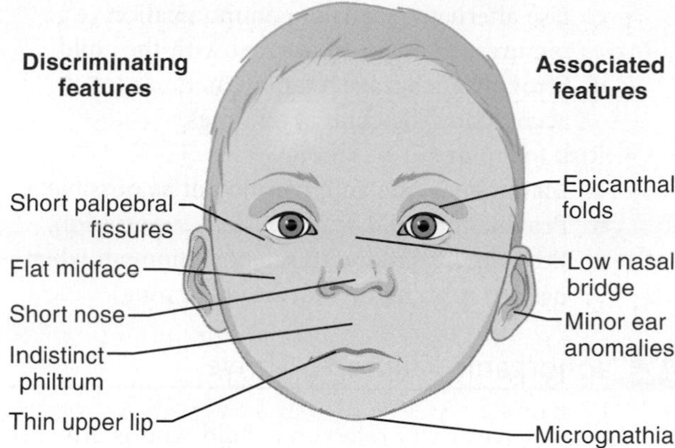

Fig 24.6 Discriminating characteristics of FASD.

A. Incidence.
1. Known incidence is approximately 1/1,000 live births, but the incidence is believed to be much higher.

B. Etiology.
1. Alcohol intake during pregnancy.
2. There is no known safe level of alcohol intake during pregnancy.

C. Pathophysiology.
1. May occur with daily alcohol consumption or with binge drinking.
2. There are a myriad of physiological and psychological signs and symptoms associated with FASD.
   a. Physiological.
      i. Head and facial anomalies (Fig. 24.6).
         (1) Smooth philtrum.
         (2) Microcephaly.
         (3) Short palpebral fissures.
         (4) Hypoplastic upper lip.
      ii. Small for gestational age.
      iii. Organ defects, including:
         (1) Cardiac, especially septal, defects.
         (2) Vertebral malformations.
         (3) Cleft lip and/or palate.
         (4) Renal anomalies.
         (5) Short fingers.
         (6) Sensory deficits.
   b. Psychological and behavioral.
      i. Low IQ.
      ii. Hyperactivity.
      iii. Learning disabilities.
      iv. Poor reasoning abilities.

D. Diagnosis.
1. Absence of a genetic defect that would explain the disorder. Evidence of alcohol consumption during pregnancy, either by self-report, third-party report, and/or toxicology report in combination with clinical evidence (see earlier).

E. Treatment.
1. Prevention.
   a. Preconception counseling regarding the need to abstain from any alcohol while trying to become pregnant until the birth of the baby.
2. Substance abuse counseling for women of childbearing age regarding the need to change behavior:
   a. To prevent FASD.
   b. In order to provide optimal parenting of the FASD child.
3. Treatment of the injured child.
   a. Surgery to correct any congenital defects.
   b. Repeated growth and development screenings.
   c. Early intervention to promote learning and optimal social and behavioral skills.

F. Nursing considerations.
1. Deficient Knowledge.
   a. Provide preconception counseling regarding the importance of avoiding all alcohol from the cessation of use of birth control until the birth of the baby.
2. Impaired Growth and Development.
   a. At each well-child visit, it is essential to assess the child's growth and development.
   b. Report any deviations from normal to the primary health-care provider.
   c. Refer the family for expert intervention, as needed.
3. Impaired Social Interaction/Impaired Verbal Communication, especially important during hospitalizations.
   a. Have the same nurse care for the child as much as possible.
   b. Establish a routine that is as close to the child's normal as possible.

c. Use alternate means of communication (e.g., pictures) as a way to interact with the child.
d. Strongly encourage a family member to accompany the child at all times.
4. Risk for Injury.
a. Maintain as safe an environment as possible.
b. Provide the child with constant supervision.
c. Provide the child with safety equipment when needed (e.g., helmet for head banging).

V. Nonorganic Failure to Thrive

Failure to thrive (FTT) refers to a child who is growing and developing much slower than would be expected. The child's growth pattern is well below the expected curve on growth charts, and his or her developmental growth is delayed. In many cases, a physical (i.e., organic) reason is diagnosed to explain the poor growth pattern. When no physiological abnormality is present, the diagnosis of nonorganic FTT (NOFTT) is made.

A. Incidence.
1. Some experts report that as many as 10 out of every 100 children exhibit FTT.

B. Etiology.
1. Usually a combination of factors. Some experts believe that NOFTT may have both a physiological and a behavioral origin.
2. Less than optimal care provided by the baby's primary caregiver, characterized by unresponsiveness to the baby's feeding cues and needs and/or failure to provide stimulation or opportunities to achieve normal behavioral milestones, are factors in the problem's etiology.
a. Behaviors often exhibited by the caregiver include:
i. Depression.
ii. Substance abuse.
iii. Lack of knowledge regarding childrearing skills.
iv. Lack of resources.
v. Poor bonding.

C. Pathophysiology.
1. Physiological indicators.
a. Below the 5th percentile for height and/or weight on growth charts or a marked drop in physiological growth.
b. Failure to achieve standard developmental milestones.
c. Poor muscle tone.
d. Abdominal distension.
e. Signs of malnutrition.
2. Behavioral indicators.
a. Poor eye contact.
b. Failure to seek parental consolation.
c. Failure to exhibit age-appropriate fear of strangers.
d. Disinterest in environmental stimuli.
e. Autistic-like behaviors (e.g., hand flapping, head banging, rocking) (see the following "Autism Spectrum Disorders" section).

D. Diagnosis.
1. Clinical signs and symptoms with no organic reason for the findings.
2. Responsiveness to intervention
a. When health-care providers exhibit appropriate parenting behaviors, modeling them for the parents.

E. Treatment.
1. Provide parenting classes to primary caregivers.
a. Parenting classes can be both a prevention and a treatment strategy.
2. Improved nutrition: Affected infants are usually fed high-calorie formula (24 kcal/oz rather than 20 kcal/oz).
3. Multivitamin supplements.

F. Nursing considerations.
1. Deficient Knowledge/Impaired Parenting/Ineffective Role Performance.
a. Conduct a thorough psychosocial assessment to identify high-risk families.
b. Refer primary caregivers for needed services, optimally before the baby is born, (e.g., substance abuse counseling, financial support counseling, psychological intervention).
c. Carefully assess parenting behaviors of primary caregivers.
d. Provide parenting education prenatally and/or postpartum, as needed.
e. Role model appropriate parenting behaviors during all nurse-parent interactions.
2. Impaired Growth and Development.
a. At each well-child visit, assess the child's growth and development.
b. Report any deviations from normal to the primary health-care provider.
c. Refer the family for expert intervention, as needed.
3. Imbalanced Nutrition: Less than Body Requirements.
a. Educate the parents about the nutritional needs of the baby, especially if the mother is breastfeeding.
b. Provide a high-calorie formula at each feeding, if needed.
c. To prevent unnecessary distractions, educate the parents to feed the baby in a low-stimulation environment.

VI. Autism Spectrum Disorders

A. Incidence.
1. Estimates range widely. The highest incidence estimates of autism spectrum disorders (ASD) are 1 in 88 to 1 in 150 children.
2. Four to five times more likely in boys than in girls (many have fragile X syndrome—see earlier).

B. Etiology.
1. Other than those with fragile X syndrome, the etiologies are unknown.
   a. Very strong belief that most autism develops as a result of a multifactorial etiology.
2. Genetic basis for some cases is likely, but other than in the case of fragile X, no genetic markers have been identified.
3. Maternal ingestion of valproic acid or thalidomide during pregnancy increases the child's risk of developing autism.

C. Pathophysiology.
1. Wide range of pathology, with many variations, including any or all of the following behaviors:
   a. Inability to understand and engage in normal social interactions.
   b. Inability to form any meaningful relationships, including with the child's own parents.
   c. Inability to communicate effectively.
   d. Inability to engage in any type of play activities.
2. Often, the child develops normally, then abnormal behaviors appear when the child reaches 2 to 3 years of age.
3. Signs and symptoms vary widely.
   a. Social impairment (e.g., ignores the existence of others, plays alone, either doesn't seek comfort when injured or doesn't even acknowledge an injury when it occurs).
   b. Language impairment (e.g., fails to engage in conversations or monopolizes conversations with topics of interest only to themselves; exhibits flat or inappropriate affect when speaking; or fails to engage in any interactive play).
   c. Behavioral impairment (e.g., engages in repetitive behaviors, such as hand flapping or head banging; has tantrums over minor changes in the environment or in daily routines; obsesses about following detailed schedules; engages in self-mutilation; exhibits marked sensitivity to sounds or light).
   d. Cognitive impairment: most have distinct cognitive deficits, although the same child may also have areas of marked intelligence (e.g., "Rain Man").

D. Diagnosis.
1. Screening tool.
   a. The American Academy of Pediatrics recommends that all children be screened for ASD between the ages of 18 and 30 months using the Modified Checklist for Autism in Toddlers, Revised (M-CHAT-R) (2009).
   b. Clinical picture: (the diagnostic signs are usually evident by the age of 3) as defined in the DSM-V.

DID YOU KNOW?

The Diagnostic and Statistical Manual of Mental Disorders is the official diagnostic reference of the American Psychiatric Association. The DSM-IV, published in 1994, referenced a diverse definition of autism, including grades of the disorder: autism disorder, Asperger's syndrome, and pervasive developmental disorder. The authors of the fifth edition of the manual, published in 2013, deleted the gradations, preferring to define autism as one problem they call "autism spectrum disorder." Some parents and professionals who work with autistic children are concerned that some children will not be diagnosed properly because of the generalized definition of the disorder now used in the manual.

E. Treatment.
1. Early diagnosis is essential, with interventions designed for each child's specific needs.
2. Behavioral therapies are most frequently employed.
3. Lifelong intervention is often required; autistic individuals have normal life spans.

F. Nursing considerations (merely a suggested list the child may require fewer or more nursing interventions).
1. Deficient Knowledge/Anxiety/Fear/Anger/Grieving/Impaired Growth and Development.
   a. Educate the parents and others regarding the child's diagnosis.
   b. Allow the parents to express grief, anger, and/or frustration regarding the child's diagnosis.
   c. At each well-child visit, the child's growth and development should be assessed.
   d. Report any deviations from normal to the primary health-care provider.
2. Impaired Social Interaction/Impaired Verbal Communication (especially important during hospitalizations).
   a. Have the same nurse care for the child as much as possible or, if the child ever needs a babysitter, encourage the parents to employ the same person each time.

b. Encourage the parents to establish a strict routine at home and maintain the routine that is as close to the child's normal as possible during hospitalizations.
c. Use alternate means of communication (e.g., pictures) as a way to interact with the child.
d. Strongly encourage a family member to accompany the child at all times.
e. Refer the child and family to educational resources specifically geared to autistic children.
f. Refer the child and family to community resources (e.g., American Autism Society, American Autism Association).

3. Risk for Injury.
   a. Maintain as safe an environment as possible.
   b. Provide the child with constant supervision.
   c. Provide the child with safety equipment when needed (e.g., helmet for head banging).

CASE STUDY: Putting It All Together

2-year, 7-month-old male who has been in daycare since 3 months of age

Subjective Data

- The child has met normal growth and development milestones to date.
- The daycare teacher notified the nurse at the facility because for the past 1 to 2 months, the teacher has noticed:
  - "He doesn't look at me when he comes into the classroom anymore."
  - "He doesn't seem very happy. I rarely see him smile, and he never laughs."
  - "The other children try to play with him, but he walks away and plays by himself."
  - "He often sits alone and rocks back and forth."

Objective Data

Nursing Assessment by Daycare Nurse

- According to the records at the daycare, the M-CHAT-R was never completed by the child's parents.
- Child's parents.
  - Both are well-educated and employed.
  - Appear to be loving parents, attentive to the child's needs, and actively involved in the child's progress at daycare.
- DDST (Denver Developmental Screening Test) administered.
  - Personal-social: fails
    - Exhibits no independent behaviors, never attempts to remove clothing and rarely attempts to use utensils when eating.
    - Parents state that the behavior is consistent with what they see at home.
  - Fine motor: passes
    - Can build a tower of four blocks but only when playing alone.
  - Language: fails
    - Speaks very little and never in response to a request.
    - Will not identify or point to any body parts, animals, colors, or any other items on request.
    - Parents state that, although their child used to be interested in books and learning, they have noticed a decline in that behavior in recent months.
  - Gross motor: passes
    - Walks up stairs, does not use alternating feet.
    - Kicks a ball but only when playing alone.
- Physical findings
  - All within normal limits, including height, weight, and vital signs.

Health-Care Provider's Orders (parents took the child to the child's primary-care provider in response to concerns expressed by the nurse and teacher at the child's daycare.)

- Referred the child for in-depth psychological testing by an expert in the field who diagnosed the child with autism spectrum disorder based on the following findings:
  - Exhibits deficits in social interaction behavior
  - Exhibits repetitive behaviors
  - Started to exhibit the abnormal behaviors between 2 and 3 years of age
  - Is unable to meet normal growth and development milestones because of the abnormal behaviors
- Based on the evidence supplied by the expert,
  - Recommend moving the child to an early intervention daycare program for autistic children
  - Refer the family to community resources for support and guidance

CASE STUDY: Putting It All Together

cont'd

Case Study Questions

A. What *subjective* assessments indicate that this client is experiencing a health alteration? Based on observations by daycare teacher and parents:

1. ____
2. ____
3. ____
4. ____
5. ____
6. ____
7. ____

B. What *objective* assessments indicate that this client is experiencing a health alteration?

1. ____
2. ____

C. After analyzing the data that has been collected, what **primary** nursing diagnosis should the nurse assign to this client?

1. ____

D. What interventions should the nurse plan and/or implement to meet this child's and his family's needs?

1. ____
2. ____
3. ____
4. ____
5. ____
6. ____

E. What client outcomes should the nurse evaluate regarding the effectiveness of the nursing interventions?

1. ____
2. ____
3. ____

F. What physiological characteristics should the child exhibit before being discharged home?

1. ____

REVIEW QUESTIONS

1. The nurse notes the following genomic nomenclature and karyotype in the amniocentesis report. Which of the following interpretations of the report is appropriate for the nurse to make?

   Nomenclature: 47, XX, +21

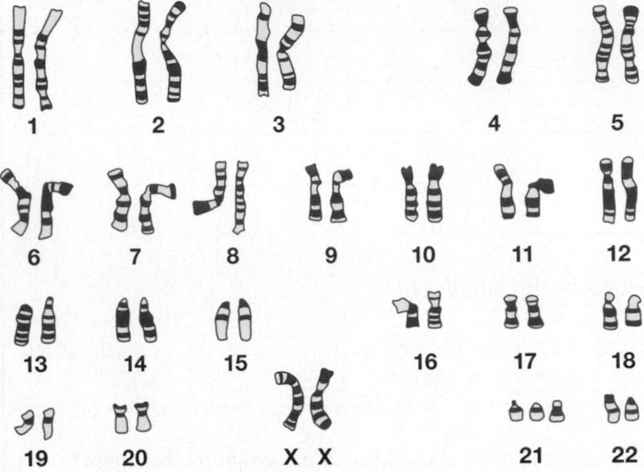

   1. The fetus has Down syndrome.
   2. The fetus has fragile X syndrome.
   3. The fetus will be born with shortened palpebral fissures and hypoplastic upper lip.
   4. The fetus will be born with hypertonic reflexes and spastic posturing.

2. A couple is being discharged from the hospital with their 2-day-old Down syndrome baby. The nurse is providing discharge teaching. The nurse should include in the teaching information regarding which of the following physiological characteristics of the syndrome?
   1. Small cerebral ventricles
   2. Weak musculature
   3. Inability to feel pain
   4. Low glomerular filtration rate

3. A baby with trisomy 21 is admitted to the newborn nursery. The baby should be assessed for which of the following features?
   1. Simian crease
   2. Polydactyly
   3. Harlequin sign
   4. Mongolian spots

4. A nurse suspects that a newly delivered baby has Down syndrome. The nurse noted that the baby exhibited which of the following physiological characteristics? **Select all that apply.**
   1. Elongated face
   2. Protruding tongue
   3. Large, high-set ears
   4. Wide, flat nasal bridge
   5. Asymmetric Moro reflex

5. A nurse working in a preschool has just been advised that a toddler with fragile X syndrome has been admitted to the school. The nurse should advise the teacher that the child may exhibit which of the following characteristics?
   1. Lordotic posturing
   2. Aggressive behavior
   3. Two different eye colors
   4. Asynchronous breathing

6. A nurse is admitting a 10-year-old child with an intellectual disability to the hospital for surgery. Before providing the child with preoperative teaching, the nurse must determine which of the following?
   1. Type of intravenous fluid the surgeon plans to order.
   2. Child's preoperative medication order.
   3. Length of time the child will likely be in the recovery room.
   4. Child's diagnosed developmental age.

7. A 9-year-old child is admitted to the hospital with a primary diagnosis of fractured femur and a secondary diagnosis of intellectual disability. Which of the following patient-care goals is appropriate for the child's nursing diagnosis of Deficient Knowledge related to the medical diagnosis?
   1. The child will write a story about a child who has broken a leg.
   2. The child will name the bones of the leg and tell the nurse which bone was broken.
   3. The child will draw a picture of a child who is in the hospital in traction.
   4. The child will complete a science project for school about how traction weights work.

8. A child has been diagnosed with fragile X syndrome. The nurse would predict that the child may exhibit which of the following signs/symptoms?
   1. Strabismus
   2. Arm flapping
   3. Vision deficit
   4. Nevus flammeus

9. The nurse is providing preconception counseling to a young woman regarding alcohol consumption during pregnancy. Which of the following information should be included in the teaching session?
   1. The alcohol content in beer is safe to consume during pregnancy.
   2. Once she learns that she is pregnant, she should stop drinking alcohol.
   3. It is safe to drink alcohol after the first trimester of pregnancy.
   4. Alcohol is contraindicated from conception to the end of pregnancy.

10. A child has been diagnosed with nonorganic failure to thrive (NOFTT). The nurse would predict that the mother may exhibit which of the following characteristics? **Select all that apply.**
    1. Abuses addictive substances
    2. Owns a number of domesticated animals
    3. Expresses disinterest in caring for her baby
    4. Misunderstands the feeding needs of babies
    5. Lacks the money needed to buy baby supplies

11. A child has been diagnosed with nonorganic failure to thrive (NOFTT). The nurse would expect the child to exhibit which of the following characteristics?
    1. Early onset stranger anxiety
    2. Fascination with lights and sounds
    3. Excessive parental attachment
    4. Failure to make eye contact

12. A child with nonorganic failure to thrive (NOFTT) is being discharged from the hospital. The baby's mother, who is now exhibiting appropriate parenting behaviors, is providing the baby with needed nutritional supplementation. In addition, the mother does which of the following?
    1. Feeds the baby through an enlarged hole in the nipple
    2. Faces a blank wall while feeding the baby
    3. Adds rice cereal to the baby's formula
    4. Puts the baby to bed with a bottle of formula

13. A school nurse suspects that a 5-year-old child has autism spectrum disorder. The nurse's suspicion is based on which of the following observations? The nurse noted that the child: **Select all that apply.**
    1. has yet to learn his colors or the names of animals.
    2. becomes upset each time the teacher asks the child to stop what he is doing.
    3. is the first in line when it is time to go out to play in the playground.
    4. runs to the teacher to get a kiss whenever he gets hurt while playing.
    5. covers his ears whenever the school principal makes an announcement on the loud speaker.

14. A 9-year-old child with autism spectrum disorder has been admitted to the hospital. Which of the following interventions is important for the nurse to perform during the child's stay?
    1. Follow a strict schedule for all medicines and treatments.
    2. Take the child to the playroom at least twice a day.
    3. Keep all of the room lights on throughout the night.
    4. Provide the child with sugar-free juice at snack time.

REVIEW ANSWERS

1. ANSWER: 1
Rationale:
1. The fetus has Down syndrome.
2. The fetus does not have fragile X syndrome.
3. Babies exposed to alcohol in utero are born with shortened palpebral fissures and hypoplastic upper lip.
4. Babies who have kernicterus, a disease seen in the neonatal period that is caused by excessive quantities of bilirubin in the bloodstream, develop hypertonic reflexes and spastic posturing.
TEST-TAKING TIP: The nomenclature connotes a fetus with 47 chromosomes, including an extra number 21 chromosome. The karyotype shows three number 21 chromosomes. Down syndrome is most frequently caused by trisomy 21.
Content Area: Maternity—Antepartum
Integrated Processes: Nursing Process: Analysis
Client Need: Health Promotion and Maintenance: Ante/Intra/Postpartum and Newborn Care
Cognitive Level: Application

2. ANSWER: 2
Rationale:
1. The child's cerebral ventricles are normal.
2. The child does have weak musculature.
3. The child does feel pain.
4. The child's glomerular filtration rate is normal.
TEST-TAKING TIP: The nurse should educate the parents regarding the child's weak musculature because the child will be at high risk for a number of problems, including upper respiratory infections, pendulous abdominal muscles, and lumbering gait.
Content Area: Pediatrics
Integrated Processes: Nursing Process: Implementation; Teaching/Learning
Client Need: Physiological Integrity: Physiological Adaptation: Alteration in Body Systems
Cognitive Level: Application

3. ANSWER: 1
Rationale:
1. Simian crease is associated with Down syndrome.
2. Polydactyly is a relatively common birth anomaly that is not directly associated with Down syndrome.
3. Harlequin sign is a normal variation in neonatal skin color.
4. Mongolian spots are a normal variation in neonatal skin color, most commonly seen in babies of color.
TEST-TAKING TIP: It is important to remember that chromosomal syndrome diseases are usually associated with a number of characteristics. In addition to features such as simian creases seen in children with Down syndrome, the babies may exhibit life-threatening anomalies, including cardiac and gastrointestinal defects.
Content Area: Pediatrics
Integrated Processes: Nursing Process: Assessment
Client Need: Physiological Integrity: Physiological Adaptation: Alteration in Body Systems
Cognitive Level: Application

4. ANSWER: 2 and 4
Rationale:
1. Elongated face is a characteristic of children with fragile X syndrome.
2. Protruding tongue is associated with Down syndrome.
3. Low-set ears are associated with Down syndrome.
4. Wide, flat nasal bridge is associated with Down syndrome.
5. Asymmetric Moro reflex is seen in children with, for example, Erb's palsy characterized by one extremity that lacks enervation.
TEST-TAKING TIP: The protruding tongue of the Down syndrome baby is not related to the fact that the tongue is enlarged but rather to the poor muscle tone of the baby. Ear height is determined by drawing and extending an imaginary line from the inner canthus to the outer canthus of the eye. The top of the ear should be found at or slightly above the imaginary line. In Down syndrome babies, the top of the ear falls below the imaginary line.
Content Area: Pediatrics
Integrated Processes: Nursing Process: Assessment
Client Need: Physiological Integrity: Physiological Adaptation: Alteration in Body Systems
Cognitive Level: Application

5. ANSWER: 2
Rationale:
1. Lordotic posturing (i.e., swayback) is not associated with fragile X syndrome.
2. Aggressive behavior is associated with fragile X syndrome.
3. Two different eye colors is not associated with fragile X syndrome.
4. Asynchronous breathing is seen in infants who are in respiratory distress.
TEST-TAKING TIP: In addition to physical characteristics and cognitive deficits, children with fragile X syndrome exhibit a number of behavioral traits, including autistic and hyperactive behaviors.
Content Area: Pediatrics
Integrated Processes: Nursing Process: Implementation; Teaching/Learning
Client Need: Physiological Integrity: Physiological Adaptation: Alteration in Body Systems
Cognitive Level: Application

6. ANSWER: 4
Rationale:
1. It is not essential for the nurse to know the type of IV fluid the surgeon plans to order.
2. It is not essential for the nurse to know the child's preoperative medication order.
3. It is not essential for the nurse to know the length of time the child will likely be in the recovery room.
4. It is essential for the nurse to know the child's diagnosed developmental age.
TEST-TAKING TIP: Even though the child is chronologically 10 years of age, the child may have a development age that is much younger. When providing

preoperative teaching, the nurse should adapt his or her teaching to the child's developmental age.
Content Area: *Pediatrics*
Integrated Processes: *Nursing Process: Assessment*
Client Need: *Health Promotion and Maintenance: Health Promotion/Disease Prevention*
Cognitive Level: *Application*

7. ANSWER: 3
Rationale:
1. With an intellectual disability, it is unlikely that the child would be able to write a story about a child who has broken a leg.
2. With an intellectual disability, it is unlikely that the child would be able to name the bones of the leg and tell the nurse which bone was broken.
3. Children with intellectual disabilities are usually able to draw pictures and should be able to draw a picture of a child who is in a hospital in traction.
4. With an intellectual disability, it is unlikely that the child could complete a science project for school about how traction weights work.
TEST-TAKING TIP: Because a child with an intellectual disability has a developmental age that is likely very different from his or her chronological age, it is very important for the nurse to determine the child's developmental age. The nurse will then be able to alter his or her care appropriately.
Content Area: *Pediatrics*
Integrated Processes: *Nursing Process: Analysis*
Client Need: *Health Promotion and Maintenance: Health Promotion/Disease Prevention*
Cognitive Level: *Application*

8. ANSWER: 2
Rationale:
1. Strabismus is not associated with fragile X syndrome.
2. Children with fragile X syndrome often exhibit arm flapping.
3. Vision deficit is not associated with fragile X syndrome, although children whose cognitive function was altered secondary to a perinatal hypoxic insult may also exhibit vision deficits.
4. Nevus flammeus, or port-wine stain, is not associated with fragile X syndrome.
TEST-TAKING TIP: Many children with fragile X syndrome exhibit autistic behaviors, including arm flapping.
Content Area: *Pediatrics*
Integrated Processes: *Nursing Process: Assessment*
Client Need: *Physiological Integrity: Physiological Adaptation: Alteration in Body Systems*
Cognitive Level: *Application*

9. ANSWER: 4
Rationale:
1. Alcohol is contraindicated from conception to the end of pregnancy.
2. Alcohol is contraindicated from conception to the end of pregnancy.
3. Alcohol is contraindicated from conception to the end of pregnancy.
4. Alcohol is contraindicated from conception to the end of pregnancy.
TEST-TAKING TIP: Although the most sensitive period of the organ development of the fetus occurs during the first trimester, the CNS is sensitive to insults throughout the entire pregnancy. Alcohol is teratogenic to the fetus during all three trimesters of pregnancy and can lead to ID even if consumed late in the pregnancy.
Content Area: *Maternity, Antepartum*
Integrated Processes: *Nursing Process: Implementation; Teaching/Learning*
Client Need: *Health Promotion and Maintenance: Ante/Intra/Postpartum and Newborn Care*
Cognitive Level: *Application*

10. ANSWER: 1, 3, 4, and 5
Rationale:
1. Mothers who abuse substances are at high risk for having a child with NOFTT.
2. Women who own a number of animals are not at high risk for having a child with NOFTT.
3. Mothers who express disinterest in caring for their babies are at high risk for having a child with NOFTT.
4. Mothers who have little knowledge of baby care are at high risk for having a child with NOFTT.
5. Mothers who live in poverty are at high risk for having a child with NOFTT.
TEST-TAKING TIP: The etiology of NOFTT in babies is related to a deficit in care by the primary-care provider. The practitioner should perform an excellent psychosocial assessment of a NOFTT child's parents to determine the underlying cause of the baby's problem.
Content Area: *Pediatrics*
Integrated Processes: *Nursing Process: Assessment*
Client Need: *Physiological Integrity: Physiological Adaptation: Alteration in Body Systems*
Cognitive Level: *Application*

11. ANSWER: 4
Rationale:
1. Babies with NOFTT often exhibit no age-appropriate stranger anxiety.
2. Babies with NOFTT often show no interest in their environment.
3. Babies with NOFTT often exhibit no need to be consoled by their parents.
4. Babies with NOFTT often fail to make eye contact.
TEST-TAKING TIP: Babies with NOFTT have missed the bonding and personal interaction with their primary caregivers during the newborn and early infancy periods that is so important for normal growth and development. Consequently, they exhibit disinterest and apathy in interacting with others.
Content Area: *Pediatrics*
Integrated Processes: *Nursing Process: Assessment*
Client Need: *Physiological Integrity: Physiological Adaptation: Alteration in Body Systems*
Cognitive Level: *Application*

12. ANSWER: 2

Rationale:

1. It is not recommended to feed babies with FTT through an enlarged hole in the nipple.
2. **It is recommended to face a blank wall while feeding babies with NOFTT.**
3. It is not recommended to add rice to a baby's bottle of formula because they can choke on the mixture.
4. It is not recommended to put babies to bed with a bottle of formula because they will be at high risk for developing dental caries.

TEST-TAKING TIP: Some babies with NOFTT eat poorly because they become distracted by external stimuli and fail to attend to the primary caregiver who is feeding them. By facing a blank wall, distractions are markedly reduced.

Content Area: *Pediatrics*

Integrated Processes: *Nursing Process: Evaluation*

Client Need: *Health Promotion and Maintenance: Health Promotion/Disease Prevention*

Cognitive Level: *Application*

13. ANSWER: 1, 2, and 5

Rationale:

1. **The child should know his or her colors and the names of animals by 5 years of age.**
2. **Autistic children often have difficulty dealing with change.**
3. Autistic children do not exhibit an involvement in group activities.
4. Autistic children rarely seek comfort and often do not even acknowledge pain.
5. **Autistic children are often very sensitive to bright lights and to loud sounds.**

TEST-TAKING TIP: Autism, usually identified by the late toddler or early preschool period, is exemplified by a variety of factors related to social, language, and/or behavioral issues.

Content Area: *Pediatrics*

Integrated Processes: *Nursing Process: Assessment*

Client Need: *Physiological Integrity: Physiological Adaptation: Alteration in Body Systems*

Cognitive Level: *Application*

14. ANSWER: 1

Rationale:

1. **It is important for the nurse to follow a strict schedule for all medicines and treatments. Autistic children are often obsessive about following schedules.**
2. Autistic children rarely engage in play activities.
3. Autistic children are often very sensitive to bright lights and to loud sounds.
4. Sugar intake has not been shown to alter autistic children's behaviors.

TEST-TAKING TIP: To reduce the stress of hospitalization for children with autism, the nurse must meet the child's needs. Maintaining strict schedules is one of those needs.

Content Area: *Pediatrics*

Integrated Processes: *Nursing Process: Implementation*

Client Need: *Physiological Integrity: Physiological Adaptation: Alteration in Body Systems*

Cognitive Level: *Application*

Nursing Care of the Child With Sensory Problems

KEY TERMS

Amblyopia—"Lazy eye," or the brain ignoring the image from the weaker of a child's eyes.
Conjunctiva—The translucent mucous membrane covering the eye and the under portion of the eyelid.
Conjunctivitis—"Pink eye," or inflammation of the conjunctiva of the eye.
Decibel (db)—The loudness of a sound.
Enucleation—Surgical removal of the eye.
Frequency—The pitch of a sound.
Occlusive therapy—Patching of a child's normally functioning eye to force the use of the weaker eye.
Ophthalmia neonatorum—A serious conjunctivitis that neonates can acquire if they are exposed to gonorrhea or chlamydia during birth.
Penalization therapy—Blurring the vision of a child's normally functioning eye to force the use of the weaker eye.
Retinoblastoma—Mutation of the cells of the retina, resulting in a malignant tumor.
Strabismus—"Cross eyes," or the misalignment of the eyes as a result of a lack of coordination between and among the muscles that control eye movement, all of which lie outside of the orbit of the eye.
White reflex—The appearance of a white (rather than red) reflection in the eye during ophthalmoscopy, a sign of retinoblastoma.

I. Description

From birth, the healthy child has very well-established sensory function—sight, hearing, smell, taste, and touch. Indeed, it is rare for children to experience deficits in any of the senses, especially smell, taste, and touch. Some children, however, do exhibit vision problems, including, of course, the ubiquitous issues of hyperopia and myopia. Vision assessments, as discussed in the growth and development chapters, are essential for screening for those problems, especially because children rarely realize when their vision is poor. Any child who does not pass the screening tests should be referred to an ophthalmic specialist for diagnostic assessments and for corrective lenses. Vision problems that are pediatric specific are discussed in this chapter: strabismus, amblyopia, and one of the few solid cancers seen in children, retinoblastoma. When auditory deficits exist, they may have been present at birth or they may result during childhood from medical or environmental causes.

II. Strabismus

A. Incidence.
  1. **Strabismus** (colloquially called "cross eyes") is present in about 5% to 6% of children.

B. Etiology.
  1. Strabismus may be present at birth as a result of a genetic cause or an environmental insult during pregnancy.

2. The problem may develop after birth from a number of causes, including extraocular tumors and infections.

C. Pathophysiology.

1. Eyes are misaligned as a result of a lack of coordination between and among the muscles that control eye movement, all of which lie outside of the orbit of the eye.
2. Signs and symptoms.
   a. In addition to eye misalignment, double vision, squinting, eye fatigue, headaches, loss of depth perception, and odd movements when attempting to focus on a specific image.

D. Diagnosis.

1. Clinical picture (i.e., the eyes do not appear to be looking at the same image) and the results of routine ophthalmic assessments are highly suggestive.
   a. Corneal light reflex test.
      i. Using the ophthalmoscope, the light is projected onto the corneas of both eyes simultaneously. The nurse should see the reflection of the light at the same place on each cornea.
      ii. If the reflection is asymmetric, strabismus should be suspected.
   b. Red reflex tests.
      i. First test:
         (1) Looking through the pupil of each eye independently using the ophthalmoscope from a short distance to determine that the reflex is present in each eye. This test assesses the ability of the retina to receive visual images.
      ii. Second test:
         (1) Holding the ophthalmoscope 2 to 3 ft from the child, the nurse should observe both red reflexes at the same time.
         (2) If the scope must be moved from side to side in order to view both red reflexes, strabismus should be suspected.
   c. Cover-uncover test.
      i. This test is not as reliable as the corneal light and red reflex tests, especially when the child is very young or uncooperative.
      ii. The child is asked to look at an object or a toy from a distance. While the child is looking with both eyes, the nurse covers one of the child's eyes and watches for any movement in the uncovered eye. The nurse repeats the process in the other eye.
      iii. Strabismus is suspected when movement is noted in the uncovered eye.
2. Specialized assessments performed by ophthalmic specialists are diagnostic.

E. Treatment.

1. In most cases, corrective lenses and eye exercises are prescribed.
2. Botox injections.
   a. Paralyzes strong muscles, allowing weaker muscles to strengthen.
3. Surgery, in extreme cases, is performed to tighten the weakened muscles.

F. Nursing considerations.

1. Risk for Disproportionate Growth/Risk for Ineffective Coping/Anxiety/Fear/Anger/Grieving/Deficient Knowledge.
   a. Provide parents the opportunity to verbalize grief, anger, and frustration over birthing a child with a physical defect.
   b. Educate the parents and child, if appropriate, regarding the pathophysiology of strabismus.
   c. Educate the parents and child, if appropriate, regarding the therapeutic management of strabismus.
      i. Temporary eyelid droop is sometimes noted with Botox injections.
   d. If indicated, provide preoperative teaching to the parents and child, if appropriate, regarding the surgical procedure.
   e. If indicated, allow the child and parents to express their anxieties, fears, and anger regarding the need for surgery.

III. Amblyopia

A. Incidence.

1. About 2% to 3% of children.
2. **Amblyopia** (often called "lazy eye") is frequently seen in children with strabismus.

B. Etiology.

1. Can result from any condition in which binocular vision is affected, as in strabismus.

C. Pathophysiology.

1. When binocular vision is affected, the brain reduces the image from the weaker eye and only attends to the image from the stronger eye.
2. Eventually, if not corrected, the weaker eye no longer sends an image to the brain (i.e., the child becomes blind in the weaker eye).
3. Signs and symptoms.
   a. Often, no symptoms are evident, but, if they are, symptoms often mimic strabismus, including:
      i. Squinting.
      ii. Odd movements when looking closely at an object.

iii. Crossing of the eyes.
iv. Loss of depth perception.

D. Diagnosis.
1. To enable the child to retain vision in both eyes, amblyopia must be diagnosed before the child enters the preschool period.
2. Specialized assessments performed by ophthalmic specialists are diagnostic.

E. Treatment.
1. **Occlusive therapy** (i.e., patching) or **penalization therapy** (i.e., blurring the vision) of the normally functioning eye. Because the child is no longer able to see from the well-functioning eye, he or she is forced to use the weaker eye to see.
   a. A drop of atropine ophthalmic 1% solution is usually prescribed for penalization therapy.
   b. The length of time each day and the number of years that the eye must be treated is determined individually.
2. Corrective lenses may also be prescribed.

F. Nursing considerations.
1. Risk for Disproportionate Growth/Risk for Ineffective Coping/Deficient Knowledge.
   a. Educate the parents and child, if appropriate, regarding the pathophysiology of amblyopia.
   b. Educate the parents and child, if appropriate, regarding the therapeutic regimen, including the rationale for the treatment, the exact intervention that has been prescribed, and the importance of following the prescribed timing of the intervention.
   c. Provide parents and child, if appropriate, with the opportunity to verbalize grief, anger, and frustration over the diagnosis and required therapy.
   d. If feasible, the child may be able to wear a patch or eyeglass lens that incorporates a design or image that is attractive to the child and will motivate the child to cooperate with the therapy.

IV. Conjunctivitis

A. Incidence.
1. **Conjunctivitis** (often called "pink eye") is the most common eye disease in children.

B. Etiology.
1. Bacteria.
   a. Chlamydia and gonorrhea, resulting in **ophthalmia neonatorum** in neonates.
   b. *Haemophilus influenzae* and *Streptococcus pneumoniae*, although the incidence of these bacteria has dropped with the addition of the Hib and pneumococcal vaccines to the childhood vaccination schedule.
2. Many viruses.
3. Allergies.
4. Injury (e.g., secondary to contact lens irritation).

C. Pathophysiology.
1. Inflammation of the **conjunctiva** of the eye (i.e., the translucent mucous membrane covering the eye and the under portion of the eyelid).

D. Diagnosis (Table 25.1).
1. Usually diagnosed on clinical evidence.
2. A culture of the discharge may be obtained.

E. Treatment (Table 25.1).

F. Nursing considerations.
1. Infection/Deficient Knowledge if viral or bacterial conjunctivitis.
   a. Educate the parents and child, if appropriate, regarding the markedly contagious nature of the disease.
      i. Meticulous handwashing should be maintained.
      ii. Transmission.
         (1) If problem starts in one eye, it is highly probable that it also will develop in the second eye.
         (2) Transmission to other family members is very possible.

Table 25.1 Clinical Evidence of Conjunctivitis

Origin	Signs/Symptoms	Classic Treatments
Bacterial	Child is concurrently experiencing a bacterial illness and/or the discharge from the eye is cloudy and pussy	*Prevention of ophthalmia neonatorum in neonates: either tetracycline (1%) or erythromycin (0.5%) ophthalmic ointment is administered within 1 hr of delivery* *Treatment of acute infection: ophthalmic antibiotic medication*
Viral	Child is concurrently experiencing a viral illness and/or the discharge from the eye is clear	*Ophthalmic antiviral medication*
Allergic	Child is concurrently experiencing allergic symptoms (e.g., seasonal symptoms, asthma)	*Ophthalmic antihistamine or, if needed, steroid medication*

(3) Child should be kept out of school until medication has been administered for a minimum of 24 hr.
(4) Towels, washcloths, medication bottles, and other such items should not be shared with other members of the family.

iii. Educate the parents and child, if appropriate, regarding the potential injury to the eye.
(1) Young child should be kept from rubbing his or her eyes by applying cotton mittens to the hands, by distracting the child, and through other such measures.
(2) If child wears contact lenses, the lenses should be removed and not worn until the infection is eradicated.
(3) If child wears eye makeup, it should be disposed of, replaced, and not worn until the infection is eradicated.

b. Educate the parents and child, if appropriate, regarding the therapeutic management.
i. Teach the parents to remove exudate from the eye using warm, wet cotton balls and wiping from the inner canthus to the outer canthus.
(1) Cotton balls should not be used more than once (i.e., a new cotton ball should be used for each swipe over the eye).
ii. Teach the parents to instill medication drops or ointment into the lower conjunctival sac at prescribed times.
iii. To prevent contaminating the medication, teach the parents the importance of preventing the medication container from touching any surface, especially the eye.

2. Impaired Tissue Integrity if allergic conjunctivitis.
a. Educate the parents and child, if appropriate, regarding medication administration.
b. Advise the parents and child, if appropriate, to soothe the eyes with cool, wet compresses.

V. Retinoblastoma

Solid tumor cancers are rare in children, but **retinoblastoma** (Fig. 25.1), although still rare, is seen in children.

A. Incidence.
1. Diagnosis is usually made during toddlerhood.
2. Fewer than 5% of all childhood cancers are retinoblastomas.

B. Etiology.
1. Genetic mutations.

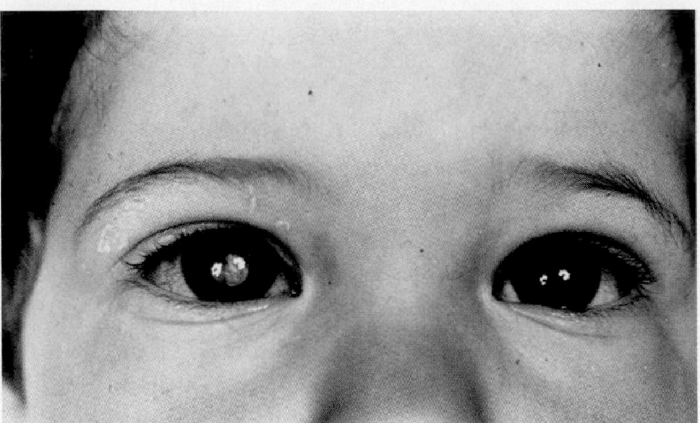

Fig 25.1 Young child with retinoblastoma.

a. Retinoblastoma is caused by genetic mutations in one or more cells in the retina of the eye.
b. Both spontaneous mutations and hereditary mutations are possible.
i. Hereditary retinoblastoma is transmitted via an autosomal dominant pattern.

C. Pathophysiology.
1. Mutation of one or more cells in the retina slowly increase in number, resulting in a malignant tumor of the retina.
2. The malignancy can metastasize to other areas of the eye as well as to the central nervous system, most notably the optic nerve and brain.
3. The tumor may be either unilateral or bilateral.
4. Children with retinoblastoma have a genetic predisposition for developing osteosarcoma, a form of bone cancer.
5. Signs and symptoms.
a. **White reflex** instead of the red reflex.

DID YOU KNOW?

Parents whose children have been diagnosed with retinoblastoma often report the abnormal appearance of white instead of red in their children's eyes in family photographs.

b. Strabismus.
c. Altered vision.
i. Although present, children rarely realize when their vision deteriorates.

D. Diagnosis.
1. When the white reflex is first seen, a thorough retinal examination is performed—usually under anesthesia—by an ophthalmologist.
2. Diagnosis is confirmed by ultrasound, CT, and/or MRI examination.

E. Treatment is dependent on the size of the tumor and the extent of metastasis, if any.
1. Laser therapy, cryotherapy, heat therapy, and/or radiation are being used to treat localized tumors.

a. Eyesight is often preserved with these interventions.
2. **Enucleation** (i.e., surgical removal of the eye) may be performed, especially if the eyesight is lost.
3. Chemotherapy is often administered before or in addition to other interventions.
a. If the eye is removed and the tumor has not metastasized, chemotherapy may not be indicated.
4. If metastasis has not occurred, prognosis is excellent.

F. Nursing considerations.
1. Anxiety/Fear/Pain.
a. Allow the child and parents to discuss their fears and concerns, including the fear of dying, although the likelihood of death is remote.
b. Query the parents/family about the use of complementary and alternative therapies, which may be beneficial or harmful.
c. Advise the parents and child, if appropriate, that when the eye is removed, a prosthetic eye will be prescribed after the site heals.
d. Provide needed care, employing principles of asepsis, following surgery:
i. Monitor the site for signs of bleeding, infection, and/or edema.
ii. Position eye patch over the operative site and educate the parents regarding actions to prevent possible injury and other complications.
iii. When the temporary and permanent prostheses are inserted into the socket, educate the parents regarding their care, including times and methods of removal and reinsertion, as well as cleaning methods.
e. Use age-appropriate pain assessment tools and assess pain on a regular basis.
f. Provide safe dosages of pain medication, as prescribed and as needed.
i. Narcotic analgesics should be administered following surgery.
g. Use nonpharmacological pain remedies in conjunction with pharmacological methods, if appropriate.
2. Deficient Knowledge/Risk for Injury.
a. Use pictures and models of the eye to provide the parents and child, if appropriate, with as complete an understanding as possible of where the tumor is located and how the tumor developed.
b. Keep the parents and child, if appropriate, informed regarding the prescribed treatments, including side effects of treatments.
c. Allow for need for repeated discussions related to the disease process and treatment needs.
d. Advise the family that children usually adapt easily to vision changes, including adapting to sight in one eye.
e. Advise the parents that the child should receive thorough eye and vision examinations yearly.
i. The child should be fitted with and wear corrective lenses, as needed.
3. Risk for Injury.
a. Parents should be encouraged to seek genetic counseling.
b. Child should be monitored closely for signs/symptoms of osteosarcoma or, if original tumor was unilateral, for signs/symptoms of retinoblastoma in the second eye.
4. If chemotherapeutic agents are administered, additional nursing diagnoses must be considered: Infection or Risk for Infection; Bleeding or Risk for Bleeding; Activity Intolerance/Fatigue; Risk for Imbalanced Nutrition: Less than Body Requirements; Risk for Deficient Fluid Volume; and Risk for Injury.
a. See the "Nursing considerations" section of acute lymphoblastic leukemia (ALL) in Chapter 18, "Nursing Care of the Child With Hematologic Illnesses."

VI. Hearing Deficit

A. Incidence.
1. Between 1 and 6 out of every 1,000 neonates is born with a hearing deficit.
2. Of the approximately three-quarters of a million Americans with hearing loss, about 8% are 18 years of age or younger.
3. The incidence of hearing loss among Americans is on the increase.

B. Etiology.
1. Congenital hearing loss can be caused by a number of factors, including genetic defects and environmental insults (e.g., prenatal rubella infection, maternal diabetes, birth trauma, prematurity).
2. Hearing loss that develops after birth also has a number of etiologies, including central nervous system infection, head trauma, medication toxicity, and exposure to loud sounds.

C. Pathophysiology: there are three main types of hearing loss.
1. Conductive: because of injury, inflammation, or blockage, sound is unable to be transmitted from the outer to the inner ear. Causes of conductive loss are often reversible, such as:

MAKING THE CONNECTION

One's ability to hear is measured on two different dimensions:

Decibel (db) level, or the loudness of a sound. Healthy individuals can hear sounds at a variety of db levels, from a faint whisper at 30 db to an extremely loud sound at over 150 db.

Frequency is measured in Hertz (Hz), or the pitch of a sound. Healthy individuals can hear sounds at a variety of frequencies, from very high pitches, or frequencies of 20,000 Hz, to very low pitches, or frequencies as low as 20 Hz.

Acquired hearing loss may be caused by repeated exposure to loud noise, which is measured in db levels. Sounds that are considered to be especially damaging to hearing are as varied as a kitchen blender and vacuum cleaner—all labeled as very loud—to a gas lawn mower, a motorcycle engine, and the maximum output from an MP3 player—all defined as extremely loud. Acquired hearing loss usually begins by affected individuals' inability to hear high frequencies.

a. Excessive earwax (cerumen).
b. Otitis media and otitis media with effusion.
c. Foreign body inserted into the ear, which is a relatively common occurrence in childhood.

2. Sensorineural: injury or defect of the configurations of the inner ear or of the auditory nerve.
3. Mixed: a combination of the sensorineural and conductive forms.

D. Diagnosis.

1. Neonates.
   a. The American Academy of Pediatrics recommends that every neonate have his or her hearing assessed prior to discharge after delivery.
   b. The babies are assessed by auditory brainstem response (ABR), otoacoustic emissions, or automated ABR testing.
2. Older children are diagnosed using sensitive audiologic tests as well as MRI and CT scans.

E. Treatment.

1. Preventing hearing loss.
   a. Prenatal infections, otitis media, and other serious infections should be treated appropriately.
   b. Remind children, especially adolescents, to keep environmental decibel levels at a safe level:
      i. Volume of MP3 players should be kept at a low level.
      ii. Earplugs or other sound-lowering equipment should be worn when loud noises are likely (e.g., around construction equipment, at music concerts, at fireworks displays).
2. Treating hearing loss.
   a. Reversible conductive hearing loss is treated by fixing the underlying problem (e.g., removing the cerumen or the foreign objective, treating the otitis).
   b. Sensorineural deficit is treated with hearing aids that amplify sounds or cochlear implants that transmit sounds to the auditory nerve.
      i. The precise type of intervention is determined individually.
      ii. There is a great deal of controversy in the deaf community, which views those who are deaf as being members of a unique culture, regarding the ethics of cochlear implants.
3. Speech therapy.
   a. Because speech development is contingent on the ability to hear sounds, young children with hearing impairment will need speech therapy.
4. Sign language, if needed.
   a. American Sign Language (ASL) is a unique language taught to the hearing impaired and to their families.

F. Nursing considerations.

1. Risk for Delayed Development.
   a. Screen the hearing and language development of children, using objective measures, at birth and at each well-child visit.
   b. Refer all children who exhibit hearing deficits and/or delayed language on screening tests to an audiologist for a thorough diagnostic assessment.
   c. Speak slowly and directly in the child's visual space to enhance lip reading and comprehension.
      i. Educate the parents and others interacting with the child to do the same.
   d. If the child uses ASL, use either visual aids or an interpreter when interacting with the child.
      i. Educate the parents and others interacting with the child to do the same.
2. Anxiety/Fear/Anger/Deficient Knowledge.
   a. Educate the parents and child, if appropriate, regarding actions that can prevent hearing loss.
      i. Prenatal infections, otitis media, and other serious infectious should be treated appropriately.
      ii. Remind children, especially adolescents, to keep environmental decibel levels at a safe level.

(1) Volume of MP3 players should be kept at a low level.
(2) Earplugs or other sound-lowering equipment should be worn when loud noises are likely (e.g., around construction equipment, at music concerts, at fireworks displays).

b. Allow the parents and child, if appropriate, to discuss their grief, anger, and fears if hearing loss has been diagnosed.

c. Refer the parents to a genetic counselor if a genetic etiology of the hearing loss is possible.

d. Educate the parents and child, if appropriate, regarding the etiology and extent of the hearing loss.

e. Educate the parents and child, if appropriate, regarding the care and use of hearing aids, as needed.

f. Educate the parents and child, if appropriate, regarding surgical procedure for cochlear implantation, if appropriate.

CASE STUDY: Putting It All Together

Mother brings 3-year, 6-month-old female to be assessed by an ophthalmologist

Subjective Data

- Volunteer at the child's daycare center performed a vision screening on the child. The child was able to identify images of animals and objects from a distance using her right eye and when using both eyes at the same time, but she was unable to identify the images when using her left eye alone.
- Mother states,
  - "I must say, I don't quite understand what the problem is. My daughter never seems to have any difficulty seeing things, and she doesn't complain."
  - "Sometimes she does move her head a little to one side when she is looking at a picture book."

Objective Data

Nursing Assessment

- Since birth, the child's well-child checks have been within normal limits, including weight, height, and head circumferences all at the 50th percentile.
- Child is up to date on immunizations.

Complete Ophthalmic Examination

- Slight strabismus
- Marked difference in visual ability between the right and left eye
- Diagnosis: mild amblyopia

Health-Care Provider's Orders

- One percent atropine ophthalmic drops: one drop to right eye each morning
- Return for follow-up appointment in 1 month

Case Study Questions

A. What subjective assessments indicate that this client is experiencing a health alteration?

1. ______________________________
2. ______________________________

B. What *objective* assessments indicate that this client is experiencing a health alteration?

1. ______________________________
2. ______________________________

C. After analyzing the data that has been collected, what **primary** nursing diagnosis should the nurse assign to this client?

1. ______________________________

D. What interventions should the nurse plan and/or implement to meet this child's and her family's needs?

1. ______________________________
2. ______________________________
3. ______________________________

Continued

CASE STUDY: Putting It All Together *cont'd*

Case Study Questions

E. What client outcomes should the nurse evaluate regarding the effectiveness of the nursing interventions?

1. ______________________________
2. ______________________________
3. ______________________________

F. What physiological characteristics should the child exhibit after treatment?

1. ______________________________

G. What psychological characteristics should the child and family exhibit before being discharged home?

1. ______________________________

REVIEW QUESTIONS

1. The nurse in a preschool is assessing the vision and hearing of the 3- and 4-year-old children. Which of the following findings would indicate that a child may have amblyopia? The child is unable to:
1. see objects at far distances.
2. hear music played at low decibel levels.
3. hear sounds at high frequency levels.
4. see clearly out of one eye.

2. The nurse in a preschool suspects that a 3-year-old child may have mild strabismus. Which of the following signs/symptoms exhibited by the child has the nurse noted? **Select all that apply.**
1. Eye squinting
2. Complaining of headaches
3. Eyeballs protruding from the eye socket
4. White reflex on ophthalmic examination
5. Moving from side to side when looking at pictures in a book

3. A nurse is assessing a child's eyes by using the corneal light reflex test. Which of the following actions should the nurse perform?
1. Move the ophthalmoscope laterally from each ear toward the nose and observe the pupils for the corneal reflex to appear.
2. Have the child watch the light as the ophthalmoscope is moved in a figure eight pattern and observe for the corneal reflex.
3. Holding the ophthalmoscope a few feet from the child, aim the light at the corneas and observe for symmetry of the light reflections.
4. Holding the ophthalmoscope a few inches from each eye, look through the scope at the eye and observe for the corneal light reflection.

4. An ophthalmologist recommends that a young girl with strabismus receive Botox (onabotulinumtoxinA) injections. The child's mother asks the nurse, "Why does my child need Botox injections? I thought only women who want to look younger get those." Which of the following responses by the nurse is appropriate?
1. "You are correct. The physician is recommending the injection so your daughter's eyes will no longer look different from other children's eyes."
2. "Botox is administered for many reasons. In this case, the medicine will weaken the muscles around the eye that are making your daughter's eye turn."
3. "Botox is administered for many reasons. The medicine is being recommended for your daughter in order to reduce her vision in her strong eye to make her use her weak eye."
4. "You are correct. Children with strabismus often develop wrinkles around the eye that is turned, so the doctor is prescribing the medicine to prevent those wrinkles from developing."

5. A nurse is advising the parents of a child with strabismus who is to receive Botox (onabotulinumtoxinA) regarding possible side effects from the medication. Which of the following items should the nurse include?
1. Paralysis of the optic nerve
2. Drooping of the eyelid
3. Blindness in the affected eye
4. Pupillary dysfunction

6. A baby is 30 minutes old. To prevent ophthalmia neonatorum, the nurse performs which of the following actions?
1. Inserts erythromycin 0.5% eye ointment in both eyes
2. Injects ampicillin 100 mg intramuscularly in the vastus lateralis
3. Cleanses the eyes with a dilute antimicrobial wash
4. Instills sterile saline eye drops bilaterally

7. A toddler has been diagnosed with bacterial conjunctivitis. Which of the following instructions should the nurse include when teaching the parents about the diagnosis? **Select all that apply.**
   1. Child's towel and washcloth should not be shared with others.
   2. Medication should be administered into the inner canthus of the eye.
   3. Eyes should be cleansed from the outer canthus to the inner canthus.
   4. Meticulous handwashing should be performed by all family members.
   5. Child should be kept home from school until all discharge disappears from the eyes.

8. A 16-year-old adolescent has been diagnosed with viral conjunctivitis. Which of the following actions should the nurse include in the teaching session?
   1. Inform the teen that the communicability of the infection is minimal.
   2. Advise the teen that contact lenses should not be worn until the infection is fully treated.
   3. Recommend that the teen wear white cotton mittens to bed at night.
   4. Warn the teen to refrain from using any makeup on the eyes for one full month.

9. Based on which of the following comments made by a child's parents would a preschool nurse suspect that the 2½-year-old child may have retinoblastoma of the right eye?
   1. "Every time we take a picture of our child, we see a white spot in her right eye and a red spot in her left eye."
   2. "When our child looks at picture books, she always closes her right eye."
   3. "We have noticed that our child's right pupil stays dilated even when it is very sunny outside."
   4. "The white part of our child's right eye looks like it has blood in it."

10. A child has been diagnosed with retinoblastoma. The nurse should recommend that the primary health-care provider refer the family to which of the following professionals?
    1. Genetic counselor
    2. Neurosurgeon
    3. Orthopedist
    4. Clinical psychologist

11. A 2-year-old who has been diagnosed with retinoblastoma of the left eye is to have the eye removed. Which of the following statements should the nurse include in the preoperative teaching session?
    1. Child will require occupational therapy to develop normal depth perception using the remaining eye.
    2. Child will be prescribed a prosthetic eye once the child turns 6 years of age.
    3. Child will wear an eye patch over the surgical site for about 1 week.
    4. Child will have a permanent prosthetic eye sutured in place immediately following the removal.

12. Five neonates were delivered in a hospital's obstetric unit. Nurses in the neonatal nursery and in the pediatric clinic should carefully assess which of the babies for a hearing deficit? **Select all that apply.**
    1. 33 weeks' gestation, mother was diagnosed with pneumonia at time of delivery.
    2. 35 weeks' gestation, mother had rubella in the 1st trimester of her pregnancy.
    3. 37 weeks' gestation, mother has been a type I diabetic since her adolescence.
    4. 39 weeks' gestation, mother experienced shoulder dystocia during delivery.
    5. 41 weeks' gestation, mother had urinary tract infection in her 2nd trimester.

13. A 17-year-old woman is being seen in the clinic for a yearly checkup. The nurse is educating the young woman regarding actions to decrease the possibility of her developing hearing loss. Which of the following recommendations would be appropriate for the nurse to include?
    1. Only use hands-free telephoning while driving in a car.
    2. Refuse to mow the lawn for her parents.
    3. Use ear plugs when attending music concerts.
    4. Wear a safety helmet when riding on a motorcycle.

14. A nurse working on a pediatric clinical unit is assigned to care for an 11-year-old child with a profound hearing deficit who is in skeletal traction. Which of the following actions should the nurse perform?

1. Clap hands behind the child's field of vision to see whether the child responds.
2. Look directly into the child's face whenever speaking with the child.
3. Educate the child regarding the success that some realize from cochlear implant surgery.
4. Assess the tympanic membrane in each ear for redness and bulging.

15. A 3-year-old child, with a history of frequent ear infections, has been diagnosed with mixed hearing loss. For which of the following complications should the nurse carefully assess the child?

1. Inflammation of the mandible
2. Serosanguineous discharge from the ear
3. Recurring temporal headaches
4. Delayed language development

REVIEW ANSWERS

1. ANSWER: 4

Rationale:

1. Inability to see objects at far distances is consistent with a diagnosis of myopia, not amblyopia.
2. Inability to hear music played at low decibel levels is consistent with a hearing deficit, not amblyopia.
3. Inability to hear music played at high frequencies is consistent with a hearing deficit, not amblyopia.
4. **Inability to see clearly out of one of eye is consistent with a diagnosis of amblyopia.**

TEST-TAKING TIP: Amblyopia is a visual disorder of young children characterized by an inability to see, employing binocular vision. Those with amblyopia, therefore, selectively see only out of one eye, suppressing the image from the other eye.

Content Area: *Pediatrics*
Integrated Processes: *Nursing Process: Assessment*
Client Need: *Health Promotion and Maintenance: Health Screening*
Cognitive Level: *Application*

2. ANSWER: 1, 2, and 5

Rationale:

1. **Eye squinting is a symptom of strabismus.**
2. **Headaches are a symptom of strabismus.**
3. Eyeballs protruding from the eye socket are not seen in children with strabismus.
4. White reflex on ophthalmic examination is not a symptom of strabismus.
5. **Children with strabismus often do move from side to side when looking at pictures in a book.**

TEST-TAKING TIP: The orbits of the eyes of children with strabismus, or cross eyes, are misaligned. Because of the strain placed on the eyes, children exhibit a number of symptoms, including squinting, headaches, and moving in order to see an image.

Content Area: *Pediatrics*
Integrated Processes: *Nursing Process: Assessment*
Client Need: *Physiological Integrity: Physiological Adaption: Alteration of Body Systems*
Cognitive Level: *Application*

3. ANSWER: 3

Rationale:

1. This is not the correct action.
2. This is not the correct action.
3. **The nurse should hold the ophthalmoscope a few feet from the child, aim the light at the corneas, and observe for symmetry of the reflections.**
4. This is not the correct action.

TEST-TAKING TIP: When performing an ophthalmic assessment, the nurse should assess for the red reflex twice: 1) looking through the pupil of each eye independently using the ophthalmoscope from a short distance to determine that the reflex is present in each eye and 2) looking at both eyes simultaneously from a distance of a few feet to make sure that both retinas are receiving an image at the same time. In addition, the nurse should perform the corneal light reflex test to determine whether the light is reflected symmetrically for the corneas. Both the second red reflex test and the corneal reflection test are employed to assess for strabismus.

Content Area: *Pediatrics*
Integrated Processes: *Nursing Process: Assessment*
Client Need: *Physiological Integrity: Physiological Adaption: Alteration of Body Systems*
Cognitive Level: *Application*

4. ANSWER: 2

Rationale:

1. Botox is not administered to improve the appearance of the child.
2. **This statement is correct. The Botox is administered to weaken the muscles around the eye that are making the eye deviate.**
3. Botox is not administered to blur the image of the child's eye.
4. Botox is not administered to improve the appearance of the child.

TEST-TAKING TIP: The muscles of the eye are functioning asymmetrically in a child with strabismus. The muscles on one side of the eye are stronger than the muscles on the other side of the eye. Botox, a paralyzing agent, is sometimes injected into the stronger set of muscles, weakening their effect. The weaker muscles then are able to strengthen. The expectation is that once the Botox is metabolized, the muscles will function symmetrically.

Content Area: *Pediatrics*
Integrated Processes: *Nursing Process: Implementation*
Client Need: *Physiological Integrity: Pharmacological and Parenteral Therapies: Expected Actions/Outcomes*
Cognitive Level: *Application*

5. ANSWER: 2

Rationale:

1. Paralysis of the optic nerve is not an expected side effect.
2. **Drooping of the eyelid is often seen when Botox is administered for strabismus.**
3. Blindness in the affected eye is not an expected side effect.
4. Pupillary dysfunction is not an expected side effect.

TEST-TAKING TIP: Botox is a paralyzing agent. When injected into the muscles of the eye, it is not uncommon for the eyelid on the eye to droop. Once the medication is metabolized, however, the drooping usually subsides.

Content Area: *Pediatrics*
Integrated Processes: *Nursing Process: Implementation*
Client Need: *Physiological Integrity: Pharmacological and Parenteral Therapies: Adverse Effects/Contraindications/ Side Effects/Interactions*
Cognitive Level: *Application*

6. ANSWER: 1

Rationale:

1. **The nurse inserts erythromycin 0.5% eye ointment in both eyes.**

2. Ampicillin is not administered to prevent ophthalmia neonatorum.
3. Neonates' eyes are cleansed only with warm water. The cleansing will not prevent ophthalmia neonatorum.
4. Sterile saline eye drops are not administered to prevent ophthalmia neonatorum.

TEST-TAKING TIP: Ophthalmia neonatorum is characterized by conjunctivitis of the eyes of the newborn resulting from exposure either to chlamydia or to gonorrhea during the birthing process. To prevent the disorder, all babies are administered either ophthalmic erythromycin 0.5% or ophthalmic tetracycline 1% in both eyes within one hour of delivery.
Content Area: Newborn
Integrated Processes: Nursing Process: Implementation
Client Need: Physiological Integrity: Pharmacological and Parenteral Therapies: Expected Actions/Outcomes
Cognitive Level: Application

7. ANSWER: 1 and 4
Rationale:
1. The child should not share a towel or washcloth with others.
2. The medication should be administered into the lower conjunctival sac.
3. Eyes should be cleansed from the inner canthus to the outer canthus.
4. Meticulous handwashing should be performed by all family members.
5. Child should be kept home from school until the child has received medication for a full 24 hr.

TEST-TAKING TIP: Conjunctivitis is highly contagious. To decrease the potential of transmission, the child should not share a towel or other items with others in the family, and every family member should practice meticulous handwashing.
Content Area: Pediatrics
Integrated Processes: Nursing Process: Implementation; Teaching/Learning
Client Need: Physiological Integrity: Physiological Adaption: Alteration of Body Systems
Cognitive Level: Application

8. ANSWER: 2
Rationale:
1. Conjunctivitis is highly communicable.
2. This statement is correct. Contact lenses should not be worn until the infection is fully treated.
3. Because of the teen's age, this is not needed. It is recommended that young children wear white cotton mittens to bed at night to decrease the possibility of their rubbing their eyes during sleep.
4. To refrain from using eye makeup for a full month is not warranted. All eye makeup should be replaced in case it has been contaminated, and it should not be warn until the infection clears.

TEST-TAKING TIP: Because the offending bacteria or virus could be present on mascara applicators or other eye makeup, all makeup used on the eyes should be replaced if a diagnosis of conjunctivitis has been made.
Content Area: Pediatrics
Integrated Processes: Nursing Process: Implementation; Teaching/Learning
Client Need: Physiological Integrity: Physiological Adaption: Alteration of Body Systems
Cognitive Level: Application

9. ANSWER: 1
Rationale:
1. A white reflection to light rather than the normal red reflex is a strong indicator of retinoblastoma.
2. Deliberate closing of the eye is not characteristic of retinoblastoma.
3. Pupil dilation in response to sunlight is not characteristic of retinoblastoma.
4. Subconjunctival hemorrhages, hemorrhages seen on the sclera of the eye, are not characteristic of retinoblastoma.

TEST-TAKING TIP: A retinoblastoma is a solid tumor originating from abnormal cells in the retina. In response to light, the tumor reflects a white image rather than the normal red reflex of the retina.
Content Area: Pediatrics
Integrated Processes: Nursing Process: Implementation
Client Need: Physiological Integrity: Physiological Adaption: Alteration of Body Systems
Cognitive Level: Application

10. ANSWER: 1
Rationale:
1. The nurse should recommend that the primary health-care provider refer the family to a genetic counselor.
2. The family need not be referred to a neurosurgeon.
3. The family need not be referred to a plastic surgeon.
4. The family need not be referred to a clinical psychologist.

TEST-TAKING TIP: Retinoblastomas, as are all cancers, are genetic in origin. Although many of the tumors result from spontaneous mutations, some are hereditary tumors. Genetic counselors should be consulted to determine whether the parents have an increased probability of conceiving another child with a retinoblastoma.
Content Area: Pediatrics
Integrated Processes: Nursing Process: Implementation
Client Need: Health Promotion and Maintenance: Health Promotion/Disease Prevention
Cognitive Level: Application

11. ANSWER: 3
Rationale:
1. This statement is incorrect. Young children who lose sight in one eye usually adapt very easily, with no need for therapy.
2. The child will be prescribed a prosthetic eye shortly after the surgery.
3. This statement is correct. The child will wear a protective eye patch over the surgical site for about 1 week.
4. This statement is incorrect. Eye prostheses are removable.

TEST-TAKING TIP: The child will have a prosthesis designed to replicate the child's other eye and fit into the child's socket. Before the prosthesis is ready, and while the socket is healing, the child will wear a protective eye patch.
Content Area: *Pediatrics*
Integrated Processes: *Nursing Process: Implementation*
Client Need: *Physiological Integrity: Physiological Adaption: Alteration of Body Systems*
Cognitive Level: *Application*

12. ANSWER: 1, 2, 3, and 4
Rationale:
1. This baby is preterm. The baby is at high risk for a hearing deficit.
2. This baby's mother had rubella in her first trimester. The baby is at high risk for a hearing deficit.
3. This baby's mother is a type I diabetic. The baby is at high risk for a hearing deficit.
4. This baby's delivery was complicated by dystocia. The baby is likely to have experienced trauma during the delivery. The baby is at high risk for a hearing deficit.
5. This baby's gestational age is within normal limits, and, although this baby's mother had a urinary tract infection in her second trimester, the baby is not at high risk for a hearing deficit.
TEST-TAKING TIP: Neonates who are at high risk for hearing deficits should be assessed carefully at birth and in early childhood. Factors that put children at high risk include both genetic and environmental issues.
Content Area: *Pediatrics*
Integrated Processes: *Nursing Process: Assessment*
Client Need: *Physiological Integrity: Physiological Adaption: Alteration of Body Systems*
Cognitive Level: *Application*

13. ANSWER: 3
Rationale:
1. Using hands-free telephoning while driving in a car is a safety recommendation. It will not decrease the potential of her developing hearing loss.
2. Lawn mower noise can be injurious, but the young woman could use earplugs while completing the chore. She should not be advised to refuse to mow the lawn.
3. The young woman should be encouraged to use earplugs when attending music concerts.
4. Safety helmets are worn to protect the head from injury during a motorcycle accident. They are not designed to protect the wearer's hearing.
TEST-TAKING TIP: A number of everyday activities can be damaging to one's hearing. Adolescents, especially, should be encouraged to protect their ears by taking such measures as wearing ear plugs in very loud situations and keeping the volume low on their MP3 players.
Content Area: *Pediatrics*
Integrated Processes: *Nursing Process: Implementation; Teaching/Learning*
Client Need: *Health Promotion and Maintenance: Health Promotion/Disease Prevention*
Cognitive Level: *Application*

14. ANSWER: 2
Rationale:
1. There is no need to assess the child's hearing. The child has already been diagnosed with a profound hearing deficit.
2. The nurse should look directly into the child's face whenever speaking with the child. Lip reading is often employed by the hearing impaired as a means of understanding oral communication.
3. It is inappropriate for the nurse to educate the child about cochlear implant surgery.
4. There is nothing in the question that implies that the child has an ear infection.
TEST-TAKING TIP: Although this child may be a candidate for a cochlear implant, it is inappropriate for the nurse to speak with an 11-year-old child regarding an invasive intervention. The nurse could, however, discuss the therapy with the child's parents.
Content Area: *Pediatrics*
Integrated Processes: *Nursing Process: Implementation*
Client Need: *Physiological Integrity: Physiological Adaption: Alteration of Body Systems*
Cognitive Level: *Application*

15. ANSWER: 4
Rationale:
1. The child is not at high risk for inflammation of the mandible.
2. The child is not at high risk for serosanguineous discharge from the ear.
3. The child is not at high risk for recurring temporal headaches.
4. The child is at high risk for delayed language development.
TEST-TAKING TIP: Children with hearing loss, whether conductive, sensorineural, or mixed, are at high risk for language delays. To learn to speak, children must hear the sounds spoken by those around them and then learn to replicate those sounds. If the children are unable to hear the sounds, they will be unable to replicate the sounds.
Content Area: *Pediatrics*
Integrated Processes: *Nursing Process: Assessment*
Client Need: *Physiological Integrity: Physiological Adaption: Alteration of Body Systems*
Cognitive Level: *Application*

Comprehensive Final Exam

1. A 2-year-old child has been admitted to the pediatric emergency department following a head injury. The nurse should monitor the child for which of the following signs/symptoms?
   1. Bulging fontanels
   2. Vomiting
   3. Hypotension
   4. Protruding tongue

2. A nurse is educating the parents and a child regarding the actions they must take to make sure that the child's diet is gluten free. The nurse's action is based on which of the following pathophysiological changes?
   1. Elevated levels of histamine in the bloodstream
   2. Atrophy of the villi of the gastrointestinal tract
   3. Lack of enervation to the distal portion of the bowel
   4. Peritonitis secondary to perforated esophageal varices

3. A girl, 15 years old, is in the school nurse's office. The nurse queries the young woman about alcohol consumption. The teenager states, "Yeah, I drink some with my friends. Those laws that say I can't drink are lame!" Which of the following responses would be best for the nurse to reply?
   1. "You may think they're lame, but they are still the law."
   2. "I would like to know who your drinking friends are."
   3. "I should call your parents about your behavior."
   4. "It worries me that you're drinking alcohol with friends."

4. The nurse is educating the parents of a child who has just been diagnosed with phenylketonuria (PKU). Which of the following information should be included in the educational session?
   1. The child must consume a diet low in fats and cholesterol.
   2. The child will develop no secondary sex characteristics during puberty.
   3. The child must take medication at the same time each day.
   4. The child will be able to pass the recessive gene to a future child.

5. A male baby is born at 29 weeks' gestation. Which of the following complications of prematurity would the nurse expect the child to exhibit? **Select all that apply.**
   1. Simian crease
   2. Hypospadias
   3. Cryptorchidism
   4. Negative Babinski
   5. Patent ductus arteriosus

6. A 12-month-old child, whose parents have opted not to have the child immunized or to send the child to day care, has had 5 watery stools in the past 4 hours. The nurse suspects that the child is infected with which of the following pathogens?
   1. Shigella
   2. Salmonella
   3. Giardia
   4. Rotavirus

7. A 4-year-old child has just returned to the pediatric floor following a cardiac catheterization. Which of the following actions should the nurse perform at this time?
1. Administer oxygen via facemask at 8 to 10 liters per minute.
2. Assess the child's upper extremities for color change every 5 to 10 minutes.
3. Keep the child's affected extremity straight for the next 4 to 6 hours.
4. Continue the infusion of whole blood for another 1 to 2 hours.

8. A nurse is assessing a 2-month-old infant in the pediatric clinic. Which of the following behaviors would the nurse expect the child to exhibit?
1. Voluntarily grasping a rattle
2. Smiling socially
3. Cooing and babbling
4. Playing with hands and feet

9. A 6-month-old infant has been diagnosed with atopic dermatitis. The nurse educates the parents to avoid performing which of the following actions?
1. Providing the child with plastic toys for play
2. Using softeners when laundering the child's clothing
3. Introducing solid foods into the child's diet
4. Covering the crib mattress with cotton bedding

10. A nurse has identified the nursing diagnosis, Caregiver Role Strain, for a mother of a patient who has just been admitted to the pediatric floor. In which of the following patient-care situations would the nursing diagnosis be most appropriate?
1. 3-year-old child in remission from acute lymphoblastic leukemia admitted for a follow-up bone marrow biopsy
2. 6-year-old child with viral diarrhea admitted for intravenous fluid and electrolyte replacement therapy
3. 9-year-old child with cystic fibrosis and acute bacterial pneumonia admitted for intravenous antibiotics and respiratory therapy
4. 12-year-old child diagnosed with idiopathic scoliosis admitted for surgical placement of a corrective rod

11. A 5-year-old child being seen in the pediatric clinic has been diagnosed with fifth disease (erythema infectiosum). Which of the following information should the nurse convey to the parent about the disease?
1. Whenever the child plays in the sun, the child's cheeks will become redder.
2. The child must be kept home from school for the next 24 hours.
3. Mothers of infants who have been in contact with the child should be monitored very carefully for signs of the disease.
4. If the child's temperature does not return to normal within the next 24 hours, the child should return to the clinic for a blood test.

12. A nurse is counseling a woman during a preconception counseling visit regarding environmental factors that would place the child at high risk for a cognitive deficit. Which of the following situations should the nurse include in the teaching session? **Select all that apply.**
1. Alcohol consumption during pregnancy
2. Fetal hypoxia during labor and delivery
3. Neonatal febrile illness in the early neonatal period
4. Lead ingestion by the father within 1 month prior to conception
5. Cigarette smoking by the father within 1 year prior to conception

13. A 16-year-old soccer player has been diagnosed with a dislocated right shoulder. Which of the following signs/symptoms would the nurse expect to see? **Select all that apply.**
1. Pain
2. Edema
3. Bruising
4. Bleeding
5. Reduced range of motion

14. A 3-year-old child is to receive a medication that is available only as an oral tablet. Which of the following actions should the nurse perform at this time?
1. Administer the tablet, and give the child a favorite drink with which to swallow it.
2. Crush the tablet, pour the powder in a medicine cup, and give the child a favorite drink with which to swallow the powder.
3. Crush the tablet, mix it with a teaspoon of applesauce, and give the mixture to the child to swallow.
4. Crush the tablet, mix it with a juice cup filled with a favorite drink, and give the mixture to the child to swallow.

15. A 5-year-old girl is due to receive a vaccination. Which of the following statements would be appropriate for the nurse to make prior to the injection?
1. "Would you like the medicine injection in your right or left arm?"
2. "Would you like me to put the needle into your arm fast or slow?"
3. "I am going to hold your arm very tight to help you not to move."
4. "I know that you are a big girl and will be brave during the shot."

16. A child is being assessed for readiness for kindergarten by the school nurse. Which of the following gross motor skills should the 5-year-old child be expected to perform?
1. Perform the broad jump
2. Walk on tiptoes
3. Ride a tricycle
4. Skip using alternate feet

17. A school nurse suspects that a 17-year-old football player is contemplating suicide. Which of the following behaviors exhibited by the adolescent might the nurse have observed? **Select all that apply.** The adolescent:
1. has given away his favorite football jersey.
2. recently has started dating a new girlfriend.
3. brags about his football team to his brother and sister.
4. talks about actors and actresses who have recently died.
5. has stated that he has decided to play baseball in the spring.

18. A 10-month-old infant has been diagnosed with acute otitis media. The baby has had symptoms, including a temperature of 104.4°F for 36 hours. Which of the following actions would be appropriate for the nurse to educate the parents to perform? **Select all that apply**
1. Administer prescribed antibiotic via oral syringe.
2. Apply warm or cold compresses to the affected area.
3. Administer over-the-counter cough suppressant per published directions.
4. Cleanse the area with a dilute solution of hydrogen peroxide.
5. Isolate the infant from other children until the child has been on medication for 24 hr.

19. A mother telephones the school nurse and states, "This morning, my 8-year-old son told me that he never wants to go to school again. What has happened?" In response, the nurse should encourage the mother to ask the child how he feels about which of the following? **Select all that apply**
1. His teacher.
2. His performance in school.
3. His friends.
4. His bus ride to school.
5. His lunches he eats at school.

20. The nurse is advising the parents of a school-age child regarding an appropriate discipline for their child who was caught stealing candy from a neighborhood store. Which of the following actions should the nurse recommend the parents take?
1. Spank the child on the buttocks.
2. Ground the child for one week.
3. Make the child return the candy to the owner.
4. Prevent the child from eating dinner.

21. A nurse is assessing a 13-month-old child in the pediatric clinic. During the assessment, the parents comment, "Even though our child is over a year of age, she still likes to go to bed with a bottle of formula. It calms her down so that she is able to fall asleep." Which of the following responses would be most important for the nurse to make?
1. "I understand. Children this age often need something to soothe them when they are settling down to sleep."
2. "I am not surprised that your child still drinks from a bottle before sleep, but does your child drink from a cup when she eats her meals during the day?"
3. "I understand. I would, however, recommend that you put water in the bottle at bedtime rather than formula."
4. "I know how much babies love their formula, but once they reach one year of age they can start to drink cow's milk."

22. A neonate is admitted to the high-risk nursery with a diagnosis of meningomyelocele. Which of the following actions should the nurse perform at this time?
1. Position the neonate on his or her right side.
2. Cover the lumbosacrum with a moist and sterile dressing.
3. Assist with the insertion of a central line.
4. Contact respiratory therapy to intubate the newborn.

23. A 6-month-old child has just been diagnosed with congenital hypothyroidism. Which of the following signs/symptoms would the nurse expect the child to exhibit?
1. Developmental delay
2. Strabismus
3. Projectile vomiting
4. Dyspnea

24. A baby in the emergency department is in respiratory distress. Which of the following blood gas results would the nurse expect the child's laboratory report to show?
1. pO_2: 90 mm Hg
2. pCO_2: 30 mm Hg
3. HCO_3: 25 mEq/L
4. pH: 7.30

25. A child with hypospadias is post-op surgical repair. For which of the following signs/symptoms should the nurse carefully monitor the child?
1. Cloudy urine
2. Hypertension
3. Macular rash
4. Pulmonary edema

26. A nurse is educating a breastfeeding mother regarding feeding her 12-month-old daughter who has been diagnosed with mild dehydration from diarrhea. The mother states that the child's appetite has not changed significantly during the illness. Which of the following statements would be appropriate for the nurse to make to the mother during the teaching session?
1. "Pump and dump your breast milk and replace your daughter's feedings with oral rehydration therapy (ORT)."
2. "Feed your daughter oral rehydration therapy (ORT) after each breastfeeding to make sure she is getting enough protein."
3. "Have your daughter drink oral rehydration therapy (ORT), but only if she refuses to breastfeed."
4. "Give your daughter oral rehydration therapy (ORT) along with lean meats, cooked vegetables, and breast milk."

27. A 13-month-old child, whose weight is 23 lb and length is 30.5 in., is placed on ferrous sulfate 50 mg PO daily for iron-deficiency anemia. The pediatric dosage recommendation is 3 to 5 mg/kg/day either once per day or in two divided doses. The medication is available as 125 mg/1 mL. Which of the following actions by the nurse is appropriate at this time?
1. Request an order change because the order is unsafe as written.
2. Request an order change to twice a day to improve absorption of the iron.
3. Teach the mother how to draw up 0.4 mL of fluid into an oral syringe.
4. Teach the mother how to draw up 1.25 mL of fluid into a medication dropper.

28. An HIV-positive, sexually active adolescent male is being seen during a clinic visit. The young man states, "I met a friend who is also HIV positive. I am finally free to be me." Which of the following responses is appropriate for the nurse to make?
1. "I am happy for you. You must be happy not to have to worry about your disease anymore."
2. "This is good news, but I do want to remind you to continue to wear condoms when having intercourse."
3. "Congratulations. Do you know whether or not your friend has any symptoms of AIDS?"
4. "What a wonderful surprise. Did you meet your friend at an HIV awareness party?"

29. A nurse is assessing a 6-month-old infant in the pediatric clinic. Which of the following abnormal findings should the nurse report to the child's primary health-care provider?
1. Exhibits a grasp reflex
2. Falls over from a sitting position
3. Follows no commands
4. Drinks formula from a cup

30. A child has been diagnosed with impetigo. Which of the following signs/symptoms would the nurse expect to see?
1. Encrusted vesicles
2. Red and scaly lesions
3. Painful abrasions
4. Alopecic scalp

31. A 17-year-old young woman is seen in the dermatology clinic with severe acne. Which of the following statements should the nurse include when educating the young woman regarding her diagnosis?
1. "You should wash your face twice daily with a dilute bleach solution."
2. "You will need to manually remove any black heads that appear on your face."
3. "Acne is caused by a virus for which there is no cure."
4. "Acne often worsens when cosmetics are worn."

32. The parent of a 2-year-old child telephones the pediatric clinic and states, "Our child has been exposed to another child with roseola. Is there anything we should know about the disease?" Which of the following information should the nurse convey to the parent regarding the disease?
1. When the rash disappears, the parent should expect the child's temperature to rise.
2. When the child's temperature rises, the parent should monitor the child carefully for febrile seizures.
3. Once a child has had roseola, he or she is at high risk for recurrences of the disease.
4. As long as the child's rash is present, he or she is highly contagious and must be kept on droplet precautions.

33. A 4-year-old with Down syndrome is being seen in the pediatric clinic. The nurse reminds the parents to seek immediate care if the child exhibits which of the following signs/symptoms?
1. Upper respiratory illness
2. Pendulous abdomen
3. Elevated temperature
4. Protruding brow

34. A 10-year-old, who has fallen while rollerblading, is seen in the emergency room complaining of pain. The nurse notes large contusions on both legs and both arms. The mother states, "I know that he has broken something!" The nurse examining the child recommends to the primary health-care provider that x-rays be taken. Which of the following is the best rationale for the nurse's action?
1. The extent of the soft tissue injuries
2. The child's complaints of pain
3. The mother's statement
4. The accuracy of the diagnostic method

35. A nurse is about to begin a physical examination of an infant who is sleeping in the mother's arms. Which of the following actions should the nurse perform first?
1. Auscultate the lung and heart sounds.
2. Palpate the fontanels.
3. Place the infant on the examining table.
4. Percuss the abdomen.

36. A nurse is questioning the parents regarding their 4-year-old's behaviors. The parents state, "Our child is great until night time when she cries because she insists that there is an alligator under the bed. She has never seen a real alligator, and we don't know where she got that crazy idea!" Which of the following statements is appropriate for the nurse to make?
1. "That is pretty unusual. Has she ever been to the zoo? Maybe she saw an alligator there that frightened her."
2. "That is pretty unusual. Does she watch television? Maybe there was a story in the news about a child being attacked by an alligator?"
3. "Many children her age have night fears. If you give into her fears, though, she will continue to have night fears well into her school-age years."
4. "Many children her age have night fears. If you look under her bed with her and give her a night light, she should go to bed more easily."

37. A child, who has been diagnosed with attention deficit hyperactivity disorder (ADHD), is being prescribed a stimulant. The child should be monitored carefully for which of the following serious side effects?
1. Jaundice
2. Arrhythmia
3. Dyspnea
4. Anasarca

38. A 2-year-old child is suspected of having acute epiglottitis. Which of the following signs/symptoms would the nurse expect to see? **Select all that apply**
1. Vomiting
2. Weight loss
3. Tachycardia
4. Nasal flaring
5. Inspiratory stridor

39. A nurse, who is caring for a chronically ill 6-year-old child in a long-term care facility, has identified the following nursing diagnosis for the child: Ineffective Coping as evidenced by detachment behaviors. When the child's parents left the hospital after a visit, which of the following assessments did the nurse observe? The child:
1. cried and begged the parents to stay.
2. waved good bye and asked the parents when they would return.
3. hugged the nurse and ignored the parents.
4. grabbed the legs of the parents and refused to let them go.

40. A baby is born with esophageal atresia with tracheoesophageal fistula. Which of the following signs/symptoms would the nurse expect to see?
1. Dyspnea
2. Coffee ground emesis
3. Bloody diarrhea
4. Lymphadenopathy

41. A nurse is taking a neonate, who was noted to have a grade 1 heart murmur during the newborn assessment, to the parents' room. It would be especially important for the nurse to advise the parents to notify the nurse if the baby exhibits which of the following signs/symptoms? The baby:
1. refuses to suckle at the breast.
2. keeps his or her eyes tightly closed.
3. spits up after each feed.
4. points his or her toes inward.

42. An 8-year-old child is post-op ventriculoperitoneal shunt revision. The nurse documents the nursing diagnosis, Excessive Fluid Volume, after noting that the child's abdomen is distended. The nurse should document that the finding is likely related to which of the following physiological changes?
1. Peritonitis
2. Drainage of cerebral spinal fluid
3. Paralytic ileus
4. Intraperitoneal hemorrhage

43. The nurse is providing nutrition education to a group of adolescent girls. Which of the following choices would best meet the mineral needs of adolescent girls?
1. Tossed salad
2. Cheeseburger
3. Fruit smoothie
4. Stuffed peppers

44. A nurse, caring for a 2-year-old child who has just been diagnosed with type 1 diabetes mellitus, is educating the child's parents regarding the values of important diagnostic tests. The nurse should include which of the following information regarding their child's illness in the teaching session?
1. Hemoglobin A1C levels should be greater than or equal to 5.5%.
2. Preprandial blood glucose levels will likely be set higher than those of older children.
3. Serum pH levels should be between 7.25 and 7.35.
4. Daily urine dipstick findings should show mild to moderate ketone levels.

45. An emergency department nurse who is assessing a school-age child reports to the primary health-care provider, "This child is exhibiting signs/symptoms of fluid overload." Which of the following signs/symptoms did the nurse assess? **Select all that apply.**
1. Ascites
2. Thready pulse
3. Desquamation
4. Elevated specific gravity
5. Adventitious lung sounds

46. A child is seen in the emergency department for suspected acute glomerular nephritis. To confirm the diagnosis, the nurse would expect to perform which of the following actions?
1. Sterile catheterization
2. Serum antibody titers
3. Urine cultures
4. Patellar reflexes

47. A one-month-old child is admitted to the emergency department with a diagnosis of pyloric stenosis. Which of the following laboratory values would be consistent with the diagnosis?
1. Hematocrit 48%
2. Potassium 5.2 mEq/L
3. White blood cell count 15,000 cells/mm^3
4. Platelet count 50,000 cell/mm^3

48. A 2-year-old child with sickle cell anemia is admitted to the emergency department in a possible sequestration crisis. For which of the following findings should the nurse carefully monitor the child?
1. Severe pain
2. Marked hypotension
3. Hyperthermia
4. Hyperkalemia

49. A 15-year-old child seen in the emergency department with dyspnea is found to have high levels of IgE in his bloodstream. As a means of determining the etiology of the finding, the nurse should ask the child which of the following questions?
1. "Are you allergic to anything?"
2. "Have you been exercising more than usual?"
3. "Are you sexually active?"
4. "Have you had any vomiting or diarrhea today?"

50. A nurse is educating a couple with a newborn regarding prevention of plagiocephaly. Which of the following actions should the nurse educate the parents to perform?
1. Keep the baby out of the sun for the first 6 months of life.
2. Provide the baby with visually stimulating items to look at.
3. Monitor the numbers of stools and wet diapers the baby has in 24 hours.
4. Place the baby on its stomach each day during supervised play.

51. A mother calls the pediatric clinic and states, "My daughter had lice last week. I washed her hair with the lice shampoo, vacuumed, and washed all the clothes, but the lice are back. What did I do wrong?" Which of the following additional information should the nurse obtain?
1. Whether the child returned to school
2. Whether the child has long or short hair
3. Whether the mother carefully combed out the child's hair after the shampooing
4. Whether the mother rinsed off the shampoo before one hour had elapsed.

52. A nurse in the newborn nursery suspects that a neonate contracted rubella via vertical transmission. Which of the following neonatal findings are consistent with the nurse's suspicions? **Select all that apply.**
1. Cataracts
2. Deafness
3. Spina bifida
4. Hyperbilirubinemia
5. Respiratory stridor

53. A child has been diagnosed with fragile X syndrome. Which of the following health-care referrals should the nurse encourage the parents to make? The nurse should encourage the parents to consult with a(n):
1. Orthopedic surgeon
2. Genetic counselor
3. Registered dietitian
4. Otolaryngologist

54. A nurse notifies the neonatal health-care provider that a newly born baby likely has a clubfoot. The nurse has noted which of the following abnormal findings?
1. Marked dorsiflexion of the big toe
2. All toes on the foot that are webbed.
3. Foot with an unusually high arch and large heel
4. Foot that is plantar flexed and turned inward

55. A nurse is preparing to administer an intravenous medication through an IV pump. The child has a saline lock in place. Please place the steps the nurse will perform in correct chronological order.
1. Wash hands.
2. Set the infusion pump to the correct rate.
3. Cleanse the saline lock with alcohol or Betadine.
4. Document on the medication administration record.
5. Calculate the safe dosage for the child and compare it with the doctor's order.

56. A nurse working in the pediatric clinic completes a report to child protective services regarding a 4-year-old child who is seen for a routine physical examination and who refuses to go to his mother for comfort. In addition, the nurse assessed which of the following physical findings?
1. Bruises on his knees and elbows
2. Bandaged laceration on his left calf
3. Burn marks on his torso
4. Brown patches on his forehead

57. A child, birthed at 24 weeks' gestation, is discharged home at 8 weeks of age. To prevent a common, but serious, respiratory illness in the baby, the public health nurse administers which of the following medications to the baby each month?
1. Pertussis immune globulin
2. Influenza immune globulin
3. Synergis (palivizumab)
4. Pulmozyme (dornase alfa)

58. A child with cleft palate is post-op reconstruction surgery. Which of the following interventions should the nurse perform?
1. Maintain total parenteral nutrition for one week following surgery.
2. Place the child with a roommate who also is not allowed to eat.
3. Feed the child without inserting any utensils into the mouth.
4. Check the position of the device protecting the sutures each hour.

59. The laboratory data on a toddler with congestive heart failure appears below.

	Date of Results		
Serum Test	**August 1**	**August 2**	**August 3**
Hematocrit	42%	43%	44%
Hemoglobin	14 G/dL	14 G/dL	15 G/dL
Potassium	3.6 mEq/L	4.0 mEq/L	4.2 mEq/L
Sodium	139 mEq/L	142 mEq/L	143 mEq/L

The child's primary health-care provider has ordered for the child to receive daily dosages of Lanoxin (digoxin) and Lasix (furosemide). On August 3, immediately before the medications are due, the nurse assesses the child's apical heart rate as 132 bpm. Which of the following actions should the nurse perform at this time?

1. Administer the medications, as ordered.
2. Administer the Lanoxin, but hold the Lasix, and inform the primary health-care provider.
3. Administer the Lasix, but hold the Lanoxin, and inform the primary health-care provider.
4. Hold both medications, and inform the primary health-care provider.

60. A 16-year-old child is seen in the pediatric clinic with signs and symptoms of the flu. To prevent further disease, the nurse educates the parents and the teenager to refrain from performing which of the following treatment practices?

1. The teenager should consume no dairy products.
2. The teenager should spend no time in the sun or under a sun lamp.
3. The teenager should perform no active range-of-motion exercises.
4. The teenager should be administered no aspirin.

61. A young woman enters the school nurse's office and states, "I've decided to get my right nipple pierced." Which of the following comments by the nurse would be most important?

1. "Before you have your nipple pierced, I would like to talk about how you will need to clean the area."
2. "Do you realize that it will hurt a great deal to have such a sensitive area pierced?"
3. "Have you gotten permission from your parents to get your nipple pierced?"
4. "I am so glad that you have decided to get pierced because, unlike a tattoo, it can be removed."

62. A 13-year-old child has just been diagnosed with type 2 diabetes. Which of the following signs/symptoms would the nurse expect the child to exhibit? **Select all that apply.**

1. Fatigue
2. Anorexia
3. Excessive thirst
4. Sweet-smelling breath
5. Darkening of the skin of the neck

63. A nurse is educating the parents of a newborn regarding the child's risk for dehydration. Which of the following information should the nurse include in the teaching session? Babies are at high risk for dehydration because:

1. they have a relatively small body surface area.
2. they retain electrolytes in high concentrations.
3. a high percentage of their weight is from fluid.
4. a low concentration of potassium is in their blood.

64. A child is admitted to the pediatric unit with a diagnosis of nephrotic syndrome. Which of the following signs/symptoms would the nurse expect to see?

1. Anasarca
2. Hyperproteinemia
3. Hypertension
4. Anemia

65. The parents of an infant in the emergency department have just been advised that their child has been diagnosed with intussusception. To help the parents to understand the pathophysiology of the illness, a nurse provides them with which of the following drawings?

1.
2.
3.
4.

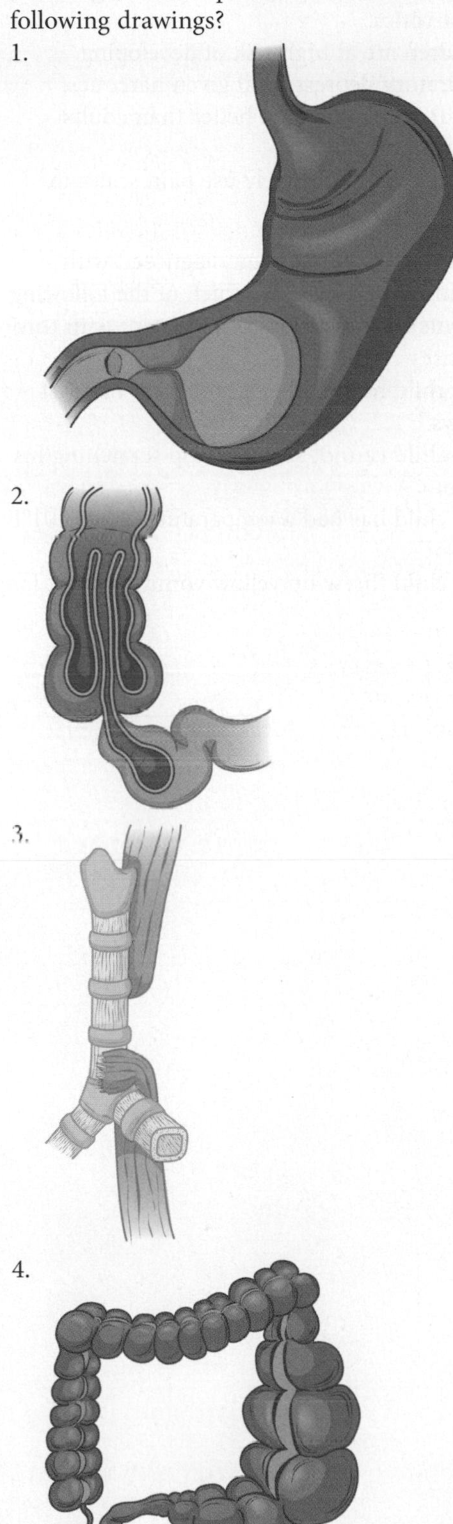

66. A child, 3 years of age, has just been diagnosed with von Willebrand's disease. Which of the following information should the nurse include in a teaching session for the child's parents?

1. Serve the child a diet that is rich in calcium.
2. Assess the child's axillary temperature each morning.
3. Avoid contact with the offending allergen.
4. Apply pressure and ice to all of the child's injuries.

67. A 13-year-old girl is seen in the pediatric clinic with painful, red joints and a macular rash over her nose and cheeks. The nurse notifies the child's primary health-care provider and requests an order for which of the following diagnostic blood tests?

1. Human chorionic gonadotropin (hCG)
2. Antinuclear antibody (ANA)
3. Partial thromboplastin time (PTT)
4. Alanine transaminase (ALT)

68. A nurse is providing an educational session for parents on burn safety. Which of the following information should be included in the educational session?

1. Parents should conduct yearly fire drills for their young children.
2. Hot water heaters should be set at no higher than 140°F.
3. Batteries in household fire alarms should be changed every 2 years.
4. No sunscreen should be put on a baby until the baby is able to crawl.

69. A nurse working in the emergency department would expect that the primary health-care provider would order a tetanus booster for previously immunized patients with which of the following admitting complaints? **Select all that apply.**

1. Tick bite
2. Viral diarrhea
3. Third-degree burn
4. Bacterial meningitis
5. Deep puncture wound

70. A baby is admitted to the pediatric unit for repair of a cleft lip. While performing the admission physical assessment, the nurse notes that the baby has a narrow distance between the inner and outer canthi of the eyes, thin upper lip, and smooth philtrum. The nurse reports to the primary health-care provider that it is likely that the mother abused which of the following substances during her pregnancy?

1. Heroin
2. Cocaine
3. Nicotine
4. Alcohol

71. A nurse, during a well-baby check, is performing Ortolani's sign. Which of the following actions is the nurse performing?

1. Externally rotating the baby's hips
2. Comparing the baby's knee heights
3. Checking the baby's plantar reflexes
4. Monitoring the baby's pedal pulses

72. A primary health-care provider has ordered a medication for a child, 48 lb and 50 in. A reliable medication reference states the safe pediatric dosage is 50 to 100 mg/kg/day in divided doses every 8 hr. Please calculate the safe dosage range of the medication for this child. If rounding is needed, please round to the nearest whole number.

__________ to __________ mg every 8 hr.

73. A 16-year-old female being examined in the pediatric clinic has a body mass index (BMI) of 16.6 kg/m^2. Which of the following questions/comments would be important for the nurse to ask the young woman? (Please refer to the growth charts in the Appendix.)

1. "Do you eat snacks between meals?"
2. "How do you feel about your body?"
3. "Let's talk about foods that are high in calories."
4. "It's important for you to start to exercise each day."

74. A nurse is providing pain medication to a 5-year-old child after abdominal surgery. Which of the following principles should provide the rationale for the nurse's action?

1. Children are at high risk of becoming addicted to narcotics.
2. Children are at high risk of developing respiratory depression if given narcotics.
3. Children tolerate pain better than adults tolerate pain.
4. Children can effectively use pain scales to measure their pain.

75. A 5-year-old child has been diagnosed with pinworms (enterobiasis). Which of the following statements by the parents is consistent with this diagnosis?

1. "My child has had black stools for the past 2 days."
2. "My child cannot seem to stop scratching his bottom."
3. "My child has had a temperature above 101°F all day."
4. "My child threw up yellow vomit all night long."

COMPREHENSIVE FINAL EXAM ANSWERS

1. ANSWER: 2
Rationale:
1. The fontanels have closed by the time a child has reached 2 years of age.
2. The nurse should monitor the child for vomiting.
3. The nurse should monitor the child for hypertension.
4. Protruding tongue is unrelated to head trauma.
TEST-TAKING TIP: If head injury results in increased intracranial pressure, the child will exhibit a number of signs/symptoms including hypertension, altered consciousness, and vomiting.
Content Area: *Pediatrics*
Integrated Processes: *Nursing Process: Assessment*
Client Need: *Physiological Integrity: Physiological Adaptation: Alterations in Body Systems*
Cognitive Level: *Application*

2. ANSWER: 2
Rationale:
1. Elevated levels of histamine in the bloodstream are noted in children exposed to allergens.
2. Children whose gastrointestinal tract villi are atrophied are maintained on gluten-free diets.
3. Lack of enervation to the distal portion of the bowel is the pathophysiology of Hirschsprung's disease.
4. Peritonitis secondary to perforated esophageal varices is unrelated to a gluten-free diet.
TEST-TAKING TIP: The gastrointestinal tract villi are atrophied in children with celiac disease. The therapeutic management of celiac disease is the consumption of a gluten-free diet.
Content Area: *Pediatrics*
Integrated Processes: *Nursing Process: Analysis*
Client Need: *Physiological Integrity: Physiological Adaptation: Alterations in Body Systems*
Cognitive Level: *Application*

3. ANSWER: 4
Rationale:
1. Although true, this statement is not the best statement for the nurse to reply.
2. Although the nurse may wish to learn which other children are consuming alcohol, this statement is not the best statement for the nurse to reply.
3. Although the nurse may wish to notify the child's parents, this statement is not the best statement for the nurse to reply.
4. This statement is the best statement for the nurse to reply.
TEST-TAKING TIP: Before a nurse can provide guidance and advice to an adolescent, the nurse must first develop a therapeutic relationship with the teen.
Content Area: *Adolescent*
Integrated Processes: *Nursing Process: Implementation*
Client Need: *Physiological Integrity: Therapeutic Communication*
Cognitive Level: *Analysis*

4. ANSWER: 4
Rationale:
1. The child must consume a diet low in phenylalanine, an essential amino acid.
2. If the child consumes large quantities of phenylalanine, the child will become intellectually disabled.
3. There is no medication for PKU.
4. This statement is true. The child will be able to pass the recessive gene to a future child.
TEST-TAKING TIP: PKU, an autosomal recessive illness, has no cure. Children with the disease are maintained on a diet low in phenylalanine. Because the amino acid is essential, they must consume some of the protein.
Content Area: *Pediatrics*
Integrated Processes: *Nursing Process: Implementation*
Client Need: *Physiological Integrity: Physiological Adaptation: Alterations in Body Systems*
Cognitive Level: *Application*

5. ANSWER: 3 and 5
Rationale:
1. Simian crease is a sign of developmental disability. It is unrelated to prematurity.
2. Hypospadias is a congenital disease of the genitourinary system. It is unrelated to prematurity.
3. Cryptorchidism, which is the medical term for undescended testes, is often seen in preterm males.
4. Negative Babinski is seen in babies with central nervous system dysfunction. It is unrelated to prematurity.
5. Patent ductus arteriosus, which refers to the fact that the fetal duct between the aorta and the pulmonary artery remains open, is often seen in preterm babies.
TEST-TAKING TIP: When a nurse assesses an infant, it is important to note not only the child's chronological age but also the child's gestational age at birth. The nurse would then be prepared to assess for alterations in the child's physiology that are consistent with prematurity.
Content Area: *Newborn-At-Risk*
Integrated Processes: *Nursing Process: Assessment*
Client Need: *Physiological Integrity: Physiological Adaptation: Alterations in Body Systems*
Cognitive Level: *Application*

6. ANSWER: 4
Rationale:
1. Although possible, it is unlikely that shigella has caused the watery stools.
2. Although possible, it is unlikely that salmonella has caused the watery stools.
3. Although possible, it is unlikely that giardia has caused the watery stools.
4. The most likely pathogen causing the watery stools is rotavirus.
TEST-TAKING TIP: Giardia is the most common pathogen causing diarrhea in nursery schools and day-care centers. Rotavirus, which can be prevented with proper immunization, is a common cause of diarrhea in young children.
Content Area: *Pediatrics*

Integrated Processes: *Nursing Process: Assessment*
Client Need: *Physiological Integrity: Physiological Adaptation: Alterations in Body Systems*
Cognitive Level: *Application*

7. ANSWER: 3
Rationale:
1. It is unnecessary to routinely administer oxygen to the child.
2. The nurse should assess the child's lower extremity distal to the insertion site for color change.
3. The nurse should keep the child's affected extremity straight for the next 4 to 6 hr.
4. Whole blood is not routinely infused after a cardiac catheterization.

TEST-TAKING TIP: To keep the child's extremity straight, it is usually best to employ the assistance of the parents. If the parents are unavailable, games and/or restraints may be utilized to keep the leg straight.
Content Area: *Pediatrics—Cardiac*
Integrated Processes: *Nursing Process: Implementation*
Client Need: *Physiological Integrity: Reduction of Risk Potential: Potential for Complications of Diagnostic Tests/Treatments/Procedures*
Cognitive Level: *Application*

8. ANSWER: 2
Rationale:
1. Voluntarily grasping a rattle is seen in babies who are 4 to 5 months of age.
2. The nurse would expect the baby to smile socially.
3. Cooing and babbling is usually seen in babies at 3 months.
4. Playing with hands and feet is seen in babies who are 4 to 5 months of age.

TEST-TAKING TIP: To determine whether infants are exhibiting normal growth and development, it is important for nurses to know normal milestones. The social smile is one of those important milestones.
Content Area: *Pediatrics—Infant*
Integrated Processes: *Nursing Process: Assessment*
Client Need: *Health Promotion and Maintenance: Developmental Stages and Transitions*
Cognitive Level: *Application*

9. ANSWER: 2
Rationale:
1. It would be appropriate to provide the child with plastic toys for play.
2. The nurse should educate the parents to avoid using softeners when laundering the child's clothing.
3. It would be appropriate to introduce solid foods into the child's diet.
4. It would be appropriate to cover the crib mattress with cotton bedding.

TEST-TAKING TIP: Children with atopic dermatitis often experience worsening of their symptoms when exposed to irritants, such as perfumed soaps, laundry softeners, and wool fabrics. The nurse should recommend that parents refrain from exposing their children to those items.
Content Area: *Pediatrics*
Integrated Processes: *Nursing Process: Implementation; Teaching/Learning*
Client Need: *Physiological Integrity: Physiological Adaptation: Illness Management*
Cognitive Level: *Application*

10. ANSWER: 3
Rationale:
1. Although this child has been ill for a period of time, the child is currently in remission, so the role strain is likely minimal.
2. This child is sick with an acute illness. The role strain is likely minimal.
3. This child has a chronic disease that requires multiple interventions throughout the day. In addition, children with CF often die from severe bacterial pneumonia. It is likely that the child's mother is suffering from caregiver role strain.
4. Although this child's illness requires surgery, the child is likely able to care for herself and, therefore, the role strain is likely minimal.

TEST-TAKING TIP: Parents of children with serious, chronic illnesses are often under a great deal of strain. Not only do many of them work outside the home, they are also responsible for the care and well-being of a chronically ill child. In addition, as is the case of CF, the parents are continually concerned that their child may die from an acute exacerbation of the illness.
Content Area: *Pediatrics—Respiratory*
Integrated Processes: *Nursing Process: Analysis*
Client Need: *Physiological Integrity: Family Dynamics*
Cognitive Level: *Analysis*

11. ANSWER: 1
Rationale:
1. This statement is correct. Whenever the child plays in the sun, the child's cheeks will become redder.
2. This statement is incorrect. There are no isolation requirements for a child with fifth disease.
3. This statement is incorrect. Pregnant women who have been in contact with the child should be monitored carefully for signs of the disease.
4. This statement is incorrect.

TEST-TAKING TIP: Children with fifth disease are no longer contagious once the rash appears; therefore, there are no isolation requirements for the disease. Fifth disease is, however, teratogenic, so any pregnant women who have been exposed to a child who has the disease should be notified.
Content Area: *Pediatrics*
Integrated Processes: *Nursing Process: Implementation*
Client Need: *Physiological Integrity: Physiological Adaptation: Alteration in Body Systems*
Cognitive Level: *Application*

12. ANSWER: 1, 2, and 3
Rationale:
1. Alcohol consumption during pregnancy would place an unborn child at high risk for a cognitive deficit.

2. Fetal hypoxia during labor and delivery would place an unborn child at high risk for a cognitive deficit.
3. Neonatal febrile illness in the early neonatal period would place the child at high risk for a cognitive deficit.
4. Maternal lead ingestion during pregnancy would place the child at risk of a cognitive deficit. A father's ingestion has not been shown to be teratogenic.
5. Cigarette smoking by the father would not place the child at risk of a cognitive deficit.

TEST-TAKING TIP: The brain is very sensitive to environmental insults throughout the pregnancy as well as during the first few years after birth.
Content Area: *Pediatrics*
Integrated Processes: *Nursing Process: Implementation; Teaching/Learning*
Client Need: *Physiological Integrity: Physiological Adaptation: Alteration in Body Systems*
Cognitive Level: *Application*

13. ANSWER: 1, 2, 3, and 5
Rationale:
1. Pain is a symptom the nurse would expect to see.
2. Edema is a symptom the nurse would expect to see.
3. Bruising is a symptom the nurse would expect to see.
4. Bleeding would not be seen.
5. Reduced range of motion is a symptom the nurse would expect to see.

TEST-TAKING TIP: Injuries to the musculoskeletal system usually result in the inflammatory response—edema, pain, heat, redness. In addition, the nurse would note ecchymosis and, in the case of a dislocation, limited range of motion.
Content Area: *Pediatrics*
Integrated Processes: *Nursing Process: Assessment*
Client Need: *Physiological Integrity: Physiological Adaptation: Alteration in Body Systems*
Cognitive Level: *Application*

14. ANSWER: 3
Rationale:
1. This action would be inappropriate. Three-year-old children are unable to swallow tablets without the potential of choking.
2. This action would be inappropriate. It is unlikely that the child would consume unmixed powder even if he or she were given a favorite drink with which to swallow the powder.
3. This action is appropriate. The nurse should crush the tablet, mix it with a teaspoon of applesauce, and give the mixture to the child to swallow.
4. This action would be inappropriate. It is unlikely that the child would consume an entire juice cup filled with fluid, even if it were his or her favorite drink.

TEST-TAKING TIP: When preparing crushed medication for children, it is important not to mix the medicine with a large amount of liquid, gelatin, or applesauce because the child will likely refuse to consume the entire amount.
Content Area: *Pediatrics—Medication*
Integrated Processes: *Nursing Process: Implementation*
Client Need: *Physiological Integrity: Pharmacological and Parenteral Therapies: Medication Administration*
Cognitive Level: *Application*

15. ANSWER: 3
Rationale:
1. Although it would be appropriate to provide the child with a choice, the child will likely not understand what the word "injection" means.
2. Although it would be appropriate to provide the child with a choice, to ask the child regarding the speed of putting a needle into his or her arm is not appropriate.
3. It would be appropriate to forewarn the child that his or her arm will be held tight, and it would be appropriate to provide the child with help in order to remain still during the procedure.
4. It would not be appropriate to pressure the child to be brave during the procedure. Children often cry during painful procedures into the school-age period and beyond.

TEST-TAKING TIP: Language is an important consideration when working with children. They are often unfamiliar with medical terms or, in some cases, may completely misinterpret the terms. The nurse must use simple, clear language, especially when conversing with young children.
Content Area: *Pediatrics—Preschool*
Integrated Processes: *Nursing Process: Implementation*
Client Need: *Health Promotion and Maintenance: Developmental Stages and Transitions*
Cognitive Level: *Application*

16. ANSWER: 4
Rationale:
1. Children usually are able to perform the broad jump at 3 years of age.
2. Children usually are able to walk on tiptoes at 3 years of age.
3. Children usually are able to ride a tricycle at 3 years of age.
4. Skipping using alternate feet is a task of 5-year-old children. It would be an indicator of readiness for the gross motor skills taught in kindergarten.

TEST-TAKING TIP: School nurses are responsible for the health and well-being of the children in their school. It is important that children be expected to perform skills safely and, when they have yet to achieve skills expected at their developmental level, that they be provided with opportunities to develop those skills. School nurses, therefore, often assess children's abilities.
Content Area: *Pediatrics—Preschool*
Integrated Processes: *Nursing Process: Assessment*
Client Need: *Health Promotion and Maintenance: Developmental Stages and Transitions*
Cognitive Level: *Application*

17. ANSWER: 1 and 4
Rationale:
1. Giving away a favored object often precedes a suicide.
2. Dating is a normal activity of adolescents.

3. Seventeen-year-old football players often brag to others about their team.
4. Talking about the death of others often precedes a suicide.
5. Changing extracurricular activities is not uncommon in adolescence.

TEST-TAKING TIP: There are a number of behaviors that may indicate that a young man or woman is contemplating suicide. If the nurse suspects that an individual is considering suicide, it is important for the nurse to ask the individual.

Content Area: *Mental Health—Suicide*
Integrated Processes: *Nursing Process: Assessment*
Client Need: *Psychosocial Integrity: Mental Health Concepts*
Cognitive Level: *Application*

18. ANSWER: 1 and 2

Rationale:
1. The nurse should educate the parents regarding the safe administration of the antibiotics.
2. The nurse should educate the parents to place warm or cold compresses on the affected area.
3. Cough suppressants should not be administered to children under 2 years of age, and they are not administered for otitis media.
4. Otitis media is an internal disorder. There is no way to cleanse the area.
5. Isolation is not indicated for a diagnosis of AOM.

TEST-TAKING TIP: The treatment of infants with AOM is dependent upon the age and health status of the baby. Because many ear infections are viral in origin, after the age of 2, practitioners are encouraged initially to provide palliative care without antibiotics. Prior to that age, antibiotics are often prescribed based on the infant's clinical signs.

Content Area: *Pediatrics*
Integrated Processes: *Nursing Process: Implementation*
Client Need: *Physiological Integrity: Physiological Adaptation: Alteration in Body Systems*
Cognitive Level: *Application*

19. ANSWER: 1, 2, 3, and 4

Rationale:
1. Fear of the teacher may be a cause of school refusal.
2. Performing poorly in school may be a cause of school refusal.
3. Bullying by classmates or a poor social experience may be a cause of school refusal.
4. Bullying often occurs on the school bus and may be a cause of school refusal.
5. Dislike of food served in the cafeteria has not been identified as a cause of school refusal.

TEST-TAKING TIP: School refusal is a common problem of the school-age period. It is important for the nurse to advise the parent to seek assistance from the school officials to determine the cause of the refusal and to have them intervene when appropriate. In addition, it is important to counsel the parents to make the child return to school as soon as possible.

Content Area: *Pediatrics—School Age*
Integrated Processes: *Nursing Process: Implementation*
Client Need: *Health Promotion and Maintenance: Developmental Stages and Transitions*
Cognitive Level: *Application*

20. ANSWER: 3

Rationale:
1. The nurse should not recommend spanking the child on the buttocks.
2. The nurse should not recommend grounding the child for 1 week.
3. The nurse should recommend making the child return the candy to the store owner.
4. The nurse should not recommend preventing the child from eating dinner.

TEST-TAKING TIP: To help children learn the difference between right and wrong, it is important that they be disciplined for improper actions. Discipline, however, should be consistent with the offense and meaningful. Requiring the child to return the candy to the owner is consistent with the offense and is a reprimand that will be remembered by the child.

Content Area: *Pediatrics—School Age*
Integrated Processes: *Nursing Process: Implementation*
Client Need: *Health Promotion and Maintenance: Developmental Stages and Transitions*
Cognitive Level: *Application*

21. ANSWER: 3

Rationale:
1. Although true, this is not the most important response for the nurse to make.
2. Although an important question to ask, this is not the most important response for the nurse to make.
3. This is the most important response for the nurse to give. Only water should be in the bottle at bed time.
4. Although true, this is not the most important response for the nurse to make.

TEST-TAKING TIP: Babies who go to bed suckling on a formula-filled bottle are at very high risk for developing dental caries. The nurse should strongly recommend that the bottle contain only water in order to decrease the potential health hazard.

Content Area: *Pediatrics—Toddler*
Integrated Processes: *Nursing Process: Implementation*
Client Need: *Health Promotion and Maintenance: Health Promotion/Disease Prevention*
Cognitive Level: *Analysis*

22. ANSWER: 2

Rationale:
1. The neonate should be placed in the prone position.
2. The nurse should cover the lumbosacrum with a moist, sterile dressing.
3. It is unlikely that a central line will be inserted.
4. It is unlikely that the newborn will need to be intubated.

TEST-TAKING TIP: To prevent injury and/or infection of the exposed sac, the nurse should cover the area with sterile, moist dressings.

Content Area: *Pediatrics*
Integrated Processes: *Nursing Process: Implementation*
Client Need: *Physiological Integrity: Physiological Adaptation: Illness Management*
Cognitive Level: *Application*

23. ANSWER: 1
Rationale:
1. **The nurse would expect the child to be developmentally delayed.**
2. The nurse would not expect the child to exhibit strabismus.
3. The nurse would not expect the child to exhibit projectile vomiting.
4. The nurse would not expect the child to be dyspneic.

TEST-TAKING TIP: To prevent developmental delay in a child with congenital hypothyroidism, a daily dosage of thyroid replacement is prescribed. The child will have to take the medication for the rest of his or her life.
Content Area: *Pediatrics*
Integrated Processes: *Nursing Process: Assessment*
Client Need: *Physiological Integrity: Physiological Adaptation: Alterations in Body Systems*
Cognitive Level: *Application*

24. ANSWER: 4
Rationale:
1. A Po_2 of 90 mm Hg is within normal limits (80 to 100 mm Hg).
2. A Pco_2 of 30 mm Hg is consistent with respiratory alkalosis caused by hyperventilation.
3. An HCO_3 of 25 mEq/L is within normal limits (22 to 26 mEq/L).
4. **A pH of 7.30 is consistent with a diagnosis of respiratory distress.**

TEST-TAKING TIP: Children who are in respiratory distress are retaining carbon dioxide. The carbon dioxide combines with water in the bloodstream and carbonic acid results. The higher the concentration of carbonic acid, the lower the pH. The normal pH is 7.35 to 7.45.
Content Area: *Pediatrics*
Integrated Processes: *Nursing Process: Assessment*
Client Need: *Physiological Integrity: Physiological Adaptation: Fluid and Electrolyte Imbalances*
Cognitive Level: *Application*

25. ANSWER: 1
Rationale:
1. **The child should be monitored for signs of urinary tract infection, including cloudy urine.**
2. The child is not at high risk for hypertension.
3. The child is not at high risk for the appearance of a macular rash.
4. The child is not at high risk for pulmonary edema.

TEST-TAKING TIP: The urethra of male children born with hypospadias is located on the underside of the penis. After the surgical repair is complete, the urethra is located at its normal site at the end of the penis.
Content Area: *Pediatrics*
Integrated Processes: *Nursing Process: Assessment*
Client Need: *Physiological Integrity: Reduction of Risk Potential: Potential for Complications from Surgical Procedures and Health Alterations*
Cognitive Level: *Application*

26. ANSWER: 4
Rationale:
1. The mother should continue to breastfeed. She should not pump and dump the breast milk and replace it with oral rehydration therapy (ORT).
2. ORT is an electrolyte solution that meets a child's fluid and electrolyte needs.
3. The child should be offered ORT after each breastfeeding session.
4. **The nurse should educate the mother to feed the child ORT along with lean meats, cooked vegetables, and breast milk.**

TEST-TAKING TIP: ORT is an important supplementation for children at high risk for severe dehydration. Children with diarrhea and mild dehydration, and who are able to eat solid foods, should be offered low-fat meats; cooked vegetables; starches, such as potatoes and rice; bananas; and yogurt with live cultures in addition to breast milk and ORT.
Content Area: *Pediatrics*
Integrated Processes: *Nursing Process: Implementation*
Client Need: *Physiological Integrity: Physiological Adaptation: Fluid and Electrolyte Imbalances*
Cognitive Level: *Application*

27. ANSWER: 3
Rationale:
1. The safe dosage range for the medication is 31.36 to 52.27 mg daily. The order is safe as written.
2. It is unnecessary to request an order change to twice a day to improve absorption of the iron.
3. **This is the correct response. The nurse should teach the mother how to draw up 0.4 mL of fluid into an oral syringe.**
4. This response is incorrect. If the parent were to administer 1.25 mL each day, the child would be markedly overdosed.

TEST-TAKING TIP: Iron is a heavy metal. The nurse must make certain that the child is receiving an appropriate dosage of the medication and that the mother safely draws up and correctly administers the medication.
Content Area: *Pediatrics—Medication*
Integrated Processes: *Nursing Process: Implementation*
Client Need: *Physiological Integrity: Pharmacological and Parenteral Therapies: Dosage Calculation*
Cognitive Level: *Application*

28. ANSWER: 2
Rationale:
1. This is not an appropriate comment for the nurse to make.
2. **This statement is appropriate. The young man should continue to wear condoms when having intercourse.**

3. This is not an appropriate comment for the nurse to make.
4. This is not an appropriate comment for the nurse to make.

TEST-TAKING TIP: It is possible to become infected with more than one strain of HIV. Those who are infected with more than one strain are at risk of developing AIDS at a younger age.

Content Area: *Adolescent; Infectious Disease*
Integrated Processes: *Nursing Process: Implementation*
Client Need: *Health Promotion and Maintenance: High-Risk Behaviors*
Cognitive Level: *Application*

29. ANSWER: 1

Rationale:
1. **The nurse should report that the child exhibits a grasp reflex.**
2. Six-month-old children do fall over from a sitting position.
3. Six-month-old children do not yet understand commands.
4. Some children begin drinking from a cup at a very young age.

TEST-TAKING TIP: The grasp reflex disappears at about 3 months of age. Children whose grasp reflex persists should be carefully assessed for other developmental delays. Many of the children with prolongation of rudimentary reflexes are diagnosed with cerebral palsy.

Content Area: *Pediatrics—Infant*
Integrated Processes: *Nursing Process: Implementation*
Client Need: *Health Promotion and Maintenance: Developmental Stages and Transitions*
Cognitive Level: *Application*

30. ANSWER: 1

Rationale:
1. **The nurse would expect to see encrusted vesicles.**
2. Red and scaly lesions are not seen in children with impetigo.
3. Painful abrasions are not seen in children with impetigo.
4. Alopecic scalp is not seen in children with impetigo.

TEST-TAKING TIP: Impetigo is characterized by pruritic lesions that begin as a macular rash and progress to vesicular. The vesicles rupture and ooze. The discharge dries into a honey-colored crust.

Content Area: *Pediatrics*
Integrated Processes: *Nursing Process: Assessment*
Client Need: *Physiological Integrity: Physiological Adaptation: Alterations in Body Systems*
Cognitive Level: *Application*

31. ANSWER: 4

Rationale:
1. This statement is incorrect. Patients with acne should not wash their faces with a dilute bleach solution.
2. This statement is incorrect. Patients with acne should not manually remove black heads that appear on their face.
3. This statement is incorrect. Acne is caused by a bacteria.
4. **This statement is correct. Acne often gets worse when cosmetics are worn.**

TEST-TAKING TIP: Acne is especially difficult for adolescents because of how it can disfigure the face. It is important for the nurse to provide those suffering with accurate information and empathy.

Content Area: *Adolescent*
Integrated Processes: *Nursing Process: Implementation*
Client Need: *Physiological Integrity: Physiological Adaptation: Illness Management*
Cognitive Level: *Application*

32. ANSWER: 2

Rationale:
1. This statement is incorrect. When the temperature returns to normal, the parents should expect the child's rash to appear.
2. **This statement is correct. When the child's temperature rises, the parents should monitor the child carefully for febrile seizures.**
3. This statement is incorrect. Once a child has had roseola, he or she is immune to the disease.
4. This statement is incorrect. There are no isolation precautions recommended for roseola.

TEST-TAKING TIP: Roseola is almost exclusively seen in very young children. Because the temperature rises so rapidly and so high, children who are prone to febrile seizures should be monitored carefully.

Content Area: *Pediatrics; Infectious Disease*
Integrated Processes: *Nursing Process: Implementation*
Client Need: *Physiological Integrity: Physiological Adaptation: Illness Management*
Cognitive Level: *Application*

33. ANSWER: 1

Rationale:
1. **The parents should seek immediate care if the child exhibits an upper respiratory illness.**
2. Because of their poor muscle tone, children with Down syndrome often have pendulous abdomens.
3. The parents need not seek immediate care if the child develops an elevated temperature.
4. The parents need not seek immediate care if the child develops a protruding brow.

TEST-TAKING TIP: Children with Down syndrome exhibit hypotonic musculature. As a result, they are unable effectively to cough or sneeze pathogens from the upper respiratory tract.

Content Area: *Pediatrics*
Integrated Processes: *Nursing Process: Implementation*
Client Need: *Physiological Integrity: Physiological Adaptation: Illness Management*
Cognitive Level: *Application*

34. ANSWER: 4

Rationale:
1. The extent of the soft tissue injuries is an important factor, but it is not the best rationale for taking x-rays.

2. The child's complaints of pain are important, but they are not the most important rationale for taking x-rays.
3. The mother's statement is an important factor, but it is not the best rationale for taking x-rays.
4. The only way to accurately diagnose a fracture is by taking an x-ray.

TEST-TAKING TIP: Whenever a child enters the health-care system after a serious accident, an x-ray must be performed to determine accurately whether he or she has fractured a bone.
Content Area: *Pediatrics*
Integrated Processes: *Nursing Process: Analysis*
Client Need: *Physiological Integrity: Physiological Adaptation: Illness Management*
Cognitive Level: *Application*

35. ANSWER: 1
Rationale:
1. The nurse should auscultate the lungs and heart sounds.
2. The nurse should palpate the fontanels after assessing the lungs and heart sounds.
3. It is not necessary to remove the infant from the mother's arms.
4. The abdomen should be percussed later in the examination.

TEST-TAKING TIP: Once a baby is disturbed, it is likely that the baby will begin to cry. If a baby is quietly sleeping, therefore, the nurse should first listen to the baby's lung and heart sounds.
Content Area: *Pediatrics*
Integrated Processes: *Nursing Process: Implementation*
Client Need: *Health Promotion and Maintenance: Techniques of Physical Assessment*
Cognitive Level: *Application*

36. ANSWER: 4
Rationale:
1. It is not unusual for preschool children to believe that there are monsters or other scary things in their rooms at night.
2. It is not unusual for preschool children to believe that there are monsters or other scary things in their rooms at night.
3. It is true that many children her age have night fears, and it is appropriate to inspect the room before bedtime and to provide the child with a nightlight to reduce the fears.
4. It is true that many children her age have night fears, and it is appropriate to inspect the room before bedtime and to provide the child with a nightlight to reduce the fears.

TEST-TAKING TIP: Preschool children are magical thinkers. They are unable to distinguish between fantasy and reality. As a result, they often truly believe that there are monsters or other scary things in their rooms at night. It is appropriate for parents to try to allay those fears by inspecting under beds and in closets before the child's bed time.
Content Area: *Pediatrics—Preschool*
Integrated Processes: *Nursing Process: Implementation*
Client Need: *Health Promotion and Maintenance: Developmental Stages and Transitions*
Cognitive Level: *Application*

37. ANSWER: 2
Rationale:
1. Jaundice is not a side effect of stimulant medications.
2. The child should be carefully monitored for arrhythmias.
3. Dyspnea is not a side effect of stimulant medications.
4. Anasarca is not a side effect of stimulant medications.

TEST-TAKING TIP: Stimulants are medications that usually increase biological functions (e.g., heart rate, respiratory rate, brain activity). In young children, however, stimulants act in a more idiosyncratic way. Instead of increasing their activity, the medications actually help the children to concentrate and to behave less impulsively.
Content Area: *Pediatrics—ADHD*
Integrated Processes: *Nursing Process: Assessment*
Client Need: *Physiological Integrity: Pharmacological and Parenteral Therapies: Adverse Effects/Contraindications/Interactions*
Cognitive Level: *Application*

38. ANSWER: 3, 4, and 5
Rationale:
1. Vomiting is not characteristic of epiglottitis.
2. Weight loss is not characteristic of epiglottitis.
3. Tachycardia is a symptom of epiglottitis.
4. Nasal flaring is a symptom of epiglottitis.
5. Inspiratory stridor is a symptom of epiglottitis.

TEST-TAKING TIP: When the epiglottis is markedly swollen, as in the case of acute epiglottitis, the airway is almost completely obstructed. The child, therefore, exhibits signs/symptoms of respiratory distress, and the heart rate increases to compensate for the poor oxygenation.
Content Area: *Pediatrics—Respiratory*
Integrated Processes: *Nursing Process: Assessment*
Client Need: *Physiological Integrity: Physiological Adaptation: Alterations in Body Systems*
Cognitive Level: *Application*

39. ANSWER: 3
Rationale:
1. Children who cry and beg to have their parents stay after a visit are exhibiting signs of protest.
2. The nurse may observe an older, school-age child or adolescent wave good-bye and ask the parents when they would return. These behaviors are less likely in a 6-year-old child.
3. Children who are exhibiting signs of detachment may hug their nurses and ignore their parents.
4. Children who grab the legs of their parents and refuse to let them go are exhibiting signs of protest.

TEST-TAKING TIP: Children who have been in the hospital for long periods of time without frequent visits from their parents often exhibit signs of detachment. The children view the nurses as their primary caregivers and sources of comfort rather than their parents.

Content Area: *Pediatrics*
Integrated Processes: *Nursing Process: Assessment*
Client Need: *Physiological Integrity: Coping Mechanisms*
Cognitive Level: *Application*

40. ANSWER: 1
Rationale:
1. Dyspnea is a symptom of esophageal atresia with tracheoesophageal fistula (TEF).
2. Coffee ground emesis is not characteristic of TEF.
3. Bloody diarrhea is not characteristic of TEF.
4. Lymphadenopathy is not characteristic of TEF.
TEST-TAKING TIP: Because a fistula is present between the esophagus and the trachea, stomach contents are able to enter the respiratory tract. As a result, the neonate exhibits signs of respiratory distress.
Content Area: *Pediatrics*
Integrated Processes: *Nursing Process: Assessment*
Client Need: *Physiological Integrity: Physiological Adaptation: Alterations in Body Systems*
Cognitive Level: *Application*

41. ANSWER: 1
Rationale:
1. The parents should advise the nurse if the baby refuses to feed.
2. Babies often keep their eyes tightly closed when they are first born.
3. Babies often spit up a small amount of milk after feeding.
4. Babies often point their toes inward as a result of their positioning in utero.
TEST-TAKING TIP: There are two activities that compel babies to utilize high levels of energy and oxygen: crying and feeding. Babies who have significant heart defects, therefore, often refuse to feed.
Content Area: *Pediatrics*
Integrated Processes: *Nursing Process: Implementation*
Client Need: *Physiological Integrity: Physiological Adaptation: Alterations in Body Systems*
Cognitive Level: *Application*

42. ANSWER: 2
Rationale:
1. The finding is unlikely related to peritonitis.
2. The finding is likely related to drainage of cerebral spinal fluid.
3. The finding is unlikely related to a paralytic ileus.
4. The finding is unlikely related to an intraperitoneal hemorrhage.
TEST-TAKING TIP: Ventriculoperitoneal (VP) shunts are inserted in children with hydrocephalus to allow excess cerebrospinal fluid to drain from the ventricles of the brain. The fluid is deposited into the peritoneal cavity.
Content Area: *Pediatrics*
Integrated Processes: *Nursing Process: Assessment*
Client Need: *Physiological Integrity: Physiological Adaptation: Illness Management*
Cognitive Level: *Application*

43. ANSWER: 2
Rationale:
1. Tossed salads are nutritious, but they are not the best choice to meet the mineral needs of adolescent girls.
2. Cheeseburgers will meet the mineral needs of adolescent girls.
3. Fruit smoothies are nutritious, but they are not the best choice to meet the mineral needs of adolescent girls.
4. Stuffed peppers are nutritious, but they are not the best choice to meet the mineral needs of adolescent girls.
TEST-TAKING TIP: Because of their rapid bone growth and because they begin to menstruate, adolescent girls need to consume foods high in calcium and iron. Cheeseburgers contain both of those minerals.
Content Area: *Adolescent*
Integrated Processes: *Nursing Process: Implementation; Teaching/Learning*
Client Need: *Health Promotion and Maintenance: Health Promotion/Disease Prevention*
Cognitive Level: *Application*

44. ANSWER: 2
Rationale:
1. Hemoglobin A1C levels should be less than or equal to 7.5%.
2. Preprandial blood glucose levels are set slightly higher for young children than for older children and adults.
3. Serum pH levels should be between 7.35 and 7.45.
4. Daily urine dipstick findings should be negative for ketones.
TEST-TAKING TIP: Hypoglycemia is a dangerous complication of type 1 diabetes, and toddlers, with their erratic eating patterns and high levels of activity, are especially at high risk for hypoglycemia. As a result, recommended preprandial blood glucose levels are usually set higher for this age group than for older children and adults.
Content Area: *Pediatrics*
Integrated Processes: *Nursing Process: Implementation; Teaching/Learning*
Client Need: *Physiological Integrity: Physiological Adaptation: Illness Management*
Cognitive Level: *Application*

45. ANSWER: 1 and 5
Rationale:
1. Ascites is a symptom of fluid overload.
2. Thready pulse is a symptom of low circulating fluid.
3. Desquamation refers to peeling of the skin.
4. Elevated specific gravity is a symptom of low circulating fluid.
5. Adventitious lung sounds are noted in children with fluid overload.
TEST-TAKING TIP: Adventitious sounds are heard when fluid enters the lung fields. Ascites is characterized by excess fluid in the abdominal cavity.
Content Area: *Pediatrics*
Integrated Processes: *Nursing Process: Assessment*

Client Need: *Physiological Integrity: Physiological Adaptation: Pathophysiology*
Cognitive Level: *Application*

46. ANSWER: 2
Rationale:
1. Sterile catheterization will not confirm the diagnosis of acute glomerular nephritis (AGN).
2. Serum antibody titers will confirm the diagnosis of AGN.
3. Urine cultures will not confirm the diagnosis of AGN.
4. Patellar reflexes will not confirm the diagnosis of AGN.
TEST-TAKING TIP: AGN is a disease that develops following an acute illness caused by group A streptococci (*S. pyogenes*). Titers are performed to assess for antistreptolysin antibodies in the bloodstream.
Content Area: *Pediatrics*
Integrated Processes: *Nursing Process: Assessment*
Client Need: *Physiological Integrity: Physiological Adaptation: Pathophysiology*
Cognitive Level: *Application*

47. ANSWER: 1
Rationale:
1. A hematocrit of 48% is consistent with the diagnosis.
2. A potassium of 5.2 mEq/L is not consistent with the diagnosis.
3. A white blood cell count of 15,000 cells/mm^3 is not consistent with the diagnosis.
4. A platelet count of 50,000 cell/mm^3 is not consistent with the diagnosis.
TEST-TAKING TIP: Because of the recurring vomiting exhibited by babies with pyloric stenosis, they become dehydrated and hemoconcentrated. An elevated hematocrit would, therefore, be consistent with the diagnosis.
Content Area: *Pediatrics*
Integrated Processes: *Nursing Process: Assessment*
Client Need: *Physiological Integrity: Physiological Adaptation: Pathophysiology*
Cognitive Level: *Application*

48. ANSWER: 2
Rationale:
1. Severe pain is noted when a child with sickle cell is in a vaso-occlusive crisis.
2. Marked hypotension is noted when a child with sickle cell is in a sequestration crisis.
3. Hyperthermia may precipitate a vaso-occlusive crisis.
4. Hyperkalemia is unrelated to a sequestration crisis.
TEST-TAKING TIP: A sequestration crisis is characterized by the marked pooling of a large quantity of blood in the spleen, resulting in hypovolemia. Tachycardia and marked hypotension, therefore, would be noted.
Content Area: *Pediatrics—Hematological*
Integrated Processes: *Nursing Process: Assessment*
Client Need: *Physiological Integrity: Physiological Adaptation: Alterations in Body Systems*
Cognitive Level: *Application*

49. ANSWER: 1
Rationale:
1. The nurse should ask the child, "Are you allergic to anything?"
2. "Have you been exercising more than usual?" is not a question that would determine the etiology of the finding.
3. "Are you sexually active?" is not a question that would determine the etiology of the finding.
4. "Have you had any vomiting or diarrhea today?" is not a question that would determine the etiology of the finding.
TEST-TAKING TIP: IgE antibodies are produced in response to exposure to an allergen.
Content Area: *Pediatrics*
Integrated Processes: *Nursing Process: Implementation*
Client Need: *Physiological Integrity: Physiological Adaptation: Alterations in Body Systems*
Cognitive Level: *Application*

50. ANSWER: 4
Rationale:
1. It is important to keep babies out of the sun for the first 6 months of their lives, but the action will not prevent plagiocephaly.
2. It is important to provide babies with visually stimulating items to look at, but the action will not prevent plagiocephaly.
3. It is important to monitor the numbers of stools and wet diapers babies have in a 24-hr period, but the action will not prevent plagiocephaly.
4. Placing the baby on its stomach each day during supervised play will help to prevent plagiocephaly.
TEST-TAKING TIP: Plagiocephaly, or flat head syndrome, develops because babies are placed on their backs so frequently, including for sleep. It is recommended, therefore, during supervised periods that babies be placed on their stomachs each day.
Content Area: *Pediatrics—Infant*
Integrated Processes: *Nursing Process: Implementation; Teaching/Learning*
Client Need: *Health Promotion and Maintenance: Health Promotion/Disease Prevention*
Cognitive Level: *Application*

51. ANSWER: 3
Rationale:
1. Whether the child returned to school is not important information.
2. Whether the child has long or short hair is not important information.
3. Whether the mother carefully combed out the child's hair after the shampooing is important for the nurse to ask.
4. Whether the mother rinsed the shampoo off before one hour had elapsed is an inappropriate question.
TEST-TAKING TIP: The nits, or lice eggs, adhere to the shafts of hair. Unless they are removed by a fine-toothed comb after the lice treatment, they will hatch approximately 1 week following lice shampooing. In addition, it is recommended that a second treatment be applied to the hair one week after the first treatment.

Content Area: *Pediatrics*
Integrated Processes: *Nursing Process: Implementation*
Client Need: *Physiological Integrity: Physiological Adaptation: Alterations in Body Systems*
Cognitive Level: *Application*

52. ANSWER: 1 and 2

Rationale:

1. Cataracts are seen in babies with congenital rubella.
2. Deafness is seen in babies with congenital rubella.
3. Spina bifida is not characteristic of congenital rubella.
4. Hyperbilirubinemia is not characteristic of congenital rubella.
5. Respiratory stridor is not characteristic of congenital rubella.

TEST-TAKING TIP: Rubella during pregnancy is highly teratogenic. In fact, if the mother contracts the illness during the first trimester, there is a 100% probability that her fetus will be adversely affected.

Content Area: *Pediatrics*
Integrated Processes: *Nursing Process: Assessment*
Client Need: *Physiological Integrity: Physiological Adaptation: Alterations in Body Systems*
Cognitive Level: *Application*

53. ANSWER: 2

Rationale:

1. It is not appropriate for the nurse to encourage the parents to consult with an orthopedic surgeon.
2. It is appropriate for the nurse to encourage the parents to consult with a genetic counselor.
3. It is not appropriate for the nurse to encourage the parents to consult a registered dietitian.
4. It is not appropriate for the nurse to encourage the parents to consult an otolaryngologist.

TEST-TAKING TIP: Fragile X syndrome is an X-linked genetic disease. The parents should be encouraged to seek genetic counseling so that they will learn about the etiology, signs, and symptoms of the disease as well as to provide them with the probability of passing the gene on to future children.

Content Area: *Pediatrics*
Integrated Processes: *Nursing Process: Implementation*
Client Need: *Safe and Effective Care Environment: Management of Care: Referrals*
Cognitive Level: *Application*

54. ANSWER: 4

Rationale:

1. Marked dorsiflexion is not characteristic of clubfoot.
2. Webbed toes are not characteristic of clubfoot.
3. A foot with an unusually high arch and large heel is not characteristic of clubfoot.
4. The nurse noted a foot that is plantar flexed and turned inward.

TEST-TAKING TIP: At birth, many babies' feet turn inward as a result of positioning in utero. When rotated manually, however, the feet return to normal positions. If the baby has a clubfoot, however, the health-care practitioner is not able manually to move the foot into proper position.

Content Area: *Pediatrics*
Integrated Processes: *Nursing Process: Implementation*
Client Need: *Physiological Integrity: Physiological Adaptation: Alterations in Body Systems*
Cognitive Level: *Application*

55. ANSWER: The order of nursing actions is: 5, 1, 3, 2, 4.

5. Calculate the safe dosage for the child and compare it with the doctor's order.
1. Wash hands.
3. Cleanse the saline lock with alcohol or Betadine.
2. Set the infusion pump to the correct rate.
4. Document on the medication administration record.

TEST-TAKING TIP: When confronted with a question that requires the test taker to place items in chronological order, he or she must realize that the question may include only some of the required steps. The test taker must simply place those that have been provided into the correct order. Note that in the question, the nurse should wash his or her hands following calculating and comparing the dosage values because the hands should be cleansed immediately before touching any equipment.

Content Area: *Pediatrics*
Integrated Processes: *Nursing Process: Implementation*
Client Need: *Physiological Integrity: Pharmacological and Parenteral Therapies: Medication Administration*
Cognitive Level: *Application*

56. ANSWER: 3

Rationale:

1. Bruises on the knees and elbows are often noted in preschool children.
2. Bandaged lacerations are not unusual in preschool children.
3. Burn marks on a child's torso are consistent with child abuse.
4. Brown patches on his forehead are likely a result of sun exposure.

TEST-TAKING TIP: Children who are cared for by loving parents seek comfort in their parents' arms when they are hurt and injured. Children who are abused often do not. One of the many findings that is consistent with child abuse is the presence of burn marks on a child's torso. Small round marks are likely caused by a lighted cigarette.

Content Area: *Child Health, Abuse*
Integrated Processes: *Nursing Process: Implementation*
Client Need: *Psychosocial Integrity: Abuse/Neglect*
Cognitive Level: *Application*

57. ANSWER: 3

Rationale:

1. Pertussis immune globulin is not administered on a monthly basis to preterm babies.
2. Influenza immune globulin is not administered on a monthly basis to preterm babies.

3. Synergis (palivizumab) is often administered on a monthly basis to preterm babies.
4. Pulmozyme (dornase alfa) is a medication for children with cystic fibrosis.
TEST-TAKING TIP: Children who are born very preterm are at high risk for bronchiolitis caused by the respiratory syncytial virus. To prevent contracting the disease, the babies are often prescribed monthly doses of Synergis.
Content Area: *Pediatrics—Respiratory*
Integrated Processes: *Nursing Process: Implementation*
Client Need: *Physiological Integrity: Pharmacological and Parenteral Therapies: Expected Actions/Outcomes*
Cognitive Level: *Application*

58. ANSWER: 3
Rationale:
1. Children following cleft palate surgery are able to consume soft foods.
2. Children following cleft palate surgery are able to consume soft foods.
3. The nurse will feed the child who is post-op cleft palate surgery without inserting any utensils into the mouth.
4. No device is left in the mouth after cleft palate surgery.
TEST-TAKING TIP: Because eating utensils could damage the cleft palate repair, the baby will be fed soft foods until the surgery is healed. The nurse and parents should feed the child using a large spoon or other device that is too large to insert into the mouth.
Content Area: *Pediatrics*
Integrated Processes: *Nursing Process: Implementation*
Client Need: *Physiological Integrity: Physiological Adaptation: Illness Management*
Cognitive Level: *Application*

59. ANSWER: 1
Rationale:
1. The nurse should administer the medications as ordered.
2. The nurse should administer the medications as ordered.
3. The nurse should administer the medications as ordered.
4. The nurse should administer the medications as ordered.
TEST-TAKING TIP: The child's heart rate is 120 bpm, and the child's potassium levels are all within normal limits. The medications should be administered as ordered.
Content Area: *Pediatrics—Cardiac*
Integrated Processes: *Nursing Process: Implementation*
Client Need: *Physiological Integrity: Pharmacological and Parenteral Therapies: Medication Administration*
Cognitive Level: *Application*

60. ANSWER: 4
Rationale:
1. The teenager may consume dairy products.
2. The teenager may spend time in the sun if sunscreen is used. It is recommended that tanning lamps never be used.
3. The teenager may perform active range-of-motion exercises.
4. The teenager should be administered no aspirin.
TEST-TAKING TIP: Reye syndrome is associated with the ingestion of aspirin during viral illnesses, most notably varicella (chicken pox) and the flu. To treat the body aches and fever associated with the flu, the teenager should be taught to take safe dosages of acetaminophen.
Content Area: *Pediatrics*
Integrated Processes: *Nursing Process: Implementation; Teaching/Learning*
Client Need: *Physiological Integrity: Pharmacological and Parenteral Therapies: Adverse Effects/Contraindications/Side Effects/Interactions*
Cognitive Level: *Application*

61. ANSWER: 1
Rationale:
1. This statement is the most appropriate comment for the nurse to make.
2. The nurse may make this statement, but it is not the most important for the nurse to make.
3. The nurse may make this statement, but it is not the most important for the nurse to make.
4. The nurse may make this statement, but it is not the most important for the nurse to make.
TEST-TAKING TIP: One of the most frequent complications of piercings is infection. To prevent infection, the teenager must be taught how to cleanse the area and to apply bactericidal medications.
Content Area: *Adolescent*
Integrated Processes: *Nursing Process: Implementation; Teaching/Learning*
Client Need: *Health Promotion and Maintenance: Health Promotion/Disease Prevention*
Cognitive Level: *Application*

62. ANSWER: 1, 3, 4, and 5
Rationale:
1. Fatigue is a symptom of diabetes.
2. Polyphagia is a symptom of diabetes.
3. Excessive thirst is a symptom of diabetes.
4. Sweet-smelling breath is a symptom of diabetes.
5. Darkening of the skin of the neck (acanthosis nigricans) is a symptom of type 2 diabetes.
TEST-TAKING TIP: Most of the signs/symptoms of type 2 diabetes are the same as those seen in type 1 diabetics. The one exception to that is acanthosis nigricans, which is only seen in those with type 2 diabetes.
Content Area: *Pediatrics*
Integrated Processes: *Nursing Process: Assessment*
Client Need: *Physiological Integrity: Physiological Adaptation: Alterations in Body Systems*
Cognitive Level: *Application*

63. ANSWER: 3
Rationale:
1. Babies have a relatively large body surface area.
2. Babies are unable to retain electrolytes in high concentrations.
3. A high percentage of babies' weight is from fluid.

4. Babies' normal potassium level is the same as the older child's and the adult's.

TEST-TAKING TIP: Up to 75% of the body of infants and young children and 60% to 65% of the body of preschoolers is comprised of fluid. Because the percentage of fluid is so high in infants and young children, they are especially at high risk for becoming dehydrated during periods of illness.

Content Area: *Pediatrics*
Integrated Processes: *Nursing Process: Implementation; Teaching/Learning*
Client Need: *Physiological Integrity: Physiological Adaptation: Alterations in Body Systems*
Cognitive Level: *Application*

64. ANSWER: 1

Rationale:

1. **The nurse would expect to see anasarca.**
2. The nurse would expect to see hypoproteinemia.
3. The nurse would expect to see a normal blood pressure.
4. The nurse would expect to see a high hematocrit resulting from hemoconcentration.

TEST-TAKING TIP: The pathophysiology of nephrotic syndrome results in the loss of large quantities of protein from the blood. The hypoproteinemia results in a drop in the colloidal pressure in the vascular tree, resulting in a fluid shift into the child's interstitial spaces, leading to anasarca and hemoconcentration.

Content Area: *Pediatrics*
Integrated Processes: *Nursing Process: Implementation*
Client Need: *Physiological Integrity: Physiological Adaptation: Alterations in Body Systems*
Cognitive Level: *Application*

65. ANSWER: 2

Rationale:

1. The image depicts a pyloric stenosis.
2. **The image depicts an intussusception.**
3. The image depicts esophageal atresia and tracheoesophageal fistula.
4. The image depicts the colon of a child with Hirschsprung's disease.

TEST-TAKING TIP: Parents of children with serious illnesses are anxious and scared. When the illnesses are described to them, they often have difficulty understanding the descriptions. When visual images are available, they help to clarify the illnesses for the family members.

Content Area: *Pediatrics*
Integrated Processes: *Nursing Process: Implementation*
Client Need: *Physiological Integrity: Physiological Adaptation: Alterations in Body Systems*
Cognitive Level: *Comprehension*

66. ANSWER: 4

Rationale:

1. A child with von Willebrand's disease does not need to consume a special diet.
2. A child with von Willebrand's disease does not need to have his or her temperature assessed.
3. A child with von Willebrand's disease does not need to avoid contact with allergens.
4. **A child with von Willebrand's disease must have pressure and ice applied to all injuries.**

TEST-TAKING TIP: Von Willebrand's disease is a hereditary bleeding disorder. To prevent excessive bleeding, a child with the disease must have pressure and ice applied to all injuries and receive DDAVP (desmopressin acetate) prior to any surgery or when seriously injured.

Content Area: *Pediatrics*
Integrated Processes: *Nursing Process: Implementation*
Client Need: *Physiological Integrity: Physiological Adaptation: Illness Management*
Cognitive Level: *Application*

67. ANSWER: 2

Rationale:

1. A human chorionic gonadotropin (hCG) assessment is a pregnancy test.
2. **Antinuclear antibody (ANA) assessment is a screening test for lupus.**
3. Partial thromboplastin time (PTT) assessment tests the clotting time of blood.
4. Alanine transaminase (ALT) assessment is a liver function test.

TEST-TAKING TIP: The macular rash over the nose and cheeks is characteristic of lupus. In addition, the girl is exhibiting arthritic changes in her joints, which are also characteristic of lupus. It would be appropriate for the nurse to request an order for an ANA test for this patient.

Content Area: *Pediatrics*
Integrated Processes: *Nursing Process: Implementation*
Client Need: *Physiological Integrity: Reduction of Risk Potential: Diagnostic Tests*
Cognitive Level: *Application*

68. ANSWER: 1

Rationale:

1. **Parents should conduct yearly fire drills for their young children.**
2. Hot water heater should be at no higher than 120°F.
3. Batteries in household fire alarms should be changed every year.
4. Sunscreen may be applied to babies of any age, but no baby should be in the direct sun until he or she is at least 6 months of age.

TEST-TAKING TIP: There are many reasons why young children become burned. Safe practices are very important as a means of preventing burns.

Content Area: *Child Health*
Integrated Processes: *Nursing Process: Implementation; Teaching/Learning*
Client Need: *Health Promotion and Maintenance: Health Promotion/Disease Prevention*
Cognitive Level: *Application*

69. ANSWER: 3 and 5

Rationale:

1. A patient with an animal bite would need to receive a tetanus booster but not with a tick bite.
2. A patient with viral diarrhea would not need to receive a tetanus booster.
3. **A patient with a third-degree burn would need to receive a tetanus booster.**
4. A patient with bacterial meningitis would not need to receive a tetanus booster.
5. **A patient with a deep puncture wound would need to receive a tetanus booster.**

TEST-TAKING TIP: *Clostridium tetani*, an anaerobic bacterium, is found everywhere in the environment. It causes a life-threatening disease, colloquially called lockjaw, that is characterized by neck stiffness, difficulty swallowing, muscle spasms, seizures, dysrhythmias, and pulmonary emboli. To prevent the illness, the DTaP and Tdap vaccinations are administered.
Content Area: *Child Health*
Integrated Processes: *Nursing Process: Analysis*
Client Need: *Health Promotion and Maintenance: Health Promotion/Disease Prevention*
Cognitive Level: *Application*

70. ANSWER: 4

Rationale:

1. The findings are characteristic of fetal alcohol syndrome.
2. The findings are characteristic of fetal alcohol syndrome.
3. The findings are characteristic of fetal alcohol syndrome.
4. **The findings are characteristic of fetal alcohol syndrome.**

TEST-TAKING TIP: There is no known safe level of alcohol consumption during pregnancy. Teratogenic changes can happen at any time during the pregnancy, with physiological changes occurring during the first trimester and cognitive changes occurring at any period of gestation. To prevent fetal alcohol syndrome, women should refrain from consuming alcohol preconceptually, while they are trying to become pregnant, as well as throughout the entire pregnancy.
Content Area: *Child Health*
Integrated Processes: *Nursing Process: Analysis*
Client Need: *Physiological Integrity: Physiological Adaptation: Alterations in Body Systems*
Cognitive Level: *Comprehension*

71. ANSWER: 1

Rationale:

1. **The nurse is assessing for developmental dysplasia of the hip (DDH) and is externally rotating the baby's hips.**
2. Comparing the baby's knee heights is another assessment to screen for DDH and is called the Galeazzi assessment.
3. Checking of the baby's plantar reflexes, also called the Babinski reflex, is unrelated to DDH.
4. Monitoring the baby's pedal pulses is unrelated to DDH.

TEST-TAKING TIP: DDH is a relatively common congenital defect that is seen most often in females, breech babies, and in conjunction with other defects (e.g., spina bifida). Because DDH may not be evident at birth, infants should be assessed for the defect at each well-baby visit.
Content Area: *Pediatrics—Infant*
Integrated Processes: *Nursing Process: Implementation*
Client Need: *Health Promotion and Maintenance: Techniques of Physical Assessment*
Cognitive Level: *Application*

72. ANSWER: 364 mg to 727 mg every 8 hr

Rationale:

Ratio and proportion method:

$$48 \text{ lb} : x \text{ kg} = 2.2 \text{ lb} : 1 \text{ kg}$$

$$2.2x = 48$$

$$x = 21.82 \text{ kg}$$

$$50 \text{ mg per day}/1 \text{ kg} = x \text{ mg per day}/21.82 \text{ kg}$$

$$x = 1091 \text{ mg per day}$$

$$x = 364 \text{ mg every 8 hr}$$

$$100 \text{ mg per day}/1 \text{ kg} = x \text{ mg per day}/21.82 \text{ kg}$$

$$x = 2182 \text{ mg per day}$$

$$x = 727 \text{ mg every 8 hr}$$

Dimensional analysis method:

50 mg	~~1 kg~~	48 ~~lb~~	~~1 day~~	= 364 mg every 8 hr
~~1 kg~~	2.2 ~~lb~~	~~1 day~~	3 (8-hr periods)	

100 mg	~~1 kg~~	48 ~~lb~~	~~1 day~~	= 727 mg every 8 hr
~~1 kg~~	2.2 ~~lb~~	~~1 day~~	3 (8-hr periods)	

TEST-TAKING TIP: There are two different methods that may be used to solve the problem: ratio and proportion method and dimensional analysis method.
Content Area: *Pediatrics—Medication*
Integrated Processes: *Nursing Process: Implementation*
Client Need: *Physiological Integrity: Pharmacological and Parenteral Therapies: Dosage Calculation*
Cognitive Level: *Synthesis*

73. ANSWER: 2

Rationale:

1. This question is not the most important for the nurse to ask the young woman.
2. **This question is the most important for the nurse to ask the young woman.**
3. This statement is not the most important for the nurse to discuss with the young woman.
4. This statement is not the most important for the nurse to discuss with the young woman.

TEST-TAKING TIP: This young woman is underweight (her BMI is below the 5th percentile) and may be anorexic. One of the characteristics of anorexia is a disturbed body

image as well as an intense fear of gaining weight. The nurse should query the young woman regarding her body image.
Content Area: Mental Health—Eating Disorders
Integrated Processes: Nursing Process: Implementation
Client Need: Psychosocial Integrity: Mental Health Concepts
Cognitive Level: Application

74. ANSWER: 4
Rationale:
1. Children are no more at high risk of becoming addicted to narcotics than are adults.
2. Children are no more at high risk of developing respiratory depression if given narcotics than are adults.
3. Children do not tolerate pain better than adults tolerate pain.
4. Children can effectively use pain scales to measure their pain.
TEST-TAKING TIP: There are excellent pain rating scales that can be used for children of all ages.
Content Area: Pediatrics—Medication
Integrated Processes: Nursing Process: Analysis
Client Need: Physiological Integrity: Pharmacological and Parenteral Therapies: Pharmacological Pain Management
Cognitive Level: Application

75. ANSWER: 2
Rationale:
1. Children with pinworms do not experience black stools.
2. Children with pinworms do scratch their anal area.
3. Children with pinworms are not febrile.
4. Children with pinworms do not vomit.
TEST-TAKING TIP: Once pinworm eggs hatch, they migrate out of the body via the anus. As a result, children with pinworms do scratch the area to relieve the itching. In addition, the children often wet the bed because of the stimulation caused by the migration of the worms.
Content Area: Pediatrics
Integrated Processes: Nursing Process: Assessment
Client Need: Physiological Integrity: Physiological Adaptation: Alterations in Body Systems
Cognitive Level: Application

Putting It All Together: Case Study Answers

Chapter 1

A. What *subjective* assessments indicate that the client is experiencing a health alteration?
   1. Family members, most notably the child's father, state that the child has injured himself.
   2. Through an interpreter, the child states that he fell while riding his bicycle.
   3. Neither the family members nor the child is aware of his immunization history.

B. What *objective* assessments indicate that the client is experiencing a health alteration?
   1. Through an interpreter, the child communicates that his pain level is 5 out of 10 on a numeric scale.
   2. Abrasion and bruise, 2 in. by 2 in. in size, noted on outer aspect of right leg distal to the knee.
   3. Abrasion is dirt covered.
   4. Negative x-rays.
   5. No immunization history.
   6. Vital signs: Temperature, 98.6°F, Heart rate: 90 bpm, Respiratory rate: 24 rpm, Blood pressure: 100/60 mm Hg

C. After analyzing the data that has been collected, what **primary** nursing diagnosis should the nurse assign to this client?
   1. Risk for Infection related to the dirt-covered abrasion and no immunization history.

D. What interventions should the nurse plan and/or implement to meet this child's and his family's needs?
   1. Provide a language interpreter throughout the emergency room visit.
   2. Allow as many family members to accompany the child during the visit as possible.
   3. Apologize to any family members who are unable to accompany the child.
   4. Educate the child and family members regarding the prescribed interventions.
   5. Administer the pain medication, as ordered, using five rights and safe administration procedures.
   6. Cleanse the wound, as ordered, encouraging the child to use guided imagery pain-reducing behavior during the procedure.
   7. Administer Tdap vaccine, as ordered, using five rights and safe administration procedures.
   8. Provide comfort measures after procedures are completed.
   9. Communicate to the family members and child the importance of follow-up care at the pediatric clinic.
   10. Educate the family members and child regarding the importance of following safety precautions and of obtaining recommended immunizations.
   11. Make the follow-up appointment for the child.

E. What client outcomes should the nurse evaluate regarding the effectiveness of the nursing interventions?
   1. Via an interpreter, the child and family members express understanding of the prescribed interventions.
   2. The child receives medication without excessive complaints.
   3. During cleansing of the wound, the child employs guided imagery, pain-reducing behavior.
   4. The family members and child state an understanding of the need to keep the follow-up appointment.

F. What physiological characteristics should the child exhibit before being discharged home?
   1. Wound is clean.

G. What psychological characteristics should the child and family exhibit before being discharged home?
   1. The child and family members state that they are pleased with the care received.
   2. The child and family members state that they will keep the follow-up appointment, obtain a bike helmet for the child, and consider returning for recommended vaccinations.

Chapter 2

A. Which *subjective* assessments are important in this scenario?
   1. The child cries when the nurse enters the room, and the mother states that he cries when approached by anyone who he does not know.
   2. The mother states that the child goes to sleep with a bottle filled with formula.
   3. The mother complains about the child's eating behavior.
   4. The mother scolds the child for "getting into things."
   5. The mother states that the child "sometimes rides on her lap" in the car.

B. Which *objective* assessments are important in this scenario?
   1. When plotted on the growth charts, the child's weight, length, and head circumference are all at approximately the same percentile. (See Growth Chart on p. 507.)
   2. The child's vital signs are all within normal limits.
   3. All other growth and development assessments are within normal limits for a child of 10 months. (Even though the child refuses to wave, the mother states that he waves to her.)
   4. The mother appears frustrated when the child refuses to wave to the nurse.

C. After analyzing the data that has been collected, what **primary** nursing diagnosis should the nurse assign to this client?
   1. Risk for Impaired Parenting related to negative statements made by the mother regarding the child's behaviors.

D. What interventions should the nurse plan and/or implement to meet this child's and his family's needs?
   1. Praise the mother for bringing in a healthy boy who is up to date on immunizations and who is exhibiting normal growth and development.
   2. Educate the mother regarding stranger anxiety—highlight the fact that fear of strangers implies that the child feels safe and secure with his mother.
   3. Educate the mother regarding dental caries and suggest that she wean him from the nighttime bottle, give him a pacifier at night instead of the bottle, or put water in the bottle at night rather than formula.
   4. Educate the mother regarding readiness for self-feeding—highlight the fact that this is normal growth and development and that the child is not trying to defy her but is simply developing and growing normally.
   5. Educate the mother regarding normal play of the 10-month-old. Highlight:
      a. The child's fine motor and gross motor movements.
      b. That he is not "getting into things" to be bad, but that that is how he is learning.
      c. That disciplining him may result in a child who is defiant and unhappy rather than obedient.
   6. Make suggestions for ways to improve the relationship between the mother and child.
      a. Toys that will enhance his development.
      b. Activities that will entertain him.
      c. Ways to divert his attention from unacceptable behavior to acceptable behavior.
   7. Educate the mother regarding unsafe car practice, and suggest that she move the car seat from her car into that of her friend when the friend is driving.
   8. Provide anticipatory guidance and safety advice regarding the changes she will see in his behavior in the future (e.g., walking independently and becoming more and more inquisitive, need for gates, move plants, lock up medicines, wash hands regularly; becoming more adept at feeding himself, need to continue to provide safe foods at all meals and snack times; becoming more independent in the bath, need never to leave the child alone near water).
   9. Provide anticipatory guidance regarding future disease prevention actions (i.e., future well-child visits, future immunizations, toilet training [to prevent possible abuse because boys are often late to train; she should not anticipate his becoming toilet trained for 18 months or even longer]).

E. What client outcomes should the nurse evaluate regarding the effectiveness of the nursing interventions?
   1. The child continues to develop and grow normally, that is:
      a. biological growth.
      b. gross motor development.
      c. fine motor development.
      d. language development.
      e. psychosocial development.
      f. cognitive development.
   2. The mother understands the normal growth and development and, therefore, interacts with the child appropriately, provides him with an appropriate and safe environment, provides him with safe and appropriate toys, and continues to seek health promotion and disease prevention health care.

Birth to 36 months: Boys
Head circumference-for-age and Weight-for-length percentiles

NAME ______________

RECORD # ______________

Date	Age	Weight	Length	Head Circ.	Comment
	Birth	3.2 kg	49 cm	34 cm	50th percentile
	10 mo	9 kg	73 cm	45.35 cm	50th percentile

Published May 30, 2000 (modified 10/16/00).
SOURCE: Developed by the National Center for Health Statistics in collaboration with the National Center for Chronic Disease Prevention and Health Promotion (2000).
http://www.cdc.gov/growthcharts

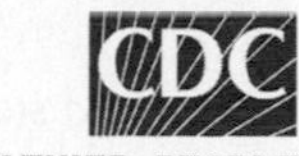

SAFER • HEALTHIER • PEOPLE™

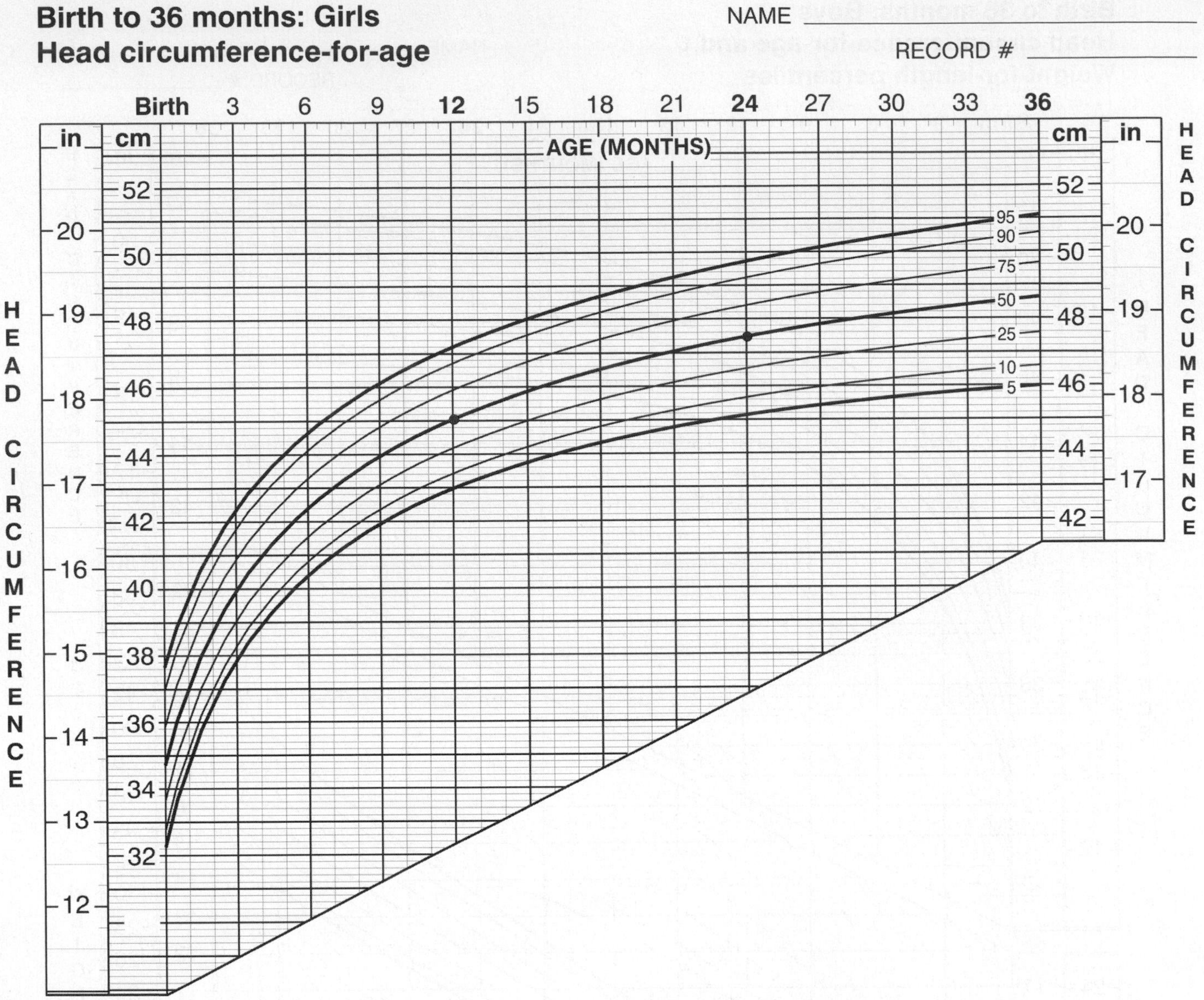

Birth to 36 months: Girls
Head circumference-for-age

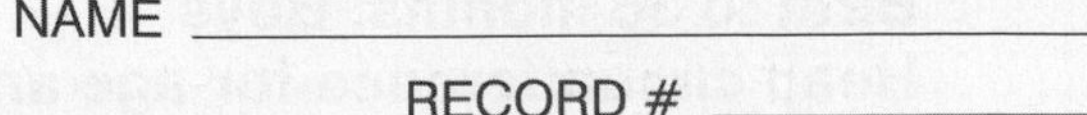

F. What physiological characteristics should the child exhibit before going home?
   1. The child hugs his mother and seeks security in her arms.
   2. The mother hugs and consoles her son.

Chapter 3

A. Which *subjective* assessments are important in this scenario?
   1. The father states that there is a new baby in the house.
   2. The child is regressing—going back to the bottle after having weaned "months ago."
   3. The child is having tantrums since the baby came home.
   4. The child is refusing to go "anywhere near a toilet."
   5. The child states, "No! No! Me do! Me do!"

B. Which *objective* assessments are important in this scenario?
   1. The child's height, weight, and head circumference were all at the 50th percentile at 1 year of age and are all at the 50th percentile at 2 years of age. (See Growth Charts above and on p. 509.)
   2. Laboratory values all within normal limits.
   3. Vital signs are all within normal limits.
   4. All other growth assessments are within normal limits. It would be best if the child could be assessed directly, but the father states that the child is exhibiting appropriate growth and development.
   5. The child has two dental cavities.

C. After analyzing the data that has been collected, what **primary** nursing diagnoses should the nurse assign to this client?
   1. Interrupted Family Processes related to regression of and tantrums by the child following the birth of a new baby.

Birth to 36 months: Girls
Length-for-age and Weight-for-age percentiles

NAME ____________________

RECORD # ____________________

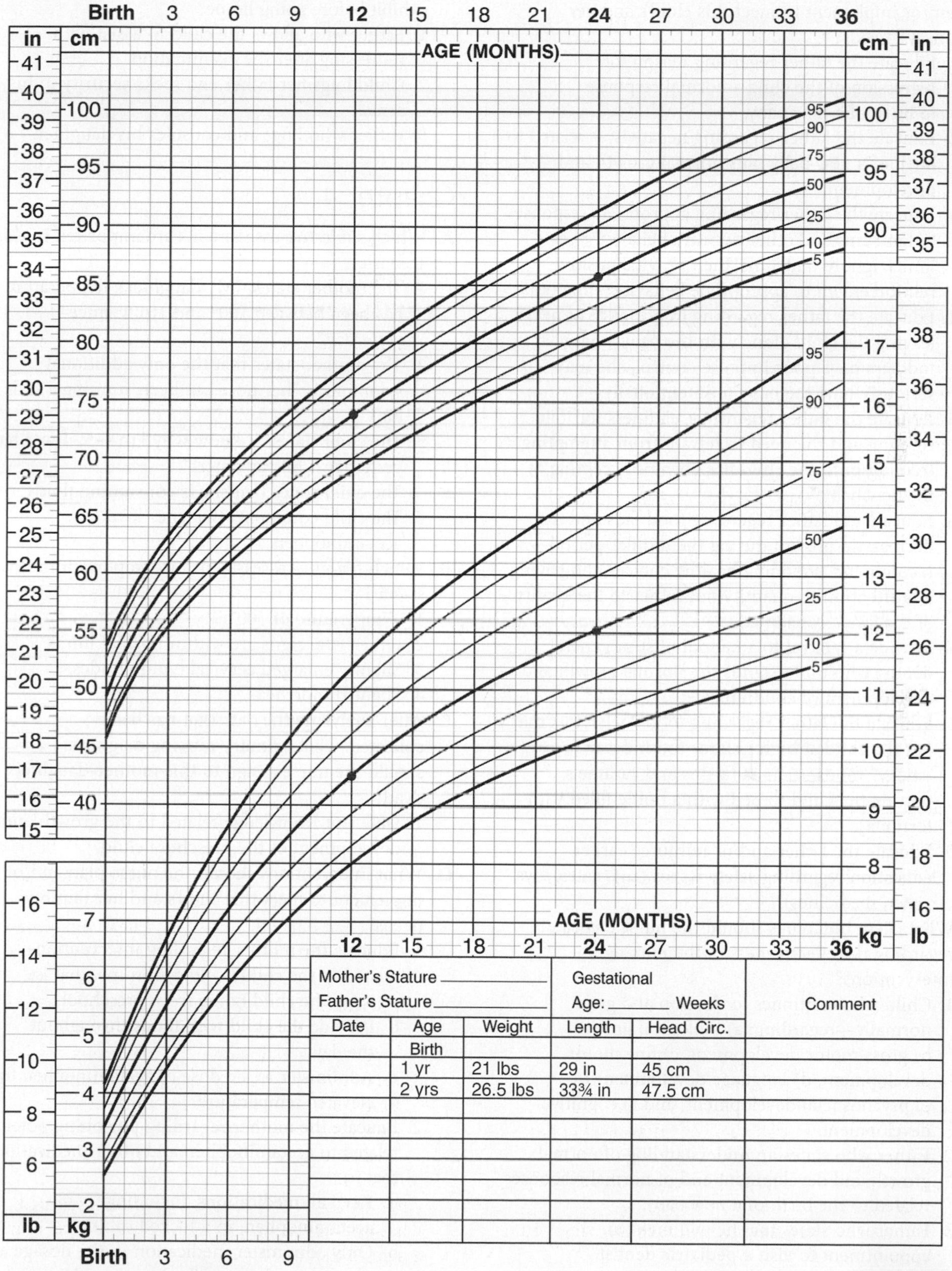

Mother's Stature ______		Gestational			Comment
Father's Stature ______		Age: ____ Weeks			
Date	Age	Weight	Length	Head Circ.	
	Birth				
	1 yr	21 lbs	29 in	45 cm	
	2 yrs	26.5 lbs	33¾ in	47.5 cm	

Published May 30, 2000 (modified 4/20/01).
SOURCE: Developed by the National Center for Health Statistics in collaboration with the National Center for Chronic Disease Prevention and Health Promotion (2000).
http://www.cdc.gov/growthcharts

CDC SAFER • HEALTHIER • PEOPLE™

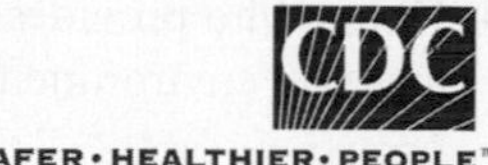

2. Deficient Knowledge related to impaired dental health of the child.

D. What interventions should the nurse plan and/or implement to meet this child's and her family's needs?
   1. Educate the father regarding reason for regression of the child—normal response to birth of a new baby.
   2. Educate the father regarding negativity—related to birth of a new baby plus normal growth and development.
   3. Educate the father regarding appropriate responses to tantrums and other negative behavior—set limits; ignore tantrums, then provide positive reinforcement to appropriate behavior; time-outs.
   4. Educate the father regarding importance of never leaving the child alone with the baby—because toddlers have poor impulse control, she may seriously hurt the baby unintentionally.
   5. Educate the father regarding readiness for toilet training and the need to refrain from attempting training until the child has become accepting of the new baby.
   6. Educate the father regarding food fads and the decrease in growth during the toddler period—recommend providing healthy choices and paying less attention to quantity but rather to the quality of the foods consumed.
   7. Provide a referral to a pedodontist or general dentist who understands the normal growth and development of children's teeth.
   8. Educate the father regarding foods/behaviors that put the child at high risk for tooth decay (e.g., "sticky" foods, such as raisins and caramels; putting the child to bed with a bottle filled with formula).
   9. Educate the father and/or reinforce earlier education regarding safety issues (e.g., gates, toys, water, medicines).

E. What client outcomes should the nurse evaluate regarding the effectiveness of the nursing interventions?
   1. Child who continues to develop and grow normally—regarding: a) biological growth, b) gross motor development, c) fine motor development, d) language development, e) psychosocial development, and f) cognitive development.
   2. Father who states an understanding of normal growth and development and of normal responses related to the birth of a new baby.
   3. Father who states that he will make an appointment to visit a pediatric dentist.
   4. Father who provides the child with an appropriate and safe environment, provides her with safe and appropriate toys, and continues to seek health promotion and disease prevention health care.

F. What physiological characteristics should the child exhibit before going home?
   1. Father who allows the child to assist with redressing after the examination.
   2. Child hugs her father and seeks security in his arms.
   3. Father who hugs and consoles his daughter.

Chapter 4

A. Which *subjective* assessments are important in this scenario?
   1. The mother states, "My daughter's temperature has been between 100° and 101°F since yesterday."
   2. The mother states that the only additional symptom is "her nose has been running a little bit."
   3. The child states, "I know why I'm sick. I was bad yesterday. I hit my sister!"
   4. The child states that she is consuming fluids.
   5. The child comments that she "love[s]" acetaminophen.

B. Which *objective* assessments are important in this scenario?
   1. Temperature of 100°F.
   2. Other vital signs are within normal limits.
   3. Slightly enlarged cervical lymph nodes.
   4. Slight rhinorrhea.

C. After analyzing the data that has been collected, what **primary** nursing diagnosis should the nurse assign to this mother-daughter dyad?
   1. Deficient Knowledge related to the growth and development of the preschool child.

D. What interventions should the nurse plan and/or implement to meet this child's and her family's needs?
   1. Educate the mother regarding interventions related to the child's cold syndrome, that is:
      a. Keep the child home from preschool.
      b. Provide the child with fluids throughout the day.
      c. Administer a safe dose of acetaminophen for elevated temperature.
   2. Educate the mother regarding poisoning potential related to acetaminophen and other medications, that is:
      a. Keep all medications, including acetaminophen, in a locked cabinet.
      b. Only administer medication in the dosage and time intervals prescribed by the primary health-care provider.

3. Educate the child regarding the importance of:
   a. Staying home from school until she is no longer sick.
   b. Drinking fluids.
   c. Only taking medicine when her mother administers it to her.
   d. Frequent hand washing to prevent the spread of the cold to others in the family.
   e. Covering her mouth and nose with her elbow or tissue when sneezing and/or coughing.
4. In simple terms, advise the child, with the mother in attendance:
   a. That colds are spread by being close to someone who has a cold.
   b. That hitting her sister may have been a "sad choice" or "sad thing to do" but that it does not make her a "bad girl" and her cold is not a punishment for the "sad choice."
5. In private, explain to the mother about the magical thinking of preschoolers and that, when disciplining the child, it is important to separate the child's actions from the child herself.

E. What client outcomes should the nurse evaluate regarding the effectiveness of the nursing interventions?
   1. The child and mother communicate an understanding of the nurse's education regarding:
      a. School attendance.
      b. Fluid intake.
      c. Medication administration.
      d. Etiology of the illness.
   2. The mother communicates an understanding of appropriate language to use when disciplining her daughter.

F. What physiological characteristics should the child exhibit before being discharged home?
   1. Child covers her mouth and nose with her elbow when she sneezes and coughs.

Chapter 5

A. Which *subjective* assessments are important in this scenario?
   1. For the past 3 days, the child has complained of a headache and stomachache.
   2. The mother has kept the child home from school for the past 3 days.
   3. The mother states that the child's symptoms resolve once the school day ends.
   4. The mother states that the child has complained about being placed in the lowest reading group in her classroom.
   5. The mother states that the child is the only Chinese immigrant in her classroom.
   6. The mother states that the child has complained that some students in the upper reading group "said something" to her.

B. Which *objective* assessments are important in this scenario?
   1. None.

C. After analyzing the data that has been collected, what **primary** nursing diagnosis should the nurse assign to this client?
   1. Altered Coping related to feelings of inferiority.

D. What interventions should the nurse plan and/or implement to meet this child's and her family's needs?
   1. Inform the mother that the child is exhibiting signs of school refusal and that it is important that the child return to school the next day.
   2. Strongly encourage the parent to meet with the teacher and school principal regarding the bullying by the students in the upper reading group.
   3. Strongly encourage the parent to meet with the teacher regarding supplementary learning experiences that the child could have to improve the child's reading level.
   4. Strongly encourage the mother to tell her daughter that she is a bright and capable young girl who does well in other school activities and in activities outside of school. The mother should give the young girl specific examples of her abilities.
   5. Strongly encourage the mother to speak with her daughter regarding the problems at school and how the mother is working hard to make the school experience a more positive one.
   6. Encourage the mother, once they are identified, to inform the child regarding the actions that will be taken to improve the school experience.
   7. Provide the mother with strategies that she can teach her child to utilize when she is being bullied by the other children, including avoiding contact with the children, affirmatively telling the children to stop bullying, and informing the teacher when the bullying occurs.

E. What client outcomes should the nurse evaluate regarding the effectiveness of the nursing interventions?
   1. The child returns to school the next day.
   2. The mother reports that the child expresses no reluctance to return to school.
   3. The mother reports that the child states that she is being bullied no longer.
   4. The mother reports that the child's reading ability is improving.

F. What physiological characteristics should the child exhibit before being discharged home?
   1. The child no longer reports headaches and/or stomachaches in the mornings before school begins.

Chapter 6

A. Which *subjective* assessments are important in this scenario?
   1. The child states that he frequently "blows off" his homework.
   2. The child states that in lieu of homework, he plays video games and watches television.
   3. The mother states that she and her husband have threatened to cancel camp for the child if he does not "do better in school."

B. Which *objective* assessments are important in the scenario?
   1. All vital signs are within normal limits (WNL).
   2. Child is at the 50th percentile for both height and weight.
   3. Normal physical examination.

C. After analyzing the data that has been collected, what **primary** nursing diagnosis should the nurse assign to this client?
   1. Deficient Knowledge of parents related to adolescent behavior, limit setting, and discipline.

D. What interventions should the nurse plan and/or implement to meet this child's and his family's needs?
   1. Educate the parent regarding adolescent behavior.
   2. Educate the parent regarding the need for limit setting.
   3. Educate the parent regarding disciplinary consequences that are appropriate and time sensitive.
   4. Educate the child regarding the importance of completing his assigned tasks.

E. What client outcomes should the nurse evaluate regarding the effectiveness of the nursing interventions?
   1. The child completes his homework prior to engaging in leisure activities (i.e., video gaming and television watching).

F. What physiological characteristics should the child exhibit before being discharged home?
   1. None. The child is physically healthy.

Chapter 7

A. What *subjective* assessments indicate that the client is a healthy child?
   1. The mother states, "She's such an angel when she's sleeping. And she is great fun when she is playing."
   2. The mother states that the child's stools are "bright yellow and loose. She stools about three or four times a day. I'm still exclusively breastfeeding her."
   3. The mother states that the child "has about six really, really wet diapers a day. And when she wakes up, her pajamas are sometimes even wet."

B. What *objective* assessments indicate that the client is a healthy child?
   1. Entire review of systems is within normal limits. Head circumference, weight, and length are all at the 50th percentile.
   2. Vital signs are all within normal limits.
   3. Child's verbalizations, "da da da," are normal for child's age.
   4. Child's reflex responses are within normal limits.
   5. Child's gross motor and fine motor development are within normal limits.

C. After analyzing the data that has been collected, what **primary** nursing diagnoses should the nurse assign to this client?
   1. Normal Health Maintenance and Normal Growth and Development.

D. What interventions should the nurse plan and/or implement to meet this child's and her family's needs?
   1. Administer 6-month vaccinations.
      a. Using appropriate method for drawing up and administering parenteral injections by locating each vastus lateralis and choosing the appropriate length and gauge needle.
      b. Separating injection sites by at least 1 in. in each thigh.
      c. Using appropriate method for oral vaccine administration.
   2. To minimize pain, either have the child suck on a sucrose soothie or have the child breastfeed while immunizations are administered. Educate the mother regarding rationale.
   3. Educate the mother regarding the method of feeding solid foods.
      a. Mix small amount of baby rice cereal with breast milk. To reduce potential for aspiration, offer the food while the baby is sitting up in an infant seat.
      b. Feed the child rice cereal two to three times each day for 4 to 7 days to observe for allergic response. If rash or other abnormal response occurs, notify the primary health-care provider.
      c. If no adverse response is noted, repeat the procedure with another cereal (e.g., barley cereal) and then another until all cereals have been offered.

d. Next, offer baby meats, vegetables, and fruits in the same 4- to 7-day format. If adverse reactions are noted, stop offering the food, and notify the primary health-care provider.
4. Reinforce the need to provide the baby with multiple forms of stimulation.

E. What client outcomes should the nurse evaluate regarding the effectiveness of the nursing interventions?
1. The baby will remain healthy.
2. The baby's growth and development will progress normally.
3. The baby will develop no allergic reactions to foods.
4. The baby will return for a follow-up assessment at 9 months of age.

F. What physiological characteristics should the child exhibit before being discharged home?
1. The child should continue to exhibit normal physiological functioning.

G. What subjective characteristics should the child exhibit before being discharged home?
1. The child should appear content in her mother's arms.

Chapter 8

A. What *subjective* assessments indicate that the client is experiencing a health alteration?
1. The mother states that the teenager has "a very high fever, and she isn't acting herself."
2. The teenager states, "I really feel awful."
3. The teenager states that she has been vomiting to lose weight.
4. The teenager asks the nurse not to tell her mother that she has been engaging in high-risk behavior.
5. When told that she needs a diagnostic procedure, the teenager states, "Do you have to do all that? I'm really okay."

B. What *objective* assessments indicate that the client is experiencing a health alteration?
1. Markedly elevated temperature, pulse, and respirations.
2. Hypotension.
3. Vomitus tinged with bright-red blood.
4. Objective assessment of pain.

C. After analyzing the data that has been collected, what **primary** nursing diagnosis should the nurse assign to this client?
1. Physiological diagnosis: Risk for Injury related to unknown pathology.
2. Psychosocial diagnosis: Risk for Altered Coping related to a history of self-induced vomiting, unknown pathology, and response to need for invasive procedure.

D. What interventions should the nurse plan and/or implement to meet this child's and her family's immediate needs?
1. After making sure that the mother has no questions regarding the rationale for and potential complications from the endoscopy, determine that the mother and a witness have signed the informed consent form.
2. Allow the teenager to express concerns regarding the endoscopy and the medications.
3. Answer questions the teenager may have regarding the primary health-care provider's orders.
4. Inform the young woman that she will receive pain medication during the endoscopy.
5. Request the teenager's assent for the procedures.
6. Ask the teen if she would like her mother to stay with her during the procedures.
7. Provide therapeutic holding, as needed, during the endoscopy.
8. The nurse recommends to the child's health care provider that a social work consult be ordered.

E. What client outcomes should the nurse evaluate regarding the effectiveness of the nursing interventions?
1. With her mother at her side, the teenager allows the nurse to administer the medications with no physical or verbal protest.
2. With her mother at her side and with the nurse providing therapeutic holding, the teenager undergoes the endoscopy procedure with no physical or verbal protest.
3. The teenager states that her pain level is below 3 on a 10-point scale.
4. The teenager's vital signs return to normal.
5. The teenager does not vomit again.

F. What physiological characteristics should the child exhibit before being discharged home?
1. Normal blood pressure, normal temperature, normal pulse, and normal respiratory rate.
2. Pain level of 0 to 2 on a 10-point, numeric pain rating scale.
3. No further episodes of blood-tinged vomitus.

G. What psychological characteristics should the child and family exhibit before being discharged home?
1. The teenager seeks comfort from her mother, and her mother provides comfort, both verbally and via touch.
2. The teenager consents to see a social worker regarding her vomiting behavior.

Chapter 9

A. What *subjective* assessments indicate that the client is experiencing a health alteration?
1. The child is crying.
2. The child is complaining of neck pain.

3. The child is complaining of photophobia.
4. The mother is stroking the child's forehead and asking for assistance.

B. What *objective* assessments indicate that the client is experiencing a health alteration?
1. The child is febrile, tachycardic, and tachypneic.
2. Positive Kernig's sign.
3. Positive Brudzinski's sign.
4. LP is abnormal, which is indicative of bacterial meningitis.
5. Positive culture for *N. meningitides.*
6. CBC shows markedly elevated white blood cell count, which is indicative of bacterial infection.

C. After analyzing the data that has been collected, what **primary** nursing diagnosis should the nurse assign to this client?
1. Risk for Injury (CNS) related to medical diagnosis and seizure potential.

D. What interventions should the nurse plan and/or implement to meet this child's and his family's needs?
1. Priority therapy: start IV and administer safe dosages of antibiotics.
   a. Insert IV using atraumatic, aseptic technique.
   b. Regulate IV pump after calculating pump rate (see "Intravenous Infusion Calculations" following the answers).
   c. Calculate safe dosages (see "Medications Calculations" following the answers).
   d. Administer medications using safe IV piggyback technique, including the five rights of medication administration.
   e. Monitor child for medication side effects.
2. Priority prevention, for contacts, is respiratory isolation.
3. Seizure precautions.
4. Dim the lights.
5. Stabilize the head to decrease pain.
6. Provide information regarding the illness and care to both the mother and the child.

E. What client outcomes should the nurse evaluate regarding the effectiveness of the nursing interventions?
1. IV site will be free from infiltration and phlebitis.
2. The child will no longer cry from neck pain or have photophobia.
3. The child will have negative Kernig's and Brudzinski's signs.
4. The child will no longer be febrile, tachycardic, or tachypneic.
5. The mother and child will verbalize an understanding of the disease process and the rationale for the therapeutic regimen.
6. The child will exhibit no side effects from the medications.

F. What physiological characteristics should the child exhibit before being discharged home?
1. Normal vital signs.
2. Normal LP.
3. Normal complete blood count (CBC).

G. What subjective characteristics should the child exhibit before being discharged home?
1. The child will be pain free.

IV Infusion Calculations

IV order reads: infuse 1,750 mL over 24 hr.

- Calculate daily maintenance volume (DMV) for child weighing 55 lb:
  - Convert pounds to kilograms:

$$1 \text{ kg}/2.2 \text{ lb} = x \text{ kg}/55 \text{ lb}$$

$$x = 25 \text{ kg}$$

  - If child weighs over 20 kg, DMV = 100 mL times 10 plus 50 mL times 10 **plus** 20 mL for every kilogram above 20 kg:

$$1{,}000 \text{ mL} + 500 \text{ mL} + (20 \text{ mL} \times 5 \text{ kg})$$
$$= 1{,}000 + 500 + 100 = 1{,}600 \text{ mL}$$

- **This child is febrile: it is appropriate to infuse additional fluids, therefore infusing 1,750 mL over 24 hr is a safe volume.**
- Calculate the pump infusion rate:
  - Ratio and proportion method:

$$1{,}750 \text{ mL}/24 \text{ hr} = 72.9 \text{ mL/hr} = 73 \text{ mL/hr}$$

  - Dimensional analysis method:

$$\frac{1{,}750 \text{ mL}}{24 \text{ hr}} = 72.9 \text{ mL/hr} = 73 \text{ mL/hr}$$

  - Infusion pump should be regulated at 73 mL/hr.

Medications Calculations

1. Physician's medication orders: Vancomycin 400 mg every 6 hr IV piggyback.
   - Recommended dosage of Vancomycin in medication reference: "children: 15 mg/kg intravenously every 6 hours." The recommended dosage is per weight.
     - Ratio and proportion method:
       - Convert pounds to kilograms:

$$1 \text{ kg}/2.2 \text{ lb} = x \text{ kg}/55 \text{ lb}$$

$$x = 25 \text{ kg}$$

       - Calculate safe dosage:

$$15 \text{ mg}/1 \text{ kg} = x \text{ mg}/25 \text{ kg}$$

$$x = 375 \text{ mg every 6 hr}$$

- Dimensional analysis method:

$$\frac{15 \text{ mg}}{\text{kg every 6 hr}} \bigg| \frac{55 \text{ lb}}{} \bigg| \frac{1 \text{ kg}}{2.2 \text{ lb}} = 375 \text{ mg every 6 hr}$$

- The primary health-care provider's order of 400 mg is higher than the calculated maximum safe dosage for this child of 375 mg.
- The nurse should request a safe order from the physician.
- The doctor changes the order to Vancomycin 350 mg every 6 hr IV piggyback.
- The nurse is now able to administer the safe dosage of the antibiotic.

2. Physician's medication orders: ceftriaxone 1.25 g every 12 hr IV piggyback.
   - Recommended dosage of ceftriaxone in medication reference: "children: 100 mg/kg/day intravenously in equal doses every 12 hours." The recommended dosage is per weight.
   - Ratio and proportion method:
     - Convert pounds to kilograms:

$$1 \text{ kg}/2.2 \text{ lb} = x \text{ kg}/55 \text{ lb}$$

$$x = 25 \text{ kg}$$

     - Calculate safe dosage:

$$100 \text{ mg}/1 \text{ kg} = x \text{ mg}/25 \text{ kg}$$

$$x = 2{,}500 \text{ mg/day}$$

     - The calculated dose must be divided by two to make the time frame the same as the doctor's order.

$$x = 2{,}500/2$$

$$x = 1{,}250 \text{ mg/12 hr}$$

     - The calculated value must be divided by 1,000 to make the units the same as the doctor's order.

$$x = 1{,}250 \text{ mg}/1{,}000$$

$$x = 1.25 \text{ g/12 hr}$$

   - Dimensional analysis method:

$$\frac{100 \text{ mg}}{\text{kg/day}} \bigg| \frac{55 \text{ lb}}{} \bigg| \frac{1 \text{ kg}}{2.2 \text{ lb}} \bigg| \frac{1 \text{ day}}{2 \text{ doses}} \bigg| \frac{1 \text{ g}}{1{,}000 \text{ mg}} = 1.25 \text{ g/2 doses}$$

     - **The order is safe because the calculated dosage and the doctor's order are the same.**
     - **The nurse can safely administer the medication every 12 hr as ordered.**

Chapter 10

A. Which *subjective* assessments are important in this scenario?
   1. The mother states that her child "started vomiting about 1 hour ago."
   2. The mother states that she "found an empty Children's Tylenol bottle on his bedroom floor."
   3. The mother states that she keeps the Tylenol bottle in her purse.
   4. The mother estimates that the child consumed the Tylenol 4 hr before the emergency department visit.

B. Which *objective* assessments are important in this scenario?
   1. The child is vomiting.
   2. Vital signs are within normal limits.
   3. CBC, ALT, and AST are all within normal limits.
   4. Serum acetaminophen concentration is 300 mcg/mL.

C. After analyzing the data that has been collected, what **primary** nursing diagnosis should the nurse assign to this client?
   1. Risk for Injury (hepatotoxicity) related to acute poisoning with Tylenol (acetaminophen).

D. What interventions should the nurse plan and/or implement to meet this child's and his family's needs?
   1. Weigh the child.
   2. Calculate the child's DMV and compare with IV order.
   3. Begin IV infusion, after requesting the primary health-care provider to provide a safe order.
   4. Input values into the applicable nomogram to confirm need for acetylcysteine.
   5. Employing the five rights of medication administration, administer IV acetylcysteine after calculating to make sure that it is a safe dosage.
   6. Employing the five rights of medication administration, administer Zofran STAT, per order.
   7. Order repeat laboratory tests, and report findings as soon as they are posted.
   8. Educate the mother regarding the poisoning potential of preschool-age children.
   9. Educate the mother regarding the importance of keeping all medications, including vitamins, in a locked medicine cabinet.

E. What client outcomes should the nurse evaluate regarding the effectiveness of the nursing interventions?
   1. Assess whether the child stops vomiting within 30 min of the administration of Zofran.
   2. Monitor for adverse responses to Zofran.
   3. Assess IV site and infusion rate hourly.
   4. Confirm that the acetylcysteine infused, as ordered.
   5. Monitor for adverse responses to acetylcysteine infusion.
   6. Monitor the child for jaundice and epigastric pain.

7. Evaluate the mother's responses to safety education.
8. Compare the repeat laboratory results with normal values.

F. What physiological characteristics should the child exhibit before being discharged home?
1. All of the child's laboratory values are within normal limits.
2. The child's skin should show no signs of jaundice.
3. The child should report no epigastric pain.

Chapter 11

A. What *subjective* assessments indicate that the client is experiencing a health alteration?
1. The patient's comments indicate that he is becoming frustrated with his diagnosis and with his medication regimen.
2. The patient states that he is sexually active.
3. The patient indicates that he inconsistently wears a condom during intercourse.
4. The patient indicates that his energy level is below normal.

B. What *objective* assessments indicate that the client is experiencing a health alteration?
1. The adolescent patient has been HIV positive since birth.
2. The patient, whose mother is deceased, lives with his grandmother.
3. The patient is currently on HAART.
4. Vital signs: blood pressure 98/50 mm Hg; temperature 100.4°F; heart rate 110 bpm, respiratory rate 20 rpm.
5. Maculopapular rash.
6. Abnormal CD4 count of 300 cells/mm^3.
7. Viral load of 1,000 copies/mL.
8. Abnormal hematocrit of 28% and hemoglobin 9 g/dL.
9. Abnormal liver function tests of AST 200 IU/L (normal 10 to 34 IU/L), ALT 250 IU/L (normal 10 to 40 IU/L), and bilirubin 6 mg/dL (normal 0 to 0.2 mg/dL).
10. Abnormal white blood cell count of 3,500 cells/mm^3.

C. After analyzing the data that has been collected, what **primary** nursing diagnosis should the nurse assign to this client?
1. Risk for Infection (opportunistic) related to current diagnosis.

D. What interventions should the nurse plan and/or implement to meet this child's and his family's needs?
1. Strongly recommend that the teenager comply with revised treatment regimen.
2. Strongly recommend that the teenager return for follow-up laboratory examinations in 1 month.
3. Counsel the teenager regarding his obligations to his girlfriend:
   a. To tell his girlfriend of his diagnosis.
   b. To wear a condom each and every time he has sexual intercourse.
   c. To encourage his girlfriend to be tested for HIV because he has confessed that there are times when he does not wear a condom during intercourse.
4. Counsel the teenager regarding the possible worsening of his condition.
   a. Low white blood cell count.
   b. Low CD4 count.
   c. Viral load of 1,000 copies/mL.
   d. Side effects of medication.
      i. Anemia, evidenced by fatigue and abnormal hematocrit and hemoglobin levels.
      ii. Hepatotoxicity, evidenced by rash and altered AST, ALT, and bilirubin levels.
5. Discuss with the teenager regarding a needed support system.
   a. His grandmother?
   b. Another family member?
   c. A teacher at his school?
   d. A mentor?
   e. His girlfriend?

E. What client outcomes should the nurse evaluate regarding the effectiveness of the nursing interventions? For the next clinic visit:
1. If the teen fails to keep his next clinic visit, call him to remind him and to set up another appointment.
2. If the teen keeps his next clinic visit:
   a. Assess all laboratory data and compare with previous findings.
   b. Assess his rash.
   c. Inquire whether his fatigue is improving or worsening.
   d. Ask whether he is following his medication regimen and about other side effects that he may be experiencing.
   e. Ask about his girlfriend and:
      i. Whether he has told his girlfriend of his diagnosis.
      ii. Whether he is wearing a condom each and every time he is having intercourse.
      iii. Whether his girlfriend has been tested for the disease.
   f. Note whether his grandmother has accompanied him to the clinic and/or whether he has identified another social support.

F. What physiological characteristics should the child exhibit before leaving the clinic?
1. None.

G. What subjective characteristics should the child exhibit before leaving the clinic?
   1. The teenager states that he will:
      a. Take his new medications each day.
      b. Report any worsening of current medication side effects and any side effects from the new medication.
      c. Return to the clinic in 1 month for a follow-up appointment.
      d. Notify his girlfriend of his diagnosis, of her risks if no condom is worn each time they have intercourse, and of her need to be tested.
      e. Advise his grandmother and/or another confidant of his changing health status.

Chapter 12

A. What *subjective* assessments indicate that the client is experiencing a health alteration?
   1. Mother states that the child is entering kindergarten in 2 months.
B. What *objective* assessments indicate that the client is experiencing a health alteration?
   1. The child's immunization record indicates that the child has yet to receive five vaccines required by the state in which the child lives.
      a. One DTaP vaccine
      b. One IPV vaccine
      c. One MMR vaccine
      d. One VAR vaccine
      e. One Hep A vaccine
C. After analyzing the data that has been collected, what **primary** nursing diagnosis should the nurse assign to this client?
   1. Ineffective Health Maintenance related to incomplete vaccination series.
D. What interventions should the nurse plan and/or implement to meet this child's and his or her family's needs?
   1. Determine which vaccinations are available in combination forms.
   2. If needed, elicit the assistance of up to three other nurses for the administration of the vaccines.
   3. With the other nurses, use the five rights of medication administration and aseptic technique to prepare injections of the vaccines needed to complete the vaccine series.
   4. Educate the mother and child regarding the injections that are required.
   5. Have the mother sign an informed consent form for the vaccine injections.
   6. Query the mother regarding any reasons why she feels the injections should not be administered at that time.
   7. Confirm that the child is not immune compromised or that there are any other contraindications to the administration of the vaccines.
   8. Question the child and mother regarding behaviors the child exhibits during painful experiences. If the mother states that the child needs to be restrained during injections, obtain additional assistance.
   9. Strongly encourage the child to utilize behaviors to mitigate the pain while the vaccines are being administered (e.g., counting to 10, utilizing guided imagery, clenching fists).
   10. Administer the injections in four different muscles (i.e., two deltoid and two vastus lateralis).
       a. If appropriate, the injections could be administered at the same time by 4 different nurses.
   11. Comfort and praise the child.
   12. Place an adhesive bandage on all injection sites.
   13. Provide the child with a prize (e.g., sticker, matchbox car, coloring book, picture book).
   14. Document the administration of the injections in the medical record.
   15. Give the parent a list of signs and symptoms to report to the primary health-care provider if the child should exhibit them.
   16. Give the parent a copy of the results of the physical assessment and the immunization record.
E. What client outcomes should the nurse evaluate regarding the effectiveness of the nursing interventions?
   1. All injections were administered using correct technique and in anatomically correct sites.
   2. All injection sites appear normal.
   3. Mother states that she will report any side effects exhibited by the child to the primary healthcare provider's office.
F. What physiological characteristics should the child exhibit after treatment?
   1. The child is composed when leaving the office.
   2. The child is walking and moving all limbs normally.

Chapter 13

A. What *subjective* assessments indicate that the client is experiencing a health alteration?
   1. The mother states, "My daughter seems to be having trouble breathing."
   2. The child's eyes are wide open, and she appears anxious.

B. What *objective* assessments indicate that the client is experiencing a health alteration?
   1. The child is sitting erect in bed and gasping for air.
   2. Pulmonary wheeze heard on auscultation.
   3. The child's fluid intake of 950 mL in 30 min (child's daily maintenance volume is 1,400 mL for the entire day).
      a. Weight on admission is 18 kg.

$$10 \text{ kg} \times 100 \text{ mL} = 1{,}000 \text{ mL}$$

$$8 \text{ kg} \times 50 \text{ mL} = 400 \text{ mL}$$

$$\text{total DMV} = 1{,}400 \text{ mL}$$

   4. Rapid, bounding pulses.
   5. Tachypnea.
   6. Elevated blood pressure.
   7. Blood gases indicate respiratory alkalosis, low oxygen saturation, and low PO2.
   8. Using ROME, the nurse determines that the pH and the pCO_2 are in opposite directions—Elevated pH and Low pCO_2
   9. High normal serum sodium related to the normal saline in the infusion.
   10. Low normal serum potassium related to the large quantity infused of IV fluid.

C. After analyzing the data that has been collected, what **primary** nursing diagnosis should the nurse assign to this client?
   1. Excess Fluid Volume related to rapid infusion of a large quantity of IV fluid.

D. What interventions should the nurse plan and/or implement to meet this child's and her family's needs?
   1. Clearly and calmly communicate to the child and mother what has happened and what actions are now being taken to rectify the problem.
   2. Administer oxygen as ordered.
   3. Raise the head of bed and maintain bedrest.
   4. Change IV infusion from gravity drip to IV pump.
   5. Calculate the safe dosage of Lasix and administer, if safe.
   6. Monitor vital signs and oxygen saturations every 15 minutes, and report any further deviations from normal.
   7. Give the child nothing by mouth.
   8. Monitor urinary output.
   9. Order repeat blood gas for 1 hr.
   10. Order repeat electrolytes for 12 hr.

E. What client outcomes should the nurse evaluate regarding the effectiveness of the nursing interventions?
   1. Auscultate the lungs for presence of abnormal breath sounds.
   2. Monitor vital signs, especially rate and depth of respirations.
   3. Monitor blood gases.
   4. Monitor urinary output.
   5. Monitor IV pump infusion.
   6. Assess serum electrolytes.
   7. Assess the child and mother for signs of fear or anxiety.

F. What physiological characteristics should the child exhibit before being discharged home?
   1. Normal pulmonary auscultation: no rales, no wheezes.
   2. All physiological functions are within normal limits, including vital signs, blood gases, and serum electrolytes.

G. What subjective characteristics should the child exhibit before being discharged home?
   1. The child and parent state that they are unafraid to return to the hospital for tonsillectomy in near future.

Chapter 14

A. What *subjective* assessments indicate that the client is experiencing a health alteration?
   1. The mother describes an unhappy, irritable child.
   2. The mother states, "I think he is having problems going to the bathroom."
   3. The child states, "My belly hurts sometimes after I eat."

B. What *objective* assessments indicate that the client is experiencing a health alteration?
   1. Weight percentile dropped from 55th percentile to 45th percentile in the past 6 months.
   2. Pale skin color.
   3. High normal heart rate.
   4. Low red blood cell count, hematocrit, and hemoglobin.
   5. Positive IgA-tTG test.
   6. Atrophy of intestinal villi on biopsy.

C. After analyzing the data that has been collected, what **primary** nursing diagnosis should the nurse assign to this client?
   1. Imbalanced Nutrition: Less than Body Requirements related to diagnosis of celiac disease.

D. What interventions should the nurse plan and/or implement to meet this child's and his family's needs?
   1. Educate the parents regarding the etiology and physical characteristics of the disease.
   2. Allow the parents and child to communicate their concerns about the child's physical and emotional health.

3. Allow the parents to communicate their concerns regarding need to supply a special diet to their son and its effects on the entire family.
4. Refer the parents to a registered dietitian and reinforce the diet education supplied by the nutritionist, including need to read the labels on all food items very carefully.
5. Inform the child that it is important for him to tell his parents if he is having abdominal pains and/or abnormal stooling patterns. Reinforce that he will not be punished or reprimanded in any way for what he will communicate to them.
6. Refer the family to the American Celiac Society.
7. Reinforce the need to bring the child back to the physician's office for a follow-up visit to assess growth patterns and blood values.

E. What client outcomes should the nurse evaluate regarding the effectiveness of the nursing interventions?
At the next pediatrician's visit:
1. Weight percentile.
2. Complete blood count.
3. Compliance with celiac diet.
4. Change in child's behavior.

F. What physiological and psychological characteristics should the child exhibit before being discharged home?
At the next pediatrician's visit, the:
1. Child is regaining his weight.
2. Child's blood values are all within normal limits.
3. Parents report that the child's behavior is "back to normal."
4. Child reports no abdominal pain after eating and no abnormal stooling patterns.
5. Mother states that she carefully reviews all labels on food items for the presence of gluten-containing products.
6. Parents and child state that maintaining the diet has not adversely affected the family.

G. What subjective characteristics should the child exhibit before being discharged home?
1. The child remarks that he no longer feels ill.

Chapter 15

A. What *subjective* assessments indicate that the client is experiencing a health alteration?
1. The mother states that the child's urine is pink.
2. The mother states that the child has had "a couple of colds" during the year.

B. What *objective* assessments indicate that the client is experiencing a health alteration?
1. Mass in left upper quadrant of the abdomen.
2. Blood pressure at the 90th percentile.
3. Serum red blood cell count below normal.
4. Hemoglobin below normal.
5. Hematocrit below normal.
6. Red blood cells in urine.
7. Mass in left kidney seen on ultrasound.

C. After analyzing the data that has been collected, what **primary** nursing diagnosis should the nurse assign to this client?
1. Risk for Injury to encapsulated Wilm's tumor related to fragility of tumor and age and activity level of the child.

D. What interventions should the nurse plan and/or implement to meet this child's and her family's needs?
1. Answer questions of parents regarding the diagnosis and clinical course.
2. Inform the parents to refrain from applying any pressure to the child's abdomen.
3. Praise the child for her behavior during the exam, and give the child a reward (e.g., sticker).
4. Inform the hospital of pending admission, and book the surgery.
5. Show the child equipment that she may see in the hospital (e.g., masks, surgical scrubs, IV tubing) and provide additional preoperative teaching care consistent with the age of the child.
6. Clearly tell the child, using age-appropriate language, that the hospitalization and surgery are not punishments but needed to make her better.
7. Using age-appropriate language, advise the child that she will have medicine after the surgery to make any pain go away.

E. What client outcomes should the nurse evaluate regarding the effectiveness of the nursing interventions?
1. The parents state that they understand the diagnosis and the rationale for hospitalization and surgery.
2. The parents freely express fear and anxiety about the child's diagnosis without frightening the child.
3. The child is familiar with items that she will see in the hospital.
4. The child does not communicate that she is sick because she has been "bad."

F. What physiological characteristics should the child exhibit before being discharged home (from hospital)?
1. Surgical incision is REEDA negative (i.e., no redness, no edema, no ecchymosis, no discharge, and the edges are well approximated).
2. The child shows no signs of infection.
3. The child shows no signs of stomatitis or vascular damage from vesicant.

4. The child's intake and output are within normal limits.
5. The child's vital signs are within normal limits, including blood pressure.
6. The child's weight is consistent with admission weight.
7. The child's laboratory data are all within normal limits.

G. What subjective characteristics should the child exhibit before being discharged home (from hospital)?
1. The child is walking, talking, and playing consistent with her growth and development.

Chapter 16

A. What *subjective* assessments indicate that the client is experiencing a health alteration?
Mother states that:
1. The child has had a cold for two days.
2. The child is having difficulty breathing through her nose.
3. The child is having "a bit of diarrhea."
4. The child awoke in the middle of night with a fever.
5. The child is irritable.
6. Mother states that child's father smokes in the house.

B. What *objective* assessments indicate that the client is experiencing a health alteration?
1. The child is crying and shaking her head back and forth while in her mother's arms.
2. The child is repeatedly tugging at her right ear.
3. Elevated temperature, heart rate, and respiratory rate.
4. Rhinorrhea.
5. Inflamed tympanic membranes.
6. The child is formula fed.

C. After analyzing the data that has been collected, what **primary** nursing diagnoses should the nurse assign to this client?
1. Infection related to physiological findings.
2. Risk for Deficient Fluid Volume related to nasal congestion and "slight diarrhea."

D. What interventions should the nurse plan and/or implement to meet this child's and her family's needs?
1. Educate the mother regarding the etiology of the otitis media.
2. Calculate the safe dosage of the medications.
3. Educate the mother regarding the safe administration of medication.
   a. Acetaminophen 80 mg PO every 6 hr is within the safe dosage range for this child.
      i. The recommended dosage range of acetaminophen for children is: 10 to 15 mg/kg PO every 6 to 8 hr prn.
      ii. This child weighs 15.5 lb or 7.05 kg.
      iii. The safe dosage every 6 to 8 hr is equal to: 70.5 mg to 105.75 mg.
   b. Ampicillin 150 mg PO every 6 hr is within the safe dosage range for this child.
      i. The recommended dosage range of ampicillin for children with AOM is: 80 to 90 mg/kg/day.
      ii. This child weighs 7.05 kg.
      iii. The safe dosage every 6 hr is equal to: 141 mg to 158.63 mg.
   c. Advise the mother regarding the milliliter equivalent to medications.
   d. Advise the mother that additional acetaminophen should not be administered because of the potential for liver damage.
   e. Advise the mother of the importance of completing the ampicillin regimen.
4. Demonstrate how to instill saline nasal drops.
5. Educate the mother regarding the need to make a follow-up appointment.
6. Educate the mother regarding administration of oral rehydration therapy, and encourage upright positioning of the baby during bottle feedings.
7. Reinforce the need for the father to smoke outside of the home.

E. What client outcomes should the nurse evaluate regarding the effectiveness of the nursing interventions?
1. The mother expresses understanding regarding the etiology of the disease, medication administration, nose drop administration, child's diet, and behaviors that may place the child at high risk for future ear infections.
2. The mother expresses understanding of need to return to pediatrician's office for a follow-up appointment or if the child's condition does not improve.

F. What physiological characteristics should the child exhibit before being discharged home?
1. Child's temperature drops to below 102°F (may be taken axillary to prevent trauma to rectum).

G. What subjective characteristics should the child exhibit before being discharged home?
1. The child's crying subsides.

Chapter 17

A. What *subjective* assessments indicate that the client is experiencing a health alteration?
1. Joint pain: joint pain is an unusual symptom in 8-year-old children. Migratory arthritis is one of the five major manifestations (Jones criteria) of rheumatic fever (RF).

2. Facial twitching: facial twitching is an unusual symptom in 8-year-old children. Chorea is one of the five major manifestations (Jones criteria) of RF.
3. Fever for 2 days: Fever indicates either the presence of an infection or an inflammatory state. It is one of the many minor manifestations (Jones criteria) of RF.
4. Sore throat 3 weeks earlier: RF usually develops approximately 2 to 3 weeks after a group A strep infection.
5. Failure to complete antibiotic course: when strep infections are incompletely eradicated from the body, the possibility of developing RF, or other serious maladies, is increased.
6. Native American family who has had inconsistent health care: in the United States, RF is seen primarily in those with poor health care.

B. What *objective* assessments indicate that the client is experiencing a health alteration?
   1. Temperature of 101.9°F.
   2. Elevated pulse and respiratory rate.
   3. Pain elicited when joints are moved.
   4. Erythematous rash on trunk: erythema marginatum is one of the five major manifestations (Jones criteria) of RF.
   5. Facial twitching: confirmation of subjective complaint of facial twitching as seen in RF.
   6. Murmur heard at the apex of the heart: new murmurs heard at the apex of the heart are evident when a child has carditis. Carditis is one of the five major manifestations (Jones criteria) of RF.
   7. Throat culture positive for group A strep.
   8. Elevated ESR: one of the many minor manifestations (Jones criteria) of RF.
   9. Elevated WBC count.
   10. Prolonged P-R interval on EKG: prolonged P-R interval is one of the many minor manifestations (Jones criteria) of RF.

C. After analyzing the data that has been collected, what **primary** nursing diagnosis should the nurse assign to this client?
   1. Risk for Injury related to the carditis of rheumatic fever.

D. What interventions should the nurse plan and/or implement to meet this child's and his family's needs?
   1. Place the child on droplet isolation, and maintain it until the child has been on antibiotic therapy for a full 24 hr.
   2. Carefully explain the disease process and the need to follow the medical management in a language that is understandable to the parents, child, and other pertinent individuals (e.g., siblings, grandparents, and, because the patient is Native American, the parents may ask the nurse to speak with a tribal shaman).
   3. Allow the child, parents, and others to express anger and fear regarding the diagnosis and medical regimen.
   4. Maintain continual cardiac monitoring.
   5. Maintain bedrest.
   6. Administer safe dose of penicillin V per physician's order: 500 mg PO tid. (Recommended dosage of penicillin V for children over 27 kg with RF is 500 mg PO bid or tid for 10 days. This child weighs 36.36 kg.)
   7. Maintain seizure precautions.
   8. Ask the child to rate his pain level from 1 to 10 every 4 hr prior to aspirin administration, and request additional pain medication, if needed
   9. Administer a safe dose of aspirin per physician's order: 325 mg PO every 4 hr. (Recommended dosage of aspirin for children with RF: 50 to 60 mg/kg/day in divided doses every 4 hr. A child weighing 36.36 kg should receive between 1,818 and 2,181.6 mg per day. When divided into doses every 4 hr, it is determined that the child should receive between 303 and 363.6 mg per dose.)
   10. Provide the child with nonpharmacological pain remedies (e.g., hot or cold compresses to his joints) as needed
   11. Provide the child with quiet activities that he finds entertaining.
   12. Begin discharge planning by educating the parents regarding the need to maintain the medical regimen at home and to administer daily antibiotics, per physician's orders.

E. What client outcomes should the nurse evaluate regarding the effectiveness of the nursing interventions? The following findings will indicate that the rheumatic fever is resolved (but they will not be evident until well after the child is discharged from the hospital):
   1. All major manifestations are no longer evident: cardiac murmur, facial twitching, arthritic joints, and erythematous rash.
   2. All minor manifestations are no longer evident: fever, prolonged P-R interval on EKG, and elevated ESR.
   3. The child no longer has a positive throat culture and white cell count is normal.

F. What physiological characteristics should the child exhibit before being discharged home?
   1. Negative throat culture and normal temperature.
   2. P-R interval on the EKG that is approaching normal.
   3. Maintenance of bedrest.
   4. Either the completion of the antibiotic course or taking prophylactic penicillin daily.

Chapter 18

A. What *subjective* assessments indicate that the client is experiencing a health alteration?
   1. The child is crying.
   2. The father states that the child has had vaso-occlusive crises since he was 2 years old.
   3. The father states that the child is not drinking well.
   4. The father states that the child has yet to receive his yearly flu shot.

B. What *objective* assessments indicate that the client is experiencing a health alteration?
   1. The child has a history of sickle cell anemia (SCA).
   2. The child chooses "hurts worse" on the Wong-Baker Pain Scale.
   3. The child is febrile.
   4. The child's elbows and knees are swollen, warm, and red.
   5. The child's spleen is enlarged.
   6. The child's O_2 saturation is 89%.
   7. The child's laboratory report shows:
      a. RBC count: 3.0 million/mm^3.
      b. Hematocrit: 28%.
      c. Hemoglobin: 9.1 g/dL.
      d. WBC: 15,500 cells/mm^3.

C. After analyzing the data that has been collected, what **primary** nursing diagnosis should the nurse assign to this client?
   1. Ineffective Peripheral Tissue Perfusion related to clumping of sickled cells.

D. What interventions should the nurse plan and/or implement to meet this child's and his family's needs?
   1. Begin IV and infuse IV D5 ¼ NS at 90 mL/hr.
      a. The nurse calculates the child's DMV as 1,400 mL/24 hr or 58.3 mL/hr (10 kg × 100 mL + 8 kg × 50 mL = 1,400 mL/24 hr). The rate of 90 mL/hr is needed to improve the child's hydration.
   2. Provide and encourage the consumption of favorite clear fluids, as tolerated.
   3. Administer morphine 3 mg IV STAT, may repeat every 2 hr, as needed.
      a. The recommended pediatric dosage of morphine sulfate for children 6 months to 12 years of age is 0.1 to 0.2 mg/kg SC/IM/IV q2 to 4h prn.
      b. The nurse calculates the safe dosage range for this child as 1.8 mg to 3.6 mg IV q2 to 4 hr prn. The ordered dosage is safe to administer.
   4. Assess pain every 30 minutes with Wong-Baker Pain Scale.
      a. If child's pain is not reduced after the initial morphine injection, the nurse should request the order be increased.
   5. Obtain and send throat culture.
   6. Administer penicillin G 600,000 units IV every 6 hr.
      a. The recommended pediatric dosage of penicillin G IV for infants and children is 100,000 to 400,000 units/kg/day IM/IV divided q4 to 6h.
      b. The nurse calculates the safe dosage range for this child as 450,000 units to 1,800,000 IV every 6 hr. The ordered dosage is safe to administer.
   7. Administer oxygen at 2 L/min.
   8. Monitor oxygen saturations.
   9. Monitor intake and output.
   10. Maintain the child on bedrest.
   11. Provide the father and child with needed emotional support.
   12. Apply warmth to enflamed joints, as needed.
   13. Provide the child with distractions/quiet activities (e.g., television, video games, books, puzzles).

E. What client outcomes should the nurse evaluate regarding the effectiveness of the nursing interventions?
   1. The child's pain level will decrease after medication administration.
   2. The child will stop crying.
   3. The child will drink fluids.
   4. The child's temperature will drop.
   5. The inflammation of the child's joints will diminish.
   6. The child will exhibit no signs of severe organ involvement (e.g., no signs of stroke, heart failure, priapism).

F. What physiological characteristics should the child exhibit before being discharged home?
   1. The child is drinking one and one-half to two times his DMV each day.
   2. The child's CBC results are stable.
   3. The child's joint involvement is minimal.
   4. Child reports that his pain level is at "no hurt" or "hurts little bit" on the Wong-Baker Pain Rating Scale without need for narcotic medications.

G. What subjective characteristics should the child exhibit before being discharged home?
   1. The child performs range of motion exercises with minimal to no complaints of pain.

Chapter 19

A. What *subjective* assessments indicate that the client is experiencing a health alteration?
   1. The mother states that "dandruff" cannot be brushed from the child's hair shafts.
   2. Daughter states that her head itches.
   3. Mother states that there is evidence that the child has been scratching her neck and behind her ears.
B. What *objective* assessments indicate that the client is experiencing a health alteration?
   1. The school nurse states that the child has lice.
C. After analyzing the data that has been collected, what **primary** nursing diagnosis should the nurse assign to this client?
   1. Infection related to lice infestation.
D. What interventions should the nurse plan and/or implement to meet this child's and her family's needs?
   1. Provide the mother with the health-care provider's prescribed medication administration procedure for the child and for all family members who have been in intimate contact with the child or with products used by the child.
   2. Provide the mother with the procedure for caring for all items that have been in contact with the child.
   3. Provide emotional support for the mother, child, and family.
E. What client outcomes should the nurse evaluate regarding the effectiveness of the nursing interventions?
   1. Eradication of signs of lice infestation from the child and all members of the family, including no evidence of nits on the hair shafts or of itching of the neck and/or behind the ears.
F. What physiological characteristics should the child exhibit after treatment?
   1. No evidence of nits on the hair shafts.
G. What subjective characteristics should the child exhibit after treatment?
   1. All complaints of itching have disappeared.

Chapter 20

A. What subjective assessments indicate that the client is experiencing a health alteration?
   1. As stated by the paramedic:
      a. History of muscular dystrophy.
      b. Dyspnea.
      c. Hyperthermia.
   2. Mother states, "He needs immediate help. He must have pneumonia. Notify his pulmonologist now!!!"
   3. Young man states, with marked difficulty, "I don't want any treatment. I am ready to die."
B. Which *objective* assessments indicate that the client is experiencing a health alteration?
   1. Gasping for breath.
   2. Rales bilaterally.
   3. Minimal intercostal retractions.
   4. Poor aeration to the bases.
   5. Marked muscular wasting.
   6. Edema of the feet and lower legs.
   7. Vitals: Temperature 102.4°F, heart rate 154 bpm, respiratory rate 60 rpm.
C. After analyzing the data that has been collected, what **primary** nursing diagnosis should the nurse assign to this client?
   1. Compromised Family Coping related to fatal illness.
D. What interventions should the nurse plan and/or implement to meet this child's and his family's needs?
   1. Elevate head of bed to 60 degrees.
   2. Administer oxygen via facemask at 2 L/min.
   3. Provide emotional support to the young man by remaining at his side at all times and acknowledging his readiness to die.
   4. Request the assistance from another nurse to provide emotional support to the patient's mother by remaining at her side and acknowledging her fear and anxiety over her son's illness and her son's readiness to die.
   5. Notify the chair of the ethics committee regarding the need for a STAT meeting regarding the patient's refusal (a minor) to give assent for medical intervention and his mother's demand (his legal guardian) that aggressive care interventions be begun.
E. What client outcomes should the nurse evaluate regarding the effectiveness of the nursing interventions?
   1. Satisfaction of the young man with the decisions made regarding his immediate and long-term care.
   2. Satisfaction of the young man's mother with the decisions made regarding her son's immediate and long-term care.
F. What physiological characteristics should the child exhibit before being discharged from the emergency department?
   1. The child's respiratory and heart rates slow.
   2. The child's core temperature remains stable or drops.

G. What subjective characteristics should the child exhibit before being discharged from the emergency department?
   1. The young man and mother verbally express satisfaction with the treatment plan developed by the ethics committee and the child's primary health-care provider.

Depending on the decision of the ethics committee and the decision of the family, the young man may remain in the hospital and receive aggressive intervention, may remain in the hospital on hospice care until his death, or may be discharged home on hospice care.

Chapter 21

A. What *subjective* assessments indicate that the client is experiencing a health alteration?
   1. The school nurse states (learned via parents' statements) that child collapsed in his classroom.
   2. The parents state that the child is a "good boy."
   3. The parents state that the child has had a cold for the past 2 days.
   4. The parents are attentive—requesting to see their son.
   5. The parents state that he has been "drinking and eating a lot lately."

B. What *objective* assessments indicate that the client is experiencing a health alteration?
   1. Glasgow Coma score of 11, including making verbal responses with inappropriate words.
   2. Elevated respiratory rate—Kussmaul-type breathing pattern.
   3. Elevated pulse rate.
   4. 8.1% weight loss since the child's last well-child check.
   5. Markedly elevated glucose.
   6. Markedly elevated hemoglobin A1C.
   7. Low potassium.
   8. Low pH.

C. After analyzing the data that has been collected, what **primary** nursing diagnosis should the nurse assign to this client?
   1. Risk for Injury related to marked hyperglycemia and diabetic ketoacidosis.

D. What interventions should the nurse plan and/or implement to meet this child's and his family's needs?
   1. Allow the parents to express anger, frustration, and guilt regarding the emergent condition of their son.
   2. Have an IV catheter inserted STAT.
   3. Begin infusion at 400 mL per hour to replace fluids because the child is severely dehydrated.
   4. Perform Glasgow Coma assessment every 15 min, and report any deterioration of response.
   5. Monitor serum glucose levels every 15 min, and report the results to the primary health-care provider.
   6. Monitor hourly potassium levels, and report to the primary health-care provider.

E. What client outcomes should the nurse evaluate regarding the effectiveness of the nursing interventions?
   1. Glasgow Coma score increasing to normal of 15, with no signs of increased intracranial pressure.
   2. Vital signs returning to normal, including normal respiratory rate and depth.
   3. Blood glucose levels dropping: initial goal 200 mg/dL
   4. Potassium levels rising to normal of 3.5 to 5 mEq/L.
   5. Urine output within normal limits.
   6. Ketones in urine dropping toward normal.
   7. Weight returning to normal.

F. What physiological characteristics should the child exhibit before being discharged home?
   1. Glasgow Coma score of 15.
   2. Vital signs within normal limits.
   3. Preprandial glucose tests between 90 and 180 mg/dL.
   4. Serum potassium 3.5 to 5 mEq/L.
   5. Urinary output within normal limits.
   6. Urine ketones are absent.
   7. Weight at or about 93 lb.

G. What psychological characteristics should the child and family exhibit before being discharged home?
   1. The child reports an understanding of the need for home blood glucose monitoring, home urine monitoring, insulin injections, diet changes, and need for routine exercise.
   2. The child demonstrates the procedure for home blood glucose monitoring, urine monitoring, and rotation of injection sites.
   3. The parents demonstrate the procedure for home blood glucose monitoring, urine monitoring, rotation of injection sites, dietary needs, administration of glucagon via injection, insulin dosaging, and subcutaneous injections.
   4. The parents and child correctly report signs and symptoms of both hyperglycemia and hypoglycemia.
   5. The parents and child correctly report treatment for both hyperglycemia and hypoglycemia.

Chapter 22

A. What *subjective* assessments indicate that the client is experiencing a health alteration?
   1. The baby's mother's aunt is wheelchair bound.
   2. The baby's mother's diet during her pregnancy was poor.

B. What *objective* assessments indicate that the client is experiencing a health alteration?
   1. Spina bifida seen on ultrasound.
   2. The mother had no prenatal care during her first trimester of pregnancy.
   3. Open sac at base of spine in lumbosacral region—likely meningomyelocele in light of other signs and symptoms.
   4. Constant dribbling of urine.
   5. Constant oozing of feces.
   6. Bilateral flaccid paralysis of both legs.
   7. Asymmetry of leg folds—likely developmental dysplasia of the hips, which commonly is seen in babies with spina bifida.
   8. Head circumference of 37 cm, chest circumference of 32 cm—likely hydrocephalus, which commonly is seen in babies with spina bifida.

C. After analyzing the data that has been collected, what **primary** nursing diagnosis should the nurse assign to this client?
   1. Risk for Infection related to presence of sacral sac.

D. What interventions should the nurse plan and/or implement to meet this child's and his or her family's needs?
   1. Meticulous handwashing and aseptic technique.
   2. Monitor for signs of infection, including elevated WBC and redness or purulent discharge at the site.
   3. Monitor vital signs every 2 hr, especially temperature for both hyper- and hypothermia.
   4. Maintain moist, sterile dressings over defect using aseptic technique, and reinforce moist dressings with dry, sterile dressing.
   5. Monitor sac for signs of rupture, CSF leakage, or drying.
   6. Accompany the baby for ultrasound of site.
   7. Maintain the baby in prone position.
   8. Change soiled diapers and underpads immediately to prevent contamination of site.
   9. Monitor for signs of pressure points on dependent surfaces.
   10. Monitor for signs of hydrocephalus, including assessing daily for increasing head circumference, bulging fontanels, separating sutures, bossing of forehead, and setting-sun sign.
   11. Only use non-latex materials when caring for the baby.
   12. Educate the mother regarding the pathophysiology of the baby's defect.
   13. Educate the mother regarding the surgery that the baby will have.
   14. Allow the mother to express her feelings regarding the baby's defect.
   15. Assess the bonding behaviors that the mother exhibits when with her baby.
   16. If appropriate, allow the mother to hold the baby prone on her lap and caress the baby.

E. What client outcomes should the nurse evaluate regarding the effectiveness of the nursing interventions?
   1. The baby shows no signs of infection.
   2. The baby's head does not increase in circumference or show any other signs of hydrocephalus.
   3. The baby's mother exhibits signs of bonding effectively with her baby (e.g., kissing and caressing the baby).
   4. The mother states a clear understanding both of the baby's diagnosis and the surgery.
   5. The mother freely expresses concern over the baby's future well-being.

F. What physiological characteristics should the child exhibit before being discharged home?
   1. Intact lumbosacral area.
   2. Functioning VP shunt.
   3. Stable vital signs with no signs of infection.
   4. Retaining feedings and gaining weight.

G. What subjective characteristics should the child exhibit before being discharged home?
   1. The child is responding appropriately to all stimuli, including hunger, touch, and sound.

Chapter 23

A. Which *subjective* assessments are important in the scenario?
   1. Marked behavioral change noted by the child's teacher from:
      a. Doing "very well on all of her assignments" and being "outgoing and talkative" to
      b. Not doing "any homework all week" and "sit[ting] alone in the corner during recess and refus[ing] to play with her friends."
      c. The mother confirming a change in behavior.
   2. The young girl states, "I really hate it when Uncle Jack visits."
   3. When queried about whether her Uncle Jack hurt her, the young girl cries and states, "I can't say. I will get into trouble."
   4. The child winces in pain when she sits.

B. Which *objective* assessments are important in the scenario?
   1. None: all vital signs are within normal limits.

C. After analyzing the data that has been collected, what **primary** nursing diagnosis should the nurse assign to this client?
   1. Ineffective Coping/Injury related to suspected sexual abuse.

D. What interventions should the nurse plan and/or implement to meet this child's and her family's needs?
   1. Notify the parents of the nurse's suspicions.
   2. Advise the parents to have their daughter seen by the primary health-care provider.
   3. Immediately report the suspicion of sexual abuse to the local office of child protective services.
E. What client outcomes should the nurse evaluate regarding the effectiveness of the nursing interventions?
   1. The parents state that they have had their daughter assessed.
   2. A formal investigation is performed by the local office of child protective services.
F. What physiological and/or psychological characteristics should the child exhibit after the child receives needed counseling?
   1. The child's behavior returns to normal.

Chapter 24

A. What *subjective* assessments indicate that the client is experiencing a health alteration?
   Based on observations by the day-care teacher and parents:
   1. The child fails to give teacher eye contact.
   2. The child "doesn't seem very happy." Teacher rarely sees the child smile.
   3. The child avoids interacting with other children; child plays alone.
   4. The child engages in repetitive behaviors.
   5. The child does not initiate independent behaviors at home, including undressing and using silverware during meals.
   6. The child rarely speaks, and his responsiveness to engage in educational interactions has declined.
   7. None of the child's behaviors can be explained by parental behavior. The parents are educated and involved in all aspects of the child's life.
B. What *objective* assessments indicate that the client is experiencing a health alteration?
   1. The child failed two scales of the DDST: personal/social and language. (Not appropriate to administer IQ tests because the child is too young.)
   2. All other data, including fine and gross motor development and all physiological parameters, are within normal limits.
C. After analyzing the data that has been collected, what **primary** nursing diagnosis should the nurse assign to this client?
   1. Impaired Social Interaction/Impaired Verbal Communication.
D. What interventions should the nurse plan and/or implement to meet this child's and his family's needs?
   1. Educate the parents and others regarding the child's diagnosis.
   2. Allow the parents to express grief, anger, and/or frustration.
   3. Refer the child and family to educational resources specifically geared to autistic children.
   4. Refer the child and family to the American Autism Society and/or American Autism Association.
   5. Strongly encourage the parents to establish a strict routine of daily activities for the child.
   6. If the child ever needs a babysitter, try to employ the same person each time.
E. What client outcomes should the nurse evaluate regarding the effectiveness of the nursing interventions?
   1. At each well-child visit, evaluate and document the child's physiological growth and development.
   2. At each well-child visit, assess and document the child's social, language, behavioral, and cognitive functioning.
   3. At each well-child visit, interview the parents to assess their individual and the family's coping.
F. What physiological characteristics should the child exhibit before being discharged home?
   1. None.

Chapter 25

A. What *subjective* assessments indicate that the client is experiencing a health alteration?
   1. A volunteer at the child's day-care center reports a disparity between the vision test results of child's left and right eyes.
   2. The mother states that she has noticed the child moving her head to one side when looking at books.
B. What *objective* assessments indicate that the client is experiencing a health alteration?
   1. Slight strabismus noted on ophthalmic examination.
   2. Marked difference in visual ability between right and left eye.
C. After analyzing the data that has been collected, what **primary** nursing diagnosis should the nurse assign to this client?
   1. Risk for Disproportionate Growth related to the diagnosis of amblyopia.

D. What interventions should the nurse plan and/or implement to meet this child's and her family's needs?
   1. Inform the mother that the child is primarily using only her right eye to see.
   2. Advise the mother that if the child continues to use the dominant eye that she will eventually become blind in the left eye.
   3. Educate the mother regarding the therapy prescribed by the ophthalmologist.
      a. One atropine drop in the right eye each morning, which will blur the image seen by that eye. Demonstrate procedure as follows:
         i. Wash hands well before administering the drop.
         ii. Maintain drops at room temperature.
         iii. Never allow the dropper to touch the eye. If it does, the mother should be advised to request a new prescription from the ophthalmologist.
         iv. Offer suggestions for distractions that the mother could use during instillation of the drop (e.g., watching television, playing handheld video games, singing songs). In addition, advise the mother that because of the child's age, she may need assistance when administering the medication.
         v. Observe a return demonstration.
      b. The intervention will require the child to use her weak eye to see. Even though she will see poorly for a while, the vision in the amblyopic eye will slowly improve.

E. What client outcomes should the nurse evaluate regarding the effectiveness of the nursing interventions?
   1. The mother communicates an understanding of the child's condition.
   2. During return demonstration, the mother uses appropriate technique when instilling eye drops into her daughter's right eye.
   3. The mother makes an appointment for a return visit in 1 month.

F. What physiological characteristics should the child exhibit before being discharged home?
   1. None.

G. What psychological characteristics should the child and family exhibit before being discharged home?
   1. The child allows her mother to instill one eye drop into her right eye with minimal complaint.

CDC Clinical Growth Charts

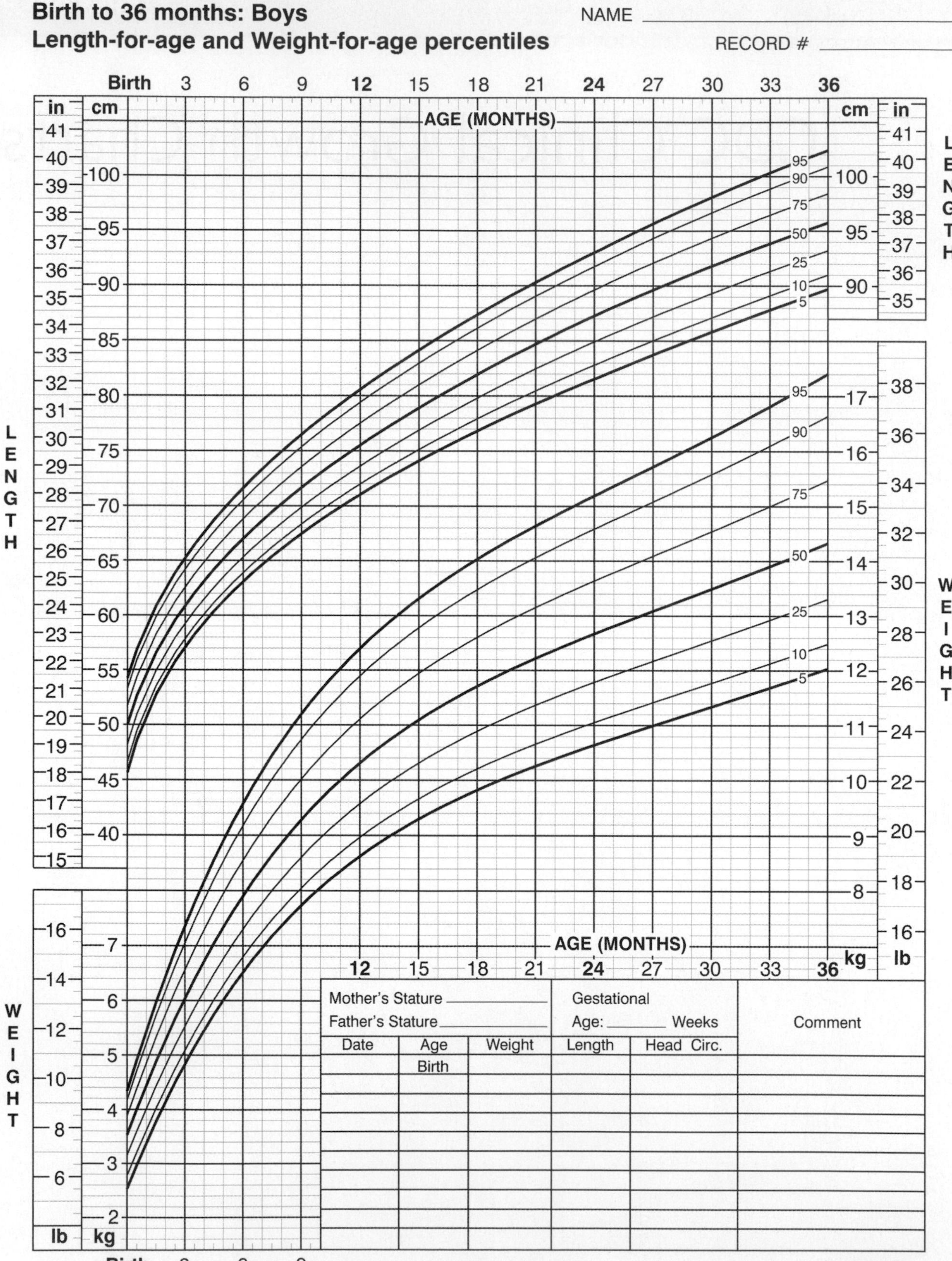

Pubished May 30, 2000 (modified 4/20/01).
SOURCE: Developed by the National Center for Health Statistics in collaboration with the National Center for Chronic Disease Prevention and Health Promotion (2000).
http://www.cdc.gov/growthcharts

CDC
SAFER • HEALTHIER • PEOPLE™

Birth to 36 months: Girls
Length-for-age and Weight-for-age percentiles

NAME ____________

RECORD # ____________

Birth 3 6 9 **12** 15 18 21 **24** 27 30 33 **36**

AGE (MONTHS)

in cm — LENGTH — cm in

in: 41 40 39 38 37 36 35 34 33 32 31 30 29 28 27 26 25 24 23 22 21 20 19 18 17 16 15

cm: 100 95 90 85 80 75 70 65 60 55 50 45 40

Length percentiles: 95 90 75 50 25 10 5

Weight percentiles: 95 90 75 50 25 10 5

WEIGHT — kg: 17 16 15 14 13 12 11 10 9 8 — lb: 38 36 34 32 30 28 26 24 22 20 18 16

WEIGHT — lb: 16 14 12 10 8 6 — kg: 7 6 5 4 3 2

AGE (MONTHS)

12 15 18 21 24 27 30 33 36 kg lb

Mother's Stature ____			Gestational		Comment
Father's Stature ____			Age: ____ Weeks		
Date	Age	Weight	Length	Head Circ.	
	Birth				

lb kg

Birth 3 6 9

Published May 30, 2000 (modified 4/20/01).
SOURCE: Developed by the National Center for Health Statistics in collaboration with the National Center for Chronic Disease Prevention and Health Promotion (2000).
http://www.cdc.gov/growthcharts

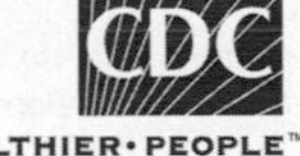

SAFER • HEALTHIER • PEOPLE™

Birth to 36 months: Boys
Head circumference-for-age and Weight-for-length percentiles

NAME ______________

RECORD # ______________

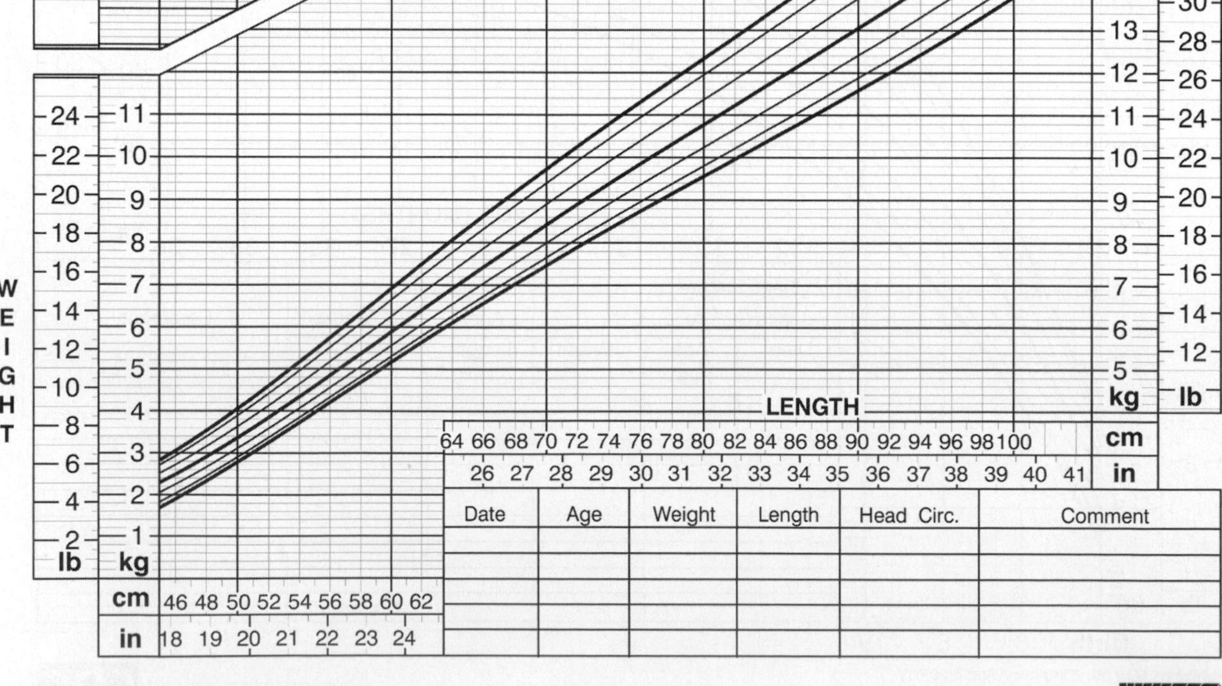

Date	Age	Weight	Length	Head Circ.	Comment

Published May 30, 2000 (modified 10/16/00).
SOURCE: Developed by the National Center for Health Statistics in collaboration with the National Center for Chronic Disease Prevention and Health Promotion (2000).
http://www.cdc.gov/growthcharts

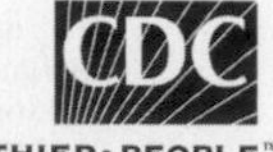

SAFER • HEALTHIER • PEOPLE™

Birth to 36 months: Girls
Head circumference-for-age and Weight-for-length percentiles

NAME ______________

RECORD # ______________

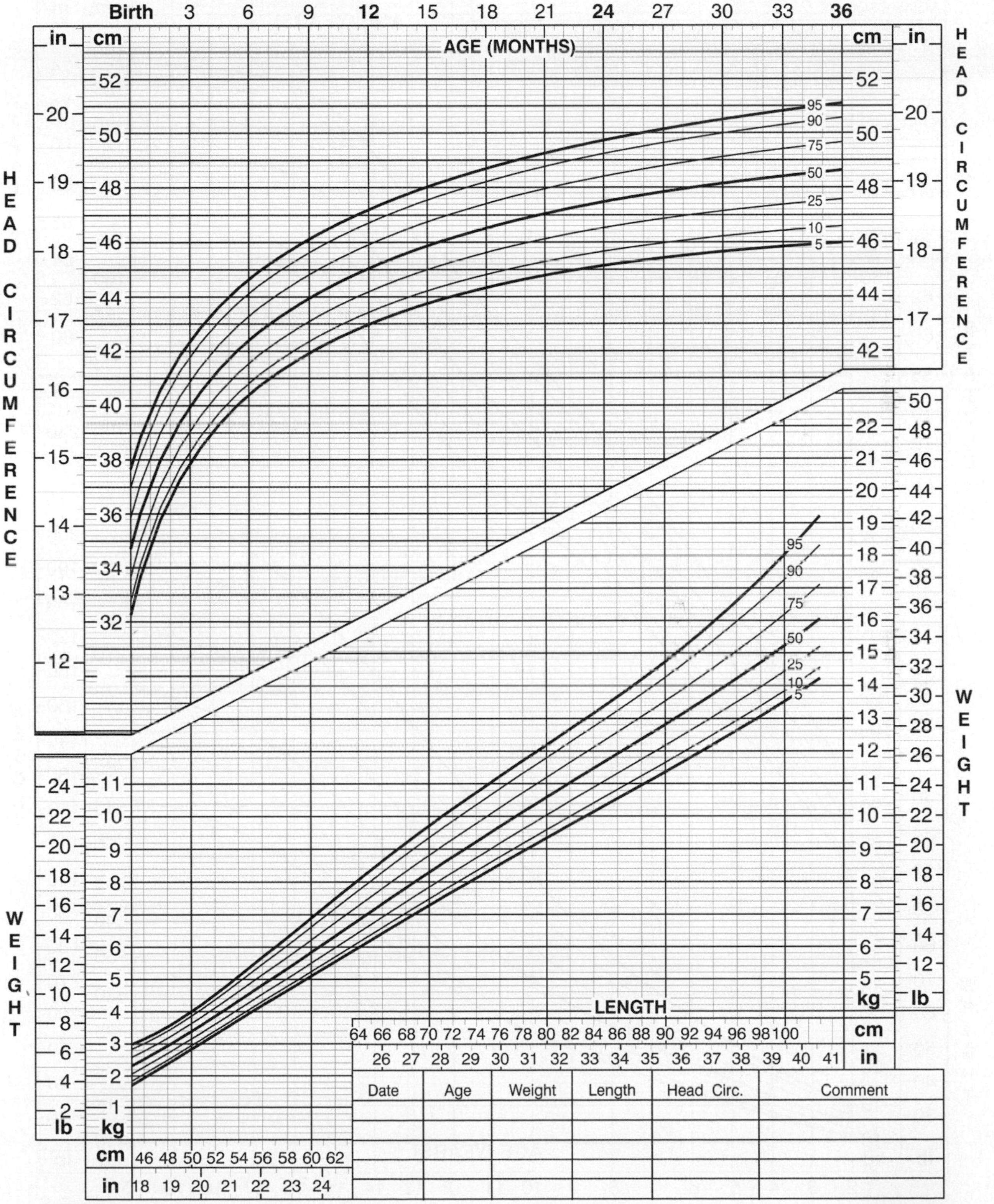

Date	Age	Weight	Length	Head Circ.	Comment

Published May 30, 2000 (modified 10/16/00).
SOURCE: Developed by the National Center for Health Statistics in collaboration with the National Center for Chronic Disease Prevention and Health Promotion (2000).
http://www.cdc.gov/growthcharts

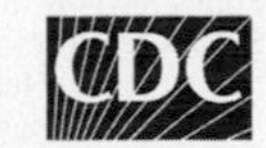

SAFER • HEALTHIER • PEOPLE™

2 to 20 years: Boys
Stature-for-age and Weight-for-age percentiles

NAME ______________

RECORD # ______________

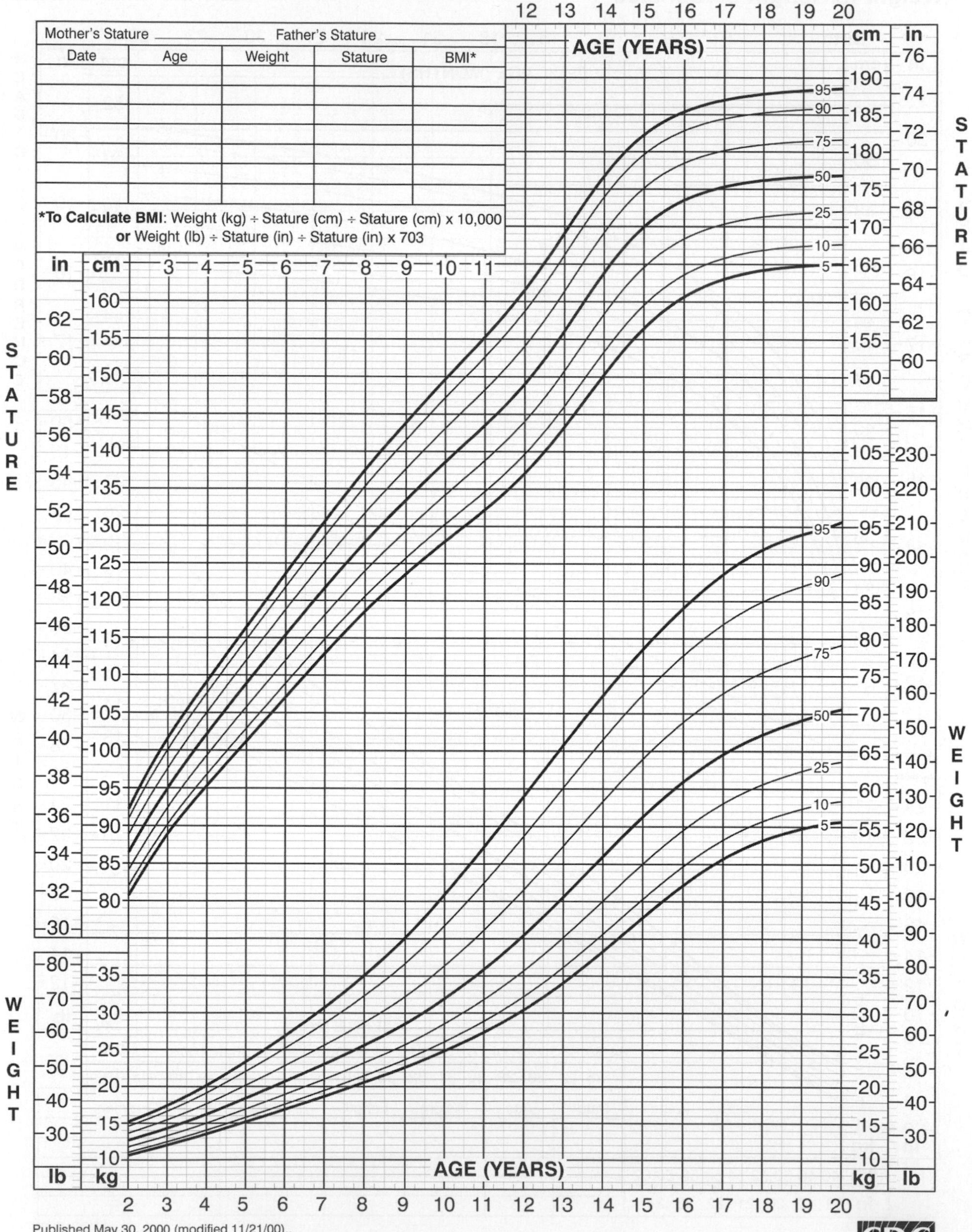

Mother's Stature ______________ Father's Stature ______________

Date	Age	Weight	Stature	BMI*

***To Calculate BMI**: Weight (kg) ÷ Stature (cm) ÷ Stature (cm) x 10,000
or Weight (lb) ÷ Stature (in) ÷ Stature (in) x 703

AGE (YEARS)

12 13 14 15 16 17 18 19 20

3 4 5 6 7 8 9 10 11

STATURE

in: 30 32 34 36 38 40 42 44 46 48 50 52 54 56 58 60 62 64 66 68 70 72 74 76

cm: 80 85 90 95 100 105 110 115 120 125 130 135 140 145 150 155 160 165 170 175 180 185 190

Percentiles: 5 10 25 50 75 90 95

WEIGHT

kg: 10 15 20 25 30 35 40 45 50 55 60 65 70 75 80 85 90 95 100 105

lb: 30 40 50 60 70 80 90 100 110 120 130 140 150 160 170 180 190 200 210 220 230

Percentiles: 5 10 25 50 75 90 95

AGE (YEARS)

2 3 4 5 6 7 8 9 10 11 12 13 14 15 16 17 18 19 20

Published May 30, 2000 (modified 11/21/00)..
SOURCE: Developed by the National Center for Health Statistics in collaboration with the National Center for Chronic Disease Prevention and Health Promotion (2000).
http://www.cdc.gov/growthcharts

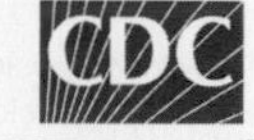

SAFER • HEALTHIER • PEOPLE™

2 to 20 years: Girls
Stature-for-age and Weight-for-age percentiles

NAME ______________

RECORD # ______________

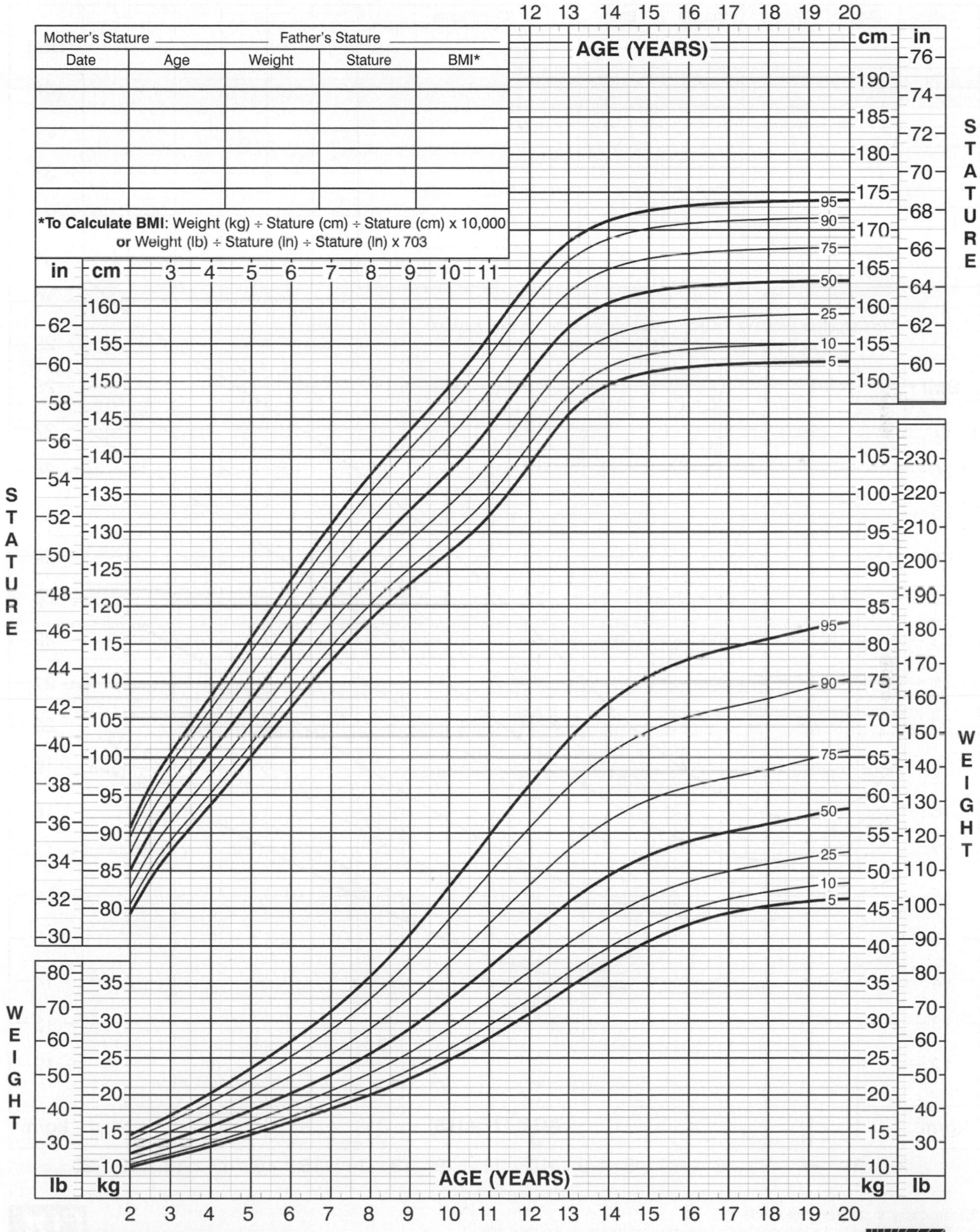

Mother's Stature ______________ Father's Stature ______________

Date	Age	Weight	Stature	BMI*

***To Calculate BMI**: Weight (kg) ÷ Stature (cm) ÷ Stature (cm) x 10,000
or Weight (lb) ÷ Stature (in) ÷ Stature (in) x 703

Published May 30, 2000 (modified 11/21/00).
SOURCE: Developed by the National Center for Health Statistics in collaboration with the National Center for Chronic Disease Prevention and Health Promotion (2000).
http://www.cdc.gov/growthcharts

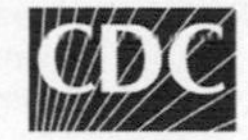

SAFER • HEALTHIER • PEOPLE™

2 to 20 years: Boys
Body mass index-for-age percentiles

NAME ______________

RECORD # ______________

Date	Age	Weight	Stature	BMI*	Comments

***To Calculate BMI**: Weight (kg) ÷ Stature (cm) ÷ Stature (cm) x 10,000
or Weight (lb) ÷ Stature (in) ÷ Stature (in) x 703

Published May 30, 2000 (modified 10/16/00).
SOURCE: Developed by the National Center for Health Statistics in collaboration with
the National Center for Chronic Disease Prevention and Health Promotion (2000).
http://www.cdc.gov/growthcharts

CDC
SAFER · HEALTHIER · PEOPLE™

2 to 20 years: Girls
Body mass index-for-age percentiles

NAME ______________________

RECORD # ____________

Date	Age	Weight	Stature	BMI*	Comments

***To Calculate BMI**: Weight (kg) ÷ Stature (cm) ÷ Stature (cm) x 10,000
or Weight (lb) ÷ Stature (in) ÷ Stature (in) x 703

BMI

35 34 33 32 31 30 29 28 27 26 25 24 23 22 21 20 19 18 17 16 15 14 13 12

95 90 85 75 50 25 10 5

kg/m² **AGE (YEARS)** **kg/m²**

2 3 4 5 6 7 8 9 10 11 12 13 14 15 16 17 18 19 20

Published May 30, 2000 (modified 10/16/00).
SOURCE: Developed by the National Center for Health Statistics in collaboration with
the National Center for Chronic Disease Prevention and Health Promotion (2000).
http://www.cdc.gov/growthcharts

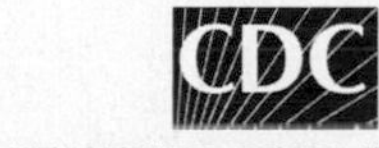

SAFER • HEALTHIER • PEOPLE™

NANDA Diagnoses

Herdman, T.H. (Ed.) *Nursing Diagnoses—Definitions and Classification 2012–2014*. Copyright © 2012, 1994–2012 NANDA International. Used by arrangement with John Wiley & Sons Limited. In order to make safe and effective judgments using NANDA-I nursing diagnoses it is essential that nurses refer to the definitions and defining characteristics of the diagnoses listed in this work.

Chapters 1–25

American Academy of Pediatrics. Available at: www.aap.org

American Cancer Society. Available at: www.cancer.org

Brown, E. (2009). Helping bereaved children and young people. *British Journal of School Nursing*, *4*(2), 69–73.

Center for Disability Resources. (2007). BabyNet diagnoses fact sheets. Retrieved from: http://uscm.med.sc.edu/tecs/babynet_covered_diagnoses.pdf

Centers for Disease Control and Prevention. Available at: www.cdc.gov

Cincinnati Children's Hospital Medical Center. Available at: www.cincinnatichildrens.org

Epocrates. Available at: www.epocrates.com

Genetics Home Reference. (2013). Newborn screening. Retrieved from: http://ghr.nlm.nih.gov/nbs

Hockenberry, M.J., & Wilson, D. (2010). *Wong's nursing care of infants and children* (9th ed.). St. Louis, MO: Elsevier/Mosby.

The Joint Commission. Available at: www.jointcommission.org

Kliegman, R.M., Stanton, B.M.D., St. Geme, J., Schor, N.F., & Behrman, R.E. (2011). *Nelson's textbook of pediatrics* (19th ed.). Philadelphia: Elsevier/Saunders.

Mayo Clinic. Available at: www.mayoclinic.com/

McKinney, E.S., James, S.R., Murray, S.S., & Ashwill, J.W. (2009). *Maternal-child nursing* (3rd ed.). St. Louis, MO: Saunders/Elsevier.

National Newborn Screening and Global Resource Center. Available at: http://genes-r-us.uthscsa.edu/

Chapter 1: The Child as a Member of the Family

Kauai's Hindu Monastery. (2014). Basics of Hinduism. Retrieved from: www.himalayanacademy.com/readlearn/basics/nine-beliefs

Islamic Bulletin. (2009). Islam beliefs and practices. Retrieved from: www.islamicbulletin.org/newsletters/issue_24/beliefs.aspx

U.S. Census Bureau. (2012). State and county quickfacts. Retrieved from: http://quickfacts.census.gov

Chapters 2–6: Normal Growth and Development

Ages and Stages Questionnaires. (2014). Available at: http://agesandstages.com/

American Academy of Pediatrics. (2011). Ultraviolet radiation: A hazard to children and adolescents. Retrieved from: http://pediatrics.aappublications.org/content/127/3/588.full.html

American Academy of Pediatrics. (2013). Ages & stages: Fluoride supplements. Retrieved from: www.healthychildren.org/English/ages-stages/baby/feeding-nutrition/Pages/Fluoride-Supplements.aspx

American Academy of Pediatrics. (2013). Safety and prevention: Car seats: Information for families for 2013. Retrieved from: www.healthychildren.org/English/safety-prevention/on-the-go/Pages/Car-Safety-Seats-Information-for-Families.aspx

American Academy of Pediatrics. (2014). Recommendations for pediatric preventive health care. *Pediatrics*, *133*, 568. DOI: 10.1542/peds.2013-4096.

American Alliance for Health, Physical Education, Recreation, and Dance. (2013). Available at: www.aahperd.org/

Burton, O.M. (2011). AAP press statement on HHS & EPA recommended change in fluoride levels in drinking water. Retrieved from: www.aap.org/en-us/about-the-aap/aap-press-room/Pages/AAP-Press-Statement-on-HHS–EPA-Recommended-Change-in-Fluoride-Levels-in-Drinking-Water.aspx

Centers for Disease Control and Prevention. (n.d.) Body mass index: Considerations for practitioners. Retrieved from: www.cdc.gov/obesity/downloads/bmiforpractitioners.pdf

Centers for Disease Control and Prevention. (2009). Growth charts: Clinical growth charts. Retrieved from: www.cdc.gov/growthcharts/clinical_charts.htm

Centers for Disease Control and Prevention. (2014). Birth–18 Years and "Catch-up" Immunization Schedules. (2104). Retrieved from: www.cdc.gov/vaccines/schedules/hcp/child-adolescent.html

Denver Developmental Screening Test II. Available at: www.denverii.com

National Highway Traffic Safety Administration. (2011). Car seat recommendations for children. Retrieved from: www.nhtsa.gov/ChildSafety/Guidance

Parents' Evaluation of Development Status. (2013). Available at: www.pedstest.com/default.aspx

U.S. Food and Drug Administration. (2012). FDA sheds light on sunscreens. Retrieved from: www.fda.gov/ForConsumers/ConsumerUpdates/ucm258416.htm

Chapter 2: Normal Growth and Development: Infancy

American Academy of Pediatrics Policy Statement. (2012). Breastfeeding and use of human milk. *Pediatrics, 129*(3), e827–e841.

American Academy of Pediatrics Task Force on Sudden Infant Death Syndrome. (2011). SIDS and other sleep-related infant deaths: Expansion of recommendations for a safe infant sleeping environment. Retrieved from: http://pediatrics.aappublications.org/content/128/5/e1341.full.html

Perrine, C.G., Sharma, A.J., Jefferds, M.E.D., Serdula, M.K., & Scanlon, K.S. (2010). Adherence to vitamin D recommendations: Among U.S. infants. *Pediatrics, 125*, 627–632. Retrieved from: http://pediatrics.aappublications.org/content/125/4/627.full.html

Chapter 3: Normal Growth and Development: Toddlerhood

Academy of Nutrition and Dietetics. (2012). It's all about eating right. Size-wise nutrition for preschool age children. Retrieved from: www.eatright.org/Public/content.aspx?id=8055

Chapter 4: Normal Growth and Development: Preschooler

Pan, Y., Tarczy-Homoch, K, Cotter, S., Wen, G., Borchert, M.S. Azen, S.P.,…& the Multi-Ethnic Pediatric Eye Disease Study Group. (2009). Visual acuity norms in preschool children: the multi-ethnic pediatric eye disease study. *Optometry and Vision Science, 86*(6), 607–612.

Chapter 5: Normal Growth and Development: The School-Age Child

Future of Sex Education Initiative. (2011). National sexuality education standards core content and skills, K–12. Retrieved from: www.futureofsexed.org/documents/josh-fose-standards-web.pdf

Chapter 6: Normal Growth and Development: Adolescence

Kann, L., Kinchen, S., Shanklin, S.L., Flint, K.H., Hawkins, J., Harris, W.A.,…Zaza, S. (2014). Youth risk behavior surveillance—United States, 2013. *MMWR Surveillance Summaries, 63*(4), 1-168.

Nerney, M.C. (2014). Personal communication: mcnerneyll@frontiernet.net.

Chapter 7: Physical Assessment of Children: From Infancy to Adolescence

Ages and Stages Questionnaires. (2014). Available at: http://agesandstages.com/

Centers for Disease Control and Prevention. (n.d.). Body mass index: Considerations for practitioners. Retrieved from: www.cdc.gov/obesity/downloads/bmiforpactitioners.pdf

Centers for Disease Control and Prevention. (2009). Growth charts: Clinical growth charts. Retrieved from: www.cdc.gov/growthcharts/clinical_charts.htm

Denver Developmental Screening Test II. (2014). Available at: www.denverii.com

Haque, I.U., & Zaritshy, A.L. (2007). Analysis of the evidence for the lower limit of systolic and mean arterial pressure in children. *Pediatric Critical Care Medicine, 8*(2), 138–144. Retrieved from: www.ncbi.nlm.nih.gov/pubmed/17273118

Kaelber, D.C., & Pickett, F. (2009). Simple table to identify children and adolescents needing further evaluation of blood pressure. *Pediatrics, 123*, e972–e974.

Parents' Evaluation of Development Status. (2013). Available at: http://www.pedstest.com/default.aspx

Chapter 8: Nursing Care of the Child in the Health-Care Setting

American Academy of Pediatrics. (1997). The use of physical restraint interventions for children and adolescents in the acute care setting. Retrieved from: http://pediatrics.aappublications.org/content/99/3/497.full.html

Brady, M. (2009). Hospitalized children's views of the good nurse. *Nursing Ethics, 16*(5), 543–560.

Gimbler-Berglund, I., Ljusegren, G., & Enskär, K. (2008). Factors influencing pain management in children. *Pediatric Nursing, 20*(10), 21–24.

Chapter 9: Pediatric Medication Administration

Buckwell, C. (2008). Administering blood transfusions. Centre for Excellence in Teaching and Learning, London. Retrieved from: www.cetl.org.uk/learning/print/blood-transfusion-print.pdf

Cook, M.C. (2010). Nurses' six rights for safe medication administration. Massachusetts Nurses' Association. Retrieved from: www.massnurses.org/nursing-resources/nursing-practice/articles/six-rights

Institute of Medicine. (2006). Preventing medication errors. Retrieved from: www.iom.edu/~/media/Files/Report%20Files/2006/Preventing-Medication-Errors-Quality-Chasm-Series/medicationerrorsnew.pdf

The Joint Commission. (2014). Facts about the official "Do Not Use" list. Retrieved from: www.jointcommission.org/assets/1/18/Do_Not_Use_List.pdf

The Joint Commission. (2008). Preventing pediatric medication errors. *Sentinel Event Alert*. Retrieved from: www.jointcommission.org/assets/1/18/SEA_39.PDF

Chapter 10: Pediatric Emergencies

Ars Informatica. (2014). Interactive Rumack-Matthew Nomogram for Acetaminophen Toxicity. Available at:

http://www.ars-informatica.ca/toxicity_nomogram.php?calc=acetamin

Ars Informatica. (2014). Interactive Done Nomogram for Salicylate Toxicity. Available at: www.ars-informatica.ca/toxicity_nomogram.php?calc=salic

Berg, M.D., Schexnayder, S.M., Chameides, L., Terry, M., Donoghue, A., Hickey, R.W.,…& Hazinski, M.F. (2010). 2010 American Heart Association guidelines for cardiopulmonary resuscitation and emergency cardiovascular care science, Part 13: Pediatric basic life support. *Circulation*, *122*, S862–S875.

Brown, M.J., & Margolis, S. (2012). Lead in drinking water and human blood lead levels in the United States. *MMWR, Supplement 61*, 1–9.

Centers for Disease Control and Prevention. (2012). Low level lead exposure harms children: A renewed call for primary prevention. Retrieved from: www.cdc.gov/nceh/lead/acclpp/final_document_030712.pdf

Children's Hospital of Pittsburgh. (2013). Mr. Yuk. Retrieved from: www.chp.edu/CHP/mryuk

Lopez, D.P. (2009). Acetaminophen poisoning. *AJN*, *109*, 48–51.

Organization of Teratology Information Specialists. (2010). Lead and pregnancy. Retrieved from: www.otispregnancy.org/lead-r108115

Schappert, S.M., & Bhuiya, F. (2012). Availability of pediatric services and equipment in emergency departments: United States, 2006. *National Health Statistics Reports*, *47*, 1–22.

Chapter 11: Nursing Care of the Child With Immunologic Alterations

AIDS.gov. Available at: http://aids.gov/

Centers for Disease Control and Prevention. (2012). HIV among pregnant women, infants and children in the United States. Retrieved from: www.cdc.gov/hiv/pdf/risk_WIC.pdf

Centers for Disease Control and Prevention. (2010). New HIV infections in the United States, 2010. Retrieved from: www.cdc.gov/hiv/pdf/HIV_infographic_11X17_HR.pdf

Centers for Disease Control and Prevention and Association of Public Health Laboratories. (2014). Laboratory testing for the diagnosis of HIV infection: Updated recommendations. Retrieved from: http://stacks.cdc.gov/view/cdc/23447

Fleischer, D.M., Spergel, J.M., Assa'ad, A.H., & Pongracic, J.A. (2013). Primary prevention of allergic disease through nutritional interventions. *The Journal of Allergy and Clinical Immunology: In Practice*, *1*(1), 29–36. Retrieved from: www.jaci-inpractice.org/article/S2213-2198(12)00014-1/fulltext

Lupus Foundation of America. Available at: www.lupus.org/

Mylan Specialty L.P. (2013). *How to use Epi-Pen Autoinjector.* Retrieved from: www.epipen.com/how-to-use-epipen

National Institute of Allergy and Infectious Diseases. Available at: www.niaid.nih.gov

U.S. Department of Health and Human Services Panel on Antiretroviral Guidelines for Adults and Adolescents, a working group of the Office of AIDS Research Advisory Council. (2012). AIDS info: HIV and its treatment. Retrieved from: http://aidsinfo.nih.gov/contentfiles/HIVandItsTreatment_cbrochure_en.pdf

Chapter 12: Nursing Care of the Child With Infectious Diseases

Centers for Disease Control and Prevention. Advisory Committee on Immunization Practices. (2014). Birth–18 Years and "Catch-up" Immunization Schedules. Retrieved from: www.cdc.gov/vaccines/schedules/hcp/child-adolescent.html

Ipp, M., Taddio, A., Gladbach, S.J., & Parkin, P.C. (2007). Vaccine-related pain: Randomized controlled trial of two injection techniques. *Archives of Disease in Childhood*, *92*(12), 1105–1108.

Siegel, J.D., Rhinehart, E., Jackson, M., Chiarello, L., & The Healthcare Infection Control Practices Advisory Committee. (2007). 2007 guideline for isolation precautions: Preventing transmission of infectious agents in healthcare settings. Retrieved from: www.cdc.gov/hicpac/pdf/isolation/Isolation2007.pdf

Chapter 13: Nursing Care of the Child With Fluid and Electrolyte Alterations

The Joint Commission. Sentinel Event Alert. (1999). High Alert Medications and Patient Safety. Retrieved from: www.jointcommission.org/assets/1/18/SEA_11.pdf

University of Connecticut. (2006). Acid base online tutorial. Retrieved from: http://fitsweb.uchc.edu/student/selectives/TimurGraham/compensatory_responses_respiratory_alkalosis.html

Chapter 14: Nursing Care of the Child With Gastrointestinal Problems

American Celiac Society. Available at: www.americanceliacsociety.org/

Carter, B., & Fedorowicz, Z. (2012). Antiemetic treatment for acute gastroenteritis in children: An updated Cochrane systematic review with meta-analysis and mixed treatment comparison in a Bayesian framework. *British Medical Journal Open*, *2*, e000622. doi: 10.1136/bmjopen-2011-000622

Celiac Disease Foundation. Available at: www.celiac.org

Children's Craniofacial Association. Available at: www.ccakids.com/

Cincinnati Children's Hospital Medical Center. Family Resource Center. Available at: www.cincinnatichildrens.org/service/f/family-resource/default/

Cleft Palate Foundation. Available at: www.cleftline.org/

EA/TEF Family Support Connection. Available at: www.eatef.org/

Intermountain Primary Children's Medical Center. (2013). Colorectal center. Retrieved from: http://intermountainhealthcare.org/hospitals/primarychildrens/services/colorectal/Pages/home.aspx

University of Chicago Celiac Disease Center. (2014). Is it fact or fiction? Retrieved from: www.cureceliacdisease.org/living-with-celiac/guide/fact-vs-fiction

University of Chicago Celiac Disease Center. (n.d.) Learn about the symptoms of celiac disease. Retrieved from: www.cureceliacdisease.org/living-with-celiac/guide/symptoms

Chapter 15: Nursing Care of the Child With Genitourinary Disorders

Thieke, C.C. (2003). Nocturnal eneuresis. *American Family Physician*, *67*(7), 1499–1506.

Chapter 16: Nursing Care of the Child With Respiratory Illnesses

American Academy of Family Physicians, American Academy of Otolaryngology-Head and Neck Surgery, and American Academy of Pediatrics. Subcommittee on Otitis Media with Effusion. (2004). Otitis media with effusion. *Pediatrics*, *113*, 1412–1429.

American Lung Association. Available at: www.lung.org/

Asthma and Allergy Foundation of America. Available at: www.aafa.org/

Bisno, A.L., Gerber, M.A., Gwaltney, J.M., Kaplan, E.L., & Schwartz, R.H. (2002). Practice guidelines for the diagnosis and management of group a *streptococcal pharyngitis*. *Clinical Infectious Diseases*, *35*, 113–125.

Cystic Fibrosis Foundation. Available at: www.cff.org/

Lieberthal, A.S., Carroll, A.E., Chonmaitree, T., Ganiats, T.G., Hoberman, A., Jackson, M.A.,...& Tunkel, D.E. (2013). The diagnosis and management of acute otitis media. *Pediatrics*, 131, e963–e999.

Pollack, A. (2012). FDA approves new cystic fibrosis drug. *New York Times*, Feb. 1, 2012, B2.

Chapter 17: Nursing Care of the Child With Cardiovascular Illnesses

American Academy of Pediatrics. Section of Cardiology and Cardiac Surgery Executive Committee. (2012). Endorsement of Health and Human Services recommendation for pulse oximetry screening for critical congenital heart disease. Retrieved from: http://pediatrics.aappublications.org/content/129/1/190.full.pdf

Berg, M.D., Schexnayder, S.M., Chameides, L., Terry, M., Donoghue, A., Hickey, R.W.,...& Hazinski, M.F. (2010). 2010 American Heart Association guidelines for cardiopulmonary resuscitation and emergency cardiovascular care science, Part 13: Pediatric basic life support. *Circulation*, *122*, S862–S875.

Kemper, A.R., Mahle, W.T., Martin, G.R., Cooley, W.C., Kumar, P., Morrow, W.R.,...& Howell, R.R. (2011). Strategies for implementing screening for critical congenital heart disease. *Pediatrics*, *132*(1), e185–e192. doi: 10.1542/peds.2011-1317

Scherf, R., & White-Reid, K. (2008). Giving intravenous immunoglobulin. *RN*, *71*(1), 29–35.

Chapter 18: Nursing Care of the Child With Hematologic Illnesses

National Hemophilia Foundation. Available at: www.hemophilia.org

National Institutes of Health. (2002). Management and therapy of sickle cell disease (4th ed.). NIH Publ. No. 96-2117. Retrieved from: www.nhlbi.nih.gov/health/prof/blood/sickle/sc_mngt.pdf

Sickle Cell Foundation. Available at: http://sicklecellfoundation.org/

Chapter 19: Nursing Care of the Child With Integumentary System Disorders

Centers for Disease Control and Prevention. (2013). Methicillin-resistant staphylococcus aureus (MRSA) infections: General information about MRSA in the community. Retrieved from: www.cdc.gov/mrsa/community/index.html

Gdalevich, M., Mimouni, D., David, M., & Mimouni, M. (2001). Breast-feeding and the onset of atopic dermatitis in childhood: A systematic review and meta-analysis of prospective studies. *American Academy of Dermatology Journal*, *45*(4), 520–528.

Greer, F.R., Sicherer, S.H., & Burks, A.W. (2008). Effects of early nutritional interventions on the development of atopic disease in infants and children: The role of maternal dietary restriction, breastfeeding, timing of introduction of complementary foods, and hydrolyzed formulas. *Pediatrics*, *121*, 183–191.

Kramer, M.S. (2011). Breastfeeding and allergy: The evidence. *Annals of Nutrition and Metabolism*, *59*(suppl 1), 20–26.

Liu, C., Bayer, A., Cosgrove, S.E., Daum, R.S., Fridkin, S.K., Gorwitz, R.J.,...& Chambers, H.F. (2011). Methicillin-resistant staphylococcus aureus infections in adults and children. *Clinical Infectious Diseases Advance Access*, *52*, 1–38.

Merck Manual for Healthcare Professionals. (2013). Burns. Retrieved from: www.merckmanuals.com/professional/injuries_poisoning/burns/burns.html

Williams, C. (2011). Assessment and management of paediatric burn injuries. *Nursing Standard*, *25*(25), 60–68.

Chapter 20: Nursing Care of the Child With Musculoskeletal Disorders

American Academy of Orthopaedic Surgeons. Available at: http://orthoinfo.aaos.org/

Children's Hospital of Philadelphia. (2011). Fetal surgery takes a huge step forward in treating children with spina bifida. Retrieved from: www.chop.edu/news/fetal-surgery-improves-outcomes-in-spina-bifida.html

Muscular Dystrophy Association. Available at: http://mda.org/

National Scoliosis Foundation. Available at: www.scoliosis.org/

Pires Prado, M.P., Moreira Mendes, A.A.M., Amodio, D.T., Camanho, G.L., Smyth, N.A., & Fernandes, T.D. (2014). A comparative, prospective, and randomized study of two conservative treatment protocols for first-episode lateral ankle ligament injuries. *Foot & Ankle International*, *35*(3), 201-6. doi: 10.1177/1071100713519776.

Chapter 21: Nursing Care of the Child With Endocrine Disorders

American Diabetes Association. Available at: www.diabetes.org/

American Thyroid Association. Available at: www.thyroid.org/

Chang, J.L., Kirkman, M.S., Laffel, L.M.B., & Peters, A.L., on behalf of the Type 1 Diabetes Sourcebook Authors. (2014). Type 1 diabetes through the life span: A position statement of the American Diabetes Association. *Diabetes Care*, 2034–2054. doi: 10.2337/dc14-1140.

Genetics Home Reference. Available at: http://ghr.nlm.nih.gov/nbs

Human Growth Foundation. Available at: www.hgfound.org

Illinois Emergency Medical Services for Children. (2012). Pediatric hyperglycemia and diabetic ketoacidosis (DKA). Retrieved from: www.luhs.org/depts/emsc/peddka_pdf.pdf

National Newborn Screening & Global Resource Center. Available at: http://genes-r-us.uthscsa.edu/

National PKU Alliance. Available at: www.npkua.org/

Chapter 22: Nursing Care of the Child With Neurological Problems

Children's Neuroblastoma Cancer Foundation. Available at: www.cncfhope.org/

Makdissi, M., Davis, G., Jordan, B., Patricios, J., Purcell, L., & Putukian, M. (2013). Revisiting the modifiers: How should the evaluation and management of acute concussions differ in specific groups? *British Journal of Sports Medicine*, *47*, 314–320. doi: 10.1136/bjsports-2013-092256

McCrory, P., Meeuwisse, W., Aubry, M., Cantu, B., Dvorák, J., Echemendia, R., . . . & Turner, M. (2013). Consensus statement on concussion in sport: The 4th international conference on concussion in sport held in Zurich, November 2012. *Physical Therapy in Sport*, *14*, e1–e13.

Neuroblastoma Children's Cancer Society. Available at: www.neuroblastomacancer.org/

Paetzold, K. (2009). The Glasgow Coma scales. Retrieved from: www.rainbowrehab.com/RainbowVisions/article_downloads/articles/Art-TECH-GComaScale.pdf

Spina Bifida Association. Available at: www.spinabifidaassociation.org

United Cerebral Palsy. Available at: http://ucp.org/

van de Beek, D., Farrar, J.J., de Gans, J., Nguyen, T.H.M., Molyneux, E.M., Peltola, H., . . . & Zwinderman, A.H. (2010). Adjunctive dexamethasone in bacterial meningitis: A meta-analysis of individual patient data. *The Lancet Neurology*, *9*(3), 254–263. doi: 10.1016/S1474-4422(10)70023-5

Chapter 23: Nursing Care of the Child With Psychosocial Disorders

American Psychiatric Association. (2013). Attention deficit/hyperactivity disorder. Retrieved from: www.dsm5.org/Documents/ADHD%20Fact%20Sheet.pdf

American Psychiatric Association. (2013). Feeding and eating disorders. Retrieved from: www.dsm5.org/Documents/Eating%20Disorders%20Fact%20Sheet.pdf

Anbarghaumi, R., Yang, L., Van Sell, S., & Miller-Anderson, M. (2007). When to suspect child abuse. *RN*, *70*(4), 34–38.

Arnsten, A.F. (2009). The emerging neurobiology of attention deficit hyperactivity disorder: The key role of the prefrontal association cortex. *The Journal of Pediatrics*, *154*(5), I–S43.

Jenny, C., Crawford-Jakubiak, J.E., & Committee on Child Abuse and Neglect. (2013). The evaluation of children in the primary care setting when sexual abuse is suspected. *Pediatrics*, *132*, e558–e567.

National Institute on Drug Abuse. Available at: www.drugabuse.gov/drugs-abuse

U.S. Department of Health and Human Services. (2013). Substance Abuse and Mental Health Services Administration Center for Behavioral Health Statistics and Quality. Results from the 2012 national survey on drug use and health: Summary of national findings. Retrieved from: http://www.samhsa.gov/data/NSDUH/2012SummNatFindDetTables/NationalFindings/NSDUHresults2012.pdf

U.S. Department of Health and Human Services. (2012). Administration for Children and Families, Administration on Children, Youth and Families, Children's Bureau. Child maltreatment 2011. Retrieved from: www.acf.hhs.gov/programs/cb/research-data-technology/statistics-research/child-maltreatment

Chapter 24: Nursing Care of the Child With Intellectual and Developmental Disabilities

American Association on Intellectual and Developmental Disabilities. Available at: http://aaidd.org/

American Autism Association. Available at: www.myautism.org/

American Autism Society. Available at: www.autism-society.org/

National Down Syndrome Society. Available at: www.ndss.org/

National Fragile X Foundation. Available at: www.fragilex.org/

Scarpinato, N., Bradley, J., Kurbjun, K., Bateman, X., Holtzer, B., & Ely, B. (2010). Caring for the child with an autism spectrum disorder in the acute care setting. *Journal for Specialists in Pediatric Nursing, 15*(3), 244–254.

Schalock, R.L. (2011). The evolving understanding of the construct of intellectual disability. *Journal of Intellectual and Developmental Disability, 36*(4), 227–237.

Chapter 25: Nursing Care of the Child With Sensory Problems

American Association for Pediatric Ophthalmology and Strabismus. Available at: www.aapos.org/

American Speech-Language-Hearing Association. (n.d.). The prevalence and incidence of hearing loss in children. Retrieved from: www.asha.org/public/hearing/disorders/children.htm

Delaney, A.M., Ruth, R.A., Faust, R.A., & Talavera, F. (2012). Newborn hearing screening. Retrieved from: http://emedicine.medscape.com/article/836646-overview

Minnesota Department of Health. (n.d.). Hearing and vision screening. www.health.state.mn.us/divs/fh/mch/hlth-vis/materials/visscreenfaq.html#12

Chapter 2

Fig 2.3. Photo courtesy of the Back to Sleep campaign, Eunice Kennedy Shriver National Institute of Child Health and Human Development, National Institutes of Health and Human Services (www.nichd.nih.gov/sids).

Review Question 9. Modified from CDC Clinical Growth Charts (www.cdc.gov/growthcharts/clinical_charts.htm).

Review Question 9 Answer. Modified from CDC Clinical Growth Charts (www.cdc.gov/growthcharts/clinical_charts.htm).

Chapter 6

Fig 6.1. Colyar, M.R. (2011). Assessment of the school-age child and adolescent. Philadelphia: F.A. Davis.

Fig 6.2. Colyar, M.R. (2011). Assessment of the school-age child and adolescent. Philadelphia: F.A. Davis.

Fig 6.3. Colyar, M.R. (2011). Assessment of the school-age child and adolescent. Philadelphia: F.A. Davis.

Review Question 2. Modified from Colyar, M.R. (2011). Assessment of the school-age child and adolescent. Philadelphia: F.A. Davis.

Chapter 7

Review Question 9. Modified from CDC Clinical Growth Charts (www.cdc.gov/growthcharts/clinical_charts.htm).

Chapter 9

Fig 9.1. From Behrman, R., Kleigman, R., & Arvin, A.M. (1996). Nelson textbook of pediatrics. Elsevier.

Box 9.1, Figs 1 and 2. Modified from Behrman, R., Kleigman, R., & Arvin, A.M. (1996). Nelson textbook of pediatrics. Elsevier.

Review Question 9. From Behrman, R., Kleigman, R., & Arvin, A.M. (1996). Nelson textbook of pediatrics. Elsevier.

Chapter 10

Fig 10.1. Berg, M.D., Schexnayder, S.M., Chameides, L., Terry, M., Donoghue, A., Hickey, R.W., ... & Hazinski, M.F. (2010). 2010 American Heart Association guidelines for cardiopulmonary resuscitation and emergency cardiovascular care science, Part 13: Pediatric basic life support. *Circulation, 122,* S862–S875.

Chapter 12

Table 12.1, Figs 1–6 and 8–9. Courtesy CDC.
Table 12.1, Fig 7. Courtesy CDC/J.D. Millar.

Chapter 16

Fig 16.3. From Dillon, P.M. (2007) Nursing health assessment: A critical thinking, case studies approach, 2nd ed. Philadelphia: F.A. Davis.

Chapter 17

Fig 17.1. Modified from Rudd, K., & Kocisko, D. (2014). Pediatric nursing: The critical components of nursing care. F.A. Davis.

Fig 17.2. Rudd, K., & Kocisko, D. (2014). Pediatric nursing: The critical components of nursing care. F.A. Davis.

Fig 17.3. Centers for Disease Control and Prevention, Department of Health and Human Services, Joe Miller, VD. (1976.). Retrieved from: http://phil.cdc.gov/Phil/details.asp, ID #6784

Table 17.1, Figs 1–10. Modiified from Ward, S.L., & Hisley, S.M. (2009). Maternal-child nursing care: Optimizing outcomes for mothers, children, and families. Philadelphia: F.A. Davis.

Chapter 19

Fig 19.1. From Dillon, P.M. (2007). Nursing health assessment: A critical thinking, case studies approach, 2nd ed. Philadelphia: F.A. Davis.

Fig 19.2. Courtesy CDC/Dr. Herman Miranda, Univ. of Trujillo, Peru; A. Chambers.

Fig 19.3. Courtesy CDC/Dr. Thomas F. Sellers/Emory University.

Fig 19.4. Courtesy CDC/Bruno Coignard, M.D.; Jeff Hageman, M.H.S.

Fig 19.5. Courtesy CDC/Dr. Lucille K. Georg.

Fig 19.6. Courtesy CDC/Frank Collins, Ph.D.

Fig 19.7. Courtesy CDC/Susan Lindsley.

Chapter 20

Fig 20.4. Rudd, K., & Kocisko, D. (2014). Pediatric nursing: The critical components of nursing care. F.A. Davis.

Fig 20.6. Rudd, K., & Kocisko, D. (2014). Pediatric nursing: The critical components of nursing care. F.A. Davis.

Fig 20.7. Rudd, K., & Kocisko, D. (2014). Pediatric nursing: The critical components of nursing care. F.A. Davis.

Fig 20.9. Dillon, P.M. (2007). Nursing health assessment: A critical thinking, case studies approach, 2nd ed. Philadelphia: F.A. Davis.

Chapter 24

Fig 24.2. De Sevo, M. (2013). Maternal and newborn success, 2nd ed. F.A. Davis.

Review Question 1. De Sevo, M. (2013). Maternal and newborn success, 2nd ed. F.A. Davis.

Chapter 25

Fig 25.1. Rudd, K., & Kocisko, D. (2014). Pediatric nursing: The critical components of nursing care. F.A. Davis.

Index

Note: Page numbers followed by *b* indicate boxes, *f* indicate figures, and *t* indicate tables.

D

E

J

K

L

R

S

X

Z